Olfaction and the Brain

Olfaction and the Brain

Editor: Hugo Ray

AMERICAN
MEDICAL PUBLISHERS
www.americanmedicalpublishers.com

AMERICAN
MEDICAL PUBLISHERS
www.americanmedicalpublishers.com

Cataloging-in-Publication Data

Olfaction and the brain / edited by Hugo Ray.
p. cm.
Includes bibliographical references and index.
ISBN 979-8-88740-349-6
1. Smell disorders. 2. Smell. 3. Brain--Physiology. 4. Developmental neurobiology.
5. Neurophysiology. I. Ray, Hugo.
QP458 .O44 2023
612.86--dc23

American Medical Publishers,
41 Flatbush Avenue,
1st Floor, New York,
NY 11217, USA

ISBN 979-8-88740-349-6 (Hardback)

Contents

Preface

Every book is initially just a concept; it takes months of research and hard work to give it the final shape in which the readers receive it. In its early stages, this book also went through rigorous reviewing. The notable contributions made by experts from across the globe were first molded into patterned chapters and then arranged in a sensibly sequential manner to bring out the best results.

The sensory system used for smelling or olfaction is called olfactory system or sense of smell. The overall olfactory system is divided into two types, namely, the main olfactory system and the accessory olfactory system. They perform different functions. The main olfactory system detects airborne substances while the accessory olfactory system detects fluid-phase stimuli. There are various types of olfactory disorders based on the type of malfunction. These disorders include anosmia, agnosia and hyperosmia. Anosmia is the loss of smell, which may be total anosmia, incomplete anosmia (partial anosmia, hyposmia, or microsmia), and distorted anosmia (dysosmia). Agnosia refers to an inability to recognize odors despite having a normally functioning olfactory system. Hyperosmia is a rare condition characterized by an abnormally heightened sense of smell. The olfactory problems can be bilateral or unilateral, similar to the case of vision and hearing problems. Olfactory dysfunction can be caused due to age, viral infections, exposure to toxic substances, neurodegenerative diseases, and head trauma. Some of the diverse topics covered in this book address the advanced researches related to olfaction and olfactory disorders. Through case studies and examples, constant effort has been made to make the understanding of the difficult concepts as easy and informative as possible for the readers.

It has been my immense pleasure to be a part of this project and to contribute my years of learning in such a meaningful form. I would like to take this opportunity to thank all the people who have been associated with the completion of this book at any step.

Editor

1

Sensory descriptors, hedonic perception and consumer's attitudes to Sangiovese red wine deriving from organically and conventionally grown grapes

***Ella Pagliarini*[1]*, Monica Laureati*[1]* * and Davide Gaeta*[2]**

[1] *Department of Food, Environmental and Nutritional Sciences (DeFENS), Università degli Studi di Milano, Milano, Italy*
[2] *Dipartimento di Economia Aziendale, Università degli Studi di Verona, Verona, Italy*

Correspondence:
Monica Laureati, Department of Food, Environmental and Nutritional Sciences (DeFENS), Università degli Studi di Milano, Via Celoria 2, Milano 20133, Italy
e-mail:monica.laureati@unimi.it

In recent years, produce obtained from organic farming methods (i.e., a system that minimizes pollution and avoids the use of synthetic fertilizers and pesticides) has rapidly increased in developed countries. This may be explained by the fact that organic food meets the standard requirements for quality and healthiness. Among organic products, wine has greatly attracted the interest of the consumers. In the present study, trained assessors and regular wine consumers were respectively required to identify the sensory properties (e.g., odor, taste, flavor, and mouthfeel sensations) and to evaluate the hedonic dimension of red wines deriving from organically and conventionally grown grapes. Results showed differences related mainly to taste (sour and bitter) and mouthfeel (astringent) sensations, with odor and flavor playing a minor role. However, these differences did not influence liking, as organic and conventional wines were hedonically comparable. Interestingly, 61% of respondents would be willing to pay more for organically produced wines, which suggests that environmentally sustainable practices related to wine quality have good market prospects.

Keywords: odor, taste, organic wine, consumer expectation, sensory, willingness to pay

INTRODUCTION

The sensory analysis of wine has always given rise to interest both in the scientific community and among consumers. Wine is tightly tied to psychological aspects besides being purely sensory. There have been many studies carried out on different aspects connected with wine tasting such as the cognitive and perceptual processes that characterize wine expertise. Wine-tasting expertise involves advanced discriminative and descriptive abilities with respect to wine. While the basis of wine expertise remains unknown, differences in performance between experts and novices are relatively clear (Lawless, 1984; Noble et al., 1987; Solomon, 1990; Hughson and Boakes, 2002; Zucco et al., 2011). Wine-tasting experts such as sommeliers have obviously a greater sensory ability than inexperienced novices, but their knowledge of wine may sometimes lead them to misperception of the product (Pangborn et al., 1963; Morrot et al., 2001). Pangborn et al. (1963) and Morrot et al. (2001) carried out experiments in which white wines were colored to obtain rosé and red wines, respectively. Pangborn et al. (1963) found that such a modification led wine experts but not novices to judge the product as sweeter than colorless controls. Similarly, Morrot et al. (2001) showed that wine experts described the white wine with the characteristics of a red wine.

While there are several studies on wine perception, little is known about sensory characteristics of wines deriving from organically and conventionally grown grapes. Organic agriculture is a production management system that promotes and enhances biodiversity, biological cycles, and soil biological activity. The primary goal of organic agriculture is to minimize all forms of pollution and to avoid the use of synthetic fertilizers and pesticides, thus optimizing the health and productivity of soil, plants, animals, and humans.

In recent years, consumers have become increasingly concerned by the effects of conventional agricultural production practices on both human and environmental health. As a consequence, production obtained from organic farming methods has been rapidly growing in developed countries. This may be explained as organic food adequately meets all requirements for quality, genuineness, and healthiness (Forbes et al., 2009). Recent evidence has also shown an increase of the related literature, even though studies are still few in number. The studies comparing foods derived from organic and conventional growing systems focused mainly on three topics: nutritional value, sensory quality, and food safety (Bourn and Prescott, 2002).

Relative to the nutritional value of wine, its antioxidant activity and benefit on health were addressed (Renaud and De Lorgeril, 1992), showing that phenolic compounds are natural anti-inflammatory and efficient scavengers of free radicals (Akçay et al., 2004).

As to the sensory quality of food products, reports indicate that organic and conventional fruits and vegetables may differ on a variety of sensory aspects; however, findings are inconsistent (Bourn and Prescott, 2002). Therefore, the assumption of organic food having a better taste may be explained by the consumer's expectation of a healthier and safer product evoked by the label "organic food" (Deliza and MacFie, 1996). Indeed, expectations greatly influence subject responses (see e.g., Dalton et al., 1997).

Few studies compared sensory properties of wines derived from organically and conventionally grown grapes. Moyano et al. (2009) for instance, examined the aroma profile of sherry wines that had been cultivated conventionally and organically and found that organic wines had a sensory profile similar to that of the conventional ones, but lower odor intensity. The same findings were reported by Dupin et al. (2000), who examined German wines and found that organic products tended to be less aromatic than conventional ones.

"Sangiovese" (*Vitis vinifera* L.) is the most widely consumed Italian wine. It is used to produce prestigious Tuscan wines such as Chianti and Brunello di Montalcino. To our knowledge no studies are available on Sangiovese red wine sensory quality. Thus, the main aim of this work is to identify and describe the sensory properties, such as odor, taste, flavor, and mouthfeel sensations, that characterize organically and traditionally grown Romagna Sangiovese red wines. Also, as sensory properties greatly influence food preference, the hedonic dimension of organic and conventional wines was investigated.

MATERIALS AND METHODS

WINES

The red wines evaluated in the present study were produced from ripe grapes from *Vitis Vinifera* Sangiovese harvested in September 2007 and 2008 in the region of Faenza (Italy). The grapes were derived from two different farms located in adjacent areas and subjected to similar environmental conditions. For both vintages, one farm produced grapes according to organic techniques whereas the other adopted conventional agricultural techniques. At variance from conventionally cultivated grapes neither insecticides nor synthetic fertilizers were used in organic agriculture during the growth.

All wines were produced following the same process according to PDO (Protected Designation of Origin) specifications. Wines were analyzed 6 months after they were bottled. Three bottles from the organic and three from the traditional production of vintage 2007 were randomly selected to be used for sensory analysis and the same procedure was used for vintage 2008.

SENSORY ANALYSIS

PARTICIPANTS

Descriptive analysis of wines: 12 assessors (seven women and five men) aged on average 27.0 ± (SD) 3.5 years (range 23–35 years) were selected. They were trained to evaluate organic and conventional wines from vintages 2007 and 2008.

Hedonic test of wines: a second group of 100 (50 women and 50 men) regular red wine consumers (inexpert individuals with no formal wine training) aged on average 32.1 ± (SD) 9.6 years (range, 20–60 years) participated.

The participants were students and employees of the University of Milan, who reported liking red wine and consuming it more than twice a month. None of the participants had previous or present taste or smell disorders. The study was in accordance with the Declaration of Helsinki. The protocol was approved by the Institutional Ethics Committee at the study site. Informed consent was obtained from all subjects.

Descriptive analysis

Descriptive analysis (Lawless and Heymann, 1998; ISO International Organization for Standardization, 2003) was used to identify and quantify the sensory properties of organic and conventional wines from two successive vintages.

Training phase: subjects were trained over a period of 2 months. During the first part of the training, assessors tasted Romagna Sangiovese wines and set up a list of descriptors that characterized the wines. To do so, assessors wrote down as many terms as they could to describe the sensory characteristics fully. Assessors agreed through panel discussion on what terms were relevant, and arrived at definitions for each term. At this stage, a reference product was provided in order to help the assessors to understand each term.

Evaluation phase: after training was completed, the panel evaluated the two wines (organic vs. conventional) in triplicate. Judges were instructed to drink and swallow each sample and rate the intensity of each attribute using a nine-point scale (1 = absence of the sensation and 9 = maximum intensity). The sessions were performed on the same day (with a minimum 2-h break between the sessions) at the sensory laboratory of the Department of Food, Environmental and Nutritional Sciences (DeFENS, Università degli Studi di Milano) designed in accordance with ISO guidelines (ISO International Organization for Standardization, 2007). Data acquisition was done using Fizz v2.31 software (Biosystèmes, Couternon, France). Assessors were asked not to smoke, eat or drink anything, except water, at least 1 h before the tasting sessions. For each sample, judges received a 30 ml sample served in glasses coded with a three-digit number and covered with a Petri dish to avoid the escape of volatile components. Participants were provided with mineral water and unsalted crackers to clean their mouth between tastings. Wines were served at 18 ± 1°C. Presentation orders were systematically varied over assessors and replicates in order to balance the effects of serving order and carryover (MacFie et al., 1989).

Consumer's preference and attitude toward wine consumption

Since the sensory properties of a food are among the primary determinants of food preference and choice, we also investigated the hedonic qualities of organic and conventional Romagna Sangiovese wines. For this purpose, the two wines under study, organic and conventional from vintage 2008, were evaluated along with four other Romagna Sangiovese wines from the same vintage produced according to conventional agriculture techniques, which were purchased in local wineries and were comparable for price category to those under study. Due to practical constraints (i.e., no availability of wine), the wines from vintage 2007 were not included in the hedonic evaluation.

Consumers were invited to take part in a hedonic test carried out at the DeFENS sensory laboratory. Each participant received a series of six wines (20 ml for each product) served in glasses coded with three-digit numbers and covered with Petri dishes. For each sample, participants were instructed to drink and swallow the wine and rate the degree of liking using a seven-point hedonic scale (with 1 = extremely disliked and 7 = extremely liked;

Lawless and Heymann, 1998). Consumers were asked to drink mineral water and to eat a piece of unsalted cracker to clean their mouth between tastings. Also, they were asked not to smoke, eat or drink anything, except water, 1 h before the tasting session. Data were collected using Fizz v2.31g software program (Biosystemes, Couternon, France). Wines were evaluated under standard light conditions at a temperature of 18 ± 1°C. In order to balance the effects of serving order and carryover, the presentation order of the wines was randomized. After the liking test, the subjects were asked a few questions about their wine consumption habit and organic wine purchase likelihood.

RESULTS

DESCRIPTIVE ANALYSIS

The panel generated a total of 12 descriptors that characterize the sensory profile of the wines: four odor descriptors (fruity, spicy, woody, and vanilla), two taste descriptors (sour and bitter), three flavor descriptors (fruity, spicy, and woody) and three mouthfeel sensations (astringent, alcohol, and body). Complete definitions and standard products for all descriptors are listed in **Table 1**.

Mean intensity ratings of organic and conventional wines are reported in **Figures 1** and **2**. Intensity data for each sensory descriptor from the two vintages were analyzed separately through ANOVA with *Wines* (organic vs. conventional), *Judges*, *Replicates* (rep 1 vs. rep 2 vs. rep3) as factors. Relative to vintage 2007, *Wines* were significantly different for sour taste ($F = 10.31$, $p < 0.01$), bitter taste ($F = 8.87$, $p < 0.05$) and astringency ($F = 51.13$, $p < 0.001$). *Post-hoc* comparison using the Bonferroni test ($p < 0.05$) showed that organic wine was perceived as having a higher intensity of sour taste, and astringent sensation but lower bitter taste. Differences between the two wines from vintage 2008 concerned only astringency ($F = 13.66$, $p < 0.01$), with organic wine having a higher intensity. The effect of *Judges* was significant ($p < 0.05$), which is expected because individuals can of course have different sensitivities to the different descriptors. This effect can seldom be changed by

Table 1 | List of the 12 sensory descriptors of Romagna Sangiovese PDO wines with their relevant definitions and reference standards.

Descriptor	Definition	Reference standard
Odor		
Fruity	Characteristic odor of a combination of blueberry, raspberry, and blackberry perceived by means of the sense of smell (orthonasal perception)	Infusion (24 h, 4°C) of 12 blueberries, two raspberries, and one blackberry in 0.5 l of red table wine
Spicy	Characteristic odor of a combination of spices (cinnamon and clove) perceived by means of the sense of smell (orthonasal perception)	Infusion (24 h, 4°C) of 16 cloves and one cinnamon stick in 0.5 l of red table wine
Vanilla	Characteristic odor of vanilla perceived by means of the sense of smell (orthonasal perception)	Commercial liquid vanilla odorant (2 ml) dissolved in 0.5 l of red table wine
Woody	Characteristic odor of toasted wood perceived by means of the sense of smell (orthonasal perception)	Guaiacol in red table wine (2 ppb)
Taste		
Sour	One of the basic tastes, caused by solution of acidic compounds perceived in the oral cavity	Anhydrous citric acid (2 g) in 0.7 l of red table wine
Bitter	One of the basic tastes, caused by solution of bitter compounds perceived in the oral cavity	Caffeine (0.8 g) in 0.5 l of red table wine
Flavor		
Fruity	Characteristic odor of a combination of blueberry, raspberry, and blackberry perceived by means of the sense of smell during swallowing (retronasal perception)	Infusion (24 h, 4°C) of 12 blueberries, two raspberries, and one blackberry in 0.5 l of red table wine
Spicy	Characteristic odor of a combination of spices (cinnamon and clove) perceived by means of the sense of smell during swallowing (retronasal perception)	Infusion (24 h, 4°C) of 16 cloves and one cinnamon stick in 0.5 l of red table wine
Woody	Characteristic odor of toasted wood perceived by means of the sense of smell during swallowing (retronasal perception)	Guaiacol in red table wine (2 ppb)
Mouthfeel		
Astringent	Mouth dryness caused by tannins and perceived in the oral cavity	Dissolve 1.5 g of tannin in 750 ml of red table wine
Alcohol	Characteristic heat/burning sensation perceived in the oral cavity	Mix 40 ml of 95% ethyl alcohol with 500 ml of red table wine
Body	Characteristic perceived in the oral cavity, due to the friction among the molecules in a liquid, that gives to it a limited fluidity and mobility	Mix 6 ml of glycerol with 1 l of red table wine

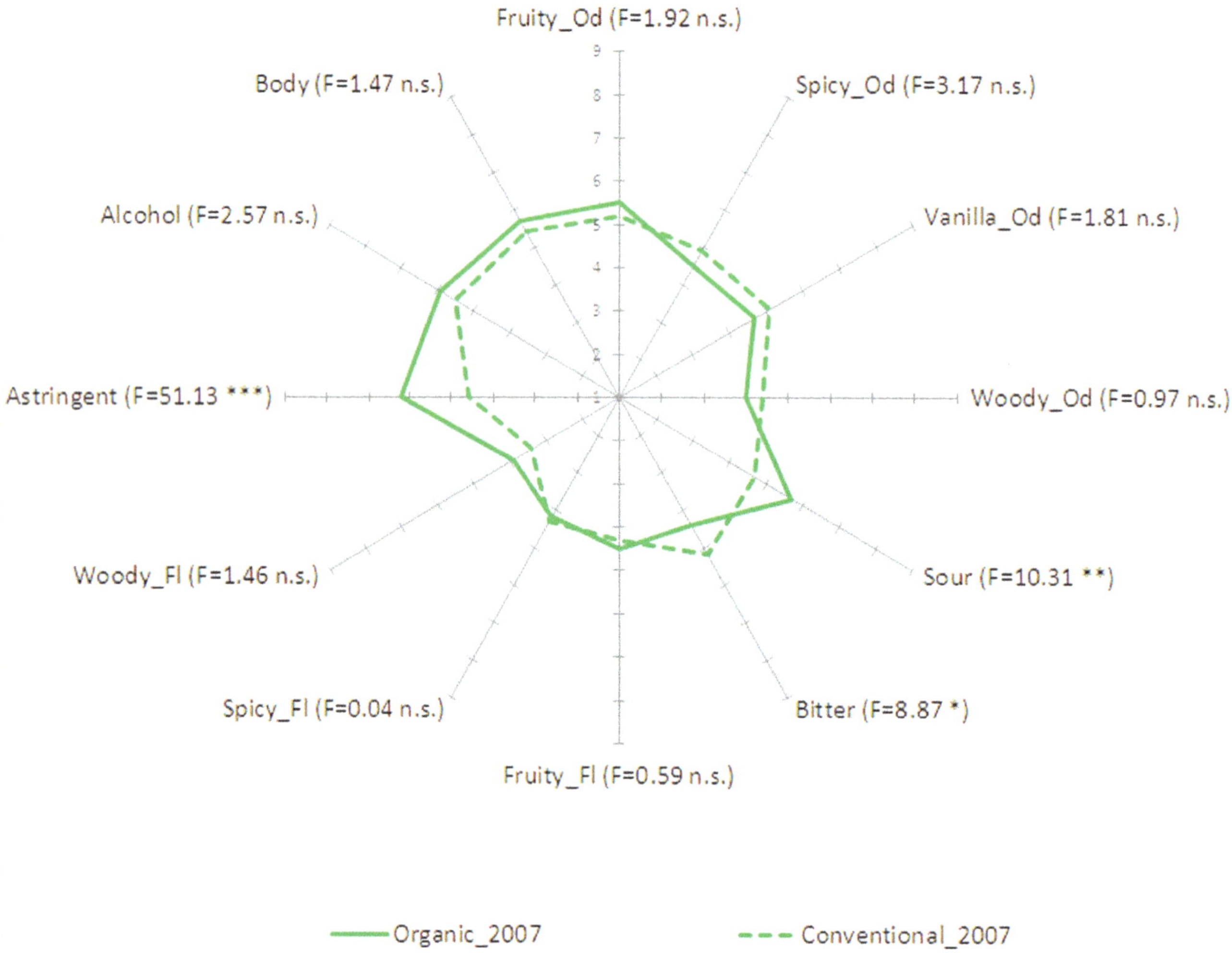

FIGURE 1 | Descriptive analysis results: mean values for each sensory descriptor by method of production (organic vs. conventional) for vintage 2007. For each descriptor the relevant significance is reported (*** $p < 0.001$, ** $p < 0.01$, * $p < 0.05$).

training (Lea et al., 1997). Also, data analysis showed that F values for *Replicates* and interactions between *Wines and Judges, Judges and Replicates* and *Wines and Replicates* were not significant ($p < 0.05$) for nearly all the attributes. These results indicated that the mean scores for each wine given by the assessors for each attribute could be assumed to be satisfactory estimates of the sensory profile of the samples (i.e., good panel reliability).

STUDY OF CONSUMER PREFERENCE AND ATTITUDE TOWARD WINE CONSUMPTION

Mean hedonic ratings and standard errors for organic and conventional Romagna Sangiovese wines are reported in **Table 2**. Data analysis by means of one-way ANOVA showed significant differences ($F = 2.42$, $p < 0.05$) between wines for liking ratings. *Post-hoc* comparison using the Bonferroni test ($p < 0.05$) showed that organic and conventional wines from vintage 2008 were not significantly different and showed liking ratings comparable to other commercial wines (Sangiovese A, B, and C).

The same subjects involved in the hedonic study were also asked to answer a few questions about their attitude toward wine consumption (see, **Table 3**). About 59% of the subjects were habitual red wine consumers. The largest part (85%) of the wine used was mostly for home consumption. Wine is purchased at retail shops (59%) and most of the consumers are used to spending no more than 7 euros for a bottle of wine. Finally, it is interesting to note that when asked about the purchase of organically produced wine, 61% of them declared they would be willing to pay more for such product.

DISCUSSION

The present study investigated the sensory and hedonic qualities of red wines derived from organically and conventionally grown grapes. The examined wines were Romagna Sangiovese red wines. The descriptive analysis identified specific olfactory properties that characterize these wines, namely fruity, spicy, vanilla, and woody odors and flavors. Odor is a relevant sensory attribute of food, as well as of wines, which lead consumer's preference and choice.

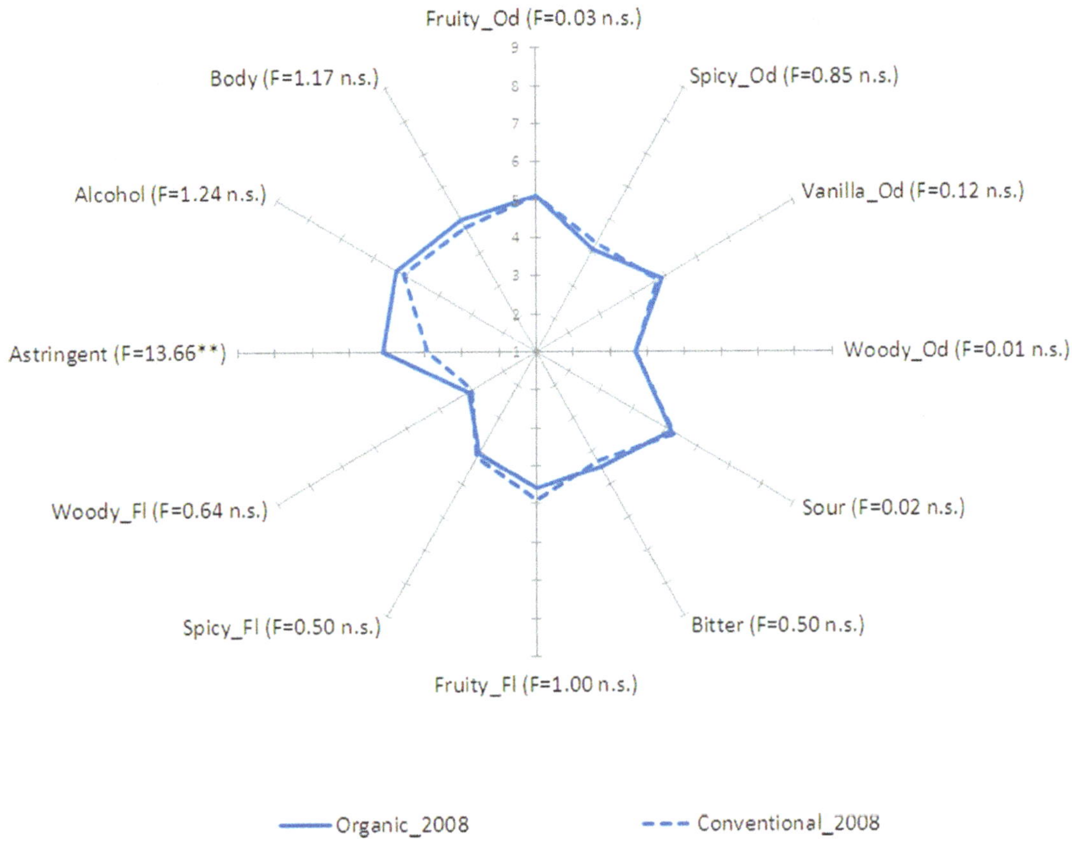

FIGURE 2 | Descriptive analysis results: mean values for each sensory descriptor by method of production (organic vs. conventional) for vintage 2008. For each descriptor the relevant significance is reported (** $p < 0.01$).

Also, the quality and specificity of each wine are associated in most cases with a specific odorant.

This study has shown that the organic and conventional wines differed marginally in the intensity of sensory descriptors. Only the properties of taste and mouthfeel sensations distinguished the two types of wine, whereas odor and flavor seemed to play a minor role. Organic wine from vintage 2007 was perceived as more sour and astringent but less bitter than its conventional counterpart, whereas differences between wines from vintage 2008 concerned only astringency.

Table 2 | Mean hedonic ratings (±STDERR) for organic and conventional Romagna Sangiovese wines from vintage 2008 and other four commercial Romagna Sangiovese wines from conventional agricultural techniques (Sangiove A–D).

Wines ($F = 2.42$; $p < 0.05$)	Hedonic rating
Sangiovese A	$4.2^{a} \pm 0.3$
Conventional 2008	$4.4^{a} \pm 0.3$
Organic 2008	$4.5^{a} \pm 0.3$
Sangiovese B	$4.8^{ab} \pm 0.3$
Sangiovese C	$4.9^{ab} \pm 0.3$
Sangiovese D	$5.3^{b} \pm 0.3$

Mean hedonic ratings with different superscripts are significantly different according to Bonferroni test ($p < 0.05$).

In addition, the differences between wines did not influence liking, as organic and conventional wines were hedonically comparable. This means that consumers are not able to discriminate among organic and conventional wines from a hedonic point of view. One reason relates to their lack of formal training in sensory evaluation, which leads them only to detect major differences among products with less sensitivity to more subtle differences. It may be assumed that differences in liking could have been perceived between organic and conventional wines from vintage 2007, which showed larger differences in the intensity of some sensory qualities (i.e., bitter taste, sour taste and astringency) than wines from vintage 2008. Unfortunately, this hypothesis could not be verified, as wines from vintage 2007 were not included in the hedonic comparison. Nevertheless, self-reported comments by the participants suggest that even though the organic wine from vintage 2007 showed a high intensity of sourness and astringency, it was judged equally liked as its conventional counterpart.

The issue of comparing the hedonic qualities of organically and conventionally produced food has been tackled by various authors

Table 3 | Results from the questionnaire related to wine consumption habit and organic wine purchase intention.

Question	Answer (%)	Items
How would you define yourself?	59	Habitual wine consumer (2 or more times a month)
	41	Occasional wine consumer (less than twice a week)
Wine purchase is mainly destined to...	85	Home consumption
	15	Restaurant consumption
Where do you usually buy wine?	12	Wine shops
	59	Retail shops
	29	Wineries
How much do you usually pay for a bottle of wine?	3	Less than 3 euros
	19	Between 3 and 5 euros
	49	Between 5 and 7 euros
	28	Between 7 and 10 euros
	2	More than 10 euros
Would you be willing to pay an extra charge for an organically produced wine?	23	Yes, less than 10%
	34	Yes, between 10 and 20%
	4	Yes, between 20 and 30%
	0	Yes, more than 30%
	39	No

with respect to different food products, e.g., yogurt (Laureati et al., 2013), cheese (Napolitano et al., 2010a), meat (Napolitano et al., 2010b), and beer (Caporale and Monteleone, 2004). Interestingly, in these studies the liking of organic and conventional products has been evaluated under different information conditions: the blind condition (i.e., consumers taste and judge the product without any kind of information); the expected condition (i.e., consumers do not taste the product and judge it only on the basis of written or visual information); and the informed condition (i.e., consumers taste and judge the product after having read written information and/or seen an image). The main outcome of these studies is that organic products are liked more than their conventional counterparts but only in informed conditions, namely when consumers knew that they were to taste an organic food. Thus, it would seem that organic products are liked more because of the "healthier" connotation they have in the consumer's mind rather than for an actual preference based on perceptual attributes. Also, the influence of information about organic production on consumers' food preferences and expectations is especially evident in the case of consumers who are more interested in and proactive for "sustainable" products (Laureati et al., 2013). This suggests that expectation plays an important role for food consumption, since it may improve or degrade the perception of a product, even before it is tasted (Deliza and MacFie, 1996; Dalton et al., 1997). In this respect, it should be pointed out that the Sangiovese wines used in the present study were evaluated under blind conditions, without any information concerning production method. Thus, consumers' liking derives mainly from the mere sensory perception of the wines without any pre-conceived ideas due to their knowledge about the product.

Finally, an interesting result is that most of the consumers declared themselves willing to pay more for organically produced wines. This result is in line with the finding of a recent study by Lockshin and Corsi (2012) who reported that consumers in European countries as well as in the United States, New Zealand and Australia are willing to pay more for organic wines mainly for health and environmental reasons but also because consumers are interested in helping producers who adopt these innovations. Of course cognitive factors as personal expectancies – addressed above – have room. Therefore, a greater predisposition to pay an additional charge for organic wine may be due to specific consumer's attitude and involvement in sustainability issues.

In conclusion, the present study evidenced the sensory properties that characterize red wines from organically and conventionally grown grapes. The differences detected from a quantitative point of view are only marginal, and do not seem to have an impact on consumer's hedonic perception. A limitation of this study may be that only two vintages of one grape variety of organic and conventional wines were considered. Further research is needed to clarify this aspect. In this context, future perspectives of study should deal with the study of sensory and hedonic qualities of wine, which are undoubtedly the strongest determinants of consumer's expectations and play a key role in consumer's purchase attitude. This aspect seems to be particularly relevant for wines deriving from organically and conventionally grapes since environmentally sustainable practices related to wine quality seem to have good market prospects.

ACKNOWLEDGMENT

The authors would like to thank professor Zucco for comments and criticisms on an early draft.

REFERENCES

Akçay, Y. D., Yıldırım, H. K., Güvenç, U., and Sözmen, E. Y. (2004). The effects of consumption of organic and nonorganic red wine on low-density lipoprotein oxidation and antioxidant capacity in humans. *Nutr. Res.* 24, 541–554. doi:10.1016/j.nutres.2004.04.004

Bourn, D., and Prescott, J. (2002). A comparison of the nutritional value, sensory qualities, and food safety of organically and conventionally produced foods. *Crit. Rev. Food Sci.* 42, 1–34. doi: 10.1080/10408690290825439

Caporale, G., and Monteleone, E. (2004). Influence of information about manufacturing process on beer acceptability. *Food Qual. Pref.* 15, 271–278. doi: 10.1016/S0950-3293(03)00067-3

Dalton, P., Wysocki, C. J., Brody, M. J., and Lawley, H. J. (1997). The influence of cognitive bias on the perceived odor, irritation and health symptoms from chemical exposure. *Int. Arch. Occup. Environ. Health* 69, 407–417. doi: 10.1007/s004200050168

Deliza, R., and MacFie, H. J. H. (1996). The generation of sensory expectation by external cues and its effect on sensory perception and hedonic ratings: a review. *J. Sens. Stud.* 7, 253–277. doi: 10.1111/j.1745-459X.1996.tb00036.x

Dupin, I., Schlich, P., and Fischer, U. (2000). "Differentiation of wines produced by organic or conventional viticulture according to their sensory profiles and aroma composition," in *Proceedings of Proceedings 6th International Congress on*

Organic Viticulture, eds H. Willer and U. Meier (Bad Dürkheim, D: Print-Online), 245–251.

Forbes, S. L., Cohen, D. A., Cullen, R., Wratten, S. D., and Fountain, J. (2009). Consumer attitudes regarding environmentally sustainable wine: an exploratory study of the New Zealand marketplace. *J. Clean. Prod.* 17, 1195–1199. doi: 10.1016/j.jclepro.2009.04.008

Hughson, L., and Boakes, R. (2002). The knowing nose: the role of knowledge in wine expertise. *Food Qual. Pref.* 13, 463–472. doi: 10.1016/S0950-3293(02)00051-4

ISO International Organization for Standardization. (2003). *Sensory Analysis – Methodology – General Guidance for Establishing a Sensory Profile* (ISO 13299:2003). Geneva, Switzerland.

ISO International Organization for Standardization. (2007). *Sensory Analysis – General Guidance for the Design of Test Rooms* (ISO 8589:2007). Geneva, Switzerland.

Laureati, M., Jabes, D., Russo, V., and Pagliarini, E. (2013). Sustainability and organic production: how information influences consumer's expectation and preference for yogurt. *Food Qual. Pref.* 30, 1–8. doi: 10.1016/j.foodqual.2013.04.002

Lawless, H. T. (1984). Flavor description of white wine by expert and non-expert wine consumers. *J. Food Sci.* 49, 120–123. doi: 10.1111/j.1365-2621.1984.tb13686.x

Lawless, H. T., and Heymann, H. (1998). "Descriptive analysis," in *Sensory Evaluation of Food: Principles and Practices*, eds H. T. Lawless and H. Heymann (New York: Chapman & Hall), 341–372.

Lea, P., Næs, T., and Rødbotten, M. (1997). "Further aspects of design and modeling," in *Analysis of Variance for Sensory Data* (Chichester: John Wiley & Sons Ltd), 20–21.

Lockshin, L., and Corsi, A. M. (2012). Consumer behavior for wine 2.0: a review since 2003 and future directions. *Wine Econ. Policy* 1, 2–23. doi: 10.1016/j.wep.2012.11.003

MacFie, H. J. H., Bratchell, N., Greenhoff, K., and Vallis, L. V. (1989). Designs to balance the effect of order of presentation and first order carry-over effects in hall tests. *J. Sens. Stud.* 4, 129–148. doi: 10.1111/j.1745-459X.1989.tb00463.x

Morrot, G., Brochet, F., and Dubourdieu, D. (2001). The color of odors. *Brain Lang.* 79, 309–320. doi: 10.1006/brln.2001.2493

Moyano, L., Zea, L., Villafuerte, L., and Medina, M. (2009). Comparison of odor-active compounds in sherry wines processed from ecologically and conventionally grown pedroximenez grapes. *J. Agric. Food Chem.* 57, 968–973. doi: 10.1021/jf802252u

Napolitano, F., Braghieri, A., Piasentier, E., Favotto, S., Naspetti, S., and Zanoli, R. (2010a). Cheese liking and consumer willingness to pay as affected by information about organic production. *Food Qual. Pref.* 18, 280–286. doi: 10.1017/S0022029910000130. Epub 2010 Mar 3.

Napolitano, F., Braghieri, A., Piasentier, E., Favotto, S., Naspetti, S., and Zanoli, R. (2010b). Effect of information about organic production on beef liking and consumer willingness to pay. *Food Qual. Pref.* 21, 207–212. doi: 10.1016/j.foodqual.2009.08.007

Noble, A., Arnold, R. A., Buechsenstein, J., Leach, E. J., Schmidt, J. O., and Stern, P. M. (1987). Modification of a standardized system of wine aroma terminology. *Am. J. Enol. Vitic.* 38, 143–146.

Pangborn, R., Berg, H., and Hansen, B. (1963). The influence of color on discrimination of sweetness in dry table-wine. *Am. J. Psychol.* 76, 492–495. doi: 10.2307/1419795

Renaud, S., and De Lorgeril, M. (1992). Wine, alcohol, platelets, and the French paradox for coronary heart disease. *Lancet* 339, 1523–1526. doi: 10.1016/0140-6736(92)91277-F

Solomon, G. (1990). Psychology of novice and expert wine talk. *Am. J. Psychol.* 105, 495–517. doi: 10.2307/1423321

Zucco, G., Carassai, A., Baroni, M. R., and Stevenson, R. J. (2011). Labeling, identification, and recognition of wine-relevant odorants in expert sommeliers, intermediates, and untrained wine drinkers. *Perception* 40, 598–607. doi: 10.1068/p6972

2

Food neophobia and its relation with olfaction

M. Luisa Demattè*, Isabella Endrizzi and Flavia Gasperi

Department of Food Quality and Nutrition, Research and Innovation Centre, Fondazione Edmund Mach, San Michele all'Adige, Italy

***Correspondence:**
M. Luisa Demattè, Department of Food Quality and Nutrition, Research and Innovation Centre, Fondazione Edmund Mach, Via E. Mach 1, San Michele all'Adige, TN 38010, Italy
e-mail: luisa.dematte@fmach.it

Food neophobia, that is the reluctance to try novel foods, is an attitude that dramatically affects human feeding behavior in many different aspects among which food preferences and food choices appear to be the most thoroughly considered. This attitude has an important evolutionary meaning since it protects the individual from ingesting potentially dangerous substances. On the other hand, it fosters an avoidance behavior that can extend even toward useful food elements. A strong link exists between food neophobia and both the variety in one person's diet and previous exposures to different foods. In this review, the more recent findings about food neophobia will be concisely described. Given the suggested connection between the exposure to different foods and food neophobia, this review will focus on the relation between this attitude and human chemosensory abilities. Olfaction, in particular, is a sensory modality that has a central role in flavor perception and in food preference acquisition. Therefore, the latest evidences about its relation with food neophobia will be discussed along with the applied and cognitive implications.

Keywords: food neophobia, olfaction, food exposure, odor identification, explorative behavior

INTRODUCTION

Human feeding behavior is guided by a number of different factors relating to the properties of both food product and individual. The intrinsic sensory properties of food are fundamental in modulating the experience the individual has while approaching and consuming the product (Desor et al., 1975). On the other hand, the physiological state of the organism (e.g., hunger; Rolls, 2012) promotes or inhibits food research and consumption (Small et al., 2001; Albrecht et al., 2009; Fernandez et al., 2013). Another extremely important aspect is represented by the cognitive and motivational factors of the individual (Assanand et al., 1998), among which the tendency to avoid foods never encountered before (known as food neophobia; Pliner and Hobden, 1992) is receiving increased attention. The rationale behind this is the existence of a strong connection between new food avoidance with the successive development of unhealthy eating habits (e.g., assuming too much fats or sugars), that can have serious negative consequences on diet balancing or on body weight (e.g., obesity; Capiola and Raudenbush, 2012). Therefore, the purpose of this review is to provide an up-to-date overview of the findings in food neophobia investigation and in the study of its relationship with chemosensory perception, focusing on odor perception.

ATTITUDES TOWARD FOOD: THE CASE OF FOOD NEOPHOBIA

Among the psychological factors modulating an individual's relationship with food, the systematic reluctance to try novel or unknown foods (i.e., food neophobia; Pliner and Hobden, 1992) appears to play a critical role in the development of possible eating disorders (see Benton, 2004). From an adaptive point of view, food neophobia protects an organism (animal or human being) from ingesting potentially dangerous foods. This mechanism has a cost, though, represented by the risk of avoiding even highly nutritious foods. The balance an organism should find between these two opposite pressures is known as the "omnivore's dilemma" (Rozin and Vollmecke, 1986). Since the late 1960s, a large body of research has been produced on this behavior in animals (see e.g., Rozin, 1968; Roberts and Cheney, 1974; Mitchell et al., 1975), whilst food neophobia in humans has only been extensively investigated in the last two decades (for an earlier review, see Frank and Raudenbush, 1998).

In order to try and quantify this in human beings, over the years a number questionnaires have been developed such as the "Food Attitude Survey" (FAS; Frank and van der Klaauw, 1994; see also Frank and Raudenbush, 1998; Raudenbush et al., 1998), but it is with the publication of the "Food Neophobia Scale" (FNS; Pliner and Hobden, 1992) that a systematic way of studying food neophobia initiated. This scale has been successfully used to predict people's attitude toward new foods and the expected liking of food products, and has been adapted for children administration ("Children Food Neophobia Scale", CFNS; Pliner, 1994). It has also been translated into different languages and cultures (e.g., for Italian, see Demattè et al., 2013; for Spanish, see Fernández-Ruiz et al., 2013; for Chilean, see Schnettler et al., 2013; for Finnish, see Tuorila et al., 2001; for Japanese, see Yamada et al., 2012). Recently, the FNS has also been adapted to the fruit and vegetable domain ("Fruit and Vegetable Neophobia Instrument", FVNI; Hollar et al., 2013).

The strength of the FNS lies in the speed at which the questionnaire can be administered, by means of both paper and pencil and computerized tests, and in its repeatedly proven internal consistency (Pliner and Hobden, 1992; Tuorila et al., 1994; Raudenbush et al., 1998). A disadvantage of the scale is that, despite the increasing number of studies performed, a common reliable methodology to use to categorize people as a function of the degree of neophobia is still not available (Meiselman et al., 2010). The FNS can be used to determine neophobia classes by using one standard deviation from the group mean as the splitting criterion (Pliner and Hobden, 1992; Falciglia et al., 2000; Tuorila et al., 2001), by median split (Mustonen et al., 2012; Raudenbush and Capiola, 2012; Yamada et al., 2012), or else by tertiles split (Raudenbush et al., 2003; Tuorila and Mustonen, 2010; Capiola and Raudenbush, 2012; Fernández-Ruiz et al., 2013). Additional new approaches have also been tested recently, for example the segmentation based on Principal Component Analysis (PCA; Demattè et al., 2013; Fernández-Ruiz et al., 2013).

FOOD NEOPHOBIA AND INDIVIDUAL FACTORS

A large number of individual factors have shown to be connected to the degree of food neophobia. Knaapila et al. (2011) reported that (especially in women) this attitude appears to be strongly genetically determined. The results of the studies conducted so far on gender differences are still quite inconclusive: Some authors have found that women are more neophobic than men (Frank and van der Klaauw, 1994), some authors described instead the contrary (Tuorila et al., 2001), whilst some others failed to find any differences at all (Flight et al., 2003; Nordin et al., 2004; Meiselman et al., 2010; Demattè et al., 2013). A clearer link has instead been described between food neophobia and age. Avoidance behavior of unfamiliar foods would appear and reach its maximum between 2 and 6 years of age (Raudenbush et al., 1998; Blissett and Fogel, 2013), starting from toddlers' developmental phase of increased physical and motor skills when they gain potential access to a larger number of (possibly dangerous) food substances (Benton, 2004). From late childhood, the levels of neophobia gradually decrease until adulthood, when this tendency would reach its minimum level (Fernández-Ruiz et al., 2013; Schnettler et al., 2013). With aging, food neophobia levels slowly start to rise again (Tuorila et al., 2001), protecting the weaker elderly organism from potential poisoning (Dovey et al., 2008). From a more psychological perspective, studies have highlighted that neophobic people would be less prone to look for strong emotions and adventures (Otis, 1984), more anxious (Dovey et al., 2008), and less open (Knaapila et al., 2011).

FEEDING BEHAVIOR AND THE ROLE OF OLFACTION

Olfaction plays a crucial role in human life. It has special connections to those areas in the brain involved in the processing and encoding of emotions and memories (Royet et al., 2003), thus it is extremely relevant in human social interaction (see e.g.; Herz and Inzlicht, 2002; Schaal et al., 2004; Demattè et al., 2007). Its importance extends also to the production of adaptive behaviors in response to the environmental stimulations. Olfaction works with the double function of alerting the organism for potentially dangerous elements present in the environment and recognizing foods useful for survival (Prescott, 1999). It is extremely influential on feeding as it represents a basic piece of flavor perception (Small et al., 1997; Prescott, 2012). As a matter of fact, flavor perception (that is the multisensory experience par excellence; Small, 2012), can be disrupted by a simple cold. While perception of the different tastes remains unaltered allowing sweetness to emerge from a candy, the information about the peach flavor of that candy gets lost in the air flow that cannot reach the olfactory epithelium. Therefore, odors appear to be crucial when it comes to the sensory evaluation of a food (Yeomans, 2006).

The investigation of chemosensory functions in eating behavior has mainly taken into account the possible differences in odor functions of patients suffering from eating disorders (e.g., anorexia) and control participants. The results described so far are not always consistent as different groups of people and different methods have been used. For instance, a study reported that people suffering from anorexia nervosa (Roessner et al., 2005) had higher olfactory thresholds and poorer discrimination abilities (but preserved odor identification performance; see also Kopala et al., 1995) than controls. On the contrary in a more recent work, anorectic patients showed to have impaired odor identification abilities (Rapps et al., 2010) with preserved olfactory thresholds. Additionally, there exist other studies targeting obese participants while focusing on taste perception rather than on olfaction. Some of the basic tastes (e.g., salty) seem to have significantly higher thresholds in obese than control participants (Overberg et al., 2012), even though others failed to show any variations (for a review, see Donaldson et al., 2009). However, for odors, there is still no evidence of the existence of reliable differences in perception in obese patients.

A different area of investigation in the field of feeding considers instead the existence of differences in the hedonic evaluation of target stimuli. The evidences indicate that people suffering from anorexia consistently perceive both odors and tastes as less pleasant than control participants (Simon et al., 1993; Jiang et al., 2010). Obese people instead do not seem to show any consistent variations in the hedonic evaluation of chemosensory stimuli (Thompson et al., 1977; Malcolm et al., 1980; though see Drewnowski et al., 1985). A significant difference seems to emerge when looking at the rewarding value of such stimuli during real food consumption. As a matter of fact in a fMRI study, a group of obese girls showed, during both food consumption and anticipation of intake, more neuronal activity than controls in those areas of the brain deputed to the encoding of reward (e.g., insula; Stice et al., 2008). This suggests that cognitive and motivational aspects might have a stronger influence on people suffering from eating disorders than purely perceptual mechanisms.

FOOD NEOPHOBIA, TASTE, AND OLFACTION

While a number of investigations have been made on the existence of systematic links between individual factors (psychological, demographical, etc.) and levels of food neophobia, others have turned their attention toward the role of sensory functions. For instance starting from the observation that neophobic children mainly refuse fruit and vegetables rather than other food categories (Wardle and Cooke, 2008), Coulthard and Blissett (2009) hypothesized that the rationale behind that could be a higher sensitivity to taste, and to bitter in particular. Using indirect measurements (i.e., parental proxy questionnaires), they highlighted that high taste sensitivity negatively correlated with the amount and variety of consumed fruit and vegetables and with the levels of food neophobia. Adults tested for their sensitivity to phenylthiocarbamide (PTC) or quinine hemisulfate (i.e., bitter substances) revealed though not to differ as a function of their attitude toward novel foods (Frank and van der Klaauw, 1994). Willingness to try unfamiliar foods, rather than having direct effects on sensory perception, influenced the hedonic evaluation of a series of food-related and food-unrelated odors. Almost all odors were judged as being less pleasant and less intense by people reluctant to try new foods supporting the notion of an important role of olfaction in food preferences and eating behavior. Interestingly, neophobic people tend to use smaller sniff magnitudes than non-neophobics, as measured during an odor detection task (Raudenbush et al., 1998), and this has been interpreted as an index of an attempt made by neophobics to avoid any possible bad odor-related experiences (Prescott et al., 2010). This would be consistent with the hypothesis that food neophobia might result from the anticipation of a possible negative outcome produced by tasting the unknown product (Pliner et al., 1993). During uncertain conditions in particular (i.e., when the information available is very scant), neophobics expect to like an unfamiliar food significantly less than neophilics. Compared to this latter group, neophobics appear to feel more uncertain about the identity of the unknown product. They are also less willing to try unfamiliar foods even when a future hypothetical situation is considered (Tuorila et al., 1994; see also Frank and Raudenbush, 1998).

Active exploration of the environment through sniffing is reckoned to be a key factor for odor detection. Frasnelli et al. (2009) described that the ability to localize a pure odorant (that is an odor that does not stimulate the trigeminal system, such as the rose-like odor of phenyl ethyl alcohol) by discriminating the stimulated nostril (right vs. left) varies as a function of the stimulus being actively sniffed or passively perceived (i.e., mechanically delivered into the nostrils). Tourbier and Doty (2007), instead, demonstrated that sniff magnitude correlates with human olfactory abilities as measured by the University of Pennsylvania Smell Identification Test (UPSIT; Doty et al., 1984), with participants having a sense of smell in the normal range showing smaller magnitude sniffs than anosmic participants. In addition interestingly, these authors highlighted that the sniff magnitude ratio is strongly modulated by the hedonic value of the perceived odor (i.e., it decreases when malodor rather than a pleasant odor is used; see also Djordjevic et al., 2008), which suggests a possible important role of expectancy in olfactory behavior that would be mediated by the hedonic dimension of odors.

Odor identification seems to be positively linked to the degree of experience one person has of the olfactory world (Lehrner and Walla, 2002; see also de Wijk and Cain, 1994a; Cain et al., 1995; Lehrner et al., 1999). de Wijk and Cain, (1994b) for instance described that odor identification ability varies according to age, being poor in childhood and improving until adulthood (Cain et al., 1995). This improvement in the odor identification ability is suggested to occur throughout the whole life-span and is dependent on a learning effect induced by a repeated exposure to the different odors. Following this logic, Demattè et al. (2013) recently formulated the hypothesis that the scant exploratory behavior described in food neophobics (Raudenbush et al., 1998) could also affect the ability of finding the right name for an odor. Therefore, a group of adult volunteers were asked to identify a series of common odors and the results revealed that neophobic people were significantly worse in the identification task than non-neophobic participants. A connection thus does seem to exist between the personal attitude toward unknown foods (as measured by the FNS) and the ability to name common odors. This relation would be mediated by the different degree of exposure a person has to different odors during life. Interestingly consistently with this, familiarity appears to have an important role in different aspects of olfactory perception (for a recent review on olfactory expertise, see Royet et al., 2013). An odor never encountered before is usually evaluated as being less pleasant than a more familiar odor (Delplanque et al., 2008), while repeated exposure to an odor appears to lower the threshold for its detection (Dalton et al., 2002).

THE MEDIATION OF EXPOSURE

The existence of an extremely powerful connection between food neophobia and both the variety in a person's diet and the repeated exposure to food products has been repeatedly demonstrated (for an earlier review, see Frank and Raudenbush, 1998; see also Pliner et al., 1993; Birch et al., 1998). In adults, diet variety plays a significant impact, as demonstrated by the negative correlation observed between the levels of food neophobia and the levels of both education and socio-economical status (Flight et al., 2003; Meiselman et al., 2010). This effect appears to be directly related to the frequency with which one person experiences different kinds of foods during everyday life (Knaapila et al., 2011). In particular, an increase in the exposure to new food has been proven to reduce general food neophobia levels (Pliner et al., 1993; Birch et al., 1998; Mustonen et al., 2012).

The effects of exposure to different foods on the attitude toward food choices have received special attention in the field of children's eating behavior (Benton, 2004; Wardle and Cooke, 2008; Raudenbush and Capiola, 2012). A crucial impact of parental behavior on the development of preferences and aversions has been highlighted, both during the weaning phase and later during childhood, and even during a child's prenatal life (Benton, 2004; Wardle and Cooke, 2008; Beauchamp and Mennella, 2011). Regular pre-exposure to anise flavor through mothers' diet has shown to be effective in inducing a preference for anise odor in newborn babies (Schaal et al., 2000). Some preferences are innate in nature, for example bitterness aversion or sweetness preference (Mennella et al., 2005; though see Desor et al., 1975), nevertheless prenatal life has been shown to have an impact also on later food preferences, showing the importance of mothers' diet quality during gestation (Trout and Wetzel-Effinger, 2012).

Food experience in the first period after birth is critical in the learning of food likes and dislikes, as such experiences are considered to drive the following development and expression of human behavior toward food (Beauchamp and Mennella, 2009). Sullivan et al. (1991) for instance have described that 1 day after birth, newborns can already learn to associate pairs of simultaneous olfactory and tactile stimuli, showing a conditioned response for the single conditioned odor experienced before. Later on during weaning, the repeated exposure to a food dramatically influences its acceptance (Nicklaus, 2011). This seems to be true if the food is actually tasted, as mere visual exposure is not sufficient to shape that preference. Other studies have highlighted the importance of parental eating style, that can influence children's food preferences by determining the ease with which they have access to a sufficiently varied diet (Finistrella et al., 2012) and by means of the powerful mechanism of parental modeling (Benton, 2004; Wardle and Cooke, 2008). In this view, it is not surprising that children's preferences strongly correlates with those of their mothers (Howard et al., 2012).

CONCLUSION

Food preferences and aversions are mediated by the chemosensory system, which underlies flavor perception (Frank and van der Klaauw, 1994). The mechanism through which food likes and dislikes are learned and modulated is represented by repeated exposure, but only if it includes actual tasting (Benton, 2004; Wardle and Cooke, 2008). Food neophobia appears to be an extremely complex attitude, its strength fluctuates during lifespan and is modulated by a number of different factors (Otis, 1984; Frank and Raudenbush, 1998; Howard et al., 2012). An individual's diet quality is strongly influenced by the attitude toward food (and novel food in particular) and it has a dramatic impact on her/his health and well-being (Falciglia et al., 2000; Capiola and Raudenbush, 2012). Therefore, an increase in the understanding of the mechanisms underlying food neophobia acquisition and modulation appears to be a critical issue for future investigations.

ACKNOWLEDGMENTS

This research was supported by Provincia Autonoma di Trento (AP 2009/2011). The authors would like to thank Valentina Ting, Eugenio Aprea, Franco Biasioli, and Maria Laura Corollaro for their valuable contribution to this work.

REFERENCES

Albrecht, J., Schreder, T., Kleemann, A. M., Schöpf, V., Kopietz, R., Anzinger, A., et al. (2009). Olfactory detection thresholds and pleasantness of a food-related and a non-food odour in hunger and satiety. *Rhinology* 47, 160–165.

Assanand, S., Pinel, J. P., and Lehman, D. R. (1998). Personal theories of hunger and eating. *J. Appl. Soc. Psychol.* 28, 998–1015. doi: 10.1111/j.1559-1816.1998.tb01664.x

Beauchamp, G. K., and Mennella, J. A. (2009). Early flavor learning and its impact on later feeding behavior. *J. Pediatr. Gastroenterol. Nutr.* 48, S25–S30. doi: 10.1097/MPG.0b013e31819774a5

Beauchamp, G. K., and Mennella, J. A. (2011). Flavor perception in human infants: development and functional significance. *Digestion* 83, 1–6. doi: 10.1159/000323397

Benton, D. (2004). Role of parents in the determination of the food preferences of children and the development of obesity. *Int. J. Obes. Rel. Metabol. Dis.* 28, 858–869. doi: 10.1038/sj.ijo.0802532

Birch, L. L., Gunder, L., and Grimm-Thomas, K. (1998). Infants' consumption of a new food enhances acceptance of similar foods. *Appetite* 30, 283–295. doi: 10.1006/appe.1997.0146

Blissett, J., and Fogel, A. (2013). Intrinsic and extrinsic influences on children's acceptance of new foods. *Physiol. Behav.* 121, 89–95. doi: 10.1016/j.physbeh.2013.02.013

Cain, W. S., Stevens, J. C., Nickou, C. M., Giles, A., Johnston, I., and Garcia-Medina, M. R. (1995). Life-span development of odor identification, learning, and olfactory sensitivity. *Perception* 24, 1457–1472. doi: 10.1068/p241457

Capiola, A., and Raudenbush, B. (2012). The effects of food neophobia and food neophilia on diet and metabolic processing. *Food Nutr. Sci.* 3, 1397–1403. doi: 10.4236/fns.2012.310183

Coulthard, H., and Blissett, J. (2009). Fruit and vegetable consumption in children and their mothers. Moderating effects of child sensory sensitivity. *Appetite* 52, 410–415. doi: 10.1016/j.appet.2008.11.015

Dalton, P., Doolittle, N., and Breslin, P. A. S. (2002). Gender-specific induction of enhanced sensitivity to odors. *Nat. Neurosci.* 5, 199–200. doi: 10.1038/nn803

de Wijk, R. A., and Cain, W. S. (1994a). Odor quality: discrimination versus free and cued identification. *Percep. Psychophys.* 56, 12–18. doi: 10.3758/BF03211686

de Wijk, R. A., and Cain, W. S. (1994b). Odor identification by name and by edibility: life-span development and safety. *Hum. Factors* 36, 182–187. doi: 10.1177/001872089403600112

Delplanque, S., Grandjean, D., Chrea, C., Aymard, L., Cayeux, I., Le Calvé, B., et al. (2008). Emotional processing of odors: evidence for a nonlinear relation between pleasantness and familiarity evaluations. *Chem. Senses* 33, 469–479. doi: 10.1093/chemse/bjn014

Demattè, M. L., Endrizzi, I., Biasioli, F., Corollaro, M. L., Pojer, N., Zampini, M., et al. (2013). Food neophobia and its relation with olfactory ability in common odour identification. *Appetite* 68, 112–117. doi: 10.1016/j.appet.2013.04.021

Demattè, M. L., Österbauer, R. A., and Spence, C. (2007). Olfactory cues modulate facial attractiveness. *Chem. Senses* 32, 603–610. doi: 10.1093/chemse/bjm030

Desor, J. A., Maller, O., and Andrews, K. (1975). Ingestive responses of human newborns to salty, sour, and bitter stimuli. *J. Compar. Physiol. Psychol.* 89, 966–970. doi: 10.1037/h0077171

Djordjevic, J., Lundstrom, J. N., Clément, F., Boyle, J. A., Pouliot, S., and Jones-Gotman, M. (2008). A rose by any other name: would it smell as sweet? *J. Neurophysiol.* 99, 386–393. doi: 10.1152/jn.00896.2007

Donaldson, L. F., Bennett, L., Baic, S., and Melichar, J. K. (2009). Taste and weight: is there a link? *Am. J. Clin. Nutr.* 90, S800–S803. doi: 10.3945/ajcn.2009.27462Q

Doty, R. L., Shaman, P., and Dann, M. (1984). Development of the University of Pennsylvania Smell Identification Test: a standardized microencapsulated test of olfactory function. *Physiol. Behav.* 32, 489–502. doi: 10.1016/0031-9384(84)90269-5

Dovey, T. M., Staples, P. A., Gibson, E. L., and Halford, J. C. G. (2008). Food neophobia and "picky/fussy" eating in children: a review. *Appetite* 50, 181–193. doi: 10.1016/j.appet.2007.09.009

Drewnowski, A., Brunzell, J. D., Sande, K., Iverius, P. H., and Greenwood, M. R. (1985). Sweet tooth reconsidered: taste responsiveness in human obesity. *Physiol. Behav.* 35, 617–622. doi: 10.1016/0031-9384(85)90150-7

Falciglia, G. A., Couch, S. C., Gribble, L. S., Pabst, S. M., and Frank, R. A. (2000). Food neophobia in childhood affects dietary variety. *J. Am. Diet. Assoc.* 100, 1474–1481. doi: 10.1016/S0002-8223(00)00412-0

Fernandez, P., Bensafi, M., Rouby, C., and Giboreau, A. (2013). Does olfactory specific satiety take place in a natural setting? *Appetite* 60, 1–4. doi: 10.1016/j.appet.2012.10.006

Fernández-Ruiz, V., Claret, A., and Chaya, C. (2013). Testing a Spanish-version of the Food Neophobia Scale. *Food Qual. Prefer.* 28, 222–225. doi: 10.1016/j.foodqual.2012.09.007

Finistrella, V., Manco, M., Ferrara, A., Rustico, C., Presaghi, F., and Morino, G. (2012). Cross-sectional exploration of maternal reports of food neophobia and pickiness in preschooler-mother dyads. *J. Am. Coll. Nutr.* 31, 152–159. doi: 10.1080/07315724.2012.10720022

Flight, I., Leppard, P., and Cox, D. N. (2003). Food neophobia and associations with cultural diversity and socio-economic status amongst rural and urban Australian adolescents. *Appetite* 41, 51–59. doi: 10.1016/S0195-6663(03)00039-4

Frank, R. A., and Raudenbush, B. (1998). "Individual differences in approach to novelty: the case of human food neophobia," in *Viewing Psychology as a Whole: The Integrative Science of William N. Dember*, eds R. R. Hoffman, M. F. Sherrick, and J. S. Warm (Washington, DC: American Psychological Association), 227–245. doi: 10.1037/10290-010

Frank, R. A., and van der Klaauw, N. J. (1994). The contribution of chemosensory factors to individual differences in reported food preferences. *Appetite* 22, 101–123. doi: 10.1006/appe.1994.1011

Frasnelli, J., Charbonneau, G., Collignon, O., and Lepore, F. (2009). Odor localization and sniffing. *Chem. Senses* 34, 139–144. doi: 10.1093/chemse/bjn068

Herz, R. S., and Inzlicht, M. (2002). Sex differences in response to physical and social factors involved in human mate selection: the importance of smell for women. *Evol. Hum. Behav.* 23, 359–364. doi: 10.1016/S1090-5138(02)00095-8

Hollar, D., Paxton-Aiken, A., and Fleming, P. (2013). Exploratory validation of the fruit and vegetable neophobia instrument among third- to fifth-grade students. *Appetite* 60, 226–230. doi: 10.1016/j.appet.2012.09.030

Howard, A. J., Mallan, K. M., Byrne, R., Magarey, A., and Daniels, L. A. (2012). Toddlers' food preferences. The impact of novel food exposure, maternal preferences and food neophobia. *Appetite* 59, 818–825. doi: 10.1016/j.appet.2012.08.022

Jiang, T., Soussignan, R., Rigaud, D., and Schaal, B. (2010). Pleasure for visual and olfactory stimuli evoking energy-dense foods is decreased in anorexia nervosa. *Psychiatry Res.* 180, 42–47. doi: 10.1016/j.psychres.2010.04.041

Knaapila, A., Silventoinen, K., Broms, U., Rose, R. J., Perola, M., Kaprio, J., et al. (2011). Food neophobia in young adults: genetic architecture and relation to personality, pleasantness and use frequency of foods, and Body Mass Index. A twin study. *Behav. Genet.* 41, 512–521. doi: 10.1007/s10519-010-9403-8

Kopala, L. C., Good, K., Goldner, E. M., and Birmingham, C. L. (1995). Olfactory identification ability in anorexia nervosa. *J. Psychiatry Neurosci.* 20, 283–286.

Lehrner, J. P., Glück, J., and Laska, M. (1999). Odor identification, consistency of label use, olfactory threshold and their relationships to odor memory over the human lifespan. *Chem. Senses* 24, 337–346. doi: 10.1093/chemse/24.3.337

Lehrner, J. P., and Walla, P. (2002). "Development of odor naming and odor memory from childhood to young adulthood," in *Olfaction, Taste, and Cognition*, eds C. Rouby, B. Schaal, D. Dubois, R. Gervais, and A. Holley (Cambridge, UK: Cambridge University Press), 278–289.

Malcolm, R., O'Neil, P. M., Hirsch, A. A., Currey, H. S., and Moskowitz, G. (1980). Taste hedonics and thresholds in obesity. *Int. J. Obes.* 4, 203–212.

Meiselman, H. L., King, S. C., and Gillette, M. (2010). The demographics of neophobia in a large commercial US sample. *Food Qual. Prefer.* 21, 893–897. doi: 10.1016/j.foodqual.2010.05.009

Mennella, J. A., Pepino, M. Y., and Reed, D. R. (2005). Genetic and environmental determinants of bitter perception and sweet preferences. *Pediatrics* 115, e216–e222. doi: 10.1542/peds.2004-1582

Mitchell, D., Kirschbaum, E. H., and Perry, R. L. (1975). Effect of neophobia and habituation on poison-induced avoidance of exteroceptive stimuli in rat. *J. Exp. Psychol.* 104, 47–55. doi: 10.1037//0097-7403.1.1.47

Mustonen, S., Oerlemans, P., and Tuorila, H. M. (2012). Familiarity with and affective responses to foods in 8-11-year-old children. The role of food neophobia and parental education. *Appetite* 58, 777–780. doi: 10.1016/j.appet.2012.01.027

Nicklaus, S. (2011). Children's acceptance of new foods at weaning. Role of practices of weaning and of food sensory properties. *Appetite* 57, 812–815. doi: 10.1016/j.appet.2011.05.321

Nordin, S., Broman, D. A., Garvill, J., and Nyroos, M. (2004). Gender differences in factors affecting rejection of food in healthy young Swedish adults. *Appetite* 43, 295–301. doi: 10.1016/j.appet.2004.07.002

Otis, L. P. (1984). Factors influencing the willingness to taste unusual foods. *Psychol. Rep.* 54, 739–745. doi: 10.2466/pr0.1984.54.3.739

Overberg, J., Hummel, T., Krude, H., and Wiegand, S. (2012). Differences in taste sensitivity between obese and non-obese children and adolescents. *Arch. Dis. Child.* 97, 1048–1052. doi: 10.1136/archdischild-2011-301189

Pliner, P. (1994). Development of measures of food neophobia in children. *Appetite* 23, 147–163. doi: 10.1006/appe.1994.1043

Pliner, P., and Hobden, K. (1992). Development of a scale to measure the trait of food neophobia in humans. *Appetite* 19, 105–120. doi: 10.1016/0195-6663(92)90014-W

Pliner, P., Pelchat, M. L., and Grabski, M. (1993). Reduction of neophobia in humans by exposure to novel foods. *Appetite* 20, 111–123. doi: 10.1006/appe.1993.1013

Prescott, J. (1999). Flavour as a psychological construct: implications for perceiving and measuring the sensory qualities of foods. *Food Qual. Prefer.* 10, 349–356. doi: 10.1016/S0950-3293(98)00048-2

Prescott, J. (2012). Chemosensory learning and flavour: perception, preference and intake. *Physiol. Behav.* 107, 553–559. doi: 10.1016/j.physbeh.2012.04.008 doi: 10.1016/j.physbeh.2012.04.008

Prescott, J., Burns, J., and Frank, R. A. (2010). Influence of odor hedonics, food-relatedness, and motivational state on human sniffing. *Chemosens. Percept.* 3, 85–90. doi: 10.1007/s12078-010-9073-1

Rapps, N., Giel, K. E., Söhngen, E., Salini, A., Enck, P., Bischoff, S. C., et al. (2010). Olfactory deficits in patients with anorexia nervosa. *Eur. Eat. Disord. Rev.* 18, 385–389. doi: 10.1002/erv.1010

Raudenbush, B., and Capiola, A. (2012). Physiological responses of food neophobics and food neophilics to food and non-food stimuli. *Appetite* 58, 1106–1108. doi: 10.1016/j.appet.2012.02.042

Raudenbush, B., Corley, N., Flower, N. R., Kozlowski, A., and Meyer, B. (2003). Cephalic phase salivary response differences characterize level of food neophobia. *Appetite* 41, 211–212. doi: 10.1016/S0195-6663(03)00059-X

Raudenbush, B., Schroth, F., Reilley, S., and Frank, R. A. (1998). Food neophobia, odor evaluation and exploratory sniffing behavior. *Appetite* 31, 171–183. doi: 10.1006/appe.1998.0161

Roberts, B., and Cheney, C. (1974). Food neophobia and taste aversion in tropical fish. *Proc. Utah Acad. Sci. Arts Lett.* 51, 201.

Roessner, V., Bleich, S., Banaschewski, T., and Rothenberger, A. (2005). Olfactory deficits in anorexia nervosa. *Eur. Arch. Psychiatry Clin. Neurosci.* 255, 6–9. doi: 10.1007/s00406-004-0525-y

Rolls, E. T. (2012). Taste, olfactory and food texture reward processing in the brain and the control of appetite. *Proc. Nutr. Soc.* 71, 488–501. doi: 10.1017/S0029665112000821

Royet, J. -P., Plailly, J., Delon-Martin, C., Kareken, D. A., and Segebarth, C. (2003). fMRI of emotional responses to odors: influence of hedonic valence and judgment, handedness, and gender. *Neuroimage* 20, 713–728. doi: 10.1016/S1053-8119(03)00388-4

Royet, J. -P., Plailly, J., Saive, A. -L., Veyrac, A., and Delon-Martin, C. (2013). The impact of expertise in olfaction. *Front. Psychol.* 4:928. doi: 10.3389/fpsyg.2013.00928

Rozin, P. (1968). Specific aversions and neophobia resulting from vitamin deficiency or poisoning in half-wild and domestic rats. *J. Compar. Physiol. Psychol.* 66, 82–88. doi: 10.1037/h0025974

Rozin, P., and Vollmecke, T. A. (1986). Food likes and dislikes. *Annu. Rev. Nutr.* 6, 433–456. doi: 10.1146/annurev.nu.06.070186.002245

Schaal, B., Hummel, T., and Soussignan, R. (2004). Olfaction in the fetal and premature infant: functional status and clinical implications. *Clin. Perinatol.* 31, 261–285. doi: 10.1016/j.clp.2004.04.003

Schaal, B., Marlier, L., and Soussignan, R. (2000). Human foetuses learn odours from their pregnant mother's diet. *Chem. Senses* 25, 729–737. doi: 10.1093/chemse/25.6.729

Schnettler, B., Crisóstomo, G., Sepúlveda, J., Mora, M., Lobos, G., Miranda, H., et al. (2013). Food neophobia, nanotechnology and satisfaction with life. *Appetite* 69, 71–79. doi: 10.1016/j.appet.2013.05.014

Simon, Y., Bellisle, F., Monneuse, M. O., Samuel-Lajeunesse, B., and Drewnowski, A. (1993). Taste responsiveness in anorexia-nervosa. *Br. J. Psychiatry* 162, 244–246. doi: 10.1192/bjp.162.2.244

Small, D. M. (2012). Flavor is in the brain. *Physiol. Behav.* 107, 540–552. doi: 10.1016/j.physbeh.2012.04.011

Small, D. M., Jones-Gotman, M., Zatorre, R. J., Petrides, M., and Evans, A. C. (1997). Flavor processing: more than the sum of its parts. *Neuroreport* 8, 3913–3917. doi: 10.1097/00001756-199712220-00014

Small, D. M., Zatorre, R. J., Dagher, A., Evans, A. C., and Jones-Gotman, M. (2001). Changes in brain activity related to eating chocolate: from pleasure to aversion. *Brain* 124, 1720–1733. doi: 10.1093/brain/124.9.1720

Stice, E., Spoor, S., Bohon, C., Veldhuizen, M. G., and Small, D. M. (2008). Relation of reward from food intake and anticipated food intake to obesity: a functional magnetic resonance imaging study. *J. Abnorm. Psychol.* 117, 924–935. doi: 10.1037/a0013600

Sullivan, R. M., Taborsky-Barba, S., Mendoza, R., Itano, A., Leon, M., Cotman, C., et al. (1991). Olfactory classical conditioning in neonates. *Pediatrics* 87, 511–518.

Thompson, D. A., Moskowitz, H. R., and Campbell, R. G. (1977). Taste and olfaction in human obesity. *Physiol. Behav.* 19, 335–337. doi: 10.1016/0031-9384(77)90348-1

Tourbier, I. A., and Doty, R. L. (2007). Sniff magnitude test: relationship to odor identification, detection, and memory tests in a clinic population. *Chem. Senses* 32, 515–523. doi: 10.1093/chemse/bjm020

Trout, K., and Wetzel-Effinger, L. (2012). Flavor learning in utero and its implications for future obesity and diabetes. *Curr. Diab. Rep.* 12, 60–66. doi: 10.1007/s11892-011-0237-4

Tuorila, H. M., Lähteenmäki, L., Pohjalainen, L., and Lotti, L. (2001). Food neophobia among the Finns and related responses to familiar and unfamiliar foods. *Food Qual. Prefer.* 12, 29–37. doi: 10.1016/S0950-3293(00)00025-2

Tuorila, H. M., Meiselman, H. L., Bell, R., Cardello, A. V., and Johnson, W. (1994). Role of sensory and cognitive information in the enhancement of certainty and linking for novel and familiar foods. *Appetite* 23, 231–246. doi: 10.1006/appe.1994.1056

Tuorila, H. M., and Mustonen, S. (2010). Reluctant trying of an unfamiliar food induces negative affection for the food. *Appetite* 54, 418–421. doi: 10.1016/j.appet.2010.01.010

Wardle, J., and Cooke, L. (2008). Genetic and environmental determinants of children's food preferences. *Br. J. Nutr.* 99, S15–S21. doi: 10.1017/S000711450889246X

Yamada, Y., Kawabe, T., and Ihaya, K. (2012). Can you eat it? A link between categorization difficulty and food likability. *Adv. Cogn. Psychol.* 8, 248–254. doi: 10.2478/v10053-008-0120-2

Yeomans, M. R. (2006). Olfactory influences on appetite and satiety in humans. *Physiol. Behav.* 87, 800–804. doi: 10.1016/j.physbeh.2006.01.029

3

A pleasant familiar odor influences perceived stress and peripheral nervous system activity during normal aging

Pauline Joussain, Catherine Rouby and Moustafa Bensafi*

Lyon Neuroscience Research Center, CNRS UMR5292, INSERM U1028, University of Lyon, Lyon, France

Correspondence:
Moustafa Bensafi, Lyon Neuroscience Research Center, CNRS UMR5292, INSERM U1028, University of Lyon, 50 Avenue Tony Garnier, F-69366 Lyon, France
e-mail: bensafi@olfac.univ-lyon1.fr

Effects of smells on stress have been demonstrated in animals and humans, suggesting that inhaling certain odorants may counteract the negative effects of stress. Because stress plays a key role in cerebral aging, the present study set out to examine whether positive odor effects on perceived stress can be achieved in elderly individuals. To this end, two groups of aged individuals ($n = 36$ women, aged from 55 to 65 years), were tested. The first group was exposed for 5 days to a pleasant and, by end of exposure, familiar odor ("exposure odor"), whereas the other was exposed to a non-scented control stimulus. Stress and mood states were assessed before and after the 5-day odor exposure period. Psychophysiological markers were also assessed at the end of exposure, in response to the "exposure odor" and to a "new odor." Results revealed that stress on this second exposure was decreased and zygomatic electromyogram activity was increased specifically in the group previously exposed to the odor ($p < 0.05$). Taken as a whole, these findings offer a new look at the relationship between perceived stress, olfaction and normal aging, opening up new research perspectives on the effect of olfaction on quality of life and well-being in aged individuals.

Keywords: olfaction, exposure, stress, mood, physiology, aging

INTRODUCTION

In daily life, odors influence behavior and affective states: toxic substances are avoided thanks to the sense of smell, whereas smells are prominent keys to the hedonic pleasure provided by food or perfumes. The relationships between olfaction and affects have been extensively studied in the last decade. This recent research showed that the effects of odors on affective behavior are partly predisposed (Khan et al., 2007; Mandairon et al., 2009; Poncelet et al., 2010b; Joussain et al., 2011; Zarzo, 2011), but are also tuned by learning mechanisms, whether associative learning or mere exposure (Cain and Johnson, 1978; Rouby et al., 2009b; Poncelet et al., 2010a). These affective states influence behavior and mood to the extent that 12 days' exposure to pleasant odors improved mood in females at midlife, opening new perspectives on the beneficial effect of odor exposure during normal aging (Schiffman et al., 1995). These effects were documented by Schiffman et al. (1995) for specific mood states (tension and depression), and very little is known about odor effects on other individual psychological and physiological responses such as stress. The aim of the present study was to test the effect of odor exposure on perceived stress during normal aging.

Studying the effect of odors on stress during normal aging would be particularly valuable because stress plays a key role in brain aging: reduced resilience in response to changes produced by exposure to a chronic stressor could explain some of the morphological, hormonal and behavioral changes observed in the aged brain (Garrido, 2011). Moreover, focusing on older people is of interest because, despite age-related loss of olfactory function in terms of detection, discrimination, pleasantness and identification (Doty, 1989; Hummel et al., 2007; Joussain et al., 2013), the subjective importance of olfaction remains unchanged (Croy et al., 2010).

Positive effects of odorants on stress were demonstrated in rats and mice and also in young adult humans (Fukada et al., 2007; Oka et al., 2008; Ito et al., 2009; Nikaido and Nakashima, 2009; Mezzacappa et al., 2010), suggesting that inhaling certain odorants may counteract the negative effects of stress. The present study tested the general hypothesis that odor exposure decreases stress in aged individuals. Women around the menopause in particular were chosen because changes around the menopause induce both physiological and social stress, added to aging effects as such [see (Pouliot et al., 2008)]. A second reason for limiting the study to women was that choosing female subjects also allowed the olfactory exposure procedure to be hidden inside an everyday activity that is far more frequent in women: a skin care routine. Finally, because stress is a multidimensional state including psychological and physiological components, both perceived stress and peripheral nervous system activity [heart rate, respiration and facial electromyogram (EMG)] were recorded.

Participants were randomly assigned to either a "test group," in which the odorized source object consisted of scented cosmetic creams, or a "control group" in which similar but unscented creams were used. Participants were not aware of this difference and no mention was made of the presence of a perfume. They were tested in two separate sessions. In the first session, on arrival in the laboratory they were asked to complete a subjective questionnaire comprising perceived stress and mood items. They were then given the cosmetics, and the procedure to be followed during a week of application was explained to them. After 5-days' exposure, they came back to the lab for a second session and completed the subjective questionnaire again. Afterward, a within-subject design was used such that each subject (in either group) was tested with the "exposure-odor" (which had been present in the cosmetic cream of the "test group" but not in that of the controls) and a "new-odor" (not present in either of the cosmetics) while physiological parameters were recorded.

Specific hypotheses were that: (i) odor exposure should decrease stress and modulate mood (increase positive mood and decrease negative mood); (ii) odor exposure should reduce the physiological response associated with stressful situations or aversive events (decrease heart rate and respiratory rhythm) and increase physiological response to positive affects [increase zygomatic activity, since a positive correlation between the activity of this facial muscle and sensorial pleasure was observed in past studies (Lang et al., 1993; Sloan et al., 2002)]; and (iii) the odor used in the exposure procedure should become more pleasant and more familiar in the "test group".

MATERIALS AND METHODS

SUBJECTS

Forty-eight women aged between 55 and 65 years participated in the experiment after giving informed consent to procedures that had been approved by the Lyon Committee for the Protection of Human Subjects and conducted in accordance with the Declaration of Helsinki. They were screened for history of neurological disease or injury and of nasal insult. They were randomly assigned to either a "test group" in which the effect of an odorized stimulus (exposure-odor) was evaluated, or a "control group" using the same (but unscented) stimulus. Only 36 of the original 48 subjects (17 from the test group and 19 from the control group) could be analyzed, due to missing questionnaire data and/or problems in recording physiological data. The two groups did not differ in age [mean+/−SEM: test group, 58.6+/−0.9 years; control group, 59.8+/−0.7 years; $F(1,34) = 1.255$, $p > 0.05$]. It is noteworthy that all the women reported menopausal symptoms but none were currently under hormonal replacement therapy. Menopausal age did not differ between groups [mean+/−SEM: test group, 7.3+/−1.3 years; control group, 9.2+/−0.7 years; $F(1,34) = 1.873$, $p > 0.05$].

Because anhedonia may influence hedonic perception of odors (Pouliot et al., 2008), the anhedonia level of each woman was assessed on the Physical Anhedonia Scale (Chapman et al., 1976), a 61-item true/false inventory. Anhedonia is measured from assertions about stimuli and situations which are socially recognized as pleasant. Thus, the anhedonia scale measures disagreement with the positive semantic encoding of sensory experience, or how much subjects distance themselves from positive emotional stimuli. The questionnaire shows significant reliability and has been validated in previous non-olfactory studies (Loas et al., 1996; Dubal et al., 2000). Possible scores range from 0 to 61 (a low score corresponding to a low degree of anhedonia). Anhedonia scores did not differ between the two groups [mean+/−SEM: test group, 13.5+/−1.4; control group, 14.5+/−1.5; $F(1,34) = 0.251$, $p > 0.05$], Finally, subjects' olfactory performance was estimated on the ETOC (Thomas-Danguin et al., 2003). The ETOC comprises 16 blocks of four flasks. Only one flask per block contains an odorant. For each block, participants are asked firstly to detect which flask contains an odorant and secondly to identify the detected smell. Identification is assessed by a multiple-choice procedure in which participants must select the correct descriptor out of four. Detection scores range from 0 to 16 and are an indicator of sensitivity; identification scores also range from 0 to 16, but only odors that have been correctly detected are taken into account, thus reducing the probability of fortuitous correct identification. Neither detection [mean+/−SEM: test group, 14.9+/−0.4; control group, 14.5+/−0.3; $F(1,34) = 0.627$, $p > 0.05$] nor identification scores [mean+/−SEM: test group, 12.8+/−0.4; control group, 11.9+/−0.4; $F(1,34) = 1.959$, $p > 0.05$] differed between groups.

PROCEDURE

Participants were tested in two separate sessions. In the first session, on arrival in the laboratory they were asked to complete a subjective questionnaire combining perceived stress assessment and positive and negative mood items. Practically, they were asked to rate what degree of stress they perceived on a single 9-point visual scale from 1 ("not at all stressed") to 9 ("very strongly stressed"). In addition, they were asked to rate how strongly they were experiencing each of a number of positive (amused, calm, confident, content, happy, interested) and negative emotional states (afraid, angry, annoyed, anxious, bored, contemptuous, disgusted, sad), using the same 9-point scales from 1 ("not at all amused," etc.) to 9 ("very strongly amused," etc.). "Sexually aroused" was also added as an item and used as a descriptor. This questionnaire was validated in previous olfactory studies (Bensafi et al., 2003, 2004).

The procedure to be followed during the week of exposure was then detailed. Practically, they were first given two cosmetic creams (one for the face and one for the body). They were explained that the main aim of the study was to assess the impact of these creams on mood and emotion. They were instructed to use the creams each morning for 5 days; they were not allowed to use their normal scented cosmetics during that week and were restricted to non-perfumed toiletries during the course of the study. They were not asked to assess any physical or sensory attributes of the creams. However, they were asked to assess their mood (on the subjective questionnaire used in the first session) every morning before and after application of the cosmetics. Participants who did not fill in all questionnaires during the 5 days were excluded from analysis. In the test group, the cosmetics were odorized with a pleasant floral odor ("exposure odor": citrus, resinous notes, Symrise®), but were non-odorized in the control group. It is noteworthy here that the cover story was exactly the same in both groups: the smell of the cosmetics was never mentioned in any instructions, whichever the group.®

After the week of exposure, subjects came back to the lab for a second session and completed the subjective questionnaire again. A within-subject design was then implemented such that each subject (in either group) was tested with the "exposure odor" (that had been present in the test group's but not the control group's cosmetics) and another pleasant floral odor ("new odor": green, woody notes, Firmenich®) while physiological parameters were recorded. It is noteworthy that both, the "exposure odor" and the "new odor" were selected because they were a priori pleasant and included olfactory notes used in perfumery (e.g., floral, citrus, resinous, green, woody notes).

All testing was performed in a ventilated room designed specifically for olfactory experiments. The experimenter fitted the subject with the peripheral nervous system recording and odor diffusion equipment. Once peripheral nervous system measurements stabilized, recording was initiated to obtain a psychophysiological baseline. The two odor conditions ("exposure odor" and "new odor") were presented randomly (i.e., individual order for each subject) via an olfactometer (Rouby et al., 2009a). There was no verbal interaction between investigator and subject during the recording session and participants were asked to relax as much as possible. At the end of the session, they were asked to rate the intensity, familiarity, and pleasantness of both odors on a scale from 1 (not at all intense, pleasant, familiar) to 9 (very intense, pleasant, familiar).

ODOR DIFFUSION AND OLFACTOMETRY

Pure air was delivered by a compressor and cleaned by an active carbon filter, then carried to the olfactometer input line (6 mm diameter, 5 m length tube). A manometer allowed selection of air input pressure. The air then entered two channels: (1) the air-carrier channel and (2) the odorized channels (one channel per odorant). Each odorized channel contained a glass tube with polypropylene marbles, in which one of the two odorants was adsorbed. Thus, at the exit from each channel, an electric valve could be programmed closed or open in order to determine which odorant would be pushed into the airflow, and for how long. This allowed opening/closure of each valve, and thus stimulus duration (60 s, two presentations of each odor), to be controlled. The interstimulus interval (ISI) was between 60 and 120 s. Odor concentration was 0.5% vol/vol in the cosmetic creams, and a similar perceived intensity was set for the smell diffused from the olfactometer. Carrier airflow was constant, at 1,500 ml/min, and the flow rate of each electric valve was set at 100 ml/min; output odorous air was led through a 4 mm tube (20 cm length) into the nasal mask; both nostrils were stimulated.

The ventilated and refreshed experimental room comprised two spaces: one for the experimenter and one for the subject. The experimenter's space contained the computer controlling the olfactometer's physiological parameters; the subject's space included the output part of the olfactometer and a computer screen and mouse to read instructions and give responses after the session.

PHYSIOLOGICAL PARAMETERS

In previous studies, olfactory compounds induced psychophysiological responses related to changes in electrodermal response, systolic blood pressure, EMG, respiration, and finger pulse rate (Alaoui-Ismaili et al., 1997a,b; Bensafi et al., 2002; Delplanque et al., 2009; Croy et al., 2013). In the present study, psychophysiological effects were measured on three parameters that were simultaneously and continuously recorded and displayed during the experiment: facial zygomatic EMG, Finger pulse frequency (FPF) and respiratory rate (RR). Electrodermal response magnitude was not used, because it is highly variable in the elderly, some aged subjects showing great variation and others no significant response (Abriat et al., 2007). All parameters were sampled and recorded at 32 Hz. Data were converted and amplified via a 8-channel Procomp+ amplifier (Thought Technology, Montreal, QC, Canada), and displayed, stored, reduced and analyzed off-line.

Facial EMG, expressed in microvolts (μV), was measured using miniature Ag/AgCl electrodes (diameter, 0.8 cm) placed on the zygomatic muscle after cleaning the skin with alcohol. The electrodes were filled with electrode paste and attached with adhesive disks. EMG activity was measured on a PROCOMP+ amplifier (Thought Technology), with band pass filtered from 20 to 1,000 Hz. Data were reduced to EMG area under the curve, calculated during a time window of 10 s after odor diffusion. This time window was chosen to limit analysis to facial mimics induced by the olfactory stimuli.

Changes in abdominal circumference with respiration were measured using a respiratory belt transducer (100 cm rest length, 10 cm maximum elongation, 3.5 cm width), responding linearly to changes in length. Data were reduced to RR, calculated during both 60-s periods of odor diffusion.

Finger pulse frequency was measured using a photoplethysmographic probe (3.2 cm/1.8 cm, LED type photodetector) placed on the thumb of the non-dominant (i.e., left) hand. Data were reduced to pulse rate in beats per minute (BPM).

DATA ANALYSIS

Stress and mood data were analyzed in two ways. First, they were expressed as differences in rating between sessions 1 and 2 (session 2 minus session 1: "long-term effect" analysis). Second, stress and mood data during the week of application were expressed as differences in rating before and after daily use of cosmetics (after minus before: "application effect" analysis) and averaged across the 5 days. In both analyzes, stress and mood data were compared on one-way ANOVA, with group ("test group" vs. "control group") as between-subjects factor.

Physiological data compared on ANOVA for each physiological parameter, with condition ("exposure odor" and "new odor") and time ("first presentation" and "second presentation") as within-subject factors and group ("test group" vs. "control group") as between-subjects factor. For physiological data, if significant "group"*"condition" or "group"*"condition"*"time" interactions were observed, the analysis was followed by paired comparisons (without setting corrections for multiple comparison, since the hypotheses were specific).

RESULTS

EFFECTS ON STRESS AND MOOD

During the week of application, a significant effect of group on mood was observed: negative mood decreased in the test group compared to the control group [$F(1,34) = 5.036$, $p = 0.03$]. This effect was accompanied by an effect on stress: perceived stress decreased in the test group compared to the control group [$F(1,34) = 4.018$, $p = 0.05$]. No effect of group was observed for positive mood [$F(1,34) = 0.584$, $p > 0.05$] or sexual arousal [$F(1,34) = 1.718$, $p > 0.05$] (**Figure 1A**; **Table 1**).

After the week of exposure, the group effect for stress was replicated [$F(1,34) = 5.040$, $p = 0.03$]: the test group felt less stress than the control group. However, no significant differences between groups were observed for sexual arousal [$F(1,34) = 0.497$, $p > 0.05$], negative mood [$F(1,34) = 1.534$, $p > 0.05$] or positive mood [$F(1,34) = 0.461$, $p > 0.05$] (**Figure 1B**; **Table 2**).

EFFECTS ON PERIPHERAL NERVOUS SYSTEM ACTIVITY

Finger pulse frequency showed a significant effect of time [$F(1,34) = 5.455$, $p = 0.0256$] reflecting a general decrease of FPF from the first presentation (mean+/−SEM: 67.85+/−1.922) to the second presentation (mean+/−SEM: 66.79 +/−1.81). However, no significant effects of group [$F(1,34) = 0.089$, $p > 0.05$] and odor [$F(1,34) = 1.161$, $p > 0.05$] and no significant odor*group or odor*group*time interactions were observed (**Figure 2B**). RR showed no significant effect of group [$F(1,34) = 4.021$, $p > 0.05$], odor [$F(1,34) = 1.321$, $p > 0.05$] and time [$F(1,34) = 0.322$, $p > 0.05$], and no significant odor*group or odor*group*time interaction (**Figures 2A,B**; **Table 3**).

For EMG, however, a significant odor*group interaction [$F(1,34) = 16.555$, $p = 0.0003$], but no significant group [$F(1,34) = 0.823$, $p > 0.05$], odor [$F(1,34) = 2.744$, $p > 0.05$] or time [$F(1,34) = 0.757$, $p > 0.05$] effect, was observed: EMG activity was greater for the exposure odor than for the new odor in the test group ($p = 0.003$) but not in the control group ($p > 0.05$; **Figure 2C**; **Table 3**). It is noteworthy here that these EMG effects were accompanied by perceptual differences in each group: (i) in the test group, the exposure odor was perceived as more pleasant ($p = 0.042$), more familiar ($p = 0.041$) but not more intense ($p > 0.05$) than the new odor, (ii) and as more familiar ($p = 0.010$), but not more pleasant ($p > 0.05$) and more intense ($p > 0.05$) in the control group (**Table 4**).

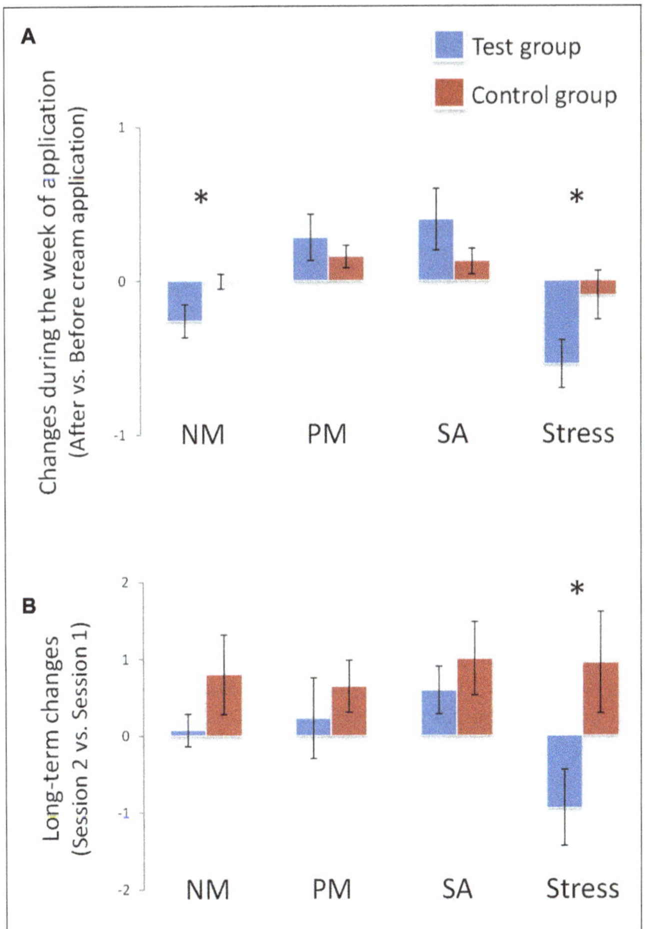

FIGURE 1 | Effects on mood, sexual arousal, and stress. (**A**) During the week of application, negative mood and stress decreased significantly (*) in the test group vs. the control group. Stress decreased significantly (*) in the test group vs. the control group at end of the week of application (long-term changes, **B**). NM, PM, SA: respectively, negative mood, positive mood and sexual arousal. *$p < 0.05$. Data are expressed as means and SEM.

Table 1 | Mood, sexual arousal, and stress changes (mean and SEM) during the week of application (after vs. before the daily application of the odorized cosmetics (test group) and non-odorized cosmetics (control group).

	Test group		Control group	
	Mean	**SEM**	**Mean**	**SEM**
Negative mood	−0.26	0.11	0.00	0.05
Positive mood	0.28	0.15	0.16	0.07
Sexual arousal	0.40	0.20	0.13	0.08
Stress	−0.54	0.16	−0.09	0.16

Table 2 | Mood, sexual arousal, and stress changes (mean and SEM) between the second session and the first session in the test group and the control group.

	Test group		Control group	
	Mean	**SEM**	**Mean**	**SEM**
Negative mood	0.07	0.21	0.80	0.52
Positive mood	0.23	0.52	0.64	0.34
Sexual arousal	0.59	0.31	1.00	0.48
Stress	−0.94	0.50	0.95	0.66

DISCUSSION

The present study tested the hypothesis that regular exposure to an odor in a natural setting decreases stress and modulates peripheral nervous system response in aged women. Daily olfactory exposure did indeed modify perceived stress: compared to controls, test group subjects showed decreased negative mood and stress during the week of regular exposure. Although the effect on mood was not confirmed one week later, the stress effect persisted at the second session: the test group showed less stress than the control group after the week of exposure. These findings are in line with animal and human studies showing an influence of odors on stress: for example, "green odors"

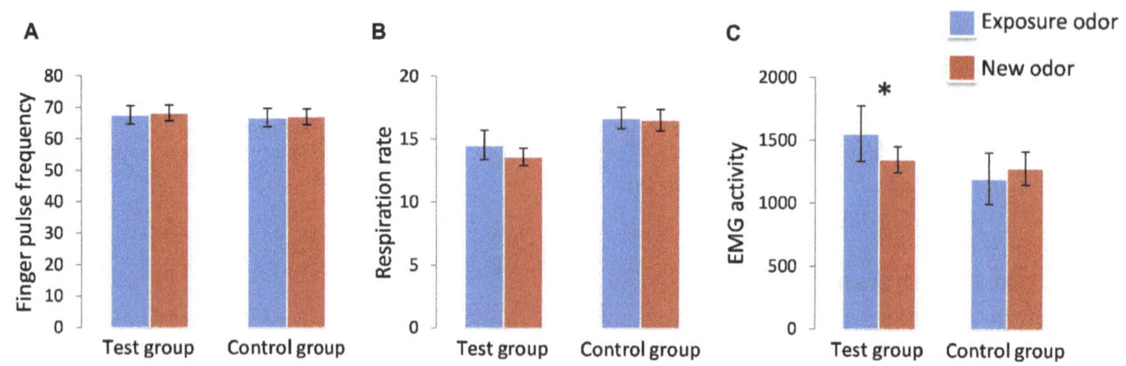

FIGURE 2 | Effects on Finger Pulse (A), Respiration (B), and EMG activity (C). Zygomatic EMG increased significantly (*) in response to the exposure odor vs. the new odor in the test group but not in the control group. Finger pulse and respiration activities did not change as a function of odor type (exposure odor vs. new odor) in the test group or the control group. *$p < 0.05$. Data are expressed as means and SEM.

Table 3 | Physiological responses to the exposure odor and the new odor (mean and SEM of EMG area under the curve, Respiratory rate or RR and Finger pulse frequency or FPF) in the test group and the control group.

		Test group		Control group	
		Mean	**SEM**	**Mean**	**SEM**
EMG	"Exposure odor"	1555.31	220.43	1200.19	103.11
	"New odor"	1350.77	204.93	1284.55	131.01
RR	"Exposure odor"	14.56	1.17	16.72	0.69
	"New odor"	13.62	0.85	16.55	0.86
FPR	"Exposure odor"	67.62	2.92	66.78	2.54
	"New odor"	68.21	2.89	67.05	2.47

Table 4 | Intensity, pleasantness, and familiarity ratings (mean and SEM) of the exposure odor and the new odor in the test group and the control group.

		Test group		Control group	
		Mean	**SEM**	**Mean**	**SEM**
Intensity	"Exposure odor"	5.94	0.42	6.84	0.38
	"New odor"	4.88	0.51	6.32	0.50
Pleasantness	"Exposure odor"	6.53	0.34	6.58	0.33
	"New odor"	5.41	0.43	6.05	0.44
Familiarity	"Exposure odor"	6.35	0.49	7.03	0.30
	"New odor"	4.79	0.59	5.47	0.61

have been shown to exert anxiolytic and stress-reducing effects in human subjects (Oka et al., 2008) and also to alleviate stress-induced cardiovascular, hormonal, and behavioral responses in rats (Ito et al., 2009; Nikaido and Nakashima, 2009). Similar effects were recently reported for coconut (Mezzacappa et al., 2010) and rose odors (Fukada et al., 2007). Because stress plays a key role in brain aging, not only exercise but also environmental stimulation can contribute to protecting the aging brain against stressors (Garrido, 2011). In line with this, animal and human studies (van Praag et al., 2000; Mahncke et al., 2006) suggest that there is significant benefit in repeatedly exposing human subjects to sensory cues. The present study extended these findings to olfaction on the one hand and perceived stress on the other.

Interestingly, the observed modulation of stress was accompanied by modified psychophysiological patterns: following stimulation with the test odor (unlike the control odor), zygomatic EMG activity increased in the test group but not in the control group. This effect on facial EMG activity was associated with a modulation of odor hedonic response: the exposure odor was perceived as more pleasant than the new odor in the test group but not in the control group, in agreement with the literature on exposure effects in the visual domain (Monahan et al., 2000). It is noteworthy that our study was conducted in women, with results in line with data showing that, in terms of emotional response to odors, women report more frequent evocations of emotional memories by odors and stronger feelings of happiness, sadness and well-being, and reduced stress as a consequence of smelling odors (Martin et al., 2001).

Another result of interest was the greater familiarity of the exposure odor compared to the control odor in both groups. Although it was expected that the exposure odor would be rated as more familiar than the control odor in the test group, this was not assumed for the control group. This reflects the fact that, overall, the exposure odor was perceived as more familiar, raising the question as to whether the present effect on stress and physiology could be obtained with an unfamiliar odor. This greater familiarity does not, however, weaken the strength of our finding, but leads us to consider the exposure odor as being a familiar odor. In sum, the present study suggests that stress (and at least negative mood during the week of exposure) and physiology in elderly people can be influenced by repeated exposure to a pleasant and familiar odor in a natural setting.

That a pleasant familiar odor influenced stress and physiological response in aged women is a novel finding. The question arises as to the route by which this effect is produced. One possibility would involve a direct effect on neural activity in the substrates of mood and stress, but mediated by the olfactory system. Such a path may reflect a privileged relationship between the neural substrates of olfaction and regions of the brain involved in affective processing (Gottfried et al., 2002; Anderson et al., 2003; Rolls et al., 2003; Bensafi et al., 2012).

The present study thus provides the first evidence for an influence of exposure to a familiar odor on perceived stress and facial electromyographic activity in aged women in a natural setting. It is important to mention here that other sensory influences may have accompanied the effect of odor exposure. Indeed, an associative learning linking the exposure odor with a supposedly pleasant touch (tactile stimulation during application of body and facial cosmetics) may have occurred. This possibility is not unlikely since our ecological situation was multimodal, involving olfactory but also visual and tactile stimuli. In such natural settings, it is not easy to isolate the specific influence of touch and smell on stress, and physiology. However, our data shows that the same situation without smell (e.g., control group), did not impact stress and physiology, reflecting that the smell used was a prominent driver of the observed effect.

Besides the above, another question that may be raised concerns potential inter-group differences in individual factors such as age, impaired sensory pleasure or hormonal status. Olfactory function is known to be impaired with age (Doty, 1989; Hummel et al., 2007), and odor hedonic perception was also found to be modified in aged people (Joussain et al., 2013). However, this possibility is ruled out in the present case by the fact that the two groups of aged women did not differ in mean chronological age or anhedonia level. Moreover, although we cannot confirm that the hormonal status of the women in the two groups was equivalent, as we did not measure it, no women in either group were taking hormonal replacement therapy and there was no difference in mean menopausal age.

In conclusion, notwithstanding the above reserves, the present study offers new insight into the effect of exposure to a familiar pleasant odor on perceived stress and physiology. The effects observed here cannot be explained adequately by age, menopausal age or differential impairment of sensory pleasure. The present study demonstrates for the first time that a 1-week odor exposure procedure in an ecological setting can modulate stress, and opens up new research perspectives on the effect of olfaction on quality of life and well-being.

REFERENCES

Abriat, A., Barkat, S., Bensafi, M., Rouby, C., and Fanchon, C. (2007). Psychological and physiological evaluation of emotional effects of a perfume in menopausal women. *Int. J. Cosmet. Sci.* 29, 399–408. doi: 10.1111/j.1468-2494.2007.00398.x

Alaoui-Ismaili, O., Robin, O., Rada, H., Dittmar, A., and Vernet-Maury, E. (1997a). Basic emotions evoked by odorants: comparison between autonomic responses and self-evaluation. *Physiol. Behav.* 62, 713–720. doi: 10.1016/S0031-9384(97)90016-0

Alaoui-Ismaili, O., Vernet-Maury, E., Dittmar, A., Delhomme, G., and Chanel, J. (1997b). Odor hedonics: connection with emotional response estimated by autonomic parameters. *Chem. Senses* 22, 237–248. doi: 10.1093/chemse/22.3.237

Anderson, A. K., Christoff, K., Stappen, I., Panitz, D., Ghahremani, D. G., Glover, G., et al. (2003). Dissociated neural representations of intensity and valence in human olfaction. *Nat. Neurosci.* 6, 196–202. doi: 10.1038/nn1001

Bensafi, M., Brown, W. M., Khan, R., Levenson, B., and Sobel, N. (2004). Sniffing human sex-steroid derived compounds modulates mood, memory and autonomic nervous system function in specific behavioral contexts. *Behav. Brain Res.* 152, 11–22.

Bensafi, M., Brown, W. M., Tsutsui, T., Mainland, J. D., Johnson, B. N., Bremner, E. A., et al. (2003). Sex-steroid derived compounds induce sex-specific effects on autonomic nervous system function in humans. *Behav. Neurosci.* 117, 1125–1134. doi: 10.1037/0735-7044.117.6.1125

Bensafi, M., Iannilli, E., Poncelet, J., Seo, H. S., Gerber, J., Rouby, C., et al. (2012). Dissociated representations of pleasant and unpleasant olfacto-trigeminal mixtures: an FMRI study. *PLoS ONE* 7:e38358. doi: 10.1371/journal.pone.0038358

Bensafi, M., Rouby, C., Farget, V., Bertrand, B., Vigouroux, M., and Holley, A. (2002). Psychophysiological correlates of affects in human olfaction. *Neurophysiol. Clin.* 32, 326–332. doi: 10.1016/S0987-7053(02)00339-8

Cain, W. S., and Johnson, F. Jr. (1978). Lability of odor pleasantness: influence of mere exposure. *Perception* 7, 459–465. doi: 10.1068/p070459

Chapman, L. J., Chapman, J. P., and Raulin, M. L. (1976). Scales for physical and social anhedonia. *J. Abnorm. Psychol.* 85, 374–382. doi: 10.1037/0021-843X.85.4.374

Croy, I., Buschhüter, D., Seo, H., Negoias, S., and Hummel, T. (2010). Individual significance of olfaction: development of a questionnaire. *Eur. Arch. Otorhinolaryngol.* 267, 67–71. doi: 10.1007/s00405-009-1054-0

Croy, I., Laqua, K., Süß, F., Joraschky, P., Ziemssen, T., and Hummel, T. (2013). The sensory channel of presentation alters subjective ratings and autonomic responses toward disgusting stimuli-Blood pressure, heart rate and skin conductance in response to visual, auditory, haptic and olfactory presented disgusting stimuli. *Front. Hum. Neurosci.* 7:510. doi: 10.3389/fnhum.2013.00510

Delplanque, S., Grandjean, D., Chrea, C., Coppin, G., Aymard, L., Cayeux, I., et al. (2009). Sequential unfolding of novelty and pleasantness appraisals of odors: evidence from facial electromyography and autonomic reactions. *Emotion* 9, 316–328. doi: 10.1037/a0015369

Doty, R. L. (1989). Influence of age and age-related diseases on olfactory function. *Ann. N. Y. Acad. Sci.* 561, 76–86. doi: 10.1111/j.1749-6632.1989.tb20971.x

Dubal, S., Pierson, A., and Jouvent, R. (2000). Focused attention in anhedonia: a P3 study. *Psychophysiology* 37, 711–714. doi: 10.1111/1469-8986.3750711

Fukada, M., Kaidoh, T., Ito, A., Yano, T., Hayashibara, C., and Watanabe, T. (2007). "Green odor" inhalation reduces the skin-barrier disruption induced by chronic restraint stress in rats: physiological and histological examinations. *Chem. Senses* 32, 633–639. doi: 10.1093/chemse/bjm031

Garrido, P. (2011). Aging and stress: past hypotheses, present approaches and perspectives. *Aging Dis.* 2, 80–99. doi: 10.1007./s12160-010-9224-2

Gottfried, J. A., Deichmann, R., Winston, J. S., and Dolan, R. J. (2002). Functional heterogeneity in human olfactory cortex : an event-related functional magnetic resonance imaging study. *J. Neurosci.* 22, 10819–10828.

Hummel, T., Kobal, G., Gudziol, H., and Mackay-Sim, A. (2007). Normative data for the "Sniffin' Sticks" including tests of odor identification, odor discrimination, and olfactory thresholds: an upgrade based on a group of more than 3,000 subjects. *Eur. Arch. Otorhinolaryngol.* 264, 237–243. doi: 10.1007/s00405-006-0173-0

Ito, A., Miyoshi, M., Ueki, S., Fukada, M., Komaki, R., and Watanabe, T. (2009). "Green odor" inhalation by rats down-regulates stress-induced increases in fos expression in stress-related forebrain regions. *Neurosci. Res.* 65, 166–174. doi: 10.1016/j.neures.2009.06.012

Joussain, P., Chakirian, A., Kermen, F., Rouby, C., and Bensafi, M. (2011). Physicochemical influence on odor hedonics: where does it occur first? *Commun. Integr. Biol.* 4, 563–565. doi: 10.4161/cib.4.5.15811

Joussain, P., Thevenet, M., Rouby, C., and Bensafi, M. (2013). Effect of aging on hedonic appreciation of pleasant and unpleasant odors. *PLoS ONE* 8:e61376. doi: 10.1371/journal.pone.0061376

Khan, R. M., Luk, C. H., Flinker, A., Aggarwal, A., Lapid, H., Haddad, R., et al. (2007). Predicting odor pleasantness from odorant structure: pleasantness as a reflection of the physical world. *J. Neurosci.* 27, 10015–10023. doi: 10.1523/JNEUROSCI.1158-07.2007

Lang, P. J., Greenwald, M. K., Bradley, M. M., and Hamm, A. O. (1993). Looking at pictures: affective, facial, visceral, and behavioral reactions. *Psychophysiology* 30, 261–273. doi: 10.1111/j.1469-8986.1993.tb03352.x

Loas, G., Dubal, S., and Pierson, A. (1996). Detection of anhedonia in the normal subject. Determination of the validity of the Chapman and Chapman (1978) revised Physical Anhedonia Scale. *Encephale* 22, 301–302.

Mahncke, H. W., Connor, B. B., Appelman, J., Ahsanuddin, O. N., Hardy, J. L., Wood, R. A., et al. (2006). Memory enhancement in healthy older adults using a brain plasticity-based training program: a randomized, controlled study. *Proc. Natl. Acad. Sci. U.S.A.* 103, 12523–12528. doi: 10.1073/pnas.0605194103

Mandairon, N., Poncelet, J., Bensafi, M., and Didier, A. (2009). Humans and mice express similar olfactory preferences. *PLoS ONE* 4:e4209. doi: 10.1371/journal.pone.0004209

Martin, G., Apena, F., Chaudry, Z., Mulligan, Z., and Nixon, C. (2001). The development of an attitude towards the sense of smell questionnaire (SoSQ) and a comparison of different profession's responses. *N. Am. J. Psychol.* 3, 491–502.

Mezzacappa, E., Arumugam, U., Chen, S., Stein, T., Oz, M., and Buckle, J. (2010). Coconut fragrance and cardiovascular response to laboratory stress: results of pilot testing. *Holist. Nurs. Pract.* 24, 322–332. doi: 10.1097/HNP.0b013e3181fbb89c

Monahan, J., Murphy, S., and Zajonc, R. (2000). Subliminal mere exposure: specific, general, and diffuse effects. *Psychol. Sci.* 11, 462–466. doi: 10.1111/1467-9280.00289

Nikaido, Y., and Nakashima, T. (2009). Effects of environmental novelty on fear-related behavior and stress responses of rats to emotionally relevant odors. *Behav. Brain Res.* 199, 241–246. doi: 10.1016/j.bbr.2008.11.043

Oka, T., Hayashida, S., Kaneda, Y., Takenaga, M., Tamagawa, Y., Tsuji, S., et al. (2008). Green odor attenuates a cold pressor test-induced cardiovascular response in healthy adults. *Biopsychosoc. Med.* 2, 2. doi: 10.1186/1751-0759-2-2

Poncelet, J., Rinck, F., Bourgeat, F., Schaal, B., Rouby, C., Bensafi, M., et al. (2010a). The effect of early experience on odor perception in humans: psychological and physiological correlates. *Behav. Brain Res.* 208, 458–465. doi: 10.1016/j.bbr.2009.12.011

Poncelet, J., Rinck, F., Ziessel, A., Joussain, P., Thevenet, M., Rouby, C., et al. (2010b). Semantic knowledge influences prewired hedonic responses to odors. *PLoS ONE* 5:e13878. doi: 10.1371/journal.pone.0013878

Pouliot, S., Bourgeat, F., Barkat, S., Rouby, C., and Bensafi, M. (2008). Increase in anhedonia level in menopausal women is accompanied by a shift in olfactory function. *Chem. Percept.* 1, 43–47. doi: 10.1007/s12078-007-9001-1

Rolls, E. T., Kringelbach, M. L., and De Araujo, I. E. (2003). Different representations of pleasant and unpleasant odours in the human brain. *Eur. J. Neurosci.* 18, 695–703. doi: 10.1046/j.1460-9568.2003.02779.x

Rouby, C., Bourgeat, F., Rinck, F., Poncelet, J., and Bensafi, M. (2009a). Perceptual and sensorimotor differences between "good" and "poor" olfactory mental imagers. *Ann. N. Y. Acad. Sci.* 1170, 333–337. doi: 10.1111/j.1749-6632.2009.03915.x

Rouby, C., Pouliot, S., and Bensafi, M. (2009b). Odor hedonics and their modulators. *Food qual. prefer.* 20, 545–549. doi: 10.1016/j.foodqual.2009.05.004

Schiffman, S. S., Sattely-Miller, E. A., Suggs, M. S., and Graham, B. G. (1995). The effect of pleasant odors and hormone status on mood of women at midlife. *Brain Res. Bull.* 36, 19–29. doi: 10.1016/0361-9230(94)00133-L

Sloan, D. M., Bradley, M. M., Dimoulas, E., and Lang, P. J. (2002). Looking at facial expressions: dysphoria and facial EMG. *Biol. Psychol.* 60, 79–90. doi: 10.1016/S0301-0511(02)00044-3

Thomas-Danguin, T., Rouby, C., Sicard, G., Vigouroux, M., Farget, V., Johanson, A., et al. (2003). Development of the ETOC: a European test of olfactory capabilities. *Rhinology* 41, 142–151.

van Praag, H., Kempermann, G., and Gage, F. H. (2000). Neural consequences of environmental enrichment. *Nat. Rev. Neurosci.* 1, 191–198. doi: 10.1038/35044558

Zarzo, M. (2011). Hedonic judgments of chemical compounds are correlated with molecular size. *Sensors (Basel)* 11, 3667–3686. doi: 10.3390/s110403667

4

Relationships between personality traits and attitudes toward the sense of smell

Han-Seok Seo*, Suji Lee and Sungeun Cho

Department of Food Science, University of Arkansas, Fayetteville, AR, USA

Correspondence:
Han-Seok Seo, Department of Food Science, University of Arkansas, 2650 North Young Avenue, Fayetteville, AR 72704, USA
e-mail: hanseok@uark.edu

Olfactory perception appears to be linked to personality traits. This study aimed to determine whether personality traits influence human attitudes toward sense of smell. Two-hundred participants' attitudes toward their senses of smell and their personality traits were measured using two self-administered questionnaires: the Importance of Olfaction Questionnaire and the Eysenck Personality Questionnaire-Revised. Demographics and olfactory function were also assessed using a self-administered questionnaire. Gender-induced differences were present in attitudes toward sense of smell. Women participants were more dependent than men participants on olfactory cues for daily decision-making. In addition, as participants evaluated their own olfactory functions more positively, they relied more on olfactory information in everyday life. To determine a relationship between personality traits and attitudes toward sense of smell, Spearman partial correlation analyses were conducted, with controlling the factors that might influence attitudes with respect to sense of smell (i.e., gender and self-awareness of olfactory function) as covariates. Participants who scored high on the lie-scale (i.e., socially desirable and faking good), tended to use olfactory cues for daily decision-making related both to social communication and product purchase. In conclusion, our findings demonstrate a significant association between personality traits and attitudes toward sense of smell.

Keywords: attitude toward sense of smell, personality traits, gender, the Eysenck Personality Questionnaire-Revised, lie-scale

INTRODUCTION

Despite its important role, relatively little attention has been paid to the sense of smell compared to other senses (e.g., vision and hearing). The sense of smell is mainly associated with eating behavior, awareness of environmental hazard, and social communication (for a review, see Stevenson, 2010). Olfactory function influences appetite (De Jong et al., 1999), food perception and palatability (Aschenbrenner et al., 2008; Seo and Hummel, 2009; Novakova et al., 2012; Schubert et al., 2012), and food-related social behavior (Aschenbrenner et al., 2008). For example, people with olfactory impairment appear to be more exposed to risks of unbalanced nutritional status (Duffy et al., 1995; Schiffman and Graham, 2000) and poor food intake (Aschenbrenner et al., 2008), although these findings have not been consistently observed in previous studies (De Jong et al., 1999; Schubert et al., 2012; Smoliner et al., 2013). In addition, a sense of smell can detect not only microbial risks such as feces, decay, and spoilage (Stevenson, 2010), but also non-microbial threats such as gas leaks and smoke (Miwa et al., 2001; Santos et al., 2004; Croy et al., 2012). Finally, the major histocompatibility complex (MHC) genotype and body odors can play a critical role in mate selection, not only by avoiding inbreeding, but also by detecting fit partners (Wedekind et al., 1995; Gangestad and Thornhill, 1998; Herz and Inzlicht, 2002; Croy et al., 2013; for a review, see Yamazaki and Beauchamp, 2007; Stevenson, 2010). For example, women students rated body odors of T-shirts worn by men different from themselves with respect to MHC alleles significantly more pleasant than body odors of T-shirts worn by men with similar MHC alleles (Wedekind et al., 1995). Olfactory signals can also deliver individual identity (Olsson et al., 2006; Lundström et al., 2008), emotional states (Chen and Haviland-Jones, 2000; Prehn-Kristensen et al., 2009; Croy et al., 2011a), age-related information (Mitro et al., 2012), and sexual interests (Croy et al., 2013). Croy et al. (2013) demonstrated an interesting relationship between sense of smell and sexual relationships in people diagnosed with isolated congenital anosmia. Men born without a sense of smell reported significantly fewer sexual relationships compared to age-matched healthy men. Also, women born without a sense of smell appeared to feel less secure about sexual partnership compared to healthy women in a control group.

Although the sense of smell plays a significant role in modulating eating behavior, hazard detection, and social communication (Stevenson, 2010), people's attitudes toward sense of smell vary as a function of olfactory performance (Frasnelli and Hummel, 2005; Shu et al., 2011), gender (Frasnelli and Hummel, 2005; Ferdenzi et al., 2008; Havlicek et al., 2008; Croy et al., 2010; Seo et al., 2011), and culture (Schleidt et al., 1981; Schaal et al., 1997; Ferdenzi et al., 2008; Seo et al., 2011). For example, patients with olfactory impairments tend to complain more strongly about their decreased quality of life than people with normal olfactory function (Frasnelli and Hummel, 2005). Furthermore, women patients consider olfactory impairment-decreased quality of life more negatively than do men patients (Frasnelli and Hummel, 2005). Gender-induced difference in attitudes toward olfaction is also observed in people with a normal sense of smell (Ferdenzi et al., 2008; Havlicek et al., 2008; Croy et al., 2010). It seems that women are more attentive than men to olfactory cues (Ferdenzi et al., 2008; Havlicek et al., 2008; Croy et al., 2010; Seo et al., 2011).

Personality is another potential factor in modulating olfactory perception (Koelega, 1970, 1994; Filsinger et al., 1987; Pause et al., 1998; Larsson et al., 2000; Chen and Dalton, 2005; Havlíček et al., 2012; La Buissonnière-Ariza et al., 2013). Earlier research demonstrated plausible relationships between olfactory sensitivity and personality traits such as extraversion/introversion; the results, however, are controversial. Koelega (1970) reported that olfactory sensitivity was positively correlated with degree of extraversion but not with degree of neuroticism. In contrast, another study by Herberner et al. (1989) demonstrated that, in comparison to extremely sociable participants, extremely shy participants were significantly more sensitive to odors. Furthermore, several studies reported no significant relationship between olfactory sensitivity and extraversion/introversion (Filsinger et al., 1987; Koelega, 1994; Pause et al., 1998; Larsson et al., 2000; Havlíček et al., 2012). Pause et al. (1998) found that neuroticism, when compared to extraversion, has a stronger impact in determination of olfactory sensitivity. Havlíček et al. (2012) also reported that olfactory sensitivity correlated with neuroticism, but not with other personality traits such as extraversion, openness, and agreeability (but see also Croy et al., 2011b). In addition, personality traits may alter a participant's ability to identify odors (Larsson et al., 2000; Havlíček et al., 2012). For example, participants who scored high in neuroticism (i.e., more emotional and anxious) identified odors more correctly (Larsson et al., 2000). In contrast, participants with high degrees of impulsiveness and assertiveness identified odors less correctly (Larsson et al., 2000). A recent study conducted by Havlíček et al. (2012) found a significant correlation between participants' anxiety traits (a neuroticism facet) and their ability to discriminate odors. That is, as participants were more anxious, they discriminated odors more correctly. Finally, personality modulates participants' reaction speed with respect to olfactory cues (Chen and Dalton, 2005). Chen and Dalton (2005) demonstrated that both neurotic and anxious men detected pleasant/unpleasant odors more quickly than emotionally neutral odors, while stable and calm men detected both odors equally quickly (i.e., no significant differences in reaction time to both pleasant/unpleasant and neutral odors). In a more recent study, La Buissonnière-Ariza et al. (2013) compared response times of both high- and low-trait anxiety adults to pleasant- and unpleasant-smelling food odors (i.e., strawberry and fish odors, respectively). Similarly to previous findings of Chen and Dalton (2005), they found that, regardless of whether odors were pleasant or unpleasant, highly anxious individuals detected odors more quickly than did less anxious ones.

Likewise, earlier studies have highlighted the modulatory effects of personality traits on olfactory perceptions such as odor sensitivity, discrimination, and identification. In addition, previous research has demonstrated that people's attitudes toward sense of smell can vary as a function of olfactory performance (Frasnelli and Hummel, 2005; Shu et al., 2011). Given the two ideas that (1) personality traits influence olfactory performance and (2) olfactory performance appears to be closely related to attitudes toward olfaction, we hypothesized that personality traits could be related to attitudes toward sense of smell. Up to now, little has been known about a potential connection between personality traits and attitudes toward sense of smell. To build on previous findings, this study has aimed to determine whether human attitudes toward sense of smell can be related to personality traits.

MATERIALS AND METHODS

This study was conducted in conformance with the Declaration of Helsinki for studies on human subjects. The protocol was approved by the University Institutional Review Board of the University of Arkansas (Fayetteville, AR, USA).

PARTICIPANTS

A total number of 207 volunteers (73 men and 134 women) representing an age range of 18–73 years [mean age ± standard deviation (SD) = 39 ± 14 years] took part in this study. Data from seven volunteers (four men and three women) who had either clinical histories of major diseases (e.g., diabetes and cancer) or olfactory impairment were discarded. The olfactory impairment was determined based on results obtained through a "Sniffin' Sticks" screening test (Burghart Instruments, Wedel, Germany; for details, see Hummel et al., 2001). Accordingly, data from a total of 200 respondents (69 men and 131 women) were analyzed. **Table 1** shows the demographic details of the respondents. The experimental procedure was thoroughly explained to all participants and a written informed consent was obtained from each prior to participation.

QUESTIONNAIRES

Participants' attitudes toward sense of smell, personality traits, and their demographics and self-ratings with respect to olfactory function were measured using self-administered questionnaires.

Attitudes toward sense of smell

To assess participants' attitudes toward sense of smell, we used the "Importance of Olfaction Questionnaire" (IOQ) designed by Croy et al. (2010). The IOQ includes three subscales: "association," "application," and "consequence." Each subscale is in turn composed of six questions to be answered with a 4-point category scale (1 = I totally disagree to 4 = I totally agree). The association-subscale indicates emotion, memory, and episode triggered by a sense of smell. The application-subscale reflects the extent to which people use sense of smell in their daily activities. Finally, the consequence-subscale reflects the extent to which people rely on sense of smell for daily decision-making. The additional subscale of "aggravation" developed for clinical applications (Croy et al., 2010) was not used because this study was designed for a general population.

Personality

Participants' personality traits were assessed using the "Eysenck Personality Questionnaire-Revised" (EPQ-R; Eysenck et al., 1985). The EPQ-R, a 48-question self-reporting questionnaire, examines four major dimensions of personality trait: "psychoticism"

Table 1 | Participants' demographic profiles and self-ratings of olfactory function.

		(N = 200)	
Categories	**Subcategories**	**Frequency**	**%**
Gender	Men	69	34.5
	Women	131	65.5
Age group	18–24 years	27	13.5
	25–44 years	107	53.5
	45–64 years	59	29.5
	65 years and over	7	3.5
Body mass index	Underweight (less than 18.5)	6	3.0
	Normal weight (18.5–24.9)	77	38.5
	Overweight (25.0–29.9)	46	23.0
	Obese (more than 30.0)	70	35.0
Ethnicity background	Caucasian	193	96.5
	African-American	1	0.5
	Asian	6	3.0
Annual household income	Under $15,000	29	14.5
	$15,000 to $34,999	46	23.0
	$35,000 to $54,999	36	18.0
	$55,000 to $74,999	31	15.5
	$75,000 to $94,999	27	13.5
	More than $95,000	31	15.5
Education level	High school	62	31.0
	2-year college	28	14.0
	4-year college	62	31.0
	Graduate school	48	24.0
Self-ratings of olfactory function	Very bad	2	1.0
	Bad	0	0.0
	Moderate	15	7.5
	Good	106	53.0
	Very good	77	38.5

(P: 12 questions), "extraversion" (E: 12 questions), "neuroticism" (N: 12 questions), and "lie-scale" (L: 12 questions). The psychoticism-subscale assesses behavior patterns used to characterize psychotic individuals or psychoses (Eysenck, 1997; Weiner and Craighead, 2010). The extraversion-subscale measures the extent to which individuals are sociable and active (Eysenck, 1997; Weiner and Craighead, 2010). The neuroticism-subscale assesses the extent to which individuals are predisposed to experience negative emotion (Eysenck, 1997; Weiner and Craighead, 2010). Finally, the lie-scale subscale reflects individuals' socially conforming behaviors or their tendency to "fake good" (Weiner and Craighead, 2010).

Demographics and self-ratings of olfactory function

Participants' demographics, such as gender, age, height, weight, ethnic background, annual household income, and education level, were assessed through a self-administered questionnaire. **Table 1** shows the participants' demographic profiles. In addition, participants were asked to evaluate their own olfactory functions on a 5-point Likert scale ranging from 1 (very bad) to 5 (very good).

DATA ANALYSIS

Data analysis was conducted using SPSS 21.0 for Windows^{TM} (IBM SPSS Inc., Chicago, IL, USA). Not all participants answered all questions (i.e., several participants did not complete all subscales; one for the association-subscale, two for the consequence-subscale, and two for the lie-scale subscale). Because the Shapiro–Wilk test (Shapiro and Wilk, 1965) revealed that the IOQ and the EPQ-R data were not normally distributed (**Table 2**), non-parametric statistical methods were used for data analysis. Mann–Whitney and Kruskal–Wallis tests were used to determine whether participants' attitudes toward sense of smell varied as a function of demographic variables like gender, age, body mass index, annual household income, and education level. Spearman correlation coefficients were used to determine whether attitudes toward sense of smell were related to self-ratings of olfactory function. A relationship between participants' personality traits and their attitudes toward sense of smell can be mediated by other factors that may possibly influence attitudes toward sense of smell, i.e., demographics and self-ratings of olfactory function (Croy et al., 2010; Seo et al., 2011). Therefore, to determine whether there is a relationship between personality traits and attitudes toward sense of smell, we used partial Spearman correlation analyses with treating potential factors to affect attitudes toward sense of smell as covariates. Calculating multiple correlations between personality traits and attitudes toward sense of smell can increase the risk of a type I error. That is, multiple correlation tests increase the probability of erroneously rejecting even one of the true null hypotheses (i.e., correlation coefficient is 0) when there is no significant correlation (Benjamini and Hochberg, 1995; Curtin and Schulz, 1998; Benjamini and Yekutieli, 2001). To avoid the risk of multiple correlation tests, the level of statistical significance of correlation coefficients was adjusted using Bonferroni's correction (Curtin and Schulz, 1998). To keep the overall level of significance at 5% in this study, the level of significance for each correlation was divided by 12 (i.e., 4 dimensions of the EPQ-R by 3 subscales of the IOQ); the adjusted level of significance was set at $P < 0.0042$.

RESULTS

Table 2 presents the results of descriptive analysis for personality traits (EPQ-R) and attitudes toward sense of smell (IOQ). As previously mentioned, the data of the IOQ and the EPQ-R were not normally distributed (**Table 2**), so non-parametric statistical methods were used for data analysis. Before examining the relationship between participants' personality traits and their attitudes toward sense of smell, potential factors that might possibly mediate the relationship, i.e., demographics and self-ratings of olfactory function, were determined.

INFLUENCES OF DEMOGRAPHICS ON ATTITUDES TOWARD SENSE OF SMELL

Mann–Whitney U-tests revealed that women participants used olfactory cues for daily decision-making more often than men

Table 2 | Descriptive analysis results for ratings of personality traits and attitudes toward sense of smell.

	Mean	Median	Standard deviation	Skewness	Kurtosis	($N = 200$ [A]) Normality of data[B]
Attitudes toward sense of smell[C]						
Association	19.0	19.0	2.4	−0.5	0.5	$W = 0.97$ ($P < 0.001$)
Application	17.6	18.0	2.9	−0.3	0.0	$W = 0.98$ ($P = 0.012$)
Consequence	17.4	18.0	2.6	−0.4	0.4	$W = 0.98$ ($P = 0.001$)
Personality traits[D]						
Psychoticism	1.8	2.0	1.5	1.0	2.4	$W = 0.89$ ($P < 0.001$)
Extraversion	8.0	9.0	3.6	−0.6	−0.8	$W = 0.90$ ($P < 0.001$)
Neuroticism	4.5	4.5	3.2	0.3	−1.0	$W = 0.95$ ($P < 0.001$)
Lie-scale	4.7	4.0	2.6	0.3	−0.7	$W = 0.95$ ($P < 0.001$)

[A] *Not all participants answered all questions (i.e., several participants did not complete all subscales; one for the association-subscale, two for the consequence-subscale, and two for the lie-scale subscale).*
[B] *Normality of data was determined by Shapiro–Wilk test (Shapiro and Wilk, 1965).*
[C] *Attitudes toward sense of smell were assessed by the Importance of Olfaction Questionnaire (IOQ; Croy et al., 2010).*
[D] *Personality traits were assessed by the Eysenck Personality Questionnaire-Revised (EPQ-R; Eysenck et al., 1985).*

participants ($P < 0.001$), as shown in **Figure 1**. However, there was no significant gender-induced difference in the ratings of association-subscale ($P = 0.15$) and application-subscale ($P = 0.23$).

The Kruskal–Wallis tests found that the ratings of three subscales (i.e., "association," "application," and "consequence") in the IOQ were not significantly different as a function of age groups ($P > 0.05$), body mass index ($P > 0.05$), education level ($P > 0.05$), and annual household income ($P > 0.05$).

RELATIONSHIPS BETWEEN SELF-RATINGS OF OLFACTORY FUNCTION AND ATTITUDES TOWARD A SENSE OF SMELL

Spearman correlation analyses showed that participants' self-ratings of olfactory function were positively correlated with the ratings of application-subscale ($\rho_{200} = 0.17$, $P = 0.02$) and consequence-subscale ($\rho_{198} = 0.15$, $P = 0.03$). For example, when participants judged their olfactory function to be more positive, they more frequently used their sense of smell in everyday life and for daily decision-making. Additionally, the self-ratings of olfactory function showed a marginally significant correlation with the ratings of association-subscale ($\rho_{199} = 0.14$, $P = 0.05$).

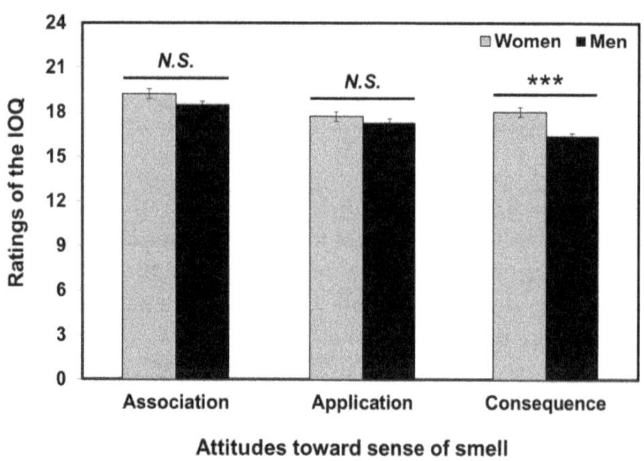

FIGURE 1 | Gender differences in the attitudes toward sense of smell. Mann–Whitney *U*-tests revealed that women participants rated consequence-subscale of the IOQ (Importance of Olfaction Questionnaire) significantly higher than men participants. The asterisks (***) indicate significance at $P < 0.001$. Error bars represent standard error of the means.

RELATIONSHIPS BETWEEN PERSONALITY TRAITS AND ATTITUDES TOWARD A SENSE OF SMELL

As previously mentioned, we controlled potential factors that might mediate the relationship between personality traits and attitudes toward sense of smell. Based on these above results, participants' gender and self-ratings of olfactory function were controlled in determining the relationship between their personality traits and attitudes toward sense of smell.

Table 3 shows partial Spearman's correlation coefficients (ρ) for the relationships between personality traits and attitudes toward a sense of smell. The ratings of consequence-subscale of the IOQ significantly correlated with the lie-scale scores at the Bonferroni-adjusted level of significance ($\rho_{191} = 0.21$, $P = 0.0038$). In other words, as participants showed socially conforming behaviors (e.g., fake good), they were more dependent on olfactory cues for daily decision-making.

However, no other significant relationships among individual ratings of the IOQ and the EPQ-R were found at the Bonferroni-adjusted level of significance ($P > 0.0042$).

DISCUSSION

INFLUENCES OF DEMOGRAPHICS ON THE ATTITUDES TOWARD A SENSE OF SMELL

The current study shows gender-induced differences in attitudes toward sense of smell; compared to men, women participants reported that they use olfactory cues more often for daily decision-making. Although the gender difference was not apparent in all

Table 3 | Partial Spearman correlation coefficients for the relationships between personality traits and attitudes toward sense of smell [A].

(N = 200)

		Attitudes toward sense of smell[B]		
		Association	**Application**	**Consequence**
Personality traits[C]	Psychoticism	$\rho_{191} = -0.06^{N.S.}$	$\rho_{191} = -0.01^{N.S.}$	$\rho_{191} = -0.001^{N.S.}$
	Extraversion	$\rho_{191} = 0.10^{N.S.}$	$\rho_{191} = 0.05^{N.S.}$	$\rho_{191} = -0.08^{N.S.}$
	Neuroticism	$\rho_{191} = 0.11^{N.S.}$	$\rho_{191} = -0.01^{N.S.}$	$\rho_{191} = 0.03^{N.S.}$
	Lie-scale	$\rho_{191} = -0.02^{N.S.}$	$\rho_{191} = 0.09^{N.S.}$	$\rho_{191} = 0.21$*

[A] *When determining correlation between a dimension of the EPQ-R and a subscale of the IOQ, participants' gender and self-ratings of olfactory function were treated as covariates.*
[B] *Attitudes toward sense of smell were assessed by the Importance of Olfaction Questionnaire (IOQ; Croy et al., 2010).*
[C] *Personality traits were assessed by the Eysenck Personality Questionnaire-Revised (EPQ-R; Eysenck et al., 1985).*
The level of significance for each correlation coefficient was adjusted using Bonferroni's correction (Curtin and Schulz, 1998).
The N.S. indicates no significance at $P < 0.0042$.
The asterisk (*) indicates significance at $P < 0.0042$.

three subscales, our results are in agreement with earlier studies using the IOQ (Croy et al., 2010; Seo et al., 2011). Similarly, Croy et al. (2010) reported that the gender difference was obtained in the consequence-subscale, but not in the association- and application-subscales. More recently, Seo et al. (2011) reported that more women than men in four different regions: Mexico, Germany, Czech, and Korea, have attentive and positive attitudes toward sense of smell. For mate selection, men usually consider women's visual appearance most important, while women tend to evaluate men's body odors in determining superiority (Herz and Inzlicht, 2002; Havlicek et al., 2008). There are three possible explanations for gender-related differences in attitudes toward sense of smell. First, women's superior olfactory performance (e.g., odor sensitivity, discrimination, identification; Doty et al., 1984; Hummel et al., 2007) may lead them to be more attentive and reactive to olfactory cues (Croy et al., 2010). Second, the proxemics theory of Hall (1966) might account for gender-induced attitudes toward sense of smell. Hall (1963) argued that people can establish interpersonal distances in eight different dimensions, including olfactory code. Generally, women stay closer to each other (i.e., smaller interpersonal distance) than men, which may provide them with more chances for judging other peoples' body odors, identities, and emotional states (Seo et al., 2011). Finally, it should be noted that women participants in this study tended to be more neurotic and emotional than men participants (Mann–Whitney U-tests, $P < 0.001$). Considering the significant influence of neuroticism not only on olfactory performance, but also on attitudes toward sense of smell, women's higher scores in neuroticism might result in more attentive attitudes to olfactory cues. However, because no significant correlation was found between ratings of neuroticism and the consequence-subscale exhibiting gender differences, further study should be conducted to support this assertion.

RELATIONSHIPS BETWEEN SELF-RATINGS OF OLFACTORY FUNCTION AND ATTITUDES TOWARD SENSE OF SMELL

In this study, participants who judged their olfactory function more positively relied on olfactory cues in daily decision-making. These results are consistent with previous findings demonstrating a positive correlation between self-rating of olfactory sensitivity and general attitudes toward sense of smell (Seo et al., 2011). Self-assessment of olfactory function seems to be related to self-rating of nasal patency (Landis et al., 2003) or odor annoyance (Knaapila et al., 2008) rather than to olfactory perceptions such as odor sensitivity and discrimination (Landis et al., 2003). This result reflects the fact that individuals regarding their olfactory function more positively tend to be more attentive and reactive to the sense of smell regardless of olfactory sensitivity.

RELATIONSHIPS BETWEEN PERSONALITY TRAITS AND ATTITUDES TOWARD SENSE OF SMELL

The above results demonstrate that gender and self-ratings of olfactory function may be associated with attitudes toward sense of smell. Therefore, factors such as gender and self-ratings of olfactory function were controlled as covariates when determining relationships between personality traits and attitudes toward sense of smell.

Previous research has focused on the idea that personality traits influence olfactory perceptions such as odor sensitivity (Koelega, 1970, 1994; Filsinger et al., 1987; Pause et al., 1998; Larsson et al., 2000; Croy et al., 2011b; Havlíček et al., 2012), odor intensity (Chen and Dalton, 2005), odor discrimination (Havlíček et al., 2012), odor identification (Larsson et al., 2000), and odor reaction time (Chen and Dalton, 2005; La Buissonnière-Ariza et al., 2013). Specifically, as people are more neurotic and anxious, they show better performance in detection (Pause et al., 1998; Chen and Dalton, 2005; Havlíček et al., 2012; La Buissonnière-Ariza et al., 2013), discrimination (Havlíček et al., 2012), and identification (Larsson et al., 2000) of olfactory cues. Based on previous research, it was expected that participants who scoring high in neuroticism (i.e., more anxious and emotional) would be prone to have more memory, episode, and emotion triggered by olfactory cues. According to Eysenck's (1967) hypothesis, it is assumed that individuals high in neuroticism are more sensitive to emotional cues, especially aversive and negative stimuli, and this may be related to greater activation of the limbic system. Spearman correlation analysis showed that the scores of neuroticism-subscale significantly correlated with ratings of association-subscale of the IOQ at $P < 0.05$, but the significant relationship was not obtained at the Bonferroni-adjusted level of significance used in this study ($P < 0.0042$).

The lie-scale of the EPQ-R was designed to measure the tendency of respondents to lie or to fake effectively, thereby reflecting their acquiescence or conformity to social rules and pressures (Powell, 1977; Francis and Pearson, 1983). Interestingly, the current study demonstrated that participants scoring high in the lie-scale also showed high ratings in the consequence-subscale of the IOQ. In other words, individuals more constrained by social desirability (e.g., faking good) appear to rely more on olfactory cues when making daily-life decisions. A number of studies have elucidated that sense of smell is closely related to social communication and behavior (Wedekind et al., 1995; Gangestad and Thornhill, 1998; Chen and Haviland-Jones, 2000; Herz and Inzlicht, 2002; Olsson et al., 2006; Yamazaki and Beauchamp, 2007; Lundström et al., 2008; Prehn-Kristensen et al., 2009; Stevenson, 2010; Croy et al., 2011a, 2013; Mitro et al., 2012). Olfactory cues such as body odors reflect emotional state (Prehn-Kristensen et al., 2009; Croy et al., 2011a), individual identity (Olsson et al., 2006; Lundström et al., 2008), and sexual interests (Wedekind et al., 1995; Gangestad and Thornhill, 1998; Herz and Inzlicht, 2002; Croy et al., 2013; for review, see Yamazaki and Beauchamp, 2007; Stevenson, 2010). Olsson et al. (2006) asked participants to sniff the contents of five zip-lock bags containing both T-shirts worn by themselves, their friends, two strangers of opposite sex, and unworn T-shirts. They were then asked to identify the two shirts worn by themselves and their friends. Participants were able to determine not only their own T-shirts (51.6%), but also the T-shirts worn by their friends (38.7%). In addition, it is known that many people have the ability to recognize others' emotional states such as happiness, fear, and anxiety (Chen and Haviland-Jones, 2000; Prehn-Kristensen et al., 2009) by smelling their body odors. A functional brain-imaging study demonstrated that body odors related to anxiety (produced during academic examination), in contrast to control group body odors (produced during bicycling), activated brain areas associated with the processing of social-anxiety information (e.g., fusiform gyrus) and the regulation of empathic feelings (e.g., insula, cingulate cortex, and precuneus). These findings reflect the fact that olfactory signals can play a key role in social communication in our society. Accordingly, it is thought that individuals more constrained by social desirability (i.e., high scores in lie-scale of the EPQ-R) tend to pay more attention to their own body odors, the better to provide positive and favorable impressions to others. In addition, they appear to judge other people's identities, emotions, and personalities based on their body odors. In a similar vein, Croy et al. (2011b) demonstrated that agreeable participants, who tend to have greater concern for social harmony and cooperative nature (Rothmann and Coetzer, 2003), have higher sensitivities to odors. Furthermore, several studies have found that individuals with social deficits (e.g., autism and schizophrenia) have lower olfactory performances in areas like odor sensitivity (Dudova et al., 2011) and odor identification (Malaspina and Coleman, 2003). These findings support possible associations of social desirability (herein, lie-scale) not with only olfactory perceptions, but also with attitudes toward olfaction.

A plausible explanation for the relationship between smelling behavior and personality traits, especially social desirability, can be found in a neuroanatomical convergence of olfactory and emotional information in the limbic system, orbitofrontal cortex, insula, and anterior cingulate cortex (for a review, see Soudry et al., 2011). Functional brain-imaging studies have revealed that the limbic and paralimbic areas are involved in regulation of emotional and social desirability (Haas et al., 2010; Boehme et al., 2013) as well as in the processing of odor valence, odor memory, and odor-induced emotion (for review, see Gottfried, 2006; Soudry et al., 2011). Based on neuroanatomical convergence, it is to be expected that individuals who are faking good are vulnerable to emotional olfactory signals, possibly leading them to rely on olfactory cues for social communication and daily decision-making.

Since this research is a questionnaire-based study, a phenomenon known as the "extreme response style" (Hamilton, 1968; Greenleaf, 1992) should be noted. In other words, in questionnaire-based studies, regardless of specific item content, up to 30% of respondents are likely to consistently favor extreme response categories (Eid and Rauber, 2000; Austin et al., 2006; Naemi et al., 2009). Previous studies demonstrated that women and younger respondents tend to prefer extreme response categories compared to men and older respondents (Austin et al., 2006). In addition, respondents who scored high on extraversion and conscientiousness are likely to show a preference for extreme response categories (Austin et al., 2006). Because an extreme response style might result in a correlation between the ratings, the outcomes must be carefully interpreted. As seen in **Table 2**, both ratings of the EPQ-R and IOQ were highly skewed and, due to their non-normal distributions, non-parametric statistical methods were employed in this study, which might reduce the plausible overestimation caused by an extreme response style.

In summary, our findings provide empirical evidence that personality traits are related to attitudes toward sense of smell. Specifically, people constrained by social desirability (e.g., fake good) relied more on a sense of smell for daily decision-making. These findings provide better understanding of how personality traits are related to peoples' attitudes toward sense of smell.

ACKNOWLEDGMENT

This research was supported by start-up funding from the University of Arkansas Division of Agriculture to Han-Seok Seo.

REFERENCES

Aschenbrenner, K., Hummel, C., Teszmer, K., Krone, F., Ishimaru, T., Seo, H. S., et al. (2008). The influence of olfactory less on dietary behaviors. *Laryngoscope* 118, 135–144. doi: 10.1097/MLG.0b013e318155a4b9

Austin, E. J., Deary, I. J., and Egan, V. (2006). Individual differences in response scale use: mixed Rasch modeling of responses to NEO-FFI items. *Pers. Individ. Differ.* 40, 1235–1245. doi: 10.1016/j.paid.2005.10.018

Benjamini, Y., and Hochberg, Y. (1995). Controlling the false discovery rate: a practical and powerful approach to multiple testing. *J. R. Stat. Soc. Ser. B Stat. Methodol.* 57, 289–300. doi:10.2307/2346101

Benjamini, Y., and Yekutieli, D. (2001). The control of the false discovery rate in multiple testing under dependency. *Ann. Stat.* 29, 1165–1188. doi:10.1214/aos/1013699998

Boehme, S., Ritter, V., Tefikow, S., Stangier, U., Strauss, B., Miltner, W. H., et al. (2013). Brain activation during anticipatory anxiety in social anxiety disorder. *Soc. Cogn. Affect. Neurosci.* doi: 10.1093/scan/nst129 [Epub ahead of print].

Chen, D., and Dalton, P. (2005). The effect of emotion and personality on olfactory perception. *Chem. Senses* 30, 345–351. doi: 10.1093/chemse/bji029

Chen, D., and Haviland-Jones, J. (2000). Human olfactory communication of emotion. *Percept. Mot. Skills* 91, 771–781. doi: 10.2466/pms.2000.91.3.771

Croy, I., Bojanowski, V., and Hummel, T. (2013). Men without a sense of smell exhibit a strongly reduced number of sexual relationships, women exhibit reduced partnership security – a reanalysis of previously published data. *Biol. Psychol.* 92, 292–294. doi: 10.1016/j.biopsycho.2012.11.008

Croy, I., Buschhüter, D., Seo, H. S., Negoias, S., and Hummel, T. (2010). Individual significance of olfaction: development of a questionnaire. *Eur. Arch. Otorhinolaryngol.* 267, 67–71. doi: 10.1007/s00405-009-1054-0

Croy, I., Negoias, S., Novakova, L., Landis, B. N., and Hummel, T. (2012). Learning about the functions of the olfactory system from people without a sense of smell. *PLoS ONE* 7:e33365. doi: 10.1371/journal.pone.0033365

Croy, I., Olgun, S., and Joraschky, P. (2011a). Basic emotions elicited by odors and pictures. *Emotion* 11, 1331–1335. doi: 10.1037/a0024437

Croy, I., Springborn, M., Lötsch, J., Johnston, A. N., and Hummel, T. (2011b). Agreeable smellers and sensitivity neurotics – correlations among personality traits and sensory thresholds. *PLoS ONE* 6:e18701. doi: 10.1371/journal.pone.0018701

Curtin, F., and Schulz, P. (1998). Multiple correlations and Bonferroni's correction. *Biol. Psychiatry* 44, 775–777. doi: 10.1016/S0006-3223(98)00043-2

De Jong, N., Mulder, I., de Graaf, C., and van Staveren, W. A. (1999). Impaired sensory functioning in elders: the relation with its potential determinants and nutritional intake. *J. Gerontol. A Biol. Sci. Med. Sci.* 54, B324–B331. doi: 10.1093/gerona/54.8.B324

Doty, R. L., Shaman, P., Applebaum, S. L., Giberson, R., Siksorski, L., and Rosenberg, L. (1984). Smell identification ability: changes with age. *Science* 226, 1441–1443. doi: 10.1126/science.6505700

Dudova, I., Vodicka, J., Havlovicova, M., Sedlacek, Z., Urbanek, T., and Hrdlicka, M. (2011). Odor detection threshold, but not odor identification, is impaired in children with autism. *Eur. Child. Adolesc. Psychiatry* 20, 333–340. doi: 10.1007/s00787-011-0177-1

Duffy, V. B., Backstrant, J. R., and Ferris, A. M. (1995). Olfactory dysfunction and related nutritional risk in free-living, elderly women. *J. Am. Diet. Assoc.* 95, 879–884. doi: 10.1016/S0002-8223(95)00244-8

Eid, M., and Rauber, M. (2000). Detecting measurement invariance in organizational surveys. *Eur. J. Psychol. Assess.* 16, 20–30. doi: 10.1027//1015-5759.16.1.20

Eysenck, H. J. (1967). *The Biological Basis of Personality.* Springfield, IL: Thomas Publisher.

Eysenck, H. J. (1997). *Dimensions of Personality.* New Brunswick, NJ: Transaction Publishers.

Eysenck, S. B. G., Eysenck, H. J., and Barrett, P. (1985). A revised version of the psychoticism scale. *Pers. Individ. Differ.* 6, 21–29. doi: 10.1016/0191-8869(85)90026-1

Ferdenzi, C., Mustonen, S., Tuorila, H., and Schaal, B. (2008). Children's awareness and uses of odor cues in everyday life: a Finland–France comparison. *Chemosens. Percept.* 1, 190–198. doi: 10.1007/s12078-008-90206

Filsinger, E. K., Fabes, R. A., and Hughston, G. (1987). Introversion–extraversion and dimensions of olfactory perception. *Percept. Mot. Skills* 64, 695–699. doi: 10.2466/pms.1987.64.3.695

Francis, L. J., and Pearson, P. R. (1983). Are religious children bigger liars? *Psychol. Rep.* 52, 551–554. doi: 10.2466/pr0.1983.52.2.551

Frasnelli, J., and Hummel, T. (2005). Olfactory dysfunction and daily life. *Eur. Arch. Otorhinolaryngol.* 262, 231–235. doi: 10.1007/s00405-004-0796-y

Gangestad, S. W., and Thornhill, R. (1998). Menstrual cycle variation in women's preference for the scent of symmetrical men. *Proc. Biol. Sci.* 265, 927–933. doi: 10.1098/rspb.1998.0380

Gottfried, J. A. (2006). "Smell: central nervous processing," in *Taste and Smell: An Update*, eds T. Hummel and A. Welge-Lüssen (Basel: Karger), 44–69.

Greenleaf, E. A. (1992). Measuring extreme response style. *Public Opin. Q.* 56, 328–351. doi: 10.1086/269326

Haas, B. W., Hoeft, F., Searcy, Y. M., Mills, D., Bellugi, U., and Reiss, A. (2010). Individual differences in social behavior predict amygdala response to fearful facial expressions in Williams syndrome. *Neuropsychologia* 48, 1283–1288. doi: 10.1016/j.neuropsychologia.2009.12.030

Hall, E. T. (1963). A system for the notation of proxemics behavior. *Am. Anthropol.* 65, 1003–1026. doi: 10.1525/aa.1963.65.5.02a00020

Hall, E. T. (1966). *The Hidden Dimension.* New York: Doubleday.

Hamilton, D. L. (1968). Personality attributes associated with extreme response style. *Psychol. Bull.* 69, 192–203. doi: 10.1037/h0025606

Havlíček, J., Nováková, L., Vondrová, M., Kuběna, A. A., Valentová, J., and Roberts, S. C. (2012). Olfactory perception is positively linked to anxiety in young adults. *Perception* 41, 1246–1261. doi: 10.1068/p7244

Havlicek, J., Saxton, T. K., Roberts, S. C., Jozifkova, E., Lhota, S., Valentova, J., et al. (2008). He sees, she smells? Male and female reports of sensory reliance in mate choice and non-mate choice contexts. *Pers. Individ. Differ.* 45, 565–570. doi: 10.1016/j.paid.2008.06.019

Herberner, E. S., Kagan, J., and Cohen, M. (1989). Shyness and olfactory threshold. *Pers. Individ. Differ.* 10, 1159–1163. doi: 10.1016/0191-8869(89)90079-2

Herz, R. S., and Inzlicht, M. (2002). Sex differences in response to physical and social factors involved in human mate selection: the importance of smell for women. *Evol. Hum. Behav.* 23, 359–364. doi: 10.1016/S1090-5138(02)00095-8

Hummel, T., Kobal, G., Gudiziol, H., and Mackay-Sim, A. (2007). Normative data for the "Sniffin' Sticks" including tests of odor identification, odor discrimination, and olfactory thresholds: an upgrade based on a group of more than 3,000 subjects. *Eur. Arch. Otorhinolaryngol.* 264, 237–243. doi: 10.1007/s00405-006-0173-0

Hummel, T., Konnerth, O. G., Rosenheim, K., and Kobal, G. (2001). Screening of olfactory function with a four-minute odor identification test: reliability, normative data, and investigations in patients with olfactory loss. *Ann. Otol. Rhinol. Laryngol.* 110, 976–981.

Knaapila, A., Tuorila, H., Kyvik, K. O., Wright, M. J., Keskitalo, K., Hansen, J., et al. (2008). Self-ratings of olfactory function reflect odor annoyance rather than olfactory acuity. *Laryngoscope* 118, 2212–2217. doi: 10.1097/MLG.0b013e3181826e43

Koelega, H. S. (1970). Extraversion, sex, arousal and olfactory sensitivity. *Acta Psychol. (Amst.)* 34, 51–66. doi: 10.1016/0001-6918(70)90004-1

Koelega, H. S. (1994). Sex differences in olfactory sensitivity and the problem of the generality of smell acuity. *Percept. Mot. Skills* 78, 203–213. doi: 10.2466/pms.1994.78.1.203

La Buissonnière-Ariza, V., Lepore, F., Kojok, K. M., and Frasnelli, J. (2013). Increased odor detection speed in highly anxious healthy adults. *Chem. Senses* 38, 577–584. doi: 10.1093/chemse/bjt028

Landis, B. N., Hummel, T., Hugentobler, M., Giger, R., and Lacroix, J. S. (2003). Ratings of overall olfactory function. *Chem. Senses* 28, 691–694. doi: 10.1093/chemse/bjg061

Larsson, M., Finkel, D., and Pedersen, N. L. (2000). Odor identification: influences of age, gender, cognition, and personality. *J. Gerontol. B. Psychol. Sci. Soc. Sci.* 55, 304–310. doi: 10.1093/geronb/55.5.P304

Lundström, J. N., Boyle, J. A., Zatorre, R. J., and Jones-Gotman, M. (2008). Functional neuronal processing of body odors differs from that of similar common odors. *Cereb. Cortex* 18, 1466–1474. doi: 10.1093/cercor/bhm178

Malaspina, D., and Coleman, E. (2003). Olfaction and social drive in schizophrenia. *Arch. Gen. Psychiatry* 60, 578–584. doi: 10.1001/archpsyc.60.6.578

Mitro, S., Gordon, A. R., Olsson, M. J., and Lundström, J. N. (2012). The smell of age: perception and discrimination of body odors of different ages. *PLoS ONE* 7:e38110. doi: 10.1371/journal.pone.0038110

Miwa, T., Furukawa, M., Tsukatani, T., Constanzo, R. M., DiNardo, L. J., and Reiter, E. R. (2001). Impact of olfactory impairment on quality of life and disability. *Arch. Otolaryngol. Head Neck Surg.* 127, 497–503. doi: 10.1001/archotol.127.5.497

Naemi, B. D., Beal, D. J., and Payne, S. C. (2009). Personality predictors of extreme response style. *J. Pers.* 77, 261–286. doi: 10.1111/j.1467-6494.2008.00545

Novakova, L., Bojanowski, V., Havlíček, J., and Croy, I. (2012). Differential patterns of food appreciation during consumption of a simple food in congenitally anosmic individuals: an explorative study. *PLoS ONE* 7:e33921. doi: 10.1371/journal.pone.0033921

Olsson, S. B., Barnard, J., and Turri, L. (2006). Olfaction and identification of unrelated individuals: examination of the mysteries of human odor recognition. *J. Chem. Ecol.* 32, 1635–1645. doi: 10.1007/s10886-006-9098-8

Pause, B. M., Ferstl, R., and Fehm-Wolfsdorf, G. (1998). Personality and olfactory sensitivity. *J. Res. Person.* 32, 510–518. doi: 10.1006/jrpe.1998.2228

Powell, G. E. (1977). Psychoticism and social deviancy in children. *Adv. Behav. Res. Ther.* 1, 27–56. doi: 10.1016/0146-6402(77)90003-0

Prehn-Kristensen, A., Wiesner, C., Bergmann, T. O., Wolff, S., Jansen, O., Mehdorn, H. M., et al. (2009). Induction of empathy by the smell of anxiety. *PLoS ONE* 4:e5987. doi: 10.1371/journal.pone.0005987

Rothmann, S., and Coetzer, E. P. (2003). The big five personality dimensions and job performance. *J. Ind. Psychol.* 29, 68–74. doi: 10.4102/sajip.v29i1.88

Santos, D. V., Reiter, E. R., DiNardo, L. J., and Costanzo, R. M. (2004). Hazardous events associated with impaired olfactory function. *Arch. Otolaryngol. Head Neck Surg.* 130, 317–319. doi: 10.1001/archotol.130.3.317

Schaal, B., Soussignan, R., Marlier, L., Kontar, F., Karima, I. S., and Tremblay, R. E. (1997). Variability and invariants in early odour preferences: comparative data from children belonging to three cultures. *Chem. Senses* 22, 212.

Schiffman, S. S., and Graham, B. G. (2000). Taste and smell perception affect appetite and immunity in the elderly. *Eur. J. Clin. Nutr.* 54, S54–S63. doi: 10.1038/sj.ejcn.1601026

Schleidt, M., Hold, B., and Attili, G. (1981). A cross-cultural study on the attitude towards personal odors. *J. Chem. Ecol.* 7, 19–31. doi: 10.1007/BF00988632

Schubert, C. R., Cruickshanks, K. J., Fischer, M. E., Huang, G. H., Klein, B. E., Klein, R., et al. (2012). Olfactory impairment in an adult population: the Beaver Dam Offspring Study. *Chem. Senses* 37, 325–334. doi: 10.1093/chemse/bjr102

Seo, H. S., Guarneros, M., Hudson, R., Distel, H., Min, B. C., Kang, J. K., et al. (2011). Attitudes toward olfaction: a cross-regional study. *Chem. Senses* 36, 177–187. doi: 10.1093/chemse/bjq112

Seo, H. S., and Hummel, T. (2009). Effects of olfactory dysfunction on sensory evaluation and preparation of foods. *Appetite* 53, 314–321. doi: 10.1016/j.appet.2009.07.010

Shapiro, S. S., and Wilk, M. B. (1965). An analysis of variance test for normality (complete samples). *Biometrika* 52, 591–611.

Shu, C. H., Lee, P. O., Lan, M. Y., and Lee, Y. L. (2011). Factors affecting the impact of olfactory loss on the quality of life and emotional coping ability. *Rhinology* 49, 337–341.

Smoliner, C., Fischedick, A., Sieber, C. C., and Wirth, R. (2013). Olfactory function and malnutrition in geriatric patients. *J. Gerontol. A Biol. Sci. Med. Sci.* 68, 1582–1588. doi: 10.1093/gerona/glt085

Soudry, Y., Lemogne, C., Malinvaud, D., Consoli, S.-M., and Bonfils, P. (2011). Olfactory system and emotion: common substances. *Eur. Ann. Otorhinolaryngol. Head Neck Dis.* 128, 18–23. doi: 10.1016/j.anorl.2010.09.007

Stevenson, R. J. (2010). An initial evaluation of the function of human olfaction. *Chem. Senses* 35, 3–20. doi: 10.1093/chemse/bjp083

Wedekind, C., Seebeck, T., Betterns, F., and Paepke, A. J. (1995). MHC-dependent mate preferences in humans. *Proc. Biol. Sci.* 260, 245–249. doi: 10.1098/rspb.1995.0087

Weiner, I. B., and Craighead, W. E. (2010). *The Corsini Encyclopedia of Psychology*, Vol. 2. Hoboken, NJ: Wiley & Sons, Inc.

Yamazaki, K., and Beauchamp, G. K. (2007). Genetic basis for MHC-dependent mate choice. *Adv. Genet.* 59, 126–145. doi: 10.1016/S0065-2660(07)59005-X

5

Liking and wanting pleasant odors: different effects of repetitive exposure in men and women

Chantal Triscoli[1,2]*, Ilona Croy[1], Håkan Olausson[1] and Uta Sailer[2]

[1] Clinical Neuroscience and Rehabilitation, Institute of Neuroscience and Physiology, University of Gothenburg, Gothenburg, Sweden
[2] Department of Psychology, University of Gothenburg, Gothenburg, Sweden

Correspondence:
Chantal Triscoli, Department of Clinical Neurophysiology, Institute of Neuroscience and Physiology, Sahlgrenska University Hospital, Blå Stråket 7, Gothenburg 413 45, Sweden
e-mail: chantal.triscoli@psy.gu.se

Odors can enrich the perception of our environment and are commonly used to attract people in marketing situations. However, the perception of an odor changes over repetitions. This study investigated whether repetitive exposition to olfactory stimuli leads to a change in the perceived pleasantness ("liking") or in the wish to be further exposed to the same olfactory stimulus ("wanting"), and whether these two mechanisms show gender differences. Three different pleasant odors were each repeatedly presented for 40 times in random order with a mean inter-stimulus interval of 18 s. Eighteen participants rated both "liking" and "wanting" for each of the 120 olfactory stimuli. Wanting ratings decreased significantly over repetitions in women and men, with a steeper decrease for men during the initial trials before plateauing. In contrast, liking ratings decreased significantly over repetitions only in men, with a steeper decrease after the initial ratings, but not in women. Additionally, women scored higher in a questionnaire on reward responsiveness than men. We conclude that positive evaluation (liking) and the wish to experience more of the same (wanting) are different concepts even in the domain of olfaction. The persistence of perceived pleasantness in women may be due to the attribution of a greater subjective value to odors.

Keywords: wanting, liking, odor, pleasantness, gender, smells, odors

INTRODUCTION

The sense of smell plays an important role in everyday life. As olfactory stimuli signal the presence of food and threat, amongst other things, they affect our behavior and subsequent actions (Gottfried et al., 2002). Odors can induce subjective feelings of pleasure and make us come back for more. It has been suggested that these two aspects, the experienced pleasantness of a stimulus and the motivation to obtain the stimulus, represent two separate and independent aspects (Berridge, 2009) that have to be differentiated from each other. For example, a strong urge to obtain a certain pleasant sensory stimulus may not necessarily mean that one subsequently enjoys its consumption. These two aspects have been termed "liking" and "wanting" (Berridge, 2009) and are thought to be mediated by different brain substrates. Indeed, pharmacological manipulations of these brain areas can alter "wanting" without affecting "liking" and vice versa (Berridge, 1996, 2009; Berridge et al., 2009). There is a rich body of literature on liking and wanting relating to food (Berridge, 1996, 2009; Berridge et al., 2009; Berridge and Robinson, 2011) and to the effects of drugs (Wise, 1980, 1996; Koob, 1992; Harriet, 1996; Spanagel and Weiss, 1999; Kelley and Berridge, 2002). However, a whole range of other stimuli can also cause positive hedonic experiences, such as odors (Gottfried and Wilson, 2011; Rolls, 2014), pleasant touch (Kida and Shinohara, 2013a,b; Rolls, 2014), social connection (Morelli et al., 2014), and music (Menon and Levitin, 2005; Montag et al., 2011; Salimpoor et al., 2013), to only name a few. It is as yet unknown whether the differentiation into wanting and liking also applies to these other types of stimuli, for example, odors.

The subjective value of odors may also be processed differently depending on gender. Although men and women have been reported to have similar sensory abilities when detecting and discriminating odors (Oberg et al., 2002), there are studies showing a female advantage for familiarity and recognition of odors (Brand and Millot, 2001), remembering (Klukty, 1990; Oberg et al., 2002) and identifying odors (Doty et al., 1985; Ferdenzi et al., 2013). Women were also found to more easily associate an odor with a term, pointing at better semantic abilities linked to odors (see also Ferdenzi et al., 2013). However, because of their enhanced association ability, it is likely that women's superiority in these olfactory tasks is due to cognitive rather than sensory factors.

A further aspect of olfaction in which men and women seem to differ is the impact of the sense of smell in everyday life. This is suggested by responses in a questionnaire evaluating the subjective importance of the sense of smell (Croy et al., 2010), in which women were found to attribute a higher importance to olfaction than men did. In the same way, a different study reported a higher interest in the sense of smell for women than for men (Seo et al., 2011). This larger interest or importance can be expected to lead to gender differences in pleasantness ratings.

Furthermore, wanting and liking may change with repeated exposure. The intensity and perception of odors has been found to change due to habituation and potential desensitization processes (Andersson et al., 2013). However, changes in the subjective value of an odor may be independent of habituation. For example, it has been reported that the perceived pleasantness ("liking") of pleasant odors was maintained over repetitions, whereas the perceived unpleasantness of malodors decreased (Croy et al., 2013b). To prevent habituation, these authors used effect of habituation a long inter-stimulus interval of 22 s. Applying 96 olfactory stimuli in a row, they found no signs of habituation for pleasant odors as measured by intensity ratings and evoked potentials (Croy et al., 2013b).

The potential persistence of the experienced pleasantness of odors is relevant for marketing situations. Odors are not only ubiquitous in shops and restaurants, but are also used for shop design (Soars, 2009). The perception of diffused pleasant odors has been shown to contribute to a positive evaluation of a mall environment, and indirectly to a product's quality (Chebat and Michon, 2003). When pleasant odors were used, shoppers perceived the time spent in a store as shorter, and their overall perception of the environment, their purchase intention, and the likelihood to revisit the store were improved, irrespective of the nature and the intensity of the odor (Spangenberg et al., 1996). Another study demonstrated that lavender odor diffused in a restaurant, compared to a non-smell condition, increased the duration of stay for customers and the amount purchased (Gueguen and Petr, 2006). Finally, a study conducted in a real-life situation (a shopping mall), showed that odors positively influenced shoppers' perceptions, but only when the shop was neither crowded nor empty (Michon et al., 2005). Thus, if the perceived pleasantness of an odor would remain constant over repetitions, perfuming shops could be considered as a selling strategy to keep customers longer inside a shop.

The present study aimed to investigate whether "wanting" and "liking" of odors develop differently over repetitions. Furthermore, we expected that gender influences the wanting and liking of odors, because women have been reported to attribute greater importance to the sense of smell than men do.

METHODS

PARTICIPANTS

In total, 18 subjects, aged between 20 and 36 years ($M = 27$, $SD = 3.8$) were recruited, 9 of them were men and 9 of them were women. The majority of the participants were students; some of them had already taken part in a previous, but unrelated experiment on touch perception. The participants were asked not to join the experiment if they were suffering from a cold, in order to avoid reduced olfactory performance. All the participants signed an informed consent form and received a compensation for participating in the study (200 SEK per hour).

The study was approved by the ethics committee of the University of Gothenburg.

MATERIALS

The odor stimuli were delivered in opaque glass bottles (50 ml capacity) containing odorant diluted in propylene glycol (Sigma Aldrich, Steinheim, Germany).

A first **pre-test** served to establish concentrations that were equal in subjective intensity. The pre-test and its results are described in the following paragraph.

The sample consisted of 18 students (16 females, 2 males), aged between 19 and 42 years ($M = 28$, $SD = 6.91$), none of which participated in the later experiment. Four different odors were presented at 3 different levels of concentration. These odors were ready-made perfume mixtures (Firmenich, Kerpen, Germany) smelling of flowers (diluted to 1.8, 5.5, 16.6%), aloe (diluted to 0.49, 0.96, 1.8%), vanilla (diluted to 0.5, 0.96, 1.8%), and coconut (diluted to 1.8, 5.5, 16.6%). Two further odors not relevant for the present study were presented in 4 different levels of concentration. Thus, 20 different stimuli resulted which were presented in random order. Pleasantness and intensity were rated on an 11-point scale, pleasantness: −5 (extremely unpleasant) to 5 (extremely pleasant); intensity: 0 (not intense at all) to 10 (extremely intense). The mean ratings for all participants were then submitted to two separate repeated-measures ANOVAs with the factors concentration (low, middle, high) and odor (flower, aloe, vanilla, coconut). Based on these results, those concentrations were selected that were found to differ in perceived pleasantness, but not in intensity (for mean rating values, see **Table 1**). This was the case for coconut (16.6%), vanilla (0.9%), aloe (0.49%), and flowers (5.5%). Pairwise comparisons with Bonferroni-corrections showed that vanilla was perceived as less pleasant than both flowers ($p < 0.01$) and aloe ($p < 0.05$). Aloe was also perceived as more pleasant than coconut ($p < 0.05$). For the subsequent experiment, we decided to use the odors coconut, aloe and flowers, since these three were on average clearly experienced as pleasant, as compared to vanilla.

Experimental setting and procedure

Prior to the experiment, normal olfactory function was ascertained with the use of the "Sniffin' Sticks" odor identification test (Burghart Instruments, Wedel, Germany) (Kobal et al., 1996). The maximal score to obtain in this test is 16. In the present study, subjects were included when they had at least 10 correct answers. The probability of having 10 or more answers right by pure chance is 0.16%. All the subjects attained this criterion.

The participants were asked to sit on a comfortable chair and to make their ratings on an iPad (Apple Inc., Cupertino, USA), which was connected to a PC via iDisplay (SHAPE, Stuttgart, Germany). The participants wore headphones in order to be able to better concentrate on their sense of smell and not to be distracted. Subjects were instructed to smell the three odors flowers, aloe and coconut, in the concentrations established in the pre-test and grade their pleasantness on the iPad in front of them. The odors were contained in opaque glass bottles that were labeled X, Y, Z. Subjects were told to breathe deeply during the break between the different smells. Odor presentation was randomized

Table 1 | Mean pleasantness ratings and standard deviations in parentheses for concentrations similar in perceived intensity, but differing in perceived pleasantness.

	Coconut (16.6%)	Vanilla (0.9%)	Aloe (0.49%)	Flowers (5.5%)
Intensity	5.78 (1.99)	5.56 (1.76)	5.83 (2.01)	5.39 (3.15)
Pleasantness	1.33 (2.09)	−0.17 (2.15)	2.94 (1.11)	2.11 (1.68)

within 40 triplets (each triplet consisting of aloe, flowers, and coconut). Thus, each odor was presented 40 times, resulting in 120 trials. The whole session lasted about 36 min.

Odor presentation was guided by a computerized experimental protocol (programmed in MATLAB, Mathworks, Natick, MA) visible only to the experimenter. It showed a count-down to present the odor to the subject at the right time, the type of odor to administer (X, Y, Z) and the subsequent one. The average of the inter-stimulus interval between the presentations of each odor was 18.27 s, thus, 15 s plus the reaction times for liking and wanting. A count-down was shown on the screen. The experimenter sat next to the subject and opened the bottle indicated by the program 8 s after the count-down started. The odor was held directly under the subject's nostrils for 3 s. During the remaining 4 s the subjects waited for the rating scale to appear. We chose a duration of 4 s so that the subjects had time to think about which rating to give. The experimental procedure is illustrated in **Figure 1**.

The ratings were made on a visual analog scale (VAS) programmed in MATLAB and displayed on the iPad. Two different VAS were displayed after each other. In the first, subjects were asked to answer the question "How pleasant was the smell?" This scale had the endpoints "not at all pleasant" and "very pleasant," and was intended to measure the concept of "liking." In the second VAS, subjects were asked to answer the question "How much do you want to smell this again?" This scale had the end points "not at all" and "very much," and was intended to measure the concept of "wanting." Each VAS scale disappeared as soon as the subject had given the rating, or otherwise after 5 s.

Prior to the experiment, at least 4 practice trials without exposition to odors were done so that the subjects got familiar with making the ratings on the iPad. In the main experiment, none of the participants exhibited problems with the ratings scales.

Questionnaires

Immediately after each experiment, subjects filled in two different questionnaires assessing several hedonic subjective features, administered in English. These questionnaires were the "BIS/BAS" Scale (Carver and White, 1994) and the "TEPS" (Gard, 2006).

The BIS/BAS Scale ("Behavioral Inhibition and Activation Systems" Scale) (Carver and White, 1994) is a 24-items questionnaire on a 4-point Likert scale (from 1 = "very true for me" to 4 = "very false for me") that measures approach behavior (BAS) and avoidance/withdrawal (BIS). High BAS is generally associated with high positive affect in response to reward, while high BIS is associated with high negative affect in response to punishment (Gray and McNaughton, 1982).

The TEPS ("Temporal Experience of Pleasure Scale") (Gard, 2006) is a measure specifically designed to capture the individual trait dispositions in both Anticipatory and Consummatory experiences of pleasure. Specifically, the Anticipatory scale is related to reward responsiveness and imagery, while the Consummatory scale is related to openness to different experiences, and appreciation of positive stimuli. It contains 18 statements about different hedonic situations that may occur in everyday life and it is measured on a 6-point Likert scale (from 1 = "very false for me" to 6 = "very true for me").

For both questionnaires, participants were instructed that there were no right or wrong responses, but subjective ones related to each person's own experiences.

STATISTICAL ANALYSIS

All statistical analyses were made using SPSS Statistics version 21 (IBM, Chicago, USA). There were no specific hypotheses about how liking and wanting or sex may differentially affect the evaluation of the three odors. Therefore, the three odors were collapsed for the analyses.

Odor identification performance

The olfactory identification scores were compared between men and women using an independent samples t-test.

Analysis of change of ratings over time

First, it was investigated whether ratings could be predicted from the number of repetitions. This analysis was done separately for men and women. To this aim, linear regression analyses were performed on the single trial data with "liking" as the outcome variable and the number of repetitions per smell as the predictor. Subsequently, an analogous analysis was performed for the wanting ratings. For men, two piecewise linear regressions were performed separately for the ratings of the initial 4 trials and the remaining trials. This choice was made because the wanting ratings of men showed a steep decrease in the first trials before plateauing. For reasons of consistence, the same analysis was performed for the liking ratings.

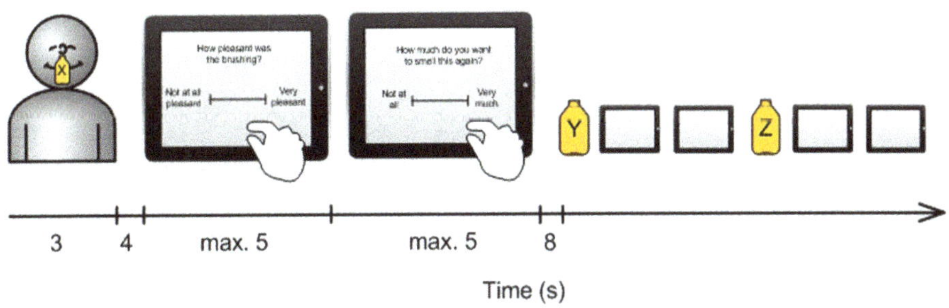

FIGURE 1 | Timeline of the experimental procedure. One trial consisted of the presentation of one smell and 2 subsequent rating scales (for explanation, see text).

Comparison of men and women

In order to determine whether the number of repetitions was a stronger predictor of the liking ratings for males than for females, a further linear regression analysis was performed with the single trials. In this analysis the regression coefficients of men and women were directly compared. We generated a dummy variable that was coded 1 for female and 0 for male (variable name "female"), one variable that contained the product of female and the liking ratings (variable name "femlike"), and a further variable that contained the product of female and the wanting ratings (variable name "femwant"). Then, "female," "femlike," and the liking ratings were used as predictors in the regression equation. In this way, the term "femlike" tests the null-hypothesis that the regression coefficients for females are the same as for men. The regression coefficients of men and women were compared twice, first between the women's slope for all trials and the men's slope for the first 4 trials (1–4), then between the women's slope for all trials and the men's slope for the remaining trials (5–40).

The same analysis was performed for wanting ratings, in order to compare the ratings between men and women. In this analysis, "female," "femwant," and the wanting ratings were used as predictors. Similar to the analysis of liking, the regression coefficients of men and women were compared twice, first between the women's slope for all trials and the men's slope for the first 4 trials (1–4), then between the women's slope for all trials and the men's slope for the remaining trials (5–40).

Whereas the regression analyses give information about the steepness of the change of ratings over time, they do not inform about the absolute rating values, i.e., whether an odor is rated as very pleasant or less pleasant in the beginning. To determine potential differences in these ratings, the second rating was selected for each subject and separately for wanting and liking ratings. The second rating was preferred to the first, because it was considered to be more reliable. The first rating may to a larger extent be influenced by novelty of the task. Also, the standard deviation of the very first rating appeared to be much higher than the standard deviation of the second rating. Moreover, despite the practice trials, subjects sometimes missed the first rating when the experiment started. Therefore, the second rating was used instead of the first.

The second rating was then submitted to a 2 × 2 repeated measures ANOVA with "evaluated aspect" (and the levels liking and wanting) as within-subjects factor and "sex" as between-subjects factor. Greenhouse-Geisser correction was used to adjust for violations of sphericity.

Questionnaires analyses

In order to determine whether there were any gender differences in the questionnaires results, a One-Way ANOVA between the scores of the questionnaires scales was computed. Level of significance was set to $p < 0.05$ for all analyses.

Spearman's correlations were computed separately for liking and wanting between the regression slopes, the second rating and the scores of the questionnaires scales. This procedure was done separately for men and women.

RESULTS

ODOR IDENTIFICATION PERFORMANCE

Women had a higher sniffing sticks score than men, obtaining a mean sniffing sticks' score of 13.6 ($SD = 1.4$) and 12.6 ($SD = 1.9$), respectively. However, the difference between men and women was not significant ($t = -1.27$; $p = 0.221$).

ANALYSIS OF CHANGE OF RATINGS OVER TIME

On average, subjects missed answering 1.3 liking ratings and 1.9 wanting ratings within 120 trials.

The *liking ratings* of women did not decrease with the number of repetitions ($t = -1.52$, $SE = 0.01$, $R = 0.05$, Beta $= -0.05$, $B = -0.01$, $p = 0.128$) (**Figure 2**). The liking ratings of men did not decrease significantly in trials 1–4 ($t = -0.66$, $SE = 0.71$, Beta $= -0.11$, $B = -0.47$, $p = 0.516$), but in the subsequent trials 5–40 ($t = -6.43$, $SE = 0.01$, Beta $= -0.20$, $B = -0.04$, $p < 0.001$). Thus, the liking ratings of men decreased significantly over repetitions from the 5th trial and could be predicted from the number of repetitions, whereas they maintained constant in women.

The *wanting ratings* of women decreased with the number of repetitions ($t = -3.26$, $SE = 0.01$, $R = 0.10$, Beta $= -0.10$, $B = -0.02$, $p = 0.001$). The wanting ratings of men decreased in trials 1–4 ($t = -3.19$, $SE = 0.17$, Beta $= -0.30$, $B = -0.54$, $p = 0.002$), but not in the trials 5–40 ($t = -1.34$, $SE = 0.01$, Beta $= -0.04$, $B = -0.01$, $p = 0.182$). Thus, after an initial steep decrease, wanting ratings maintained constant over repetitions.

COMPARISON OF MEN AND WOMEN

Regarding *gender* differences, women's liking rating slopes did not significantly differ from that of men for trials 1–4 ($t = -1.53$, $SE = 0.01$, Beta $= -0.05$, $B = -0.01$, $p = 0.127$). Therefore, in the beginning of the experiment, liking ratings showed a similar pattern over repetitions for both sexes. However, liking ratings differed significantly between men and women in trials 5–40 ($t = 4.08$, $SE = 0.01$, Beta $= 0.20$, $B = 0.03$, $p < 0.001$). Thus, as the stimulation progressed, liking decreased more in men than in women, and the number of repetitions was a stronger predictor for liking in men than in women (**Figure 2**).

For the wanting ratings, men and women also showed different results, but in the opposite direction than for the liking ratings. The slope of women differed significantly from that of men for the trials 1–4 ($t = 2.37$, $SE = 0.22$, Beta $= 2.60$, $B = 0.52$, $p = 0.018$); decreasing at a steeper rate in men than women,

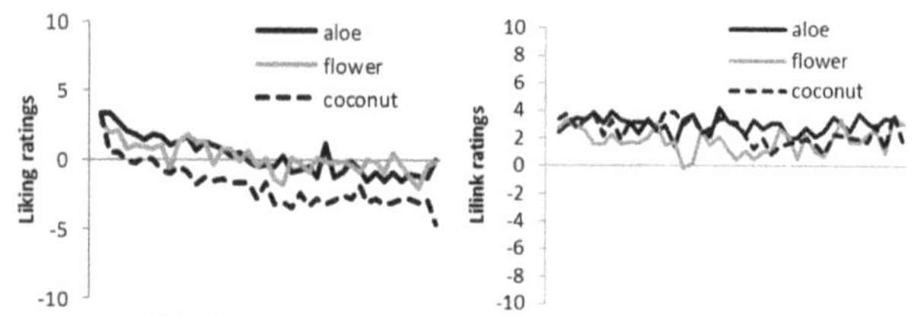

FIGURE 2 | Mean liking ratings of men (left) and women (right) across the number of repetitions.

but not for the trials 5–40 ($t = -1.41$, $SE = 0.01$, Beta $= -0.08$, $B = -0.01, p = 0.159$). Thus, after the first fast decrease in men, the wanting ratings showed a similar pattern over repetitions for both sexes (see **Figure 3**, for all trials).

The comparison of the second wanting and liking ratings showed a main effect with tendency toward significance of "evaluated aspects" [$F_{(1, 16)} = 3.55$; $p = 0.078$] but neither a significant main effect of "sex" [$F_{(1, 16)} = 0.02$; $p = 0.881$], nor a significant interaction between these two factors [$F_{(1, 16)} = 0.22$; $p = 0.648$]. This means that the second liking rating was slightly higher than the second wanting rating in both men and women (compare **Table 2**).

QUESTIONNAIRES ANALYSES

Significant sex differences were found for BAS Reward Responsiveness [One-Way ANOVA: $F_{(1, 16)} = 8.33$, $p = 0.011$] and BIS [$F_{(1, 16)} = 9.45$, $p = 0.007$] (compare **Table 2**). Women were found to be more sensitive to reward than men and also to be more oriented toward avoidance or withdrawal from negative stimuli.

No significant correlations were found between the second ratings and the slopes, neither for liking nor for wanting.

Correlations with the questionnaires scales, performed separately for men and women, showed significant correlations for both sexes (**Table 3**). In men, the slopes of the liking ratings 1–4 and BAS Reward Responsiveness ($r = -0.68$, $p = 0.043$) were significantly negatively correlated, as were the slopes 5–40 with BAS Reward Responsiveness ($r = -0.72$, $p = 0.029$), BIS ($r = -0.71, p = 0.034$) and TEPS Anticipatory scale ($r = -0.82$, $p = 0.007$). This means that the steeper the slope, the smaller men's reward responsiveness and reward anticipation. The slopes

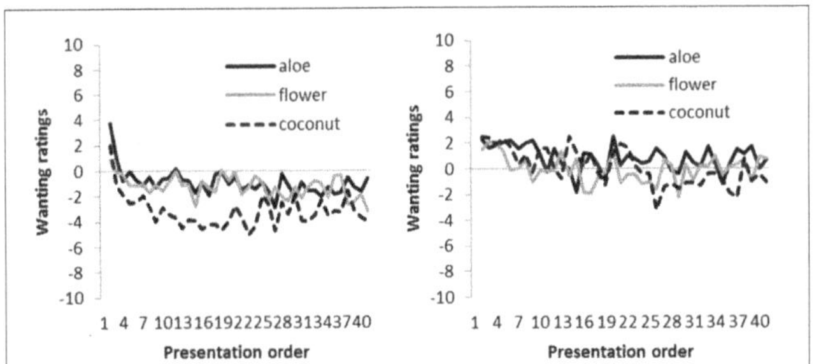

FIGURE 3 | Mean wanting ratings men (left) and women (right) across the number of repetitions.

Table 2 | Mean values and standard deviations (*SD*) for questionnaire scales and ratings.

	Men		Women	
	Mean	***SD***	**Mean**	***SD***
Liking ratings	4.76	2.39	6.22	1.98
Wanting ratings	4.10	2.06	5.14	2.53
BAS reward responsiveness	3.27	0.24	3.60	0.24
BIS	2.71	0.53	3.38	0.38
Initial liking ratings	6.28	2.00	6.69	1.67
Initial wanting ratings	5.66	1.91	6.24	2.17

1–4 of the wanting ratings were also negatively correlated with the BIS ($r = -0.79, p = 0.012$).

In women, no correlation between any slope and a questionnaire score was observed. However, women's second liking rating and the TEPS Anticipatory ($r = 0.74$, $p = 0.023$) and Consummatory ($r = 0.78$, $p = 0.014$) scales were significantly positively correlated. That means, the more women were reward-responsive, open to different experiences and appreciated positive stimuli, the higher their pleasantness ratings were at the beginning of the experiment. Moreover, in women, there were two significant positive correlations between the second wanting ratings and the TEPS Anticipatory ($r = 0.71$, $p = 0.031$) and Consummatory ($r = 0.77$, $p = 0.016$) scales: the more women were reward-responsive, open to different experiences and appreciating positive stimuli, the higher their wanting ratings were at the beginning.

DISCUSSION

It has been suggested that "liking," the actual affective or hedonic experience, differs from "wanting," the motivation or urge to make such experiences (Berridge and Robinson, 2003). The present study aimed to determine whether such a difference could also be observed for olfactory stimuli, i.e., pleasant odors. In addition, we were interested in whether there are potential gender differences in the appreciation of pleasant odors over repetitions.

Our results suggest that wanting and liking are different concepts also in the domain of olfaction. Firstly, at the first contact with the olfactory stimulus, the degree of pleasantness is evaluated slightly higher than the willingness to be exposed further to it. More importantly, liking and wanting changed differently over time. Women "liked," i.e., continued to find the odors pleasant during the entire experiment, although they did not wish ("want") to smell the odors again after a while. Thus, liking persisted in women even after 120 odor presentations in total (40 repetitions per odor), but wanting decreased.

Differently to women, men's liking decreased only slightly during the first 4 expositions, but more steeply afterwards. This fast decrease in liking after the first 4 trials in men was related to both reward responsiveness and reward anticipation. The steeper the slope with which ratings decreased, the less the individual was responsive to reward. Wanting, in contrast, decreased steeply during the first 4 expositions, but to a much lesser extent for the remaining trials. Thus for men, the very initial ratings are enough in order not to want being exposed to the same olfactory stimulation again, while afterwards the ratings are still maintained low but constant. Altogether, wanting and liking developed differently across repetitions in both men and women.

DIFFERENCES BETWEEN MEN AND WOMEN

In addition to these differences between wanting and liking that were observed in both men and women, there were also sex differences for liking and wanting. Women showed a smaller decrease in liking over repetitions than men. This may be due to the fact that smells are more important for women than for men (Croy et al., 2010), or to the fact that women are more interested in odors than men (Seo et al., 2011). This may be related to the finding that women's second liking and wanting ratings

Table 3 | Correlations between ratings and questionnaires.

	Men ($N = 9$)					
	Second liking	**Slope liking 1–4**	**Slope liking 5–40**	**Second wanting**	**Slope wanting 1–4**	**Slope wanting 5–40**
BAS drive	$r = -0.01$, $p = 0.983$	$r = 0.15$, $p = 0.695$	$r = -0.14$, $p = 0.719$	$r = 0.23$, $p = 0.560$	$r = -0.07$, $p = 0.862$	$r = -0.01$, $p = 0.974$
BAS Fun Seeking	$r = -0.08$, $p = 0.841$	$r = 0.47$, $p = 0.199$	$r = 0.02$, $p = 0.964$	$r = -0.09$, $p = 0.822$	$r = -0.15$, $p = 0.702$	$r = 0.51$, $p = 0.161$
BAS reward responsiveness	$r = 0.34$, $p = 0.369$	$r = -0.68$, $p = 0.043$	$r = -0.72$, $p = 0.029$	$r = -0.09$, $p = 0.814$	$r = -0.62$, $p = 0.075$	$r = -0.32$, $p = 0.400$
BIS	$r = 0.34$, $p = 0.370$	$r = -0.62$, $p = 0.074$	$r = -0.71$, $p = 0.034$	$r = -0.12$, $p = 0.751$	$r = -0.79$, $p = 0.012$	$r = -0.19$, $p = 0.620$
TEPS anticipatory	$r = 0.22$, $p = 0.574$	$r = -0.41$, $p = 0.273$	$r = -0.82$, $p = 0.007$	$r = -0.01$, $p = 0.974$	$r = -0.41$, $p = 0.271$	$r = -0.27$, $p = 0.491$
TEPS consummatory	$r = -0.23$, $p = 0.544$	$r = 0.47$, $p = 0.203$	$r = 0.11$, $p = 0.788$	$r = -0.26$, $p = 0.498$	$r = 0.45$, $p = 0.220$	$r = -0.02$, $p = 0.966$

	Women ($N = 9$)			
	Second liking	**Slope liking**	**Second wanting**	**Slope wanting**
BAS drive	$r = 0.09$, $p = 0.811$	$r = 0.02$, $p = 0.965$	$r = -0.06$, $p = 0.879$	$r = -0.55$, $p = 0.129$
BAS fun seeking	$r = 0.16$, $p = 0.690$	$r = -0.44$, $p = 0.238$	$r = -0.04$, $p = 0.930$	$r = -0.07$, $p = 0.859$
BAS reward responsiveness	$r = -0.10$, $p = 0.793$	$r = 0.44$, $p = 0.232$	$r = -0.06$, $p = 0.878$	$r = -0.03$, $p = 0.947$
BIS	$r = -0.15$, $p = 0.699$	$r = 0.26$, $p = 0.507$	$r = -0.04$, $p = 0.915$	$r = 0.41$, $p = 0.279$
TEPS anticipatory	$r = 0.74$, $p = 0.023$	$r = -0.44$, $p = 0.241$	$r = 0.71$, $p = 0.031$	$r = -0.25$, $p = 0.509$
TEPS consummatory	$r = 0.78$, $p = 0.014$	$r = -0.26$, $p = 0.500$	$r = 0.77$, $p = 0.016$	$r = -0.04$, $p = 0.921$

were significantly correlated to anticipatory and consummatory experiences of pleasure in the current study. We speculate that, when approaching pleasant odors, the anticipatory pleasure of those women who are more reward sensitive may have led to high expectations, thus, high initial liking and wanting ratings, and to their constant maintenance over repetitions. However, replications with a larger number of subjects would be required.

It has also been suggested that women are more attentive to odors than men from an early age (Ferdenzi et al., 2008), and that women evaluate odors as more important than men, for example when selecting a potential partner (Herz and Inzlicht, 2002). Moreover, hormonal factors associated with gender differences may also modulate the perceived pleasantness of odors (Rouby et al., 2009).

Women and men also differed regarding wanting. Wanting is conceptualized as the consequence of a process that assigns value to perceptual events (Berridge and Robinson, 2003). During this process, sensory and cognitive information is transformed into attractive and desirable entities. The fact that liking changed in a different way for men and women may indicate that the repeated stimulation leads to different hedonic experiences in women and men, but only after relatively long periods of time. Indeed, at the very beginning of the stimulation, both men and women liked the odors to the same degree, whereas after a short while only the men did not like the odors anymore. On the contrary, wanting was processed differently only at the beginning of the stimulation, with men showing a sort of "instantaneous rejection" which settled down afterwards, while women showed a more constant decrease. Thus, after the initial ratings, men and women behaved in the same way: they did not wish to smell the odors again and this feeling maintained constant until the end of the experiment. These results support the idea that liking and wanting are two related but different concepts which also act differently between sexes. In an applied context, women may continue to experience the repeated exposure to a perfume in odorized shop as pleasant. In the same way, the repeated smell of a perfume may decrease the wish to buy it, and this may take much less time in men than women, both because men start experiencing the smell as less and less pleasant already after the very first expositions and because they would avoid to smell it again already after a short while.

In addition to the small sample size, the present study is limited by the lack of an intensity measure which makes it difficult to estimate the influence of habituation. However, we assume that habituation was unlikely to induce the observed variation of pleasantness, since we had an ISI of 18 s, and long ISIs have previously been found to prevent habituation (Croy et al., 2013a). Moreover, the different odors were always presented alternatingly, thereby further disrupting a possible process of habituation. Moreover, habituation does not imply that perception disappears. If an odor would not be detectable (perceivable) anymore, its rated pleasantness should be at around 0, which is the neutral baseline. This was not the case in the present study, which suggests that the change in pleasantness ratings cannot solely be attributed to a decrease in detectability.

Finally, the constant order of the "liking" and "wanting" scales may have induced effects of the first on the second evaluation. Nevertheless, the ratings for liking and wanting were significantly different. Thus, even though we cannot exclude an influence of the liking ratings on the wanting ratings, we still found evidence for the two concepts being different, even in the domain of olfaction.

Summing up, the experienced pleasantness for olfactory stimuli showed a steeper decrease over repetitions for men than women. Further studies should investigate whether liking and wanting also differ in other sensory modalities than taste and smell, and possibly also between men and women.

ACKNOWLEDGMENTS

This study was supported by the Swedish Research Council (grant 2011-1529) and a fellowship of the German Research Foundation (DFG; CR 479/1-1) to Ilona Croy. We thank Firmenich GmbH, Germany, for providing the odors. We also thank Lukas Rotter for assisting with data collection.

REFERENCES

Andersson, L., Claeson, A. S., Ledin, L., Wisting, F., and Nordin, S. (2013). The influence of health-risk perception and distress on reactions to low-level chemical exposure. *Front. Psychol.* 4:816. doi: 10.3389/fpsyg.2013.00816

Berridge, K. C. (1996). Food reward: brain substrates of wanting and liking. *Neurosci. Biobehav. Rev.* 20, 1–25. doi: 10.1016/0149-7634(95)00033-B

Berridge, K. C. (2009). "Liking" and "wanting" food rewards: brain substrates and roles in eating disorders. *Physiol. Behav.* 97, 537–550. doi: 10.1016/j.physbeh.2009.02.044

Berridge, K. C., and Robinson, T. E. (2003). Parsing reward. *Trends Neurosci.* 26, 507–513. doi: 10.1016/S0166-2236(03)00233-9

Berridge, K. C., and Robinson, T. E. (2011). What is the role of dopamine in reward: hedonic impact, reward learning, or incentive salience? *Brain Res. Brain Res. Rev.* 3, 309–369. doi: 10.1016/S0165-0173(98)00019-8

Berridge, K. C., Robinson, T. E., and Aldridge, J. W. (2009). Dissecting components of reward: "liking," "wanting" and learning. *Curr. Opin. Pharmacol.* 9, 65–73. doi: 10.1016/j.coph.2008.12.014

Brand, G., and Millot, J. L. (2001). Sex differences in human olfaction: between evidence and enigma. *Q. J. Exp. Psychol. B* 54, 259–270. doi: 10.1080/713932757

Carver, C. S., and White, T. L. (1994). Behavioral inhibition, behavioral activation, and affective responses to impending reward and punishment: the BIS/BAS Scales. *J. Pers. Soc. Psychol.* 67, 319–333. doi: 10.1037/0022-3514.67.2.319

Chebat, J. C., and Michon, R. (2003). Impact of ambient odors on mall shoppers' emotions, cognition, and spending. A test of competitive causal theories. *J. Bus. Res.* 56, 529–539. doi: 10.1016/S0148-2963(01)00247-8

Croy, I., Buschhüter, D., Seo, H. S., Negoias, S., and Hummel, T. (2010). Individual significance of olfaction: development of a questionnaire. *Eur. Arch. Otorhinolaryngol.* 267, 67–71. doi: 10.1007/s00405-009-1054-0

Croy, I., Laqua, K., Suss, F., Joraschky, P., Ziemssen, T., and Hummel, T. (2013a). The sensory channel of presentation alters subjective ratings and autonomic responses toward disgusting stimuli-blood pressure, heart rate and skin conductance in response to visual, auditory, haptic and olfactory presented disgusting stimuli. *Front. Hum. Neurosci.* 7:510. doi: 10.3389/fnhum.2013.00510

Croy, I., Maboshe, W., and Hummel, T. (2013b). Habituation effects of pleasant and unpleasant odors. *Int. J. Psychophysiol.* 88, 104–108. doi: 10.1016/j.ijpsycho.2013.02.005

Doty, R. L., Applebaum, S., Zusho, H., and Settle, R. G. (1985). Sex differences in odor identification ability: a cross-cultural analysis. *Neuropsychologia* 23, 667–672. doi: 10.1016/0028-3932(85)90067-3

Ferdenzi, C., Coureaud, G., Camos, V., and Schaal, B. (2008). Human awareness and uses of odor cues in everyday life: results from a questionnaire study in children. *Int. J. Behav. Dev.* 32, 422–431. doi: 10.1177/0165025408093661

Ferdenzi, C., Roberts, S. C., Schirmer, A., Delplanque, S., Cekic, S., Porcherot, C., et al. (2013). Variability of affective responses to odors: culture, gender, and olfactory knowledge. *Chem. Senses* 38, 175–186. doi: 10.1093/chemse/bjs083

Gard, D. E. (2006). Anticipatory and consummatory components of the experience of pleasure: a scale development study. *J. Res. Pers.* 40, 1086–1102. doi: 10.1016/j.jrp.2005.11.001

Gottfried, J. A., O'Doherty, J., and Dolan, R. J. (2002). Appetitive and aversive olfactory learning in humans studied using event-related functional magnetic resonance imaging. *J. Neurosci.* 22, 10829–10837. Available online at: http://www.jneurosci.org/content/22/24/10829.long

Gottfried, J. A., and Wilson, D. A. (2011). "Smell," in *Neurobiology of Sensation and Reward*, ed J. A. Gottfried (Boca Raton, FL: CRC Press), 99–125. doi: 10.1201/b10776-8

Gray, J. A., and McNaughton, N. (1982). *The Neuropsychology of Anxiety: An Enquiry into the Functions of the Septo-Hippocampal System.* Oxford, UK: Oxford University Press.

Gueguen, N., and Petr, C. (2006). Odors and consumer behavior in a restaurant. *Hosp. Manag.* 25, 335–339. doi: 10.1016/j.ijhm.2005.04.007

Harriet, W. (1996). Priming effects with drugs and other reinforcers. *Exp. Clin. Psychopharmacol.* 4, 5–10. doi: 10.1037/1064-1297.4.1.5

Herz, R. S., and Inzlicht, M. (2002). Sex differences in response to physical and social factors involved in human mate selection: the importance of smell for women. *Evol. Hum. Behav.* 23, 359–364. doi: 10.1016/S1090-5138(02)00095-8

Kelley, A. E., and Berridge, K. C. (2002). The neuroscience of natural rewards: relevance to addictive drugs. *J. Neurosci.* 22, 3306–3311. Available online at: http://www.jneurosci.org/content/22/9/3306.full

Kida, T., and Shinohara, K. (2013a). Gentle touch activates the anterior prefrontal cortex: an NIRS study. *Neurosci. Res.* 76, 76–82. doi: 10.1016/j.neures.2013.03.006

Kida, T., and Shinohara, K. (2013b). Gentle touch activates the prefrontal cortex in infancy: an NIRS study. *Neurosci. Lett.* 541, 63–66. doi: 10.1016/j.neulet.2013.01.048

Klukty, N. (1990). Geschlechtsunterschiede in der Gedachtnisleistung für Geruche, Tonfolgen und Farben. *Z. Exp. Angew. Psychol.* 37, 437–446.

Kobal, G., Hummel, T., Sekinger, B., Barz, S., Roscher, S., and Wolf, S. (1996). Sniffin' sticks: screening of olfactory performance. *Rhinology* 34, 222–226.

Koob, G. F. (1992). Drugs of abuse: anatomy, pharmacology and function of reward pathways. *Trends Pharmacol. Sci.* 13, 177–184. doi: 10.1016/0165-6147(92)90060-J

Menon, V., and Levitin, D. J. (2005). The rewards of music listening: response and physiological connectivity of the mesolimbic system. *Neuroimage* 28, 175–184. doi: 10.1016/j.neuroimage.2005.05.053

Michon, R., Chebat, J. C., and Turley, W. L. (2005). Mall atmospherics: the interaction effects of the mall environment on shopping behavior. *J. Bus. Res.* 58, 576–583. doi: 10.1016/j.jbusres.2003.07.004

Montag, C., Reutera, M., and Axmacherc, N. (2011). How one's favorite song activates the reward circuitry of the brain: personality matters! *Behav. Brain Res.* 225, 511–514. doi: 10.1016/j.bbr.2011.08.012

Morelli, S. A., Torre, J. B., and Eisenberger, N. I. (2014). The neural bases of feeling understood and not understood. *Soc. Cogn. Affect. Neurosci.* doi: 10.1093/scan/nst191. [Epub ahead of print].

Oberg, C., Larsson, M., and Backman, L. (2002). Differential sex effects in olfactory functioning: the role of verbal processing. *J. Int. Neuropsychol. Soc.* 8, 691–698. doi: 10.1017/S1355617702801424

Rolls, E. T. (2014). *Emotion and Decision-Making Explained.* Oxford, UK: Oxford University Press.

Rouby, C., Pouliot, S., and Bensafi, M. (2009). Odor hedonics and their modulators. *Food Qual. Prefer.* 20, 545–549. doi: 10.1016/j.foodqual.2009.05.004

Salimpoor, V. N., Van den Bosch, I., Kovacevic, N., McIntosh, A. R., Dagher, A., and Zatorre, R. J. (2013). Interactions between the nucleus accumbens and auditory cortices predict music reward value. *Science* 340, 216–219. doi: 10.1126/science.1231059

Seo, H. S., Guarneros, M., Hudson, R., Distel, H., Min, B. C., Kang, J. K., et al. (2011). Attitudes toward olfaction: a cross-regional study. *Chem. Senses* 36, 177–187. doi: 10.1093/chemse/bjq112

Soars, B. (2009). Driving sales through shoppers' sense of sound, sight, smell and touch. *J. Retail Distrib. Manag.* 37, 286–298. doi: 10.1108/09590550910941535

Spanagel, R., and Weiss, F. (1999). The dopamine hypothesis of reward: past and current status. *Trends Neurosci.* 22, 521–527. doi: 10.1016/S0166-2236(99)01447-2

Spangenberg, E. R., Crowley, A. E., and Henderson, P. W. (1996). Improving the store environment: do olfactory cues affect evaluations and behaviors? *J. Mark.* 60, 67–80. doi: 10.2307/1251931

Wise, R. A. (1980). Action of drugs of abuse on brain reward systems. *Pharmacol. Biochem. Behav.* 13(Suppl. 1), 213–223. doi: 10.1016/S0091-3057(80)80033-5

Wise, R. A. (1996). Addictive drugs and brain stimulation reward. *Annu. Rev. Neurosci.* 19, 319–340. doi: 10.1146/annurev.ne.19.030196.001535

6

The perception of odor objects in everyday life: a review on the processing of odor mixtures

Thierry Thomas-Danguin[1]*, Charlotte Sinding[2], Sébastien Romagny[1], Fouzia El Mountassir[1], Boriana Atanasova[3], Elodie Le Berre[4], Anne-Marie Le Bon[1] and Gérard Coureaud[1]*

[1] Centre des Sciences du Goût et de l'Alimentation, CNRS UMR6265, INRA UMR1324, Université de Bourgogne, Dijon, France
[2] Smell and Taste Clinic, Department of Otorhinolaryngoly, TU Dresden, Dresden, Germany
[3] INSERM U930, Université François Rabelais, Tours, France
[4] Unilever R&D, Vlaardingen, Netherlands

****Correspondence:***
Thierry Thomas-Danguin, Centre des Sciences du Goût et de l'Alimentation, INRA, 17 rue Sully, F-21000 Dijon, France
e-mail: thierry.thomas-danguin@dijon.inra.fr;
Gérard Coureaud, Centre des Sciences du Goût et de l'Alimentation, 9E boulevard Jeanne d'Arc, F-21000 Dijon, France
e-mail: gerard.coureaud@u-bourgogne.fr

Smelling monomolecular odors hardly ever occurs in everyday life, and the daily functioning of the sense of smell relies primarily on the processing of complex mixtures of volatiles that are present in the environment (e.g., emanating from food or conspecifics). Such processing allows for the instantaneous recognition and categorization of smells and also for the discrimination of odors among others to extract relevant information and to adapt efficiently in different contexts. The neurophysiological mechanisms underpinning this highly efficient analysis of complex mixtures of odorants is beginning to be unraveled and support the idea that olfaction, as vision and audition, relies on odor-objects encoding. This configural processing of odor mixtures, which is empirically subject to important applications in our societies (e.g., the art of perfumers, flavorists, and wine makers), has been scientifically studied only during the last decades. This processing depends on many individual factors, among which are the developmental stage, lifestyle, physiological and mood state, and cognitive skills; this processing also presents striking similarities between species. The present review gathers the recent findings, as observed in animals, healthy subjects, and/or individuals with affective disorders, supporting the perception of complex odor stimuli as odor objects. It also discusses peripheral to central processing, and cognitive and behavioral significance. Finally, this review highlights that the study of odor mixtures is an original window allowing for the investigation of daily olfaction and emphasizes the need for knowledge about the underlying biological processes, which appear to be crucial for our representation and adaptation to the chemical environment.

Keywords: odor mixture, perception, interactions, configural, elemental, animal behavior, human applications

INTRODUCTION

The way human beings map their environment as a brain representation is a cornerstone to the interactions they can develop with their surroundings and thus determines their fitness to the world they live in. This representation is built on the basis of sensory cues provided by sensory organs and gathered in the brain. The environment is particularly rich in volatile chemical compounds emitted from a large variety of natural and unnatural sources (e.g., plants, food, conspecifics, organisms, perfumes, human activities). The olfactory system must compute this mixture of volatiles, all day long at a certain distance from the sources and in a timescale reconcilable with fast but relevant behaviors. This is the challenge of the sense of smell, which has to extract relevant information from highly complex chemical mixtures. For humans and other organisms, the success of this computation is a prerequisite to a reliable mental representation of the olfactory environment, which is essential for maximizing adapted behaviors throughout life. Conversely, impaired olfactory processing may affect health and/or well-being and can even lead to death in certain species.

Efficient processing of odorants mixtures should allow for not only the instantaneous recognition and categorization of smells but also the discrimination of odors among others (e.g., background). The different ways in which the olfactory system processes an odor mixture relative to its components contributes to this discrimination. Nevertheless, though olfaction has been the subject of numerous studies, most of them used so-called "monomolecular odors" (i.e., they were based on single odorants as stimuli). As a consequence, the psychophysiological and neurobiological mechanisms that govern the perception of complex odor stimuli, namely the daily functioning of the sense of smell, remain poorly understood. In this context, the present review aims to depict the current knowledge on the perception of odor mixtures. The main guideline of this review is to gather and discuss the results of very recent as well as major studies on the processing of odor mixtures whatever they focused on cellular, neurobiological, behavioral or psychological aspects, and to take into consideration studies conducted both in humans and animals. Considering that olfactory neuroanatomy is remarkably conserved among animals (Ache and Young, 2005), we especially took advantage of studies in non-human species to highlight the ongoing research on the mechanisms of peripheral and central processing specific to complex odor stimuli. Then we discuss the implications of these mechanisms in relation to the perception of odor objects and the cognitive and behavioral significance of such a processing. Finally we consider the applied consequences and benefits that research on odor mixture perception may have for clinical approaches in individuals with mood disorder and for formulation approaches in the field of flavors and fragrances.

THE SPECIFICITY OF ODOR MIXTURES PROCESSING: PERCEPTUAL INTERACTIONS

The main features of monomolecular odor processing are well characterized. Odor intensity is mainly driven by the odorant concentration (Stevens, 1960; Berglund et al., 1971; Chastrette et al., 1998; Devos et al., 2002). Odor quality is mainly related to the odorant chemical structure (Chastrette, 1997; Gaudin et al., 2007; Sanz et al., 2008; Kaeppler and Mueller, 2013; Snitz et al., 2013). Odor pleasantness is highly correlated to odor quality (Kermen et al., 2011) and largely depends on the molecular structure (Khan et al., 2007); odor intensity (Doty, 1975) and individual cognitive factors (e.g., Rouby et al., 2009) also impact pleasantness. However, in the case of odor mixtures, everything becomes more complicated due to the perceptual interactions that arise from the complex chemical signal encoding and processing within the olfactory system.

As defined by Berglund et al. (1976), a mixture percept can be homogeneous when a single odor is perceived from the mixture or heterogeneous when several odors are perceived from the mixture. A homogeneous percept first arises when the odors of the mixed odorants blend into a new odor perceived as an entity. In that case, the mixture is called a blending mixture (Thomas-Danguin et al., 2007) and the perception may be considered configural (or robust configural; Kay et al., 2005) or synthetic (Berglund and Olsson, 1993; Laing, 1994). Second, the odor mixture could also be considered homogeneous when one mixture component has a strong intensity and thus completely covers the quality of the other components; in that case, one speaks about complete overshadowing (Kay et al., 2005) or masking (Cain and Drexler, 1974). When the percept induced by the mixture is heterogeneous, at least some of the component odors can be perceived within the mixture. This refers to the analytical processing of olfactory information (Berglund and Olsson, 1993) also qualified as elemental (Kay et al., 2005). In that case, the odor quality of the mixture can be predicted based on the odor intensity of the components (Laing and Willcox, 1983; Olsson, 1998; Wise and Cain, 2000), but some perceptual interactions may be observed, such as perceptual dominance or partial overshadowing (Atanasova et al., 2005a; Kay et al., 2005; Brodin et al., 2009; Kurtz et al., 2009; Ferreira, 2012b). In many cases, the mixture can have blending properties that lead to the perception of a specific odor for the mixture, on top of the odors of the odorants, which are still perceived (weak configural; Kay et al., 2005). **Figure 1A** illustrates all of the theoretical interactions for odor quality in binary mixtures. In the case of more complex mixtures, it has been suggested that the odor quality of the mixture is more frequently different from the quality of their constituting odorants. In other words, complex mixtures are more inclined to evoke the perception of a new odor (Livermore and Laing, 1998b; Ferreira, 2012b; Lindqvist et al., 2012).

Regarding odor intensity, perceptual interactions induced by the mixing of at least two odors can lead to several effects that can be categorized depending on whether the mixture quality is homogeneous or heterogeneous (Cain and Drexler, 1974; Berglund et al., 1976; Thomas-Danguin, 1997; Ferreira, 2012a; Thomas-Danguin and Dumont, 2012). To demonstrate the perceptual effect of mixing odors, the mixture intensity is compared to the intensities of the single components or their sum (Cain, 1975; Patte and Laffort, 1979; Berglund and Olsson, 1993; Thomas-Danguin and Chastrette, 2002); all of the theoretical possibilities are summarized in **Figure 1B**. For homogeneous percepts, hyper-addition, complete addition, or hypo-addition can arise. In the case of hypo-addition, depending on whether the mixture intensity is higher or lower than the single components' odor intensities, one can observe partial addition, compromise, or subtraction (**Figure 1B**). In the case of heterogeneous percept, it is possible to differentiate among synergy, independence, or masking (partial overshadowing, **Figure 1B**). In the case of complex mixtures including more than two odorants, the odor intensity of the mixture usually does not increase when increasing the number of components (Berglund, 1974; Laffort and Dravnieks, 1982; Miyazawa et al., 2009; Ferreira, 2012a).

Pleasantness is another key feature of odors, but the perceived pleasantness of mixtures has been poorly studied. The available results on binary mixtures all suggest that the pleasantness of the mixture falls between the pleasantness of the components (Moskowitz and Barbe, 1977; Dravnieks and Jarke, 1980). More recently, it was reported that components' odor intensity strongly contributed to the overall mixture pleasantness (Lapid et al., 2008). However, for greater than binary-order mixtures, pleasantness seems to be hardly predictable (Lindqvist et al., 2012).

Perceptual interactions induced by the perception of odorants' mixtures could arise from several biochemical or neurobiological interactions during all stages of olfactory information processing within the olfactory system from the periphery to the brain, as reviewed hereafter.

INTERACTIONS AT THE PERIPHERY: CODING COMPLEX CHEMICAL INFORMATION

Interactions occurring at the peripheral level of the olfactory system play a critical role in the processing of odorants' mixture (Berglund et al., 1976; Bell et al., 1987; Derby, 2000; Kay et al., 2003; Goyert et al., 2007). In both vertebrates and invertebrates, the periphery of the olfactory system triggers the first step of olfactory information coding. At this stage, odorants are sampled by a large number of olfactory receptors (ORs) located in the cilia of olfactory sensory neurons/cells (OSNs). In mammals, each OSN expresses only one functional OR (Chess et al., 1994; Malnic et al., 1999; Serizawa et al., 2004), while insect OSNs express a conventional ligand-binding OR together with OR83b, a highly conserved member of the insect OR family (Larsson et al., 2004). Each OSN/OR typically responds to a variety of odorants so that the identity of a molecule is encoded by the combination of ORs/OSNs that recognize it (Malnic et al., 1999; Duchamp-Viret et al., 2000; Kajiya et al., 2001). The overlapping response profiles of OSNs introduce the possibility of interactions within the context of odorants' mixtures.

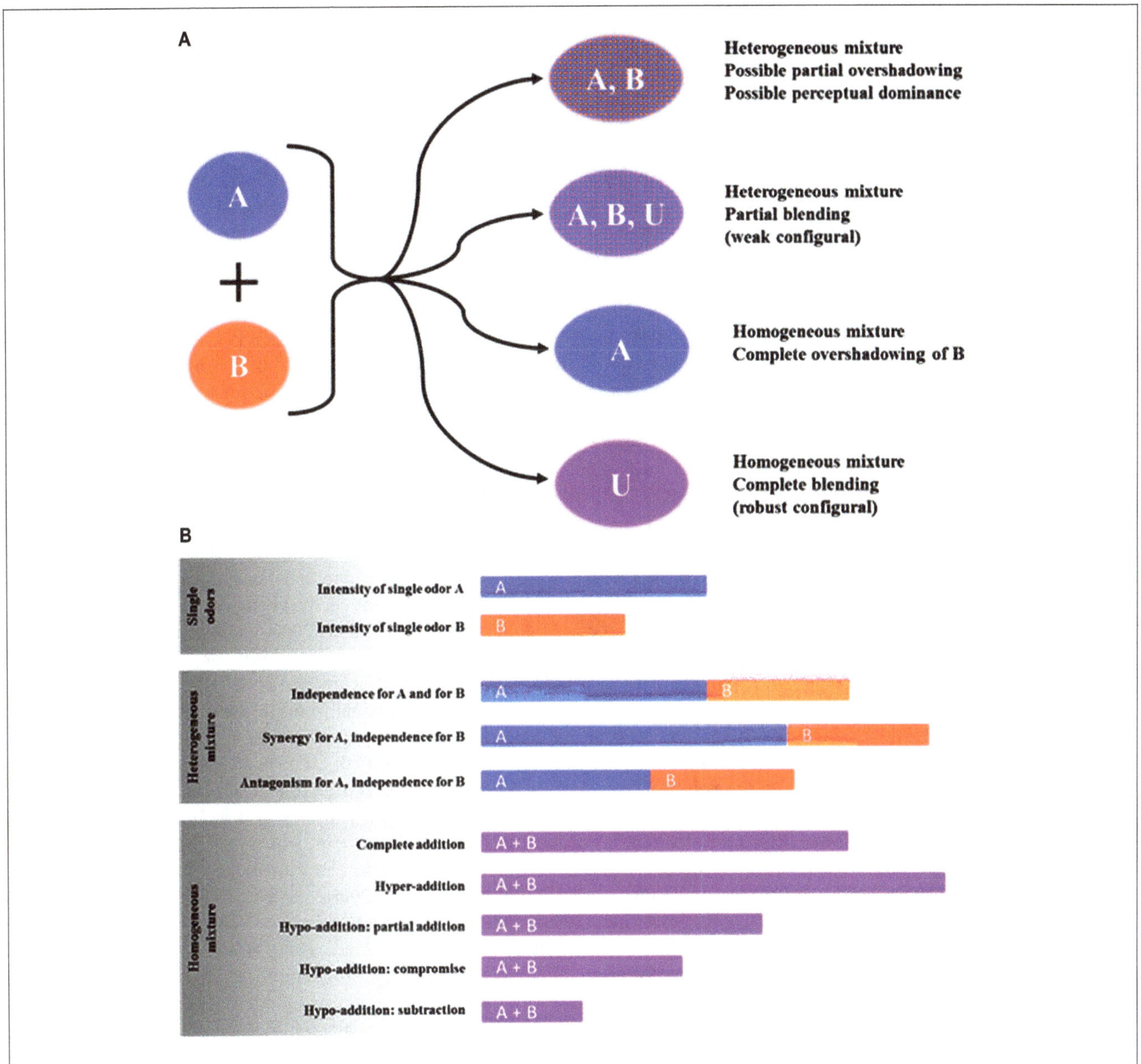

FIGURE 1 | Theoretical outcomes on odor quality (A) and odor intensity (B) when two odorants are perceived in the mixture. One odorant has an odor noted A and the other B, while odor U is specific to the mixture (Unique-cue, see section on configural processing of odorants in mixtures) (this figure was partially adapted from Thomas-Danguin (1997).

Electrophysiological studies in different vertebrate and invertebrate species have compared the responses of OSNs to binary mixtures and their components (Ache et al., 1988; Caprio, 1989; Akers and Getz, 1993; Kang and Caprio, 1997; Steullet and Derby, 1997; Carlsson and Hansson, 2002; Ochieng et al., 2002; Duchamp-Viret et al., 2003). Three types of interactions were mainly observed; they depended on the odorants included in the mixtures and their concentration ratios. In many cases, the response intensity of OSNs to the mixture is lower than the response to the most efficacious component. This phenomenon is reconcilable with the compromise or the subtraction levels of hypo-addition (**Figure 1B**; Gleeson and Ache, 1985; Ache, 1989; Steullet and Derby, 1997; Duchamp-Viret et al., 2003; Rospars et al., 2008). Conversely, the response intensity of OSNs to a mixture can be higher than that induced by the most efficacious component; this phenomenon is classified as partial addition or hyper-addition when the response to the mixture exceeds the summed responses to the components (**Figure 1B**; Akers and Getz, 1993; Kang and Caprio, 1997; Ochieng et al., 2002; Duchamp-Viret et al., 2003; Chaput et al., 2012). In most cases, a given type of interaction was observed over the whole concentration range, but in some cases, a shift to another interaction type as a function of odorant concentration was reported (Duchamp-Viret et al., 2003; Rospars et al., 2008). Data modeling suggests that both competitive and non-competitive interactions occur at the OR level and may account for the effects reported in these studies (Rospars et al., 2008; Cruz and Lowe, 2013; Münch et al., 2013). There is competitive interaction when two molecules bind to the same receptor binding site. This mechanism could involve either two agonist odorants, i.e., molecules that are able to activate the receptor, or one agonist and one antagonist (the latter being a molecule that binds to the receptor but is unable to activate it; Spehr et al., 2003; Oka et al., 2004; Sanz et al., 2005, 2008; Jacquier et al., 2006). For example, it has been shown that the odorant bourgeonal is a powerful agonist for the human receptor hOR17-4 recombinantly expressed in human embryonic kidney (HEK) 293 cells, while another odorant undecanal fails to activate this receptor (Spehr et al., 2003). However, the co-incubation of bourgeonal with undecanal strongly suppressed the hOR17-4 response, which indicates that undecanal inhibited the receptor activation by bourgeonal. The electrical activity in the human olfactory epithelium in response to bourgeonal was dramatically decreased after undecanal exposure (Spehr et al., 2004). Moreover undecanal odor exhibits a strong inhibitory effect on bourgeonal odor at the perceptual level in humans (Spehr et al., 2004; Brodin et al., 2009). A recent study (Chaput et al., 2012) gave additional evidence for a direct link between peripheral and perceptual responses to a mixture containing two odorants naturally occurring in wine, i.e., whiskey lactone and isoamyl acetate. Rat OSN responses to this mixture were enhanced or reduced depending on the OR type and/or the concentration of whiskey lactone in the mixture. Similarly, in humans, the fruity note intensity within the same mixture was increased by low concentrations of whiskey lactone and decreased by high concentrations. Thus, for a given mixture, different types of interactions can occur at the peripheral level, depending on the odorant concentration ratios, which likely govern the mixture's perceptual properties. In insects too, various types of interactions occur at the periphery after stimulation with mixtures of plant odorants and pheromones (Ochieng et al., 2002; Deisig et al., 2012). Hypo-addition-like effects have been observed in a number of cases, and inhibition caused by one molecule at the level of OSNs can modify the response to a pheromone either by reducing its magnitude or by modifying its temporal dynamics (Su et al., 2011; Deisig et al., 2012).

Overall, studies in vertebrates and invertebrates highlight the importance of peripheral interactions in the coding of odorants' mixtures. These events likely shape the odor signal, which might determine the perceptual features of complex mixtures. Nevertheless, the peripheral coding of odorants' mixtures remains poorly understood, and it is still difficult to predict the outcomes of this process though the properties of the single compounds are known.

INTERACTIONS AT HIGHER LEVELS: PROCESSING ODOR INFORMATION

The emergence of new methods of brain imaging in both humans and animals has shed new light on how odors, especially those elicited by mixtures, are encoded in the brain olfactory regions where activation or inhibition between neurons or clusters of neurons can occur. From an anatomical point of view, the OSN enters the olfactory bulb (OB, mammals) or antennal lobe (AL, insects) and connects the mitral cells (mammals) or projection neurons (insects). In mammals, OSNs expressing the same OR converge onto one glomerulus and connect one mitral cell, which is accompanied by tufted cells (Buonviso and Chaput, 1990; Mombaerts et al., 1996; Chen et al., 2009). In insects, similar OSNs also converge onto one glomerulus (Galizia and Menzel, 2000; Wang et al., 2003), but one glomerulus can connect several projection neurons (Kirschner et al., 2006). This neuronal architecture helps gather information from several similar OSNs while staying close to the combinatorial code provided by the binding odorant/OR. Nevertheless, inhibitory systems at this brain processing level can modify the output information that is projected to higher areas. A significant modification of the odor output code occurs post-synaptically and is triggered by granular cells in mammals (Wright and Smith, 2004; McGann et al., 2005; Kay and Stopfer, 2006; Abraham et al., 2010). In insects, inhibition arises from local neurons that connect glomeruli pre- and/or post-synaptically (Silbering and Galizia, 2007).

In odorants' mixture processing, perceptual interactions occurring at the OB/AL level are thought to mostly result from these inhibitory processes, which may contribute to the sparse representation of complex odor mixtures in these brain structures (Dulac, 2006). This may also lead to the apparent perceptual contribution of only a few dominant chemical cues within a complex mixture (e.g., natural scents; Dulac, 2006; Clifford and Riffell, 2013). In line with the involvement of inhibitory processes in the OB, it has also been reported that mitral/tufted cells respond to odorants presented both individually and in mixtures, although the firing rates evoked by mixtures typically showed partial suppression (i.e., hypo-addition; **Figure 1B**; Davison and Katz, 2007). However, an unanswered question is what triggers the inhibition. One hypothesis is that chemical (structural) similarity between odorants could activate overlapping patterns, which may induce perceptual similarity but may also increase the interaction potential (Linster et al., 2001; Grossman et al., 2008). Indeed, at a behavioral level, rats discriminate a binary mixture from its components better when the components are perceived as very similar (Wiltrout et al., 2003). Using a computational model Linster and Cleland (2004) went further and showed that mixing odorants with similar glomerular patterns resulted in lateral inhibition in the OB that lead to a loss of information about each single odorant. This loss of information would favor a bulbar pattern of activation specific to the mixture and contribute to a distinct code for the mixture compared to the code of each component, in line with configural processing of the mixture (but see Fletcher, 2011). However, an alternative theory was proposed to account for these results and suggests that very overlapping odorants, in terms of glomerular activation pattern, would not induce a configural perception because of their almost perfect perceptual similarity (Frederick et al., 2009). Thus, a concentration effect may be considered: mixing two odorants that are perceptually similar would be like doubling the concentration of one odorant. The change in concentration can actually modify the quality of the odor (Laing et al., 2003).

Interactions also occur at the AL level in insects. In the honeybee, the glomerular pattern activated by hexanol and citral in a mixture is different from the sum of patterns activated by each odorant (Joerges et al., 1997). This difference supposedly results from the activation/inhibition of close glomeruli via local neurons, not from the odorants' similarity (hexanol and citral are not structurally or perceptually similar), even if, as proposed in mammals, configural processing is more likely to occur in mixtures of similar odors (Deisig et al., 2002). In this species, the pre-synaptic transduction of information appears to be mainly ruled by elemental laws (Deisig et al., 2006). In contrast, because of lateral inhibition, the output from the AL to higher-order brain regions by projection neurons supports a more configural and less elemental type of processing (Deisig et al., 2010); patterns sent to superior areas would directly encode configurations. In sum, at the OB/AL processing level, lateral inhibition and mixture-specific cell activation were observed and could account for the perceptual interactions induced by the processing of odor mixture.

Beyond these primary brain structures, the olfactory information is processed in superior areas of the brain. In mammals, mitral cells project to the anterior olfactory nucleus, anterior and posterior piriform cortex (aPC and pPC), olfactory tract, lateral entorhinal cortex, and part of the amygdala, among other regions (Mori and Sakano, 2011). The piriform cortex (PC) has been the center of several investigations related to odor discrimination and representation, some of which have used mixtures of odorants (Haberly and Bower, 1984; Granger and Lynch, 1991; Litaudon et al., 1997; Haberly, 2001; Wilson and Stevenson, 2003a; Kadohisa and Wilson, 2006; Barnes et al., 2008; Howard et al., 2009; Stettler and Axel, 2009; Bekkers and Suzuki, 2013). The processing of olfactory information in the OB and the PC is highly contrasted. A study of odorants' mixture processing in mice revealed nonlinear combinatorial interactions at the PC level, as shown by a broader responsiveness of the anterior PC neurons relative to the OB mitral cells (Lei et al., 2006). From a functional point of view, it has been shown in rats that the PC can rapidly discriminate a mixture from its components, thereby producing a minimal cross-habituation to components after habituation to the mixture, while the OB still computes the mixture like the sum of odorants (Wilson, 2000, 2003). Because, the aPC and pPC are quite different in their anatomical organization, they likely have distinct roles in odor encoding: encoding of odorant identity may occur in the aPC while encoding of odor similarity or odor quality occurs in the pPC (Kadohisa and Wilson, 2006; Yoshida and Mori, 2007). These dissociated roles of the aPC and pPC were confirmed by a functional magnetic resonance imaging (fMRI) study performed in humans with single odorants (Gottfried et al., 2006; Gottfried, 2009; Howard et al., 2009). When taken together, these results suggest that the pPC is a key structure for the perception of odor mixtures since it may contribute to their configural processing, namely their putative coding as odor objects, each carrying a specific odor quality.

Higher-order cortices are also involved in olfactory information integration. In a positron emission tomography (PET) study comparing the brain processing of citral + pyridine mixtures, the odors of the single odorants and mixtures both activated the primary and secondary olfactory regions. However, the contrast between the two types of stimuli revealed activation in the middle cingulate cortex, superior frontal gyrus, and angular gyrus (Boyle et al., 2009). In this study, the lateral and anterior regions of the OFC played a distinct role in mixtures' processing and responded in a preferential manner to the binary mixtures. The anterior portion of the OFC acted such as an on-off detector for odor mixtures because it was activated in response to odor mixtures and deactivated in response to single odorants; the lateral portion of the OFC responded in a graded fashion to relatively small differences in intensity ratios of the two mixed odors (Boyle et al., 2009). Anatomically, the OFC is located at a three-synapse step from the olfactory epithelium and receives information already computed by the OB and PC/amygdala (Gottfried and Zelano, 2011). This cortex is known to encode odor identity (quality) but also odor valence (Anderson et al., 2003; Royet et al., 2003) and odor significance (acquired value; Critchley and Rolls, 1996). Therefore, this structure probably plays a major, but still unknown, role in the configural processing of complex odor stimuli. A contrasted processing of binary odor mixtures and their single odorants was also observed by fMRI in higher-order brain areas but not primary olfactory cortices (Grabenhorst et al., 2007). In this study, different parts of the OFC simultaneously and independently represented the positive and negative hedonic value of an odor mixture that contains pleasant and unpleasant components. Interestingly, the medial OFC responded more to the jasmine's pleasant odor when it is mixed with a small amount of the unpleasant odor of indole (Grabenhorst et al., 2007). This response may reflect the perceptual synergy or pleasantness enhancement of the pleasant odor sometimes observed when mixed with an unpleasant one. Such perceptual outcome could be due to an attention-capturing effect of hedonically complex mixtures that operate unconsciously and involve the superior frontal gyrus (Grabenhorst et al., 2011).

ODOR OBJECTS: CONFIGURAL PROCESSING OF ODORANTS IN MIXTURES

Perceptual interactions induced by the previously reviewed neurobiological mechanisms can be considered as an effectiveness of the olfactory system to capture the complex chemical information as a whole or as elements pertaining to the whole. Indeed, in both mammals and insects, these perceptual interactions are the basis of configural and elemental processing of mixtures of odorants, which may lead to the perception of mixtures as odor objects (configurations) or not. This section of our review focuses on the results that support the notion of odor objects perception.

THE LIMIT IN ODOR MIXTURES ANALYSIS

A key finding supporting the odor object theory is the number of odorants that can be discriminated and identified within an odorants' mixture. This is most likely one of the most investigated question in the human perceptual analysis of odor mixtures (Laing and Francis, 1989; Laska and Hudson, 1992; Jinks and Laing, 1999a,b; Laing and Jinks, 2001). The resolution of this central question should give cues about odorants (or odors) that primarily contribute to the global mixture's percept. A series of studies have shown that humans are hardly able to identify more than three odorants in a mixture that contains up to eight odorants (Laing and Francis, 1989; Laing and Livermore, 1992). This limitation is not a function of the stimulus features. Indeed, untrained subjects cannot correctly identify more than four familiar odors in a mixture containing up to eight odorants (Livermore and Laing, 1998b). Trained subjects reach the same odor identification limit when submitted to mixtures of familiar odors issued from a complex composition designed to evoke real odor sources (e.g., lavender, cheese; Livermore and Laing, 1998a). Cognitive factors play a minor role in the human in-mixture odor identification limit. Focusing subjects' attention on a specific quality to be identified in a mixture containing up to six odorants does not increase the identification rate compared to the standard identification task, in which all odors have to be identified (Laing and Glemarec, 1992). Moreover, training or expertise does not enhance the identification performance since only three or four components of a mixture containing up to five odorants can be correctly identified by either a trained panel or an expert panel (Livermore and Laing, 1996).

Considering these results, the group of D. G. Laing concluded that the human limit of identification of in-mixture odors may be imposed physiologically or by processing constraints. Even in binary mixtures, there might be a loss of the odorant's major characteristic because of inhibitory interactions within the olfactory processing pathway, especially in the OB as reviewed above, or by a limit in working memory, which likely impairs identification. Similar findings were reported in animal studies. Adult rats have difficulty identifying components within mixtures with more than three or four components (Staubli et al., 1987), but many odorants in a mixture can be more readily identified by honeybees (e.g., Reinhard et al., 2010). The interpretation of this compilation of more than 10 years of research appears to be in line with the hypothesis of configural functioning of olfaction, which is analogous to that for facial and object recognition (Jinks and Laing, 2001).

THE CONCEPT OF ODOR OBJECTS

Odor object recognition would allow for the sense of smell to perform feature extraction and object synthesis that lead to the elaboration of a stable, background-detached representation of complex signals. Due to interactions within the olfactory processing pathway, a stereotyped map could be elaborated; this map, where odor identity can be represented in spatiotemporal patterns, may be specific to a given complex stimulus and contain information about the elements of the mixture and likely about their association. The unique spatial and temporal signature could be recognized in the brain as an entity against a background of other odors and identified as an odor object (Margot, 2009). To perform this complex task, the brain could rely on rapid and specific cortical adaptation to background odors and recognition of bulbar activation patterns (Stevenson and Wilson, 2007; Frank et al., 2010). When a stimulus activates the olfactory system, the activation pattern produced at the OB level, and further processed in cortical areas, would be compared to stored ones (for details about the processing mechanisms see the previous sections on interactions at the periphery and interactions at higher levels). If there is a good match, we consciously experience a discrete odor that is distinct from the background and discriminable from other odors (Stevenson and Wilson, 2007). If there is no match between the bulbar incoming pattern and a stored one, the novel pattern may be rapidly acquired (Stevenson and Wilson, 2007). Even if alternative definitions of odor objects have been proposed (Yeshurun and Sobel, 2010), suggesting a critical role of hedonic features, the most commonly accepted definition relies on the integration of a specific blend of volatile molecules that can be separated from the surrounding clutter of volatiles to stand out as an entity reflecting a putatively unidentified specific source (e.g., a melon's odor in the market).

The principle of a unique spatial and temporal signature for complex odor stimuli, which accounts for odor object perception, is in line with configural processing of odorants' mixtures. Following Rescorla's unique-cue theory (Rescorla, 1972, 1973; Rescorla et al., 1985), an odor mixture can carry, beside the elements, another stimulus that is unique to the combination of those elements. In other words an AB binary mixture may be conceptualized as being composed of the individual A and B elements as well as a separate stimulus unique to the AB combination, usually noted U (unique-cue; **Figure 1A**). However there is an unresolved debate in the literature regarding the unique-cue theory and its consequences in complex stimuli configural learning experiments (Brandon et al., 1998; Harris, 2006). Indeed, from Rescorla's point of view, in a conditioning paradigm one can learn about the separate elements A and B but also U, and the associative strength of U is then equal to the sum of the strengths of the elements. The unique-cue stimulus is thought to occur at the level of memory representation rather than that of perceptual representation or spontaneous processing (Rescorla et al., 1985). Adopting a different point of view, Pearce's configural approach (Pearce, 1987, 1994) proposes that the unique stimulus, U, which is specific to the mixture, is represented as a configural pattern whose elements are integrated prior to any learning. Whether Rescorla's or Pearce's view of configural learning better accounts for experimental results is not resolved yet (Dreumont-Boudreau et al., 2006).

There are several lines of evidence showing that animals are able to perform configural processing of odor mixtures and thus differentiate between mixtures and their constituting monomolecular odors (insects: Chandra and Smith, 1998; Lei and Vickers, 2008; Riffell et al., 2009; Deisig et al., 2010; van Wijk et al., 2010; Riffell, 2012; Szyszka et al., 2012; aquatic animals: Derby et al., 1996; Valentincic et al., 2000; Tabor et al., 2004; mammals: Staubli et al., 1987; Kay et al., 2003; Wiltrout et al., 2003; Dreumont-Boudreau et al., 2006). This seems to be true even early in life. For instance, a binary mixture of ethyl isobutyrate and ethyl maltol is configurally processed, at least in part, by newborn rabbits. For the pups, this mixture spontaneously evokes an odor that is different from the one of its constituting odorants and provokes very contrasted behavior in a conditioning paradigm using the mammary pheromone (Coureaud et al., 2008, 2009, 2010, 2011; **Figure 2**). Similar results were obtained with a more complex mixture of six odorants (RC mixture; Sinding et al., 2013).

These results from animal studies demonstrate the possibility of specific encoding for odor mixtures compared to their constituting elements. However, it is worth noting that the nature of stimulus representation is inferred from experiments examining how the conditioned response to one odorant or a mixture of two or more odorants generalizes to another single odorant or mixture (Harris, 2006). As a consequence, whether the mixture

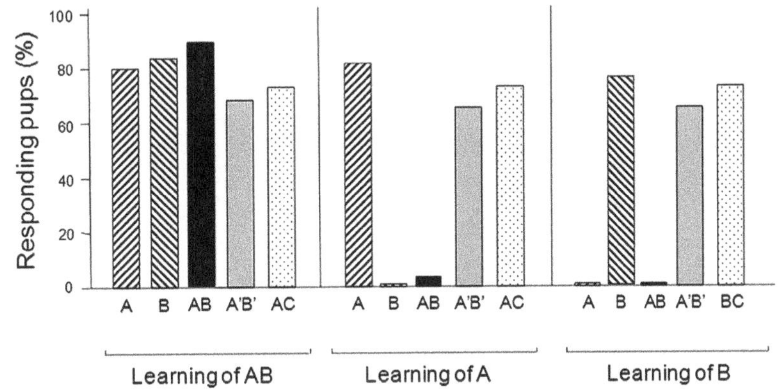

FIGURE 2 | Proportions (%) of 2- or 3-day-old newborn rabbits responding behaviorally (sucking response) to the odorant A (ethyl isobutyrate), the odorant B (ethyl maltol), their AB or A'B' mixtures (respectively, at a ratio of 30/70 and 68/32 of the two components), and the AC mixture (C: guaïacol; ratio 50/50) after a single conditioning to the AB mixture or to one of its components. The results show that after conditioning to AB, the pups respond both to the odorants and the different mixtures. Therefore they perceive the elements A and B during the learning episode. However, after conditioning to odorant A or B, they respond to the conditioned odorant but not to the AB mixture; nevertheless, they respond to the A'B' and AC mixtures. Thus, newborn rabbits perceive the odor of a configuration in the AB mixture in addition to the odors of each odorant, while they perceive only (or mainly) the elements in the A'B' and AC mixtures (adapted from Coureaud et al., 2008, 2009, 2011).

configuration is reconcilable with odor object encoding is not straightforward in animal studies. One way to circumvent this issue is to address the question in parallel in animals and humans. In humans, even if configural processing is difficult to demonstrate, it is advantageously possible to assess whether an odor mixture has a different quality from its single odorants (Livermore and Laing, 1998a; Jinks and Laing, 2001; Bott and Chambers, 2006; Weiss et al., 2012; Chambers and Koppel, 2013). Following an animal/human parallel approach, we have shown that the binary mixture of ethyl isobutyrate and ethyl maltol used in rabbit pups (Coureaud et al., 2008, 2009, 2011) evokes, in human subjects, a more typical odor of pineapple (Le Berre et al., 2008b; Barkat et al., 2012) and is more frequently identified as a pineapple odor (Le Berre et al., 2010) compared to the single odorants (**Figure 3**). Similar results were obtained with the RC mixture of six components, which is configurally perceived by newborn rabbits and specifically evokes a red cordial odor in human adults (Le Berre et al., 2008b; Sinding et al., 2013). These findings, which resulted from the combined data obtained in rabbit pups and human adults, support the idea that mixtures of odorants can be perceived as odor objects in the sense that they can be configurally processed and can evoke new percepts, different from those of the elements, and which could be attributed to unique sources (e.g., pineapple or red cordial).

THE CRITICAL IMPACT OF STIMULUS COMPOSITION

Natural chemical signals frequently undergo concentration changes that produce differences in both the level and pattern of activation of ORs. This variability makes the processing of complex stimuli even more difficult, since the olfactory system must extract perceptual constancy from inconstant input (Gottfried, 2010). It has been argued that complex stimuli recognition might be concentration-invariant and mostly results from ratio-information extraction (Cleland et al., 2007). For instance, rats can discriminate binary odor mixtures according to the molar ratios of their components, which further ensures mixture odor recognition at higher or lower concentrations (Uchida and Mainen, 2008). The ratio of odorants in binary odor mixtures was also found to be the driving factor for odor processing and perception in insects (e.g., Clifford and Riffell, 2013) and in catfish (Valentincic et al., 2000). In rats, a binary mixture of the same two odorants can be processed elementally, configurally, or induce overshadowing (Kay et al., 2003; McNamara et al., 2007). The impact of mixed odorants ratios was clearly observed at the OSN level in rats (Chaput et al., 2012). In humans, psychophysical studies have clearly shown that odorants' ratio and, more precisely, odorants' intensity proportions in a heterogeneous binary mixture, largely determine the odor quality perception (Olsson, 1994, 1998). Supporting these findings, data obtained in both rabbit pups and human adults demonstrate the influence of in-mixture odorant ratios on processing and perception. In rabbit pups, while a 30/70 ratio of ethyl isobutyrate and ethyl maltol induced the configural processing of the mixture, a reversed ratio (68/32) induced the elemental processing of this mixture (Coureaud et al., 2011; **Figure 2**). In human adults, a barely detectable variation of one odorant concentration in the same mixture (slight variation the ratio of the odorants), influenced its perception and particularly decreased its typicality toward pineapple (Le Berre et al., 2008a). A similar influence of the odorants' proportions was observed with the more complex six-odorant RC mixture since a modification of the concentration ratio resulted in a significant shift in odor quality, which depended on the extent of the proportion modification (Sinding et al., 2013, 2014). Therefore, the odorant concentration ratio in a mixture is clearly a key factor that can drive the configural versus elemental perception of the mixture.

The chemical nature, or the odor quality, of the mixed odorants is another key factor of mixture processing (Kay et al., 2003, 2005). Indeed, it is well-established from human studies dealing with food aroma analyses that there are key compounds in the

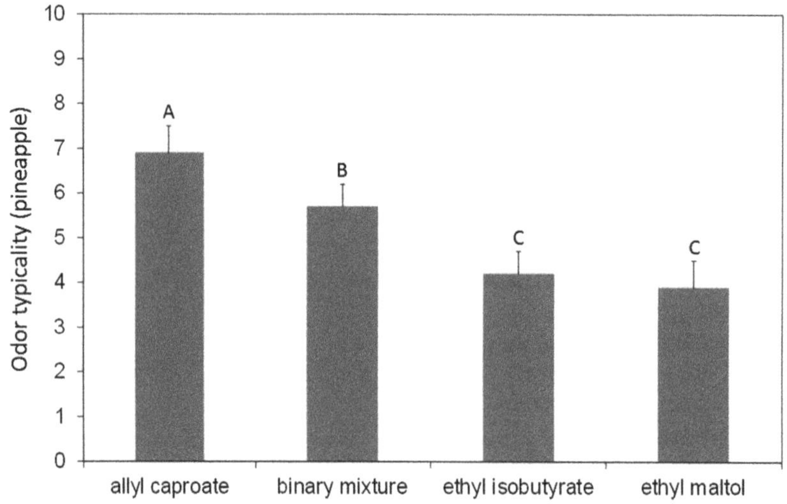

FIGURE 3 | Mean typicality ratings (gray bars) of the term pineapple obtained with a group of 20 untrained subjects for a binary mixture of ethyl isobutyrate and ethyl maltol, each single odorant and a control odorant (allyl caproate carrying a typical pineapple odor). The error bars represent the standard error of the mean. The same letters indicate that the means were not different at a significance level of 5%. The results indicated that the binary mixture carried a pineapple odor that was significantly less present in the single odorants. This finding supports the idea that the odor quality of the mixture is different from those of its components (adapted from Le Berre et al., 2008b).

complex chemical mixture of volatiles responsible for a given food aroma (e.g., Escudero et al., 2004; Falcao et al., 2012). Studies in animals have also demonstrated that certain odorants in mixtures can be more readily identifiable than others (Staubli et al., 1987; Laska and Hudson, 1993; Kay et al., 2005; Reinhard et al., 2010). Therefore these odorants can contribute more strongly to the overall perceptual quality of the whole odor mixture. For instance, in rats, the identity of the odorant removed from a complex 10-component mixture affected the discrimination between the 10-odorant mixture and the nine-odorant sub-mixtures. Nevertheless, rats had difficulty discriminating the whole mixture from the same mixture with one component missing. These results suggest that the missing component was most often "filled-in" by the olfactory system to promote perceptual stability (Barnes et al., 2008; Chen et al., 2011; Chapuis and Wilson, 2012; Lovitz et al., 2012). In contrast, rats could reliably discriminate mixtures containing even small traces of contaminants from unadulterated complex mixtures; indeed, the replacement of an odorant by another was easily detected, and in a concentration-dependent manner (Wilson and Sullivan, 2011; Lovitz et al., 2012). Data obtained in newborn rabbits have shown that once conditioned to one of the odorants, whatever the odorant, animals cannot generalize their behavioral response to a six-odorant RC mixture configurally processed. This result supports the idea that the two stimuli are discriminated. Nevertheless, animals can generalize their response to the same mixture in which one odorant is missing (five-component mixture), regardless of the odorant (Sinding et al., 2013). These last results suggest that each odorant is a key odorant for rabbit pups. In contrast, data obtained using the same mixture in human subjects have shown that the red cordial odor quality carried by this six-odorant RC mixture is significantly different from the odor quality of some, but not all, sub-mixtures in which one odorant was missing (Sinding et al., 2013). Therefore, in human adults, many components would contribute more strongly to the overall perceptual quality of the odor mixture than do others. Even at subthreshold level, many odorants can modify the perception and/or the processing of odor mixtures (Atanasova et al., 2005b; Pineau et al., 2009; Lytra et al., 2012; Hummel et al., 2013).

Interestingly, it has been recently reported that different mixtures made of 30 equally intense, non-overlapping components that span the physicochemical space of odorants, give rise to a similar odor quality for humans. This finding lead the author to term such percept as an "olfactory white" (similar to a white color or "white noise"; Weiss et al., 2012). The need to equilibrate each component intensity in this study is reconcilable with the key role of the mixture ratio; however, the absence of a link between a single odorant's odor quality and the mixture's odor is at odd with the concept of key odorants in the perception of these specific mixtures. Even if such specific mixtures would be unlikely in ecological conditions, their processing is consistent with the concept of odor objects and might be of significant value as a model to decipher the mechanisms of odor mixture perception.

THE IMPORTANCE OF INDIVIDUAL FACTORS

Individuals from the same species do not necessarily perceive the same odor in a particular odorant, and more generally, they do not present the same sensibility to odor cues (Amoore, 1967; Frumin et al., 2013). This inter-individual variability may result from many factors, e.g., genetic and/or anatomical differences; health status; ecological constraints; effects of experience; age and the abilities associated with the specific needs that characterize the successive stages of development; and semantic knowledge (in humans). For example, anosmia to certain odorants is shared between identical twins and transmitted to offspring (Wysocki et al., 1977; Wysocki and Beauchamp, 1984). Conversely, some individuals have a better sensitivity for certain odorants compared to other individuals (Keller et al., 2007; Menashe et al., 2007; Mainland et al., 2014). In this context, one may hypothesize that a contrasted sensitivity toward the components of a mixture can affect the ability to perceive odorants in mixtures and therefore directly influence the elemental vs. configural perception of the mixture. One may suggest that the ratio of the component thresholds drives the perception of the mixture by the subjects, as occurs with the ratio of concentrations. Such questions remain to be explored in detail, but preliminary results in human adults indicate that some subjects perceive the pineapple AB mixture in a more robust configural way than do others; curiously, the more the subjects have a configural perception of AB, the lower their detection thresholds of the components (Sinding, 2012; Sinding et al., in preparation).

Regarding developmental aspects, one may consider that due to the maturation of the sensory systems and brain and the change in ecological niches encountered by the organism over the development, the processing of odor mixtures may also be modified over time. In particular, around birth, the urgent need for neonates to acquire knowledge about the novel, aerial environment, could result in higher elemental abilities than in adults. Later in life, increased experience with a large variety of more or less complex odors and repeated exposure to some of the complex odors could promote their encoding as odor objects. While some results are in line with this developmental hypothesis (Sinding et al., 2013), others show that the perception of olfactory configuration is already present in young animals, and that neonate and adult mammals perceive certain mixtures of various chemical complexity in a comparable way (Coureaud et al., 2008, 2009, 2011; Sinding et al., 2013). This is consistent with the chemical complexity of early life environments (perinatal niches) from which organisms must rapidly extract salient information despite their immaturity, only relative (see the section dedicated to behavioral aspects below).

THE IMPACT OF LEARNING

In addition to the previously discussed factors that clearly influence odor mixture processing, it is crucial to emphasize that the perception of odor mixtures is under cognitive control and that learning could shape this perception, but depending on the mixture. Perceptual learning, which contributes to the improvement of an organism's ability to extract information from the environment (Gibson, 1969; Rabin et al., 1989), can affect the way in which a mixture of odorants is processed. In humans, odor-odor perceptual learning has been described and is likely comparable to odor-taste learning (Wilson and Stevenson, 2003a; Case et al., 2004; Stevenson et al., 2007). For instance, when two odorants were repeatedly experienced in a binary mixture, each odorant's odor could acquire the perceptual quality of the other. This was demonstrated in a study in which an odorant, initially perceived with a cherry odor, smelled smokier after having been repeatedly experienced in mixture with guaiacol, another odorant perceived with a smoky odor. Furthermore, guaiacol smelled more like cherry after the co-exposure (Stevenson, 2001a). Odor-odor learning is not just stimulus -or quality- specific but is also a direct consequence of the learning procedure (Stevenson, 2001a). Odors experienced in a mixture were judged to be more alike than were odors smelled an equal number of times but out of mixture. This exchange of perceptual qualities between mixed odorants is related to how similar the elements were judged (Stevenson, 2001a). These results support the idea that the representation of odor qualities can combine to form new configurations that carry their own odors. These results also indicate that cognitive processes are engaged to decrease the chemical complexity of the environment by building experience-dependent perceptual associations (Wilson and Stevenson, 2003a).

Results obtained in animal studies also demonstrate the impact of conditioning on odor mixture processing (Livermore et al., 1997; Valentincic et al., 2000; Gerber et al., 2011). For instance, one conditioning experience to the previously mentioned mixture of ethyl isobutyrate and ethyl maltol (which smells like pineapple to human adults) allowed rabbit pups to generalize their response to both odorants, something they cannot do when tested with the mixture after single conditioning to one odorant only (Coureaud et al., 2008, 2009; **Figure 2**). However, repeated conditioning to this binary mixture led to a drastic decrease of generalization and the pups became more responsive to the mixture than to the elements. This result suggests an improved configural perception of the mixture. Conversely, after repeated conditioning to a single component, the pups responded to the mixture, which suggests improved elemental perception. Interestingly, these perceptual changes greatly depend on the mixture and its components. Indeed, with a mixture of ethyl isobutyrate and guaïacol, the same paradigm of repeated conditioning had no consequence on the perception, and the mixture remained always elementally perceived (Sinding et al., 2011). These results suggest that the initial status of the mixture, either purely elementally processed or akin to configural perception (i.e., weak configural; **Figure 1A**), likely plays a critical role in further cognitive processing.

Perceptual experience can also be acquired by passive exposure to odors (Rabin, 1988). When the olfactory environment of rats was enriched, their ability to discriminate odorants in binary mixtures increased (regardless of the odorant to which the rat was exposed during the enrichment period; Mandairon et al., 2006b,c). This effect was linked to neurogenesis in the rat OB (Mandairon et al., 2006a). In human adults, the mixture of ethyl isobutyrate and ethyl maltol was less configurally processed by a group of subjects after passive exposure to the single elements compared to non-exposed subjects. Perceptual learning would then favor the elemental perception of the mixture (Le Berre et al., 2008b).

Expertise is also a cognitive factor that can influence odor mixture perception. In a typicality rating task, experts in oenology rated the pineapple typicality of the ethyl isobutyrate and ethyl maltol mixture as equivalent to that of ethyl isobutyrate, while naïve participants rated this typicality as significantly higher compared to both elements perceived out of the mixture (Barkat et al., 2012). Thus, experts would be less sensitive to the configuration induced by the mixture. One could hypothesize that due to their perceptual expertise acquired through training to single odors, experts may be more inclined to focus on the elements' odor in the mixture, which may make them more efficient in elemental processing. The ability to focus on the elements may be linked to their familiarity with the odorants, insomuch that the identification ability increases when the target is familiar (Rabin, 1988; Rabin et al., 1989). In this regard, identifying a familiar target mixed with a familiar contaminant was found to be easy (87% correct identification), while finding an unfamiliar target mixed with an unfamiliar contaminant was much more difficult (58% correct identification; Rabin et al., 1989). Nevertheless, learning, considered as perceptual training in experts, increases the absolute ability to identify odors in low but not highly complex mixtures. Indeed experts were more proficient than non-experts at discriminating and identifying odors in binary and ternary mixtures; for quaternary mixtures the correct identification rate fell below 20%, regardless of the expertise level (Livermore and Laing, 1996).

Expertise can also rely on semantic knowledge (Rabin, 1988; de Wijk and Cain, 1994; Stevenson, 2001b), which is another cognitive factor that influences odor mixture processing in humans. In a dedicated experiment assessing the impact of semantic learning on the perception of odor mixtures, it was found that exposure to the mixture target odor label (semantic learning) facilitated the perception of the configural odor of blending mixtures (Le Berre et al., 2010). Thus, verbal labels could have provided perceptually expected and reliable information regarding the frame of reference for odors (Herz and von Clef, 2001; Rouby et al., 2005), which may result in the top-down facilitation of odor recognition. A similar cognitive top-down effect, even if not directly related to semantic knowledge, could explain the results obtained in a study exploring the influence of odor context on odor mixture perception (Arao et al., 2012). Using colors that are congruent with the odor of each element of a binary mixture, it has been shown that participants judged the odor of the element congruent with the color to be more dominant in the mixture. The visual cue could have directed the participants' attention toward the color-congruent odor, which then led to an enhancement of its perceptual representation within the mixture. In line with attentional processes, perceptual processing strategies may also modify odor mixture perception. The same blending mixture was less configurally processed by a group of naïve subjects engaged in an analytical task compared to a group of subjects engaged in a configural task (Le Berre et al., 2008b).

Taken together, these results demonstrate that odor mixture perception can be modulated by cognitive and/or attentional factors. According to the high complexity of the environment, it is likely that learning and attention can fine-tune the perception by highlighting the meaningful elemental features or configural shapes from the background (Wilson and Stevenson, 2003b).

IMPLICATIONS OF ODOR MIXTURE PROCESSING ON BEHAVIOR

In the real life situation, odors are important vectors of information that elicit behavioral decisions from animals in their natural environment. For instance, odors are involved in the interaction between conspecifics, with competitors and predators, and in the selection of habitats, preys and food. Odors are never perceived alone, but among other odors, and chemical mixtures are usually the global stimuli that drive chemically mediated patterns of animal behaviors. Therefore, animals have no choice but to simplify the surrounding amount of information, which constantly varies over time. They must adapt to the chemical complexity of the environment by extracting information from this mass of molecules, especially in mixtures, by discriminating and assigning meaning to some of them and responding in a way adapted to their needs.

One strategy to reduce this complexity is to respond to certain odorants among others present in the same mixture, i.e., to focus on elements triggering behavioral responsiveness by themselves. This occurs when organisms respond to key odorants in complex odorous substrates, e.g., to components that mainly contribute to the flavor of food (Grosch, 2001; Bult et al., 2002; Reinhard et al., 2010); the odor of familiar/unfamiliar conspecifics (Breed and Julian, 1992); or more generally to pheromones (single odorants or associations of key odorants), which are sometimes carried in complex biological fluids or secretions (Schaal, 2010; Martin et al., 2013). A second strategy consists of attributing additional or unique information to the odorants forming a mixture as a whole, which carries a behavioral value that is distinct from the individual value of each component, i.e., to perceive the mixture as a single meaningful object (see previous section on odor objects and configural processing of odorants in mixture). This configural strategy is functional both in aquatic and terrestrial organisms. For instance, after food-rewarded exposures, catfish differentially modify their swimming activity in response to mixtures of amino-acids and to their elements (Valentincic et al., 2000, 2011). Spiny lobsters display food searching and exploration/avoidance responses that illustrate their ability to differentially process and perceive mixtures of odorants and odorants themselves (Fine-Levy et al., 1989; Lynn et al., 1994; Livermore et al., 1997). In a double-choice test, a mollusk, the terrestrial slug, displays a strong aversion to a binary mixture while the odor of each component remains strongly attractive (Hopfield and Gelperin, 1989). In insects, the configural perception of odor mixtures is involved in flower-foraging behaviors. For example, when exposed to flower-scents containing dozens of components, bees perceive certain mixtures of volatile molecular constituents as configurations, an ability that certainly contributes to the discrimination of flowers and expression of preferences for those offering higher quality or quantity of nectar (Deisig et al., 2001; Wright et al., 2009). In rats, the configural perception of odor mixtures influences their spatial performance, localization of reward, and digging activity related to foraging (Staubli et al., 1987; Linster and Smith, 1999). In dogs, and especially military dogs, the discrimination between complex mixtures of volatiles and their elements may be critical in the detection of explosives (Lazarowski and Dorman, 2014). In humans, odor mixture processing may support the categorization of food while simultaneously keeping the ability to differentiate between different products that belong to the same category due to the perception of inconstant elements in addition to invariant configurations (Gottfried, 2009).

The chemical environment is complex not only for adult organisms but also for young, neonates, fetuses, and embryos, even if it is more limited during earlier periods of development (e.g., when the organism is developing in the maternal body, nests, or eggs). Indeed, maternal fluids such as amniotic fluid, colostrum, or milk in mammals, and more generally the maternal body itself, generate or carry a large number of odorants (Antoshechkin et al., 1989; Schaal, 2010). Very young organisms have an urgent need to respond to some of these odors to rapidly interact with the mother; to localize the nipples and suck; and to expand their knowledge about the surroundings. Interestingly, although this remains to be more generally investigated, both elemental and configural processing appear functional early in life. Thus, newborn rabbits respond to the monomolecular mammary pheromone (2-methylbut-2-enal) carried in milk among 150 other odorants (Coureaud, 2001; Schaal et al., 2003; Coureaud et al., 2010), and they elementally process "artificial" mixtures containing up to six components. They are also able to perceive configurations in some binary and senary mixtures (Coureaud et al., 2008, 2010, 2011; Sinding et al., 2011, 2013). As in adults, the ability of very young organisms to process odor mixtures both configurally or elementally may contribute to decision making and to the discrimination between a peculiar conspecific, the mother, which carries peculiar odor elements or definite configurations, and another category of conspecifics, the lactating females, which emit the same or at least overlapping elements and configurations (Coureaud et al., 2006, 2011; Logan et al., 2012).

IMPLICATIONS OF ODOR MIXTURES PROCESSING IN INDIVIDUALS WITH MOOD DISORDERS

Olfactory dysfunction may be a prodrome of neurodegenerative diseases such as Alzheimer's and Parkinson's disease (Albers et al., 2006; Djordjevic et al., 2008). Because of the partial overlap between the brain structures involved in affective disorders, olfaction and emotion, olfactory impairments can be observed in several psychiatric diseases: major depression (Pause et al., 2001; Atanasova et al., 2010), seasonal affective disorder (Postolache et al., 1999), anorexia nervosa (Kopala et al., 1995), psychoses (Moberg and Turetsky, 2003), and obsessive compulsive disorder (Hermesh et al., 1999). These impairments affect different aspects of olfactory function (i.e., detection threshold, odor identification, discrimination, memory, intensity, familiarity, and pleasantness) and depend on the nature and extent of psychiatric and neurological involvement.

The majority of olfactory studies and mood disorders have focused on the perception of single odorants. To date, only a few studies have investigated olfactory perception in major depression using odor mixtures (Atanasova et al., 2010; Atanasova, 2012; Naudin et al., 2012). However, studies using odor mixtures are of specific interest because complex olfactory stimuli reflect daily life situations, which is important in the study of anhedonia (failure to gain pleasure from normal pleasant experiences). Anhedonia is considered as a core symptom of major depression in an objective way. Using binary mixtures of both pleasant (vanillin) and unpleasant (butyric acid) odorants at three different iso-intense concentrations, it has been shown that depressed patients perceived the majority of odor mixtures (67%) as significantly less pleasant compared to healthy subjects (Atanasova et al., 2010; Atanasova, 2012). Depressed subjects also had low performance in correctly identifying the odor of the odorants within the binary iso-intense mixture, and they more readily perceived the unpleasant compound compared to control subjects. The perception of a binary odor mixture depends on the subjects' psychological state and depressed level; a higher depression score is associated to a better perception of the unpleasant stimulus and to a lesser perception of the pleasant stimulus within a binary iso-intense mixture (Atanasova et al., 2010). These observations were confirmed and generalized in a study using an iso-intense mixture of another pleasant (2-phenylethanol) and unpleasant (isovaleric acid) odorant (Naudin et al., 2012). Since the same results were obtained in patients during a depressive episode and in remission, the authors suggested that these olfactory impairments may constitute potential trait markers of depression. These results could be explained by the cognitive bias for emotionally negative stimuli observed in depression that could persist in the remitted state (Bhalla et al., 2006).

All of the observations revealed that anhedonia can be advantageously observed in depressed patients at the olfactory level with complex olfactory stimuli. They also suggest that the loss of food cravings often described in depression could be partly explained by a modification in olfactory perception, ending in a better perception of unpleasant sensory components in food. This finding emphasizes the importance of using complex mixtures of odorants, which are more ecologically relevant stimuli, to better understand the modulation of olfactory perception in mood disorders. Future psychophysical, neurophysiological, and neuroimaging investigations are needed in this field to increase our knowledge of the etiology of the diseases and to develop the appropriate tools to better care for patients with affective disorders.

IMPLICATIONS OF ODOR MIXTURES PROCESSING IN ODOR STIMULI FORMULATION

Odors (orthonasal smell and retronasal aroma) are key perceptual characteristics to formulate in foods and in home and personal care products. It is the first chemical sense involved when a consumer is using such a product. Consumers base their opinion on the quality of a product, i.e., whether they like it and whether it is fulfilling its intended function, based partly (for food products) or completely (for perfumes) on the olfactory experience. Therefore, formulating the right olfactory experience cannot be taken lightly. Most food and beverage companies employ the services of flavor companies to create the flavors or aromas that will enter the formulation of the end product. Indeed, food and beverage companies may require flavors for their new products or for compensating changes in the formulation of their existing products.

Focusing on olfactory perception, which is largely involved in flavor (Hornung and Enns, 1989; Thomas-Danguin, 2009), we explained in the previous sections of this review that odors arise from perceptual representations of mixtures of odorants, whose construction is far from being fully understood and remains mostly impossible to predict on the basis of chemical composition. Within flavor houses, flavor formulation is thus performed by specially trained scientists called flavorists, who have empirical knowledge about the perception of chemicals in mixtures. They know a large variety of odorous raw materials but also specific mixtures' recipes to produce specific flavors and continuously create new ones. Usually, they follow a brief delivered by the client. This brief must specify the direction of flavor to be formulated (e.g., strawberry), the type of product into which the new flavor will be incorporated in (e.g., dairy product), and other requirements (e.g., all natural). It is then the role of the flavorist to use his/her expertise with the chemical ingredients at his/her disposal and his/her experience to formulate a flavor mixture that match the client's requirements. The flavor house may also seek the assistance of an application specialist to ensure that the newly formulated flavor will deliver its expected quality in the application for which it is intended. Indeed, when formulated in a complex matrix, such as a food matrix (e.g., a chocolate bar), interactions with the different components of the matrix can influence the volatility of the odorants within the mixture and, consequently, the whole headspace mixture composition (Guichard, 2002).

In perfume composition, creation also relies on empirical knowledge. For instance, it is known that adding sulfur components, which are often unpleasant (e.g., cat urine odor), could give a lift to a fruity component in a complex mixture of odorants evoking a tropical fruit odor. Indeed, we have presented several examples of the impact of an unpleasant odor mixed with a pleasant one. Synergistic effects are also extensively used in perfume design. For instance, fatty aldehydes are known to enhance many floral odors at low concentrations, even if their own odor is very different from the target one. These synthetic odorants have been used in floral-aldehydic perfumes such as the famous Chanel no.5 created by Ernest Beaux for the house of Chanel in 1921 (Chastrette, 1995). Perfume chords are also very well empirically used in this industry. The concept of perfume chords is reconcilable with configural processing of odor mixtures. Indeed, chords usually rely on mixtures of three or four odors (which are sometimes linked to pure chemicals) that are included in larger formulae. This is made possible by perfumers after a huge amount of trials following the artist's intuition (Chastrette, 1995). Moreover, as explained by the famous perfumer Edmond Roudnitska (quoted by Chastrette, 1995), a perfume composition includes not only one chord but an unknown number that are not smelled one after the other but can overlap, be enhanced, or be canceled. Therefore, the perceptual interactions that result from smelling a perfume are likely the playground of the artist and allowed him to create esthetic odor objects.

Besides the complexity of formulating a flavor or a perfume based on product properties, top-down influences also play a role in the way consumers perceive a product. Indeed, packaging (color, shape) and the type of claim made on the product can influence the consumer's perception of the product (e.g., Gatti et al., 2014). Finally, the above examples demonstrate the empirical knowledge and methods used in the formulation of aromas and fragrances but also describe how recent insights into odor processing and perception impact the development of new products.

CONCLUSION

The study of odor mixtures is an original window to investigate olfactory processes in a manner that may be more relevant to ecological perceptual contexts, which is crucial to understanding how organisms, including humans, represent and adapt to their chemical complex environment. It is also an original path to identify, characterize and further treat adaptation disorders in humans.

However, it is obvious that the scientific knowledge available on odor mixtures' perception, even the simplest ones with only two odorants, is far from being up to empirical knowledge. Yet, a better understanding of the underlying biological processes involved when organisms manage to identify an odor object based on hundreds of chemicals in a few milliseconds would likely impact many scientific fields. Indeed, deciphering what odors (elements and/or configurations) are perceived in a mixture may contribute to the efficiency of flavor analysis, the identification of key components of food acceptance or disliking, and the elaboration of food flavors and perfumes. Moreover, extending our investigations on the odor processing of natural mixtures would shed light on the ability of organisms, including humans, to code complex information in the olfactory brain and how, through development, learning, or evolution, the resulting odors are stored as perceptual objects and reused by individuals.

It appears from this review that the appropriate description of the stimulus representations is likely the most critical factor in odor mixture perception. This is fundamental and should not be overlooked since a mixture is not a simple addition of each of its component and because it is the starting point of every following process. This requires for a large part to clearly pinpoint the peripheral spatiotemporal coding processes of odorants in mixtures, which is the only way to decipher the role of mixture composition and to predict accurately odor perception on the basis of chemical composition. Nevertheless, the incoming information is highly subjected to modulations at all stages of integration. If we highlighted in this review that the processing is contrasted at each stage, the specific role of these distinct stages remains largely to be discovered. To take up these research challenges, one should favor a systemic approach that would combine several investigation levels thus gathering cellular, neurobiological and psychological aspects both in human and other animal species. That was the guideline of this review to put together the results obtained in various models in order to underline similitude and differences in perception mechanisms. Indeed multidisciplinary studies may help to tackle specific questions regarding both odor mixture coding and perception, plasticity of perception and behavioral consequences, and thus would likely bring the field forward.

ACKNOWLEDGMENTS

We would like to acknowledge support from the National Institute for Agricultural Research (INRA); the National Center for Scientific Research (CNRS); the Burgundy Regional council; the EU European Regional Development Fund (FEDER); the French National Research Agency (ANR; in particular the JC/JC ANR MEMOLAP program); The University of Burgundy (uB); The European Chemoreception Research Organization (ECRO); The Association for Chemoreception Sciences (AChemS); and The French Ministry of Higher Education and Research (MESR).

REFERENCES

Abraham, N. M., Egger, V., Shimshek, D. R., Renden, R., Fukunaga, I., Sprengel, R., et al. (2010). Synaptic inhibition in the olfactory bulb accelerates odor discrimination in mice. *Neuron* 65, 399–411. doi: 10.1016/j.neuron.2010.01.009

Ache, B. (1989). "Central and peripheral bases for mixture suppression in olfaction: a crustacean model," in *Perception of Complex Smells and Tastes*, eds D. G. Laing, W. S. Cain, R. L. McBride, and B. W. Ache (Sidney: Academic Press), 101–114.

Ache, B. W., and Young, J. M. (2005). Olfaction: diverse species, conserved principles. *Neuron* 48, 417–430. doi: 10.1016/j.neuron.2005.10.022

Ache, B. W., Gleeson, R. A., and Thompson, H. A. (1988). Mechanisms for mixture suppression in olfactory receptors of the spiny lobster. *Chem. Senses* 13, 425–434. doi: 10.1093/chemse/13.3.425

Akers, R. P., and Getz, W. M. (1993). Response of olfactory receptor neurons in honeybees to odorants and their binary mixtures. *J. Comp. Physiol. A* 173, 169–185. doi: 10.1007/BF00192976

Albers, M. W., Tabert, M. H., and Devanand, D. P. (2006). Olfactory dysfunction as a predictor of neurodegenerative disease. *Curr. Neurol. Neurosci. Rep.* 6, 379–386. doi: 10.1007/s11910-996-0018-7

Amoore, J. E. (1967). Specific anosmia: a clue to the olfactory code. *Nature* 214, 1095–1098. doi: 10.1038/2141095a0

Anderson, A. K., Christoff, K., Stappen, I., Panitz, D., Ghahremani, D. G., Glover, G., et al. (2003). Dissociated neural representations of intensity and valence in human olfaction. *Nat. Neurosci.* 6, 196–202. doi: 10.1038/nn1001

Antoshechkin, A. G., Golovkin, A. B., Maximova, L. A., and Bakharev, V. A. (1989). Screening of amniotic fluid metabolites by gas chromatography-mass spectrometry. *J. Chromatogr. B Biomed. Sci. Appl.* 489, 353–358. doi: 10.1016/S0378-4347(00)82913-8

Arao, M., Suzuki, M., Katayama, J., and Yagi, A. (2012). An odorant congruent with a colour cue is selectively perceived in an odour mixture. *Perception* 41, 474–482. doi: 10.1068/p7152

Atanasova, B. (2012). Hedonic olfactory perception in depression: relationship between self-evaluation and autonomic response. *Psychology* 3, 959–965. doi: 10.4236/psych.2012.311144

Atanasova, B., El-Hage, W., Chabanet, C., Gaillard, P., Belzung, C., and Camus, V. (2010). Olfactory anhedonia and negative olfactory alliesthesia in depressed patients. *Psychiatry Res.* 176, 190–196. doi: 10.1016/j.psychres.2008.11.016

Atanasova, B., Thomas-Danguin, T., Chabanet, C., Langlois, D., Nicklaus, S., and Etiévant, P. (2005a). Perceptual interactions in odour mixtures: odour quality in binary mixtures of woody and fruity wine odorants. *Chem. Senses* 30, 209–217. doi: 10.1093/chemse/bji016

Atanasova, B., Thomas-Danguin, T., Langlois, D., Nicklaus, S., Chabanet, C., and Etievant, P. (2005b). Perception of wine fruity and woody notes: influence of peri-threshold odorants. *Food Qual. Prefer.* 16, 504–510. doi: 10.1016/j.foodqual.2004.10.004

Barkat, S., Le Berre, E., Coureaud, G., Sicard, G., and Thomas-Danguin, T. (2012). Perceptual blending in odor mixtures depends on the nature of odorants and human olfactory expertise. *Chem. Senses* 37, 159–166. doi: 10.1093/chemse/bjr086

Barnes, D. C., Hofacer, R. D., Zaman, A. R., Rennaker, R. L., and Wilson, D. A. (2008). Olfactory perceptual stability and discrimination. *Nat. Neurosci.* 11, 1378–1380. doi: 10.1038/nn.2217

Bekkers, J. M., and Suzuki, N. (2013). Neurons and circuits for odor processing in the piriform cortex. *Trends Neurosci.* 36, 429–438. doi: 10.1016/j.tins.2013.04.005

Bell, G. A., Laing, D. G., and Panhuber, H. (1987). Odour mixture suppression: evidence for a peripheral mechanism in human and rat. *Brain Res.* 426, 8–18. doi: 10.1016/0006-8993(87)90419-7

Berglund, B. (1974). Quantitative and qualitative analysis of industrial odors with human observers. *Ann. N. Y. Acad. Sci.* 237, 35–51. doi: 10.1111/j.1749-6632.1974.tb49842.x

Berglund, B., and Olsson, M. J. (1993). Odor-intensity interaction in binary mixtures. *J. Exp. Psychol. Hum. Percept. Perform.* 19, 302–314. doi: 10.1037/0096-1523.19.2.302

Berglund, B., Berglund, U., and Lindvall, T. (1976). Psychological processing of odor mixtures. *Psychol. Rev.* 83, 432–441. doi: 10.1037/0033-295X.83.6.432

Berglund, B., Berglund, U., Ekman, G., and Engen, T. (1971). Individual psychophysical functions for 28 odorants. *Percept. Psychophys.* 9, 379–384. doi: 10.3758/BF03212672

Bhalla, R. K., Butters, M. A., Mulsant, B. H., Begley, A. E., Zmuda, M. D., Schoderbek, B., et al. (2006). Persistence of neuropsychologic deficits in the remitted state of late-life depression. *Am. J. Geriatr. Psychiatry* 14, 419–427. doi: 10.1097/01.JGP.0000203130.45421.69

Bott, L., and Chambers, E. (2006). Sensory characteristics of combinations of chemicals potentially associated with beany aroma in foods. *J. Sens. Stud.* 21, 308–321. doi: 10.1111/j.1745-459X.2006.00067.x

Boyle, J. A., Djordjevic, J., Olsson, M. J., Lundstrom, J. N., and Jones-Gotman, M. (2009). The human brain distinguishes between single odorants and binary mixtures. *Cereb. Cortex* 19, 66–71. doi: 10.1093/cercor/bhn058

Brandon, S. E., Vogel, E. H., and Wagner, A. R. (1998). "A componential view of configural cues in generalization and discrimination in Pavlovian conditioning," in *Annual Meeting of the Pavlovian-Society*, Dusseldorf, 67–72.

Breed, M. D., and Julian, G. E. (1992). Do simple rules apply in honey-bee nestmate discrimination? *Nature* 357, 685–686. doi: 10.1038/357685a0

Brodin, M., Laska, M., and Olsson, M. J. (2009). Odor interaction between bourgeonal and its antagonist undecanal. *Chem. Senses* 34, 625–630. doi: 10.1093/chemse/bjp044

Bult, J. H. F., Schifferstein, H. N. J., Roozen, J. P., Boronat, E. D., Voragen, A. G. J., and Kroeze, J. H. A. (2002). Sensory evaluation of character impact components in an apple model mixture. *Chem. Senses* 27, 485–494. doi: 10.1093/chemse/27.6.485

Buonviso, N., and Chaput, M. A. (1990). Response similarity to odors in olfactory bulb output cells presumed to be connected to the same glomerulus: electrophysiological study using simultaneous single-unit recordings. *J. Neurophysiol.* 63, 447–454.

Cain, W. S. (1975). Odor intensity: mixtures and masking. *Chem. Senses Flavor* 1, 339–352. doi: 10.1093/chemse/1.3.339

Cain, W. S., and Drexler, M. (1974). Scope and evaluation of odor counteraction and masking. *Ann. N. Y. Acad. Sci.* 237, 427–439. doi: 10.1111/j.1749-6632.1974.tb49876.x

Caprio, J. (1989). Electro-olfactogram and multiunit olfactory receptor responses to binary and trinary mixtures of amino acids in the channel catfish, Ictalurus punctatus. *J. Gen. Physiol.* 93, 245–262. doi: 10.1085/jgp.93.2.245

Carlsson, M. A., and Hansson, B. S. (2002). Responses in highly selective sensory neurons to blends of pheromone components in the moth Agrotis segetum. *J. Insect Physiol.* 48, 443–451. doi: 10.1016/S0022-1910(02)00065-3

Case, T. I., Stevenson, R. J., and Dempsey, R. A. (2004). Reduced discriminability following perceptual learning with odours. *Perception* 33, 113–119. doi: 10.1068/p5044

Chambers, E., and Koppel, K. (2013). Associations of volatile compounds with sensory aroma and flavor: the complex nature of flavor. *Molecules* 18, 4887–4905. doi: 10.3390/molecules18054887

Chandra, S., and Smith, B. H. (1998). An analysis of synthetic processing of odor mixtures in the honeybee (*Apis mellifera*). *J. Exp. Biol.* 201, 3113–3121.

Chapuis, J., and Wilson, D. A. (2012). Bidirectional plasticity of cortical pattern recognition and behavioral sensory acuity. *Nat. Neurosci.* 15, 155–161. doi: 10.1038/nn.2966

Chaput, M. A., El Mountassir, F., Atanasova, B., Thomas-Danguin, T., Le Bon, A. M., Perrut, A., et al. (2012). Interactions of odorants with olfactory receptors and receptor neurons match the perceptual dynamics observed for woody and fruity odorant mixtures. *Eur. J. Neurosci.* 35, 584–597. doi: 10.1111/j.1460-9568.2011.07976.x

Chastrette, M. (1995). *L'art des parfums. Hachette.* Paris: Hachette.

Chastrette, M. (1997). Trends in structure-odor relationships. *SAR QSAR Environ. Res.* 6, 215–254. doi: 10.1080/10629369708033253

Chastrette, M., Thomas-Danguin, T., and Rallet, E. (1998). Modelling the human olfactory stimulus-response function. *Chem. Senses* 23, 181–196. doi: 10.1093/chemse/23.2.181

Chen, C. F. F., Barnes, D. C., and Wilson, D. A. (2011). Generalized vs. stimulus-specific learned fear differentially modifies stimulus encoding in primary sensory cortex of awake rats. *J. Neurophysiol.* 106, 3136–3144. doi: 10.1152/jn.00721.2011

Chen, T.-W., Lin, B.-J., and Schild, D. (2009). Odor coding by modules of coherent mitral/tufted cells in the vertebrate olfactory bulb. *Proc. Natl. Acad. Sci. U.S.A.* 106, 2401–2406. doi: 10.1073/pnas.0810151106

Chess, A., Simon, I., Cedar, H., and Axel, R. (1994). Allelic inactivation regulates olfactory receptor gene expression. *Cell* 78, 823–834. doi: 10.1016/S0092-8674(94)90562-2

Cleland, T. A., Johnson, B. A., Leon, M., and Linster, C. (2007). Relational representation in the olfactory system. *Proc. Natl. Acad. Sci. U.S.A.* 104, 1953–1958. doi: 10.1073/pnas.0608564104

Clifford, M. R., and Riffell, J. A (2013). Mixture and odorant processing in the olfactory systems of insects: a comparative perspective. *J. Comp. Physiol. A. Neuroethol. Sens. Neural. Behav. Physiol.* 199, 911–928. doi: 10.1007/s00359-013-0818-6

Coureaud, G. (2001). *Olfactory Regulation of Sucking in Newborn Rabbit: Ethological and Chemical Characterization of a Pheromonal Signal.* PhD Thesis, University Paris 13.

Coureaud, G., Charra, R., Datiche, F., Sinding, C., Thomas-Danguin, T., Languille, S., et al. (2010). A pheromone to behave, a pheromone to learn: the rabbit mammary pheromone. *J. Comp. Physiol. A Neuroethol. Sens. Neural Behav. Physiol.* 196, 779–790. doi: 10.1007/s00359-010-0548-y

Coureaud, G., Gibaud, D., Le Berre, E., Schaal, B., and Thomas-Danguin, T. (2011). Proportion of odorants impacts the configural versus elemental perception of a binary blending mixture in newborn rabbits. *Chem. Senses* 36, 693–700. doi: 10.1093/chemse/bjr049

Coureaud, G., Hamdani, Y., Schaal, B., and Thomas-Danguin, T. (2009). Elemental and configural processing of odour mixtures in the newborn rabbit. *J. Exp. Biol.* 212, 2525–2531. doi: 10.1242/jeb.032235

Coureaud, G., Langlois, D., Perrier, G., and Schaal, B. (2006). Convergent changes in the maternal emission and pup reception of the rabbit mammary pheromone. *Chemoecology* 16, 169–174. doi: 10.1007/s00049-006-0345-9

Coureaud, G., Thomas-Danguin, T., Le Berre, E., and Schaal, B. (2008). Perception of odor blending mixtures in the newborn rabbit. *Physiol. Behav.* 95, 194–199. doi: 10.1016/j.physbeh.2008.05.018

Critchley, H. D., and Rolls, E. T. (1996). Olfactory neuronal responses in the primate orbitofrontal cortex: analysis in an olfactory discrimination task. *J. Neurophysiol.* 75, 1659–1672.

Cruz, G., and Lowe, G. (2013). Neural coding of binary mixtures in a structurally related odorant pair. *Sci. Rep.* 3, 1220. doi: 10.1038/srep01220

Davison, I. G., and Katz, L. C. (2007). Sparse and selective odor coding by mitral/tufted neurons in the main olfactory bulb. *J. Neurosci.* 27, 2091–2101. doi: 10.1523/JNEUROSCI.3779-06.2007

de Wijk, R. A., and Cain, W. S. (1994). Odor quality: discrimination versus free and cued identification. *Percept. Psychophys.* 56, 12–18. doi: 10.3758/BF03211686

Deisig, N., Giurfa, M., and Sandoz, J. C. (2010). Antennal lobe processing increases separability of odor mixture representations in the honeybee. *J. Neurophysiol.* 103, 2185–2194. doi: 10.1152/jn.00342.2009

Deisig, N., Giurfa, M., Lachnit, H., and Sandoz, J. C. (2006). Neural representation of olfactory mixtures in the honeybee antennal lobe. *Eur. J. Neurosci.* 24, 1161–1174. doi: 10.1111/j.1460-9568.2006.04959.x

Deisig, N., Kropf, J., Vitecek, S., Pevergne, D., Rouyar, A., Sandoz, J.-C., et al. (2012). Differential interactions of sex pheromone and plant odour in the olfactory pathway of a male moth. *PLoS ONE* 7:e33159. doi: 10.1371/journal.pone.0033159

Deisig, N., Lachnit, H., and Giurfa, M. (2002). The effect of similarity between elemental stimuli and compounds in olfactory patterning discriminations. *Learn. Mem.* 9, 112–121. doi: 10.1101/lm.41002

Deisig, N., Lachnit, H., Giurfa, M., and Hellstern, F. (2001). Configural olfactory learning in honeybees: negative and positive patterning discrimination. *Learn. Mem.* 8, 70–78. doi: 10.1101/lm.8.2.70

Derby, C. D. (2000). Learning from spiny lobsters about chemosensory coding of mixtures. *Physiol. Behav.* 69, 203–209. doi: 10.1016/S0031-9384(00)00202-X

Derby, C. D., Hutson, M., Livermore, A., and Lynn, W. H. (1996). Generalization among related complex odorant mixtures and their components: analysis of olfactory perception in the spiny lobster. *Physiol. Behav.* 60, 87–95. doi: 10.1016/0031-9384(95)02237-6

Devos, M., Rouault, J., and Laffort, P. (2002). *Standardized olfactory power law exponents.* Dijon: Editions Universitaires de Dijon.

Djordjevic, J., Jones-Gotman, M., De Sousa, K., and Chertkow, H. (2008). Olfaction in patients with mild cognitive impairment and Alzheimer's disease. *Neurobiol. Aging* 29, 693–706. doi: 10.1016/j.neurobiolaging.2006.11.014

Doty, R. L. (1975). An examination of relationships between the pleasantness, intensity, and concentration of 10 odorous stimuli. *Percept. Psychophys.* 17, 492–496. doi: 10.3758/BF03203300

Dravnieks, A., and Jarke, F. H. (1980). "Hedonic values of odor mixtures as fuctions of hedonic values of their components," in *Olfaction and Taste VII*, ed. H. Van der Starre (London: IRL Press), 393–396.

Dreumont-Boudreau, S. E., Dingle, R. N., Alcolado, G. M., and LoLordo, V. M. (2006). An olfactory biconditional discrimination in the mouse. *Physiol. Behav.* 87, 634–640. doi: 10.1016/j.physbeh.2006.01.001

Duchamp-Viret, P., Duchamp, A., and Chaput, M. A. (2000). Peripheral odor coding in the rat and frog: quality and intensity specification. *J. Neurosci.* 20, 2383–2390.

Duchamp-Viret, P., Duchamp, A., and Chaput, M. A. (2003). Single olfactory sensory neurons simultaneously integrate the components of an odour mixture. *Eur. J. Neurosci.* 18, 2690–2696. doi: 10.1111/j.1460-9568.2003.03001.x

Dulac, C. (2006). Sparse encoding of natural scents. *Neuron* 50, 816–818. doi: 10.1016/j.neuron.2006.06.002

Escudero, A., Gogorza, B., Melus, M. A., Ortin, N., Cacho, J., and Ferreira, V. (2004). Characterization of the aroma of a wine from maccabeo. Key role played by compounds with low odor activity values. *J. Agric. Food Chem.* 52, 3516–3524. doi: 10.1021/jf035341l

Falcao, L. D., Lytra, G., Darriet, P., and Barbe, J.-C. (2012). Identification of ethyl 2-hydroxy-4-methylpentanoate in red wines, a compound involved in blackberry aroma. *Food Chem.* 132, 230–236. doi: 10.1016/j.foodchem.2011.10.061

Ferreira, V. (2012a). Revisiting psychophysical work on the quantitative and qualitative odour properties of simple odour mixtures: a flavour chemistry view. Part 1: intensity and detectability. A review. *Flavour Fragr. J.* 27, 124–140. doi: 10.1002/ffj.2090

Ferreira, V. (2012b). Revisiting psychophysical work on the quantitative and qualitative odour properties of simple odour mixtures: a flavour chemistry view. Part 2: qualitative aspects. A review. *Flavour Fragr. J.* 27, 201–215. doi: 10.1002/ffj.2091

Fine-Levy, J. B., Daniel, P. C., Girardot, M.-N., and Derby, C. D. (1989). Behavioral resolution of quality of odorant mixtures by spiny lobsters: differential aversive conditioning of olfactory responses. *Chem. Senses* 14, 503–524. doi: 10.1093/chemse/14.4.503

Fletcher, M. L. (2011). Analytical Processing of Binary Mixture Information by Olfactory Bulb Glomeruli. *PLoS ONE* 6:e29360. doi: 10.1371/journal.pone.0029360

Frank, M. E., Goyert, H. F., and Hettinger, T. P. (2010). Time and intensity factors in identification of components of odor mixtures. *Chem. Senses* 35, 777–787. doi: 10.1093/chemse/bjq078

Frederick, D. E., Barlas, L., Ievins, A., and Kay, L. M. (2009). A critical test of the overlap hypothesis for odor mixture perception. *Behav. Neurosci.* 123, 430–437. doi: 10.1037/a0014729

Frumin, I., Sobel, N., and Gilad, Y. (2013). Does a unique olfactory genome imply a unique olfactory world? *Nat. Neurosci.* 17, 6–8. doi: 10.1038/nn.3608

Galizia, C. G., and Menzel, R. (2000). Odour perception in honeybees: coding information in glomerular patterns. *Curr. Opin. Neurobiol.* 10, 504–510. doi: 10.1016/S0959-4388(00)00109-4

Gatti, E., Bordegoni, M., and Spence, C. (2014). Investigating the influence of colour, weight, and fragrance intensity on the perception of liquid bath soap: an experimental study. *Food Qual. Prefer.* 31, 56–64. doi: 10.1016/j.foodqual.2013.08.004

Gaudin, J.-M., Nikolaenko, O., de Saint Laumer, J.-Y., Winter, B., and Blanc, P.-A. (2007). Structure–activity relationship in the domain of odorants having marine notes. *Helv. Chim. Acta* 90, 1245–1265. doi: 10.1002/hlca.200790126

Gerber, B., Eschbach, C., Vogt, K., and Schmuker, M. (2011). The similarity between odors and their binary mixtures in Drosophila. *Chem. Senses* 36, 613–621. doi: 10.1093/chemse/bjr016

Gibson, E. J. (1969). *Principles of Perceptual Learning and Development*, Prentice-Hall: Prentice Hall College.

Gleeson, R. A., and Ache, B. W. (1985). Amino acid suppression of taurine-sensitive chemosensory neurons. *Brain Res.* 335, 99–107. doi: 10.1016/0006-8993(85)90280-X

Gottfried, J. A. (2009). Function follows form: ecological constraints on odor codes and olfactory percepts. *Curr. Opin. Neurobiol.* 19, 422–429. doi: 10.1016/j.conb.2009.07.012

Gottfried, J. A. (2010). Central mechanisms of odour object perception. *Nat. Rev. Neurosci.* 11, 628–641. doi: 10.1038/nrn2883

Gottfried, J. A., and Zelano, C. (2011). "The value of identity: olfactory notes on orbitofrontal cortex function," in *Critical Contributions of the Orbitofrontal Cortex to Behavior*, eds G. Schoenbaum, J. A. Gottfried, E. A. Murray, and S. J. Ramus (Oxford: Blackwell Science Publication), 138–148.

Gottfried, J. A., Winston, J. S., and Dolan, R. J. (2006). Dissociable codes of odor quality and odorant structure in human piriform cortex. *Neuron* 49, 467–479. doi: 10.1016/j.neuron.2006.01.007

Goyert, H. F., Frank, M. E., Gent, J. F., and Hettinger, T. P. (2007). Characteristic component odors emerge from mixtures after selective adaptation. *Brain Res. Bull.* 72, 1–9. doi: 10.1016/j.brainresbull.2006.12.010

Grabenhorst, F., Rolls, E. T., and Margot, C. (2011). A hedonically complex odor mixture produces an attentional capture effect in the brain. *Neuroimage* 55, 832–843. doi: 10.1016/j.neuroimage.2010.12.023

Grabenhorst, F., Rolls, E. T., Margot, C., da Silva, M., and Velazco, M. I. (2007). How pleasant and unpleasant stimuli combine in different brain regions: odor mixtures. *J. Neurosci.* 27, 13532–13540. doi: 10.1523/JNEUROSCI.3337-07.2007

Granger, R., and Lynch, G. (1991). Higher olfactory processes: perceptual learning and memory. *Curr. Opin. Neurobiol.* 1, 209–214. doi: 10.1016/0959-4388(91)90080-Q

Grosch, W. (2001). Evaluation of the key odorants of foods by dilution experiments, aroma models and omission. *Chem. Senses* 26, 533–545. doi: 10.1093/chemse/26.5.533

Grossman, K. J., Mallik, A. K., Ross, J., Kay, L. M., and Issa, N. P. (2008). Glomerular activation patterns and the perception of odor mixtures. *Eur. J. Neurosci.* 27, 2676–2685. doi: 10.1111/j.1460-9568.2008.06213.x

Guichard, E. (2002). Interactions between flavor compounds and food ingredients and their influence on flavor perception. *Food Rev. Int.* 18, 49–70. doi: 10.1081/FRI-120003417

Haberly, L. B. (2001). Parallel-distributed processing in olfactory cortex: new insights from morphological and physiological analysis of neuronal circuitry. *Chem. Senses* 26, 551–576. doi: 10.1093/chemse/26.5.551

Haberly, L. B., and Bower, J. M. (1984). Analysis of association fiber system in piriform cortex with intracellular recording and staining techniques. *J. Neurophysiol.* 51, 90–112.

Harris, J. A. (2006). Elemental representations of stimuli in associative learning. *Psychol. Rev.* 113, 584–605. doi: 10.1037/0033-295X.113.3.584

Hermesh, H., Zohar, J., Weizman, A., Voet, H., and Gross-Isseroff, R. (1999). Orbitofrontal cortex dysfunction in obsessive-compulsive disorder? II. Olfactory quality discrimination in obsessive-compulsive disorder. *Eur. Neuropsychopharmacol.* 9, 415–420. doi: 10.1016/S0924-977X(99)00018-8

Herz, R. S., and von Clef, J. (2001). The influence of verbal labeling on the perception of odors: evidence for olfactory illusions? *Perception* 30, 381–391. doi: 10.1068/p3179

Hopfield, J. F., and Gelperin, A. (1989). Differential conditioning to a compound stimulus and its components in the terrestrial mollusc Limax maximus. *Behav. Neurosci.* 103, 329–333. doi: 10.1037/0735-7044.103.2.329

Hornung, D. E., and Enns, M. P. (1989). "Separating the contributions of smells and tastes in flavor perception," in *Perception of Complex Smells and Tastes*, eds D. G. Laing, W. S. Cain, R. L. McBride, and B. Ache (Sydney: Academic Press), 285–296.

Howard, J. D., Plailly, J., Grueschow, M., Haynes, J. D., and Gottfried, J. A. (2009). Odor quality coding and categorization in human posterior piriform cortex. *Nat. Neurosci.* 12, 932–939. doi: 10.1038/nn.2324

Hummel, T., Olgun, S., Gerber, J., Huchel, U., and Frasnelli, J. (2013). Brain responses to odor mixtures with sub-threshold components. *Front. Psychol.* 4, 1–8. doi: 10.3389/fpsyg.2013.00786

Jacquier, V., Pick, H., and Vogel, H. (2006). Characterization of an extended receptive ligand repertoire of the human olfactory receptor OR17-40 comprising structurally related compounds. *J. Neurochem.* 97, 537–544. doi: 10.1111/j.1471-4159.2006.03771.x

Jinks, A., and Laing, D. G. (1999a). A limit in the processing of components in odour mixtures. *Perception* 28, 395–404. doi: 10.1068/p2898

Jinks, A., and Laing, D. G. (1999b). Temporal processing reveals a mechanism for limiting the capacity of humans to analyze odor mixtures. *Cogn. Brain Res.* 8, 311–325. doi: 10.1016/S0926-6410(99)00034-8

Jinks, A., and Laing, D. G. (2001). The analysis of odor mixtures by humans: evidence for a configurational process. *Physiol. Behav.* 72, 51–63. doi: 10.1016/S0031-9384(00)00407-8

Joerges, J., Küttner, A., Galizia, C. G., and Menzel, R. (1997). Representations of odours and odour mixtures visualized in the honeybee brain. *Nature* 387, 285–288. doi: 10.1038/387285a0

Kadohisa, M., and Wilson, D. A. (2006). Separate encoding of identity and similarity of complex familiar odors in piriform cortex. *Proc. Natl. Acad. Sci. U.S.A.* 103, 15206–15211. doi: 10.1073/pnas.0604313103

Kaeppler, K., and Mueller, F. (2013). Odor classification: a review of factors influencing perception-based odor arrangements. *Chem. Senses* 38, 189–209. doi: 10.1093/chemse/bjs141

Kajiya, K., Inaki, K., Tanaka, M., Haga, T., Kataoka, H., and Touhara, K. (2001). Molecular bases of odor discrimination: reconstitution of olfactory receptors that recognize overlapping sets of odorants. *J. Neurosci.* 21, 6018–6025.

Kang, J., and Caprio, J. (1997). In vivo responses of single olfactory receptor neurons of channel catfish to binary mixtures of amino acids. *J. Neurophysiol.* 77, 1–8.

Kay, L. M., and Stopfer, M. (2006). Information processing in the olfactory systems of insects and vertebrates. *Semin. Cell Dev. Biol.* 17, 433–442. doi: 10.1016/j.semcdb.2006.04.012

Kay, L. M., Crk, T., and Thorngate, J. (2005). A redefinition of odor mixture quality. *Behav. Neurosci.* 119, 726–733. doi: 10.1037/0735-7044.119.3.726

Kay, L. M., Lowry, C. A., and Jacobs, H. A. (2003). Receptor contributions to configural and elemental odor mixture perception. *Behav. Neurosci.* 117, 1108–1114. doi: 10.1037/0735-7044.117.5.1108

Keller, A., Zhuang, H., Chi, Q., Vosshall, L. B., and Matsunami, H. (2007). Genetic variation in a human odorant receptor alters odour perception. *Nature* 449, 468–472. doi: 10.1038/nature06162

Kermen, F., Chakirian, A., Sezille, C., Joussain, P., Le Goff, G., Ziessel, A., et al. (2011). Molecular complexity determines the number of olfactory notes and the pleasantness of smells. *Sci. Rep.* 1, 206. doi: 10.1038/srep00206

Khan, R. M., Luk, C. H., Flinker, A., Aggarwal, A., Lapid, H., Haddad, R., et al. (2007). Predicting odor pleasantness from odorant structure: pleasantness as a reflection of the physical world. *J. Neurosci.* 27, 10015–10023. doi: 10.1523/JNEUROSCI.1158-07.2007

Kirschner, S., Kleineidam, C. J., Zube, C., Rybak, J., Grünewald, B., and Rössler, W. (2006). Dual olfactory pathway in the honeybee, *Apis mellifera*. *J. Comp. Neurol.* 499, 933–952. doi: 10.1002/cne.21158

Kopala, L. C., Good, K., Goldner, E. M., and Birmingham, C. L. (1995). Olfactory identification ability in anorexia nervosa. *J. Psychiatry Neurosci.* 20, 283–286.

Kurtz, A. J., Lawless, H. T., and Acree, T. E. (2009). Reference matching of dissimilar binary odor mixtures. *Chemosens. Percept.* 2, 186–194. doi: 10.1007/s12078-009-9063-3

Laffort, P., and Dravnieks, A. (1982). Several models of suprathreshold quantitative olfactory interaction in humans applied to binary, ternary and quaternary mixtures. *Chem. Senses* 7, 153–174. doi: 10.1093/chemse/7.2.153

Laing, D. G. (1994). Perceptual odour interactions and objective mixture analysis. *Food Qual. Prefer.* 5, 75–80. doi: 10.1016/0950-3293(94)90010-8

Laing, D. G., and Francis, G. W. (1989). The capacity of humans to identify odors in mixtures. *Physiol. Behav.* 46, 809–814. doi: 10.1016/0031-9384(89)90041-3

Laing, D. G., and Glemarec, A. (1992). Selective attention and the perceptual analysis of odor mixtures. *Physiol. Behav.* 52, 1047–1053. doi: 10.1016/0031-9384(92)90458-E

Laing, D. G., and Jinks, A. L. (2001). Psychophysical analysis of complex odor mixtures. *Chimia (Aarau)*. 55, 413–420.

Laing, D. G., and Livermore, B. A. (1992). "Perceptual analysis of complex chemical signals by humans," in *Chemical Signals in Vertebrates VI*, eds R. L. Doty and D. Müller-Schwarze (New York: Plenum Press), 587–593. doi: 10.1007/978-1-4757-9655-1_90

Laing, D. G., and Willcox, M. E. (1983). Perception of components in binary odour mixtures. *Chem. Senses* 7, 249–264. doi: 10.1093/chemse/7.3-4.249

Laing, D. G., Legha, P. K., Jinks, A. L., and Hutchinson, I. (2003). Relationship between molecular structure, concentration and odor qualities of oxygenated aliphatic molecules. *Chem. Senses* 28, 57–69. doi: 10.1093/chemse/28.1.57

Lapid, H., Harel, D., and Sobel, N. (2008). Prediction models for the pleasantness of binary mixtures in olfaction. *Chem. Senses* 33, 599–609. doi: 10.1093/chemse/bjn026

Larsson, M. C., Domingos, A. I., Jones, W. D., Chiappe, M. E., Amrein, H., and Vosshall, L. B. (2004). Or83b encodes a broadly expressed odorant receptor essential for *Drosophila* olfaction. *Neuron* 43, 703–714. doi: 10.1016/j.neuron.2004.08.019

Laska, M., and Hudson, R. (1992). Ability to discriminate between related odor mixtures. *Chem. Senses* 17, 403–415. doi: 10.1093/chemse/17.4.403

Laska, M., and Hudson, R. (1993). Discriminating parts from the whole - determinants of odor mixture perception in squirrel-monkeys, Saimiri-Sciureus. *J. Comp. Physiol. Sensory Neural Behav. Physiol.* 173, 249–256. doi: 10.1007/BF00192984

Lazarowski, L., and Dorman, D. C. (2014). Explosives detection by military working dogs: olfactory generalization from components to mixtures. *Appl. Anim. Behav. Sci.* 151, 84–93. doi: 10.1016/j.applanim.2013.11.010

Le Berre, E., Béno, N., Ishii, A., Chabanet, C., Etiévant, P., and Thomas-Danguin, T. (2008a). Just noticeable differences in component concentrations modify the odor quality of a blending mixture. *Chem. Senses* 33, 389–395. doi: 10.1093/chemse/bjn006

Le Berre, E., Jarmuzek, E., Béno, N., Etiévant, P., Prescott, J., and Thomas-Danguin, T. (2010). Learning influences the perception of odor mixtures. *Chemosens. Percept.* 3, 156–166. doi: 10.1007/s12078-010-9076-y

Le Berre, E., Thomas-Danguin, T., Béno, N., Coureaud, G., Etiévant, P., and Prescott, J. (2008b). Perceptual processing strategy and exposure influence the perception of odor mixtures. *Chem. Senses* 33, 193–199. doi: 10.1093/chemse/bjm080

Lei, H. M., Mooney, R., and Katz, L. C. (2006). Synaptic integration of olfactory information in mouse anterior olfactory nucleus. *J. Neurosci.* 26, 12023–12032. doi: 10.1523/JNEUROSCI.2598-06.2006

Lei, H., and Vickers, N. (2008). Central processing of natural odor mixtures in insects. *J. Chem. Ecol.* 34, 915–927. doi: 10.1007/s10886-008-9487-2

Lindqvist, A., Höglund, A., and Berglund, B. (2012). The role of odour quality in the perception of binary and higher-order mixtures. *Perception* 41, 1373–1391. doi: 10.1068/p7267

Linster, C., and Cleland, T. A. (2004). Configurational and elemental odor mixture perception can arise from local inhibition. *J. Comput. Neurosci.* 16, 39–47. doi: 10.1023/B:JCNS.0000004840.87570.2e

Linster, C., and Smith, B. H. (1999). Generalization between binary odor mixtures and their components in the rat. *Physiol. Behav.* 66, 701–707. doi: 10.1016/S0031-9384(99)00007-4

Linster, C., Johnson, B. A., Yue, E., Morse, A., Xu, Z., Hingco, E. E., et al. (2001). Perceptual correlates of neural representations evoked by odorant enantiomers. *J. Neurosci.* 21, 9837–9843.

Litaudon, P., Datiche, F., and Cattarelli, M. (1997). Optical recording of the rat piriform cortex activity. *Prog. Neurobiol.* 52, 485–510. doi: 10.1016/S0301-0082(97)00027-0

Livermore, A., and Laing, D. G. (1996). Influence of training and experience on the perception of multicomponent odor mixtures. *J. Exp. Psychol. Hum. Percept. Perform.* 22, 267–277. doi: 10.1037/0096-1523.22.2.267

Livermore, A., and Laing, D. G. (1998a). The influence of chemical complexity on the perception of multicomponent odor mixtures. *Percept. Psychophys.* 60, 650–661. doi: 10.3758/BF03206052

Livermore, A., and Laing, D. G. (1998b). The influence of odor type on the discrimination and identification of odorants in multicomponent odor mixtures. *Physiol. Behav.* 65, 311–320. doi: 10.1016/S0031-9384(98)00168-1

Livermore, A., Hutson, M., Ngo, V., Hadjisimos, R., and Derby, C. D. (1997). Elemental and configural learning and the perception of odorant mixtures by the spiny lobster panulirus argus. *Physiol. Behav.* 62, 169–174. doi: 10.1016/S0031-9384(97)00031-0

Logan, D. W., Brunet, L. J., Webb, W. R., Cutforth, T., Ngai, J., and Stowers, L. (2012). Learned recognition of maternal signature odors mediates the first suckling episode in mice. *Curr. Biol.* 22, 1998–2007. doi: 10.1016/j.cub.2012.08.041

Lovitz, A. M., Sloan, A. M., Rennaker, R. L., and Wilson, D. A. (2012). Complex mixture discrimination and the role of contaminants. *Chem. Senses* 37, 533–540. doi: 10.1093/chemse/bjs006

Lynn, W. H., Meyer, E. A., Peppiatt, C. E., and Derby, C. D. (1994). Perception of odor mixtures by the spiny lobster *Panulirus argus*. *Chem. Senses* 19, 331–347. doi: 10.1093/chemse/19.4.331

Lytra, G., Tempere, S., de Revel, G., and Barbe, J.-C. (2012). Impact of perceptive interactions on red wine fruity aroma. *J. Agric. Food Chem.* 60, 12260–12269. doi: 10.1021/jf302918q

Mainland, J. D., Keller, A., Li, Y. R., Zhou, T., Trimmer, C., Snyder, L. L., et al. (2014). The missense of smell: functional variability in the human odorant receptor repertoire. *Nat. Neurosci.* 17, 114–120. doi: 10.1038/nn.3598

Malnic, B., Hirono, J., Sato, T., and Buck, L. B. (1999). Combinatorial receptor codes for odors. *Cell* 96, 713–723. doi: 10.1016/S0092-8674(00)80581-4

Mandairon, N., Sacquet, J., Garcia, S., Ravel, N., Jourdan, F., and Didier, A. (2006a). Neurogenic correlates of an olfactory discrimination task in the adult olfactory bulb. *Eur. J. Neurosci.* 24, 3578–3588. doi: 10.1111/j.1460-9568.2006.05235.x

Mandairon, N., Stack, C., Kiselycznyk, C., and Linster, C. (2006b). Enrichment to Odors improves olfactory discrimination in adult rats. *Behav. Neurosci.* 120, 173–179. doi: 10.1037/0735-7044.120.1.173

Mandairon, N., Stack, C., and Linster, C. (2006c). Olfactory enrichment improves the recognition of individual components in mixtures. *Physiol. Behav.* 89, 379–384. doi: 10.1016/j.physbeh.2006.07.013

Margot, C. (2009). A noseful of objects. *Nat. Neurosci.* 12, 813–814. doi: 10.1038/nn0709-813

Martin, J. P., Lei, H., Riffell, J. A., and Hildebrand, J. G. (2013). Synchronous firing of antennal-lobe projection neurons encodes the behaviorally effective ratio of sex-pheromone components in male Manduca sexta. *J. Comp. Physiol. A Neuroethol. Sens. Neural. Behav. Physiol.* 199, 963–979. doi: 10.1007/s00359-013-0849-z

McGann, J. P., Pírez, N., Gainey, M. A., Muratore, C., Elias, A. S., and Wachowiak, M. (2005). Odorant representations are modulated by intra- but not interglomerular presynaptic inhibition of olfactory sensory neurons. *Neuron* 48, 1039–1053. doi: 10.1016/j.neuron.2005.10.031

McNamara, A. M., Magidson, P. D., and Linster, C. (2007). Binary mixture perception is affected by concentration of odor components. *Behav. Neurosci.* 121, 1132–1136. doi: 10.1037/0735-7044.121.5.1132

Menashe, I., Abaffy, T., Hasin, Y., Goshen, S., Yahalom, V., Luetje, C. W., et al. (2007). Genetic elucidation of human hyperosmia to isovaleric acid. *PLoS Biol.* 5:2462–2468. doi: 10.1371/journal.pbio.0050284

Miyazawa, T., Gallagher, M., Preti, G., and Wise, P. M. (2009). Psychometric functions for ternary odor mixtures and their unmixed components. *Chem. Senses* 34, 753–761. doi: 10.1093/chemse/bjp062

Moberg, P. J., and Turetsky, B. I. (2003). Scent of a disorder: olfactory functioning in schizophrenia. *Curr. Psychiatry Rep.* 5, 311–319. doi: 10.1007/s11920-003-0061-x

Mombaerts, P., Wang, F., Dulac, C., Chao, S. K., Nemes, A., Mendelsohn, M., et al. (1996). Visualizing an olfactory sensory map. *Cell* 87, 675–686. doi: 10.1016/S0092-8674(00)81387-2

Mori, K., and Sakano, H. (2011). How is the olfactory map formed and interpreted in the mammalian brain? *Annu. Rev. Neurosci.* 34, 467–499. doi: 10.1146/annurev-neuro-112210-112917

Moskowitz, H. R., and Barbe, C. D. (1977). Profiling of odor components and their mixtures. *Sens. Processes* 1, 212–226.

Münch, D., Schmeichel, B., Silbering, A. F., and Galizia, C. G. (2013). Weaker ligands can dominate an odor blend due to syntopic interactions. *Chem. Senses* 38, 293–304. doi: 10.1093/chemse/bjs138

Naudin, M., El-Hage, W., Gomes, M., Gaillard, P., Belzung, C., and Atanasova, B. (2012). State and trait olfactory markers of major depression. *PLoS ONE* 7:e46938. doi: 10.1371/journal.pone.0046938

Ochieng, S. A., Park, K. C., and Baker, T. C. (2002). Host plant volatiles synergize responses of sex pheromone-specific olfactory receptor neurons in male *Helicoverpa zea*. *J. Comp. Physiol. A. Neuroethol. Sens. Neural. Behav. Physiol.* 188, 325–333. doi: 10.1007/s00359-002-0308-8

Oka, Y., Omura, M., Kataoka, H., and Touhara, K. (2004). Olfactory receptor antagonism between odorants. *EMBO J.* 23, 120–126. doi: 10.1038/sj.emboj.7600032

Olsson, M. J. (1994). An interaction model for odor quality and intensity. *Percept. Psychophys.* 55, 363–372. doi: 10.3758/BF03205294

Olsson, M. J. (1998). An integrated model of intensity and quality of odor mixtures. *Ann. N. Y. Acad. Sci.* 855, 837–840. doi: 10.1111/j.1749-6632.1998.tb10672.x

Patte, F., and Laffort, P. (1979). Alternative model of olfactory quantitative interaction in binary-mixtures. *Chem. Senses Flavour* 4, 267–274. doi: 10.1093/chemse/4.4.267

Pause, B. M., Miranda, A., Göder, R., Aldenhoff, J. B., and Ferstl, R. (2001). Reduced olfactory performance in patients with major depression. *J. Psychiatr. Res.* 35, 271–277. doi: 10.1016/S0022-3956(01)00029-2

Pearce, J. M. (1987). A model for stimulus generalization in Pavlovian conditioning. *Psychol. Rev.* 94, 61–73. doi: 10.1037/0033-295X.94.1.61

Pearce, J. M. (1994). Similarity and discrimination: a selective review and a connectionist model. *Psychol. Rev.* 101, 587–607. doi: 10.1037/0033-295X.101.4.587

Pineau, B., Barbe, J. C., Van Leeuwen, C., and Dubourdieu, D. (2009). Examples of perceptive interactions involved in specific "red-" and "black-berry" aromas in red wines. *J. Agric. Food Chem.* 57, 3702–3708. doi: 10.1021/jf803325v

Postolache, T. T., Doty, R. L., Wehr, T. A., Jimma, L. A., Han, L., Turner, E. H., et al. (1999). Monorhinal odor identification and depression scores in patients with seasonal affective disorder. *J. Affect. Disord.* 56, 27–35. doi: 10.1016/S0165-0327(99)00027-0

Rabin, M. D. (1988). Experience facilitates olfactory quality discrimination. *Percept. Psychophys.* 44, 532–540. doi: 10.3758/BF03207487

Rabin, M. D., Cain, W. S., and Cain, J. (1989). "Attention and learning in the perception of odor mixtures," in *Perception of Complex Smells and Tastes*, eds D. G. Laing, W. S. Cain, R. L. McBride, and B. W. Ache (Sidney: Academic Press), 173–188.

Reinhard, J., Sinclair, M., Srinivasan, M. V., and Claudianos, C. (2010). Honeybees learn odour mixtures via a selection of key odorants. *PLoS ONE* 5:e9110. doi: 10.1371/journal.pone.0009110

Rescorla, R. A. (1972). "Configural" conditioning in discrete-trial bar pressing. *J. Comp. Physiol. Psychol.* 79, 307–317. doi: 10.1037/h0032553

Rescorla, R. A. (1973). Evidence for unique stimulus account of configural conditioning. *J. Comp. Physiol. Psychol.* 85, 331–338. doi: 10.1037/h0035046

Rescorla, R. A., Gruau, J. W., and Durlach, P. J. (1985). Analysis of the unique cue in configural discriminations. *J. Exp. Psychol. Anim. Behav. Process.* 11, 356–366. doi: 10.1037/0097-7403.11.3.356

Riffell, J. A. (2012). Olfactory ecology and the processing of complex mixtures. *Curr. Opin. Neurobiol.* 22, 236–242. doi: 10.1016/j.conb.2012.02.013

Riffell, J. A., Lei, H., Christensen, T. A., and Hildebrand, J. G. (2009). Characterization and coding of behaviorally significant odor mixtures. *Curr. Biol.* 19, 335–340. doi: 10.1016/j.cub.2009.01.041

Rospars, J.-P., Lansky, P., Chaput, M., and Duchamp-Viret, P. (2008). Competitive and noncompetitive odorant interactions in the early neural coding of odorant mixtures. *J. Neurosci.* 28, 2659–2666. doi: 10.1523/JNEUROSCI.4670-07.2008

Rouby, C., Pouliot, S., and Bensafi, M. (2009). Odor hedonics and their modulators. *Food Qual. Prefer.* 20, 545–549. doi: 10.1016/j.foodqual.2009.05.004

Rouby, C., Thomas-Danguin, T., Sicard, G., Vigouroux, M., Jiang, T., Poitevineau, J., et al. (2005). Influence du contexte sémantique sur la performance d'identification d'odeurs. *Psychol. Française* 50, 225–239. doi: 10.1016/j.psfr.2004.11.003

Royet, J.-P., Plailly, J., Delon-Martin, C., Kareken, D. A., and Segebarth, C. (2003). fMRI of emotional responses to odors: influence of hedonic valence and judgment, handedness, and gender. *Neuroimage* 20, 713–728. doi: 10.1016/S1053-8119(03)00388-4

Sanz, G., Schlegel, C., Pernollet, J.-C., and Briand, L. (2005). Comparison of odorant specificity of two human olfactory receptors from different phylogenetic classes and evidence for antagonism. *Chem. Senses* 30, 69–80. doi: 10.1093/chemse/bji002

Sanz, G., Thomas-Danguin, T., Hamdani, E. H., Le Poupon, C., Briand, L., Pernollet, J.-C., et al. (2008). Relationships between molecular structure and perceived odor quality of ligands for a human olfactory receptor. *Chem. Senses* 33, 639–653. doi: 10.1093/chemse/bjn032

Schaal, B. (2010). Mammary odor cues and pheromones: mammalian infant-directed communication about maternal state, mammae, and milk. *Vitam. Horm.* 83, 83–136. doi: 10.1016/S0083-6729(10)83004-3

Schaal, B., Coureaud, G., Langlois, D., Ginies, C., Semon, E., and Perrier, G. (2003). Chemical and behavioural characterization of the rabbit mammary pheromone. *Nature* 424, 68–72. doi: 10.1038/nature01739

Serizawa, S., Miyamichi, K., and Sakano, H. (2004). One neuron-one receptor rule in the mouse olfactory system. *Trends Genet.* 20, 648–653. doi: 10.1016/j.tig.2004.09.006

Silbering, A. F., and Galizia, C. G. (2007). Processing of odor mixtures in the Drosophila antennal lobe reveals both global inhibition and glomerulus-specific interactions. *J. Neurosci.* 27, 11966–11977. doi: 10.1523/JNEUROSCI.3099-07.2007

Sinding, C. (2012). *Perception des Mélanges d'odeurs Étude Comportementale et Psychophysique Chez le Mammifère Nouveau-né et l'homme.* Ph.D. Thesis, University of Burgundy, Burgundy.

Sinding, C., Coureaud, G., Chabanet, C., Chambault, A., Béno, N., Dosne, T., et al. (2014). "Chapter 5 - perceptual interactions in complex odor mixtures: the blending effect," in *Flavour Science: Proceedings from XIII Weurman Flavour Research Symposium*, eds V. Ferreira and R. B. T.-F. S. Lopez (San Diego: Academic Press), 27–31.

Sinding, C., Thomas-Danguin, T., Chambault, A., Béno, N., Dosne, T., Chabanet, C., et al. (2013). Rabbit neonates and human adults perceive a blending 6-component odor mixture in a comparable manner. *PLoS ONE* 8:e53534. doi: 10.1371/journal.pone.0053534

Sinding, C., Thomas-Danguin, T., Crepeaux, G., Schaal, B., and Coureaud, G. (2011). Experience influences elemental and configural perception of certain binary odour mixtures in newborn rabbits. *J. Exp. Biol.* 214, 4171–4178. doi: 10.1242/jeb.063610

Snitz, K., Yablonka, A., Weiss, T., Frumin, I., Khan, R. M., and Sobel, N. (2013). Predicting odor perceptual similarity from odor Structure. *PLoS Comput. Biol.* 9:e1003184. doi: 10.1371/journal.pcbi.1003184

Spehr, M., Gisselmann, G., Poplawski, A., Riffell, J. A., Wetzel, C. H., Zimmer, R. K., et al. (2003). Identification of a testicular odorant receptor mediating human sperm chemotaxis. *Science* 299, 2054–2058. doi: 10.1126/science.1080376

Spehr, M., Schwane, K., Heilmann, S., Gisselmann, G., Hummel, T., and Hatt, H. (2004). Dual capacity of a human olfactory receptor. *Curr. Biol.* 14, R832–R833. doi: 10.1016/j.cub.2004.09.034

Staubli, U., Fraser, D., Faraday, R., and Lynch, G. (1987). Olfaction and the "data" memory system in rats. *Behav. Neurosci.* 101, 757–765. doi: 10.1037/0735-7044.101.6.757

Stettler, D. D., and Axel, R. (2009). Representations of Odor in the Piriform Cortex. *Neuron* 63, 854–864. doi: 10.1016/j.neuron.2009.09.005

Steullet, P., and Derby, C. D. (1997). Coding of blend ratios of binary mixtures by olfactory neurons in the Florida spiny lobster, Panulirus argus. *J. Comp. Physiol. A.* 180, 123–135. doi: 10.1007/s003590050033

Stevens, S. S. (1960). The psychophysics of sensory function. *Am. Sci.* 48, 226–253.

Stevenson, R. J. (2001a). Associative learning and odor quality perception: how sniffing an odor mixture can alter the smell of its parts. *Learn. Motiv.* 32, 154–177. doi: 10.1006/lmot.2000.1070

Stevenson, R. J. (2001b). Perceptual learning with odors: implications for psychological accounts of odor quality perception. *Psychon. Bull. Rev.* 8, 708–712. doi: 10.3758/BF03196207

Stevenson, R. J., and Wilson, D. A. (2007). Odour perception: an object-recognition approach. *Perception* 36, 1821–1833. doi: 10.1068/p5563

Stevenson, R. J., Case, T. I., and Tomiczek, C. (2007). Resistance to interference of olfactory perceptual learning. *Psychol. Rec.* 57, 103–116.

Su, C.-Y., Martelli, C., Emonet, T., and Carlson, J. R. (2011). Temporal coding of odor mixtures in an olfactory receptor neuron. *Proc. Natl. Acad. Sci. U.S.A.* 108, 5075–5080. doi: 10.1073/pnas.1100369108

Szyszka, P., Stierle, J. S., Biergans, S., and Galizia, C. G. (2012). The speed of smell: odor-object segregation within milliseconds. *PLoS ONE* 7:e36096. doi: 10.1371/journal.pone.0036096

Tabor, R., Yaksi, E., Weislogel, J. M., and Friedrich, R. W. (2004). Processing of odor mixtures in the zebrafish olfactory bulb. *J. Neurosci.* 24, 6611–6620. doi: 10.1523/JNEUROSCI.1834-04.2004

Thomas-Danguin, T. (1997). *Intensité olfactive de composés purs et de mélanges: application au masquage des odeurs.* Ph.D. Thesis, University of Lyon 1, Villeurbanne.

Thomas-Danguin, T. (2009). "Flavor," in *Encyclopedia of Neuroscience*, eds M. D. Binder, N. Hirokawa, and U. Windhorst (Berlin: Springer-Verlag Berlin and Heidelberg GmbH & Co. K), 1580–1582. doi: 10.1007/978-3-540-29678-2_1772

Thomas-Danguin, T., and Chastrette, M. (2002). Odour intensity of binary mixtures of odorous compounds. *C. R. Biol.* 325, 767–772. doi: 10.1016/S1631-0691(02)01485-3

Thomas-Danguin, T., and Dumont, J.-P. (2012). "Perception des Arômes en mélange: Les facettes de la Flaveur," in *Texture et Flaveur des Aliments*, eds E. Guichard, C. Genot, and A. Voilley (Dijon: FRA), 235–261.

Thomas-Danguin, T., Le Berre, E., Barkat, S., Coureaud, G., and Sicard, G. (2007). Evidence for odor blending in odorant mixtures. *Chem. Annu. Meet.* 32, A64.

Uchida, N., and Mainen, Z. F. (2008). Odor concentration invariance by chemical ratio coding. *Front. Syst. Neurosci.* 1:3. doi: 10.3389/neuro.06.003.2007

Valentincic, T., Kralj, J., Stenovec, M., Koce, A., and Caprio, J. (2000). The behavioral detection of binary mixtures of amino acids and their individual components by catfish. *J. Exp. Biol.* 203, 3307–3317.

Valentincic, T., Miklavc, P., Kralj, S., and Zgonik, V. (2011). Olfactory discrimination of complex mixtures of amino acids by the black bullhead Ameiurus melas. *J. Fish Biol.* 79, 33–52. doi: 10.1111/j.1095-8649.2011.02976.x

van Wijk, M., de Bruijn, P. J. A., and Sabelis, M. W. (2010). The predatory mite phytoseiulus persimilis does not perceive odor mixtures as strictly elemental objects. *J. Chem. Ecol.* 36, 1211–1225. doi: 10.1007/s10886-010-9858-3

Wang, J. W., Wong, A. M., Flores, J., Vosshall, L. B., and Axel, R. (2003). Two-photon calcium imaging reveals an odor-evoked map of activity in the fly brain. *Cell* 112, 271–282. doi: 10.1016/S0092-8674(03)00004-7

Weiss, T., Snitz, K., Yablonka, A., Khan, R. M., Gafsou, D., Schneidman, E., et al. (2012). Perceptual convergence of multi-component mixtures in olfaction implies an olfactory white. *Proc. Natl. Acad. Sci. U.S.A.* 1, 6. doi: 10.1073/pnas.1208110109

Wilson, D. A. (2000). Odor specificity of habituation in the rat anterior piriform cortex. *J. Neurophysiol.* 83, 139–145.

Wilson, D. A. (2003). Rapid, experience-induced enhancement in odorant discrimination by anterior piriform cortex neurons. *J. Neurophysiol.* 90, 65–72. doi: 10.1152/jn.00133.2003

Wilson, D. A., and Stevenson, R. J. (2003a). Olfactory perceptual learning: the critical role of memory in odor discrimination. *Neurosci. Biobehav. Rev.* 27, 307–328. doi: 10.1016/S0149-7634(03)00050-2

Wilson, D. A., and Stevenson, R. J. (2003b). The fundamental role of memory in olfactory perception. *Trends Neurosci.* 26, 243–247. doi: 10.1016/S0166-2236(03)00076-6

Wilson, D. A., and Sullivan, R. M. (2011). Cortical processing of odor objects. *Neuron* 72, 506–519. doi: 10.1016/j.neuron.2011.10.027

Wiltrout, C., Dogra, S., and Linster, C. (2003). Configurational and nonconfigurational interactions between odorants in binary mixtures. *Behav. Neurosci.* 117, 236–245. doi: 10.1037/0735-7044.117.2.236

Wise, P. M., and Cain, W. S. (2000). Latency and accuracy of discriminations of odor quality between binary mixtures and their components. *Chem. Senses* 25, 247–265. doi: 10.1093/chemse/25.3.247

Wright, G. A., and Smith, B. H. (2004). Variation in complex olfactory stimuli and its influence on odour recognition. *Proc. R. Soc. Lond. B Biol. Sci.* 271, 147–152. doi: 10.1098/rspb.2003.2590

Wright, G. A., Carlton, M., and Smith, B. H. (2009). A honeybee's ability to learn, recognize, and discriminate odors depends upon odor sampling time and concentration. *Behav. Neurosci.* 123, 36–43. doi: 10.1037/a0014040

Wysocki, C. J., and Beauchamp, G. K. (1984). Ability to smell androstenone is genetically determined. *Proc. Natl. Acad. Sci. U.S.A.* 81, 4899–4902. doi: 10.1073/pnas.81.15.4899

Wysocki, C. J., Whitney, G., and Tucker, D. (1977). Specific anosmia in the laboratory mouse. *Behav. Genet.* 7, 171–188. doi: 10.1007/BF01066005

Yeshurun, Y., and Sobel, N. (2010). An odor is not worth a thousand words: from multidimensional odors to unidimensional odor objects. *Annu. Rev. Psychol.* 61, 219–241. doi: 10.1146/annurev.psych.60.110707.163639

Yoshida, I., and Mori, K. (2007). Odorant category profile selectivity of olfactory cortex neurons. *J. Neurosci.* 27, 9105–9114. doi: 10.1523/JNEUROSCI.2720-07.2007

7

Genetic basis of olfactory cognition: extremely high level of DNA sequence polymorphism in promoter regions of the human olfactory receptor genes revealed using the 1000 Genomes Project dataset

Elena V. Ignatieva[1,2*†], Victor G. Levitsky[2,3†], Nikolay S. Yudin[2,4], Mikhail P. Moshkin[2,5] and Nikolay A. Kolchanov[2,6,7]

[1] Laboratory of Evolutionary Bioinformatics and Theoretical Genetics, Institute of Cytology and Genetics, Siberian Branch, Russian Academy of Sciences, Novosibirsk, Russia
[2] Department of Natural Science, Novosibirsk State University, Novosibirsk, Russia
[3] Laboratory of Molecular-Genetic Systems, Institute of Cytology and Genetics, Siberian Branch, Russian Academy of Sciences, Novosibirsk, Russia
[4] Laboratory of Human Molecular Genetics, Institute of Cytology and Genetics, Siberian Branch, Russian Academy of Sciences, Novosibirsk, Russia
[5] Laboratory of Mammalian Ecological Genetics, Institute of Cytology and Genetics, Siberian Branch, Russian Academy of Sciences, Novosibirsk, Russia
[6] Department of Systems Biology, Institute of Cytology and Genetics, Siberian Branch, Russian Academy of Sciences, Novosibirsk, Russia
[7] National Research centre "Kurchatov Institute," Moscow, Russia

Correspondence:
Elena V. Ignatieva, Laboratory of Evolutionary Bioinformatics and Theoretical Genetics, Institute of Cytology and Genetic, Siberian Branch, Russian Academy of Sciences, 10 Lavrentyev Ave., Novosibirsk 630090, Russia
e-mail: eignat@bionet.nsc.ru

The molecular mechanism of olfactory cognition is very complicated. Olfactory cognition is initiated by olfactory receptor proteins (odorant receptors), which are activated by olfactory stimuli (ligands). Olfactory receptors are the initial player in the signal transduction cascade producing a nerve impulse, which is transmitted to the brain. The sensitivity to a particular ligand depends on the expression level of multiple proteins involved in the process of olfactory cognition: olfactory receptor proteins, proteins that participate in signal transduction cascade, etc. The expression level of each gene is controlled by its regulatory regions, and especially, by the promoter [a region of DNA about 100–1000 base pairs long located upstream of the transcription start site (TSS)]. We analyzed single nucleotide polymorphisms using human whole-genome data from the 1000 Genomes Project and revealed an extremely high level of single nucleotide polymorphisms in promoter regions of olfactory receptor genes and *HLA* genes. We hypothesized that the high level of polymorphisms in olfactory receptor promoters was responsible for the diversity in regulatory mechanisms controlling the expression levels of olfactory receptor proteins. Such diversity of regulatory mechanisms may cause the great variability of olfactory cognition of numerous environmental olfactory stimuli perceived by human beings (air pollutants, human body odors, odors in culinary etc.). In turn, this variability may provide a wide range of emotional and behavioral reactions related to the vast variety of olfactory stimuli.

Keywords: olfactory cognition, olfactory receptor gene, single nucleotide polymorphism, promoter, 1000 Genomes Project

INTRODUCTION

Human olfactory perception varies enormously among individuals. People vary both in their general olfactory acuity and in perceiving specific odors. For example, according to a study of 391 adult subjects in New York, general olfactory acuity correlated with age, gender, race, smoking habits, and body type. Factors found to influence olfactory perception included race, age, and gender. Over 100 instances in which the intensity or pleasantness perception of an odor varied significantly among demographic groups were described (Keller et al., 2012). Significant differences in the perception of everyday odors were revealed in a Japanese–German cross-cultural study. A close association of pleasantness ratings and edibility judgments was found, suggesting the particular influence of eating habits on odor perception (Ayabe-Kanamura et al., 1998). Notable differences in perceived odor pleasantness were found in children with autism spectrum disorders: patients with this disorder perceived the smell of cinnamon and pineapple as significantly less pleasant compared to healthy controls, the same was true of cloves (Hrdlicka et al., 2011). Factors influencing human odor perception are extensively studied (Moshkin et al., 2011; Seo et al., 2011, 2013; Greenberg et al., 2013). Recent studies demonstrate that genetic factors may contribute to inter-individual differences in odor perception (Keller et al., 2007; Weiss et al., 2011; Knaapila et al., 2012; Mainland et al., 2014).

Abbreviations: 5′UTRs, 5′-untranslated regions; bp, base pairs; CRS, coding region start; Kb, kilobase (1000 base pairs of DNA); OR, olfactory receptor; SNP, single nucleotide polymorphism; TSS, transcription start site; Amino acids: A, Alanine; Ile, Isoleucine; Q, Glutamine; R, Arginine; T, Threonine; W, Tryptophan; M, Methionine; Thr, Threonine; Nucleotides: A, Adenine; C, Cytosine; G, Guanine; T, Thymine.

The molecular mechanism of olfactory cognition is very complex. In mammals, the cellular and molecular machinery for olfactory transduction is located in olfactory epithelium in the nasal cavity. Odorant transduction is initiated by olfactory (odorant) receptors (ORs), which are located on the membranes of the cilia that are whip-like extensions of olfactory sensory neurons.

Odorants in the mucus bind directly (or are shuttled via odorant-binding proteins) to receptor molecules located in the membranes of the cilia (Supplementary section, Figure S1). The ligand-bound receptor activates the signal transduction cascade, which involves G protein (an olfactory specific subtype, G_{olf}), adenylyl cyclase (AC), the cyclic nucleotide-gated (CNG) ion channel and several other proteins (Firestein, 2001; De Palo et al., 2012). Calmodulin (CALM), phosphodiesterase (PDE), β-arrestin2 (ARRB2), some kinases (PKA, GRK3, ORK), and RGS2 protein (regulator of G-protein signaling) participate in feedback mechanisms that olfactory sensory neurons use for adjusting their sensitivity (Boekhoff et al., 1997; Sinnarajah et al., 2001; Mashukova et al., 2006; De Palo et al., 2012). A detailed description of this complex intracellular mechanism is presented in Supplementary section (Part 1).

Mammals have 6–10 million olfactory receptor neurons, which enable organisms to detect and discriminate thousands of odors (Buck and Axel, 1991; Firestein, 2001; Glusman et al., 2001; Olender et al., 2008). There are about 1000 olfactory receptor genes and pseudogenes in the mammalian genome; thus, it is the largest gene family in the entire genome (Firestein, 2001; Menashe et al., 2006). However, in the human genome about 60% of OR genes seem to be pseudogenes (Gilad et al., 2003; Malnic et al., 2004; Hasin et al., 2008; Olender et al., 2012). Their genomic locations show that OR genes are unevenly distributed among 51 different loci on 21 human chromosomes. Sequence comparisons show that the human OR family is composed of 172 subfamilies. Types of odorant structures that can be recognized by some OR subfamilies and OR gene loci were predicted. (Malnic et al., 2004). Analysis of interaction profiles for 93 odorants against 219 murine and 245 human ORs gave rise to a predictive model relating physicochemical odorant properties, OR sequences, and their interactions (Saito et al., 2009). The model was based on 18 physicochemical odorant descriptors and properties of 16 OR amino acid residues. It provided a basis for translating odorants into receptor neuron responses.

Detection of the enormous range of odors requires a combinatorial strategy. Most odor molecules are recognized by more than one receptor (perhaps by dozens), and most receptors recognize several odors, probably related by chemical properties (Firestein, 2001). Each odorant receptor detects distinct sets of odorant molecules. Different odors activate overlapping but non-identical patterns of receptors. The cognition of each odor is based on the detection of signals from different sets of ORs. Two unique structural and functional features of the olfactory system enable an ability of the living organism to discriminate a large number of diverse stimuli. First, each mammalian olfactory sensory neuron expresses only one of ~1000 OR genes (Lewcock and Reed, 2004; Nguyen et al., 2007) In addition, axons from all the cells expressing that particular receptor (no matter where they are found on the epithelial sheet) converge to a single "target" in the olfactory bulb. These targets are glomeruli, spherical conglomerates of neuropils some 0.05–0.1 mm in diameter that consist of the incoming axons of olfactory sensory neurons and the dendrites of the main projection cell in the bulb, the mitral cell (Firestein, 2001).

The sensitivity to a particular ligand depends on the expression level of multiple proteins involved in olfactory cognition: olfactory receptors, proteins that participate in the signal transduction cascade, etc. The content of each protein in the cell is controlled by the expression level of the respective gene.

Transcription is the first step of gene expression at which a particular segment of DNA is copied into RNA by the complex enzyme, RNA polymerase. Transcription is precisely regulated depending on cellular conditions. The transcriptional activity of each gene is regulated by its promoter region which is located upstream of the transcription start site (TSS). Promoters contain specific DNA sequences (transcription factor binding sites), short regions of DNA (10-20 nucleotides) recognized by regulatory proteins (transcription factors). Specific interaction of transcription factors with DNA sequences within promoter region (alone or with other proteins in a complex) facilitates the recruitment of RNA polymerase to specific genes (Merkulova et al., 2013).

Eukaryotic gene regulatory regions may be organized in a complicated manner, so that the regulatory regions of a specific gene may contain binding sites for more than 20 different transcription factors (Kolchanov et al., 2000, 2002, 2008; Vaskin et al., 2011–2012). On the other hand, a great number of different regulatory proteins are involved in transcription regulation. For instance, according to recent data, the human genome encodes about 1500 transcription factors (Zhang et al., 2012; Wingender et al., 2013).

The human olfactory receptor promoters have not been studied sufficiently. Recently, the promoter architecture was characterized in details for 87.5% of the mouse OR genes (Plessy et al., 2012). It was found that 88.5% of OR promoters were of the sharp type with only a one dominant TSS position (a known feature of tissue-restricted transcripts). Moreover, 21% of OR promoters had a canonical TATA-box (binding site for TATA-binding protein). The binding of the TATA-binding protein (TBP), early B-cell factor 1 (EBF1), and myocyte-specific enhancer factor 2A (MEF2A) to OR promoters was confirmed by chromatin immunoprecipitation. The results of these experiments suggested that transcription factors TBP, EBF1 (OLF1), and MEF2A were involved in the regulation of OR expression.

A single nucleotide polymorphism, or SNP, is a variation at a single position in a DNA sequence among individuals. The 1000 Genomes Project characterizes human genomic variation by using next-generation sequencing strategies. At present, the project reports on genomes of 1092 individuals sampled from 14 populations drawn from Europe, East Asia, sub-Saharan Africa and the Americas. Over 38 million SNPs have been identified by the 1000 Genomes Project, 58.6% of which were previously undescribed (1000 Genomes Project Consortium et al., 2012). According to NCBI's dbSNP build 138 (http://www.ncbi.nlm.nih.gov/SNP/), more than half of the total number of SNPs (59.05%), identified by 1000 Genomes Project, are located in transcribed regions of the human genome, among which 1.07% of the total number are located in coding regions (exons). Of the total number of SNPs, 1.05% are located within the promoter regions of genes. The SNP density in the 500 base pair regions upstream of TSSs is approximately the same as in introns (3.7 SNPs per 1000 bp). It is considerably higher than in coding regions (2.4 SNPs per 1000 bp).

Many SNPs located in the upstream regions of genes are likely to be regulatory. One functional mechanism is that the genetic variants within upstream regions may influence gene transcription by altering the binding affinity of a transcription factor to the DNA (Chorley et al., 2008; Kim et al., 2008; Benson et al., 2011). For example, it was estimated that the G→T substitution (rs1271572) in the *ERβ* promoter prevented transcription factor Yin Yang 1 (YY1) binding and reduced its transcription activity. The TT genotype for rs1271572 was associated with increased risk for breast cancer in Chinese women and with unfavorable prognosis in Chinese breast cancer patients (Chen et al., 2013).

In the other study the T(−13,910) variant upstream the lactase-phlorizin hydrolase gene (*LPH*) associated with lactase persistence was found to bind the octamer transcription factor 1 (Oct-1) tighter than the C(−13,910) variant did. The data suggest that the binding of Oct-1 to the T(−13,910) variant directs elevated lactase promoter activity and this might provide an explanation for the lactase persistence phenotype in the human population (Lewinsky et al., 2005).

Two SNPs (T-1993C and T-1514C) in the promoter of the T box 21 (*TBX21*) gene involved in control of gene expression in T cells have been shown to be associated with systemic lupus erythematosus. Both promoter SNPs effect gene expression by modulating the affinity of a transcription factor binding sites. The affinity of the USF-1 transcription factor (upstream stimulatory factor 1) to the −1514C allele probe was higher than that to the −1514T allele probe. Individuals carrying the −1514C allele were found to have significantly reduced expression of *TBX21* in comparison to those with −1514T allele (Li et al., 2012). In a similar manner, an effect of the T-1993C SNP on the Yin Yang 1 transcription factor-mediated promoter activity was demonstrated (Li et al., 2011).

As discussed above, odor discrimination begins with interaction of volatile organic compounds with different types of low-selective olfactory receptors, inducing different patterns of glomerular activity. Therefore, the patterns of glomerular activity rather than the activities of individual olfactory sensory neurons enable living organisms to recognize odors. Thus, the variability in expression levels of OR genes caused by SNPs located in promoter regions may partly explain the variability of olfactory cognition of different olfactory stimuli and interindividual differences in olfactory perception that are observed in human populations.

The aim of the study was to analyze single nucleotide polymorphisms in promoter regions of human genes controlling olfactory cognition and transduction of olfactory stimuli in olfactory sensory neurons. Using data from the 1000 Genomes Project Consortium we found that 5.5% of human transcripts possessed extremely high SNPs contents in their upstream regions (six and more SNPs per 500-bp region). Functional analysis of this group of transcripts (genes) revealed a large portion of genes involved in olfactory transduction and antigen processing and presentation. Most of genes related to these two biological processes that have six or more SNPs per 500-bp upstream regions were found to belong to the olfactory receptor or HLA gene families. Then comparisons among all genes responsible for olfactory transduction (or antigen processing and presentation, or olfactory receptors only) and genes from the whole genome were done. Analysis of transcript distributions as a function of SNPs contents per 500-bp regions showed that SNP contents for all three functional groups of genes (transcripts) were higher than that for the whole genome set of transcripts. In addition, a similar analysis was performed for longer regions upstream TSSs (1000-bp long) and regions upstream coding region starts (CRSs). An increased genetic variability of upstream regions controlling olfactory transduction and antigen processing and presentation was also observed in these cases.

MATERIALS AND METHODS

The annotations of genes and SNPs for hg19 assembly of the human genome were extracted from the UCSC Table Browser (https://genome.ucsc.edu/cgi-bin/hgTables, the tracks *hg19 RefSeq genes* and *common SNPs(138)*, respectively; the latter track refers to the release 138 of dbSNP, http://www.ncbi.nlm.nih.gov/SNP). For SNP data, we used additional flags *class single* and *validation by 1000-genomes*. We chose 23,372 transcripts according to the following criteria: (a) only curated transcripts remained in analysis (accession numbers start with NM_, http://www.ncbi.nlm.nih.gov/books/NBK21091/); (b) only data mapped to chromosomes 1–22, X and Y remained in analysis; (c) if at least two transcripts have matching TSSs then only one of them is analyzed. Among selected 23,372 transcripts, 22,290 ones had annotated 5′-untranslated regions (5′UTRs), which means that for 22,290 transcripts positions of TSSs and coding region starts (CRSs) were different. Transcripts were annotated by the length of their 5′UTRs and gene names. We intentionally left in analysis transcripts with matching TSSs and CRSs (see **Table 1**, line *Whole-genome*). Finally, for each transcript the SNP content was determined as the count of SNPs in the 500 bp long region upstream of the annotated TSS.

Table 1 | The description of sequence sets used in analysis and their classification according to number of unique transcripts or genes and the presence/absence of annotated 5′-untranslated regions (5′UTRs).

Dataset of transcripts		Number of transcripts/genes		
Full name	**Short name**	**Total**	**5′UTR is annotated**	**5′UTR is not annotated**
Whole-genome		23,372/18,974	22,290/17,961	1082/1013
KEGG pathway *Olfactory transduction*	KEGG_Olf_Tr	414/399	104/92	310/307
KEGG pathway *Antigen processing and presentation*	KEGG_Ant_Pr_Pr	76/70	76/70	0/0
Olfactory receptor genes from HORDE	HORDE_ORs	375/372	62/62	313/310

The DAVID (Database for Annotation, Visualization and Integrated Discovery) web-based Functional Annotation Tool (DAVID tool) was applied (Huang da et al., 2007) to the set of 1258 transcripts, each containing at least six SNPs in the 500-bp region upstream the annotated TSS. The latter dataset will be designated below as *SNP-rich*. The DAVID tool performs functional analysis of large gene lists using information from GO (Gene Ontology) and KEGG (Kyoto Encyclopedia of Genes and Genomes) pathway databases. In GO, genes are annotated using a fixed vocabulary for the description of (a) biological processes in which a gene product is involved, (b) molecular functions which it executes, and (c) cellular compartments in which it is located. The GO vocabulary itself comprises more than 8000 explicitly defined terms and relations between them. The benefits of using the ontological and pathway analyses for functional annotation of group of genes revealed by different criteria have been presented in numerous publications (Smirnova et al., 2009; Jia and Zhao, 2012). The DAVID tool, which was applied for our purpose, allows detection of enriched functionally related gene groups for any specified gene list.

The result was obtained as a *Functional Annotation Chart*, which presents: (a) the list of enriched GO terms and KEGG pathways associated with the gene list; (b) the numbers of genes involved in each GO term or KEGG pathway; (c) fold enrichments for each GO term or KEGG pathway; and (d) the *P*-values for each GO term (or KEGG pathway). A Fold Enrichment is defined by DAVID tool as the ratio of two proportions: the proportion of genes with the GO category (or involved in the KEGG pathway) in a gene list under study, and the proportion of genes associated with the GO category (KEGG pathway) in the human genome. Usually, groups with fold enrichments 1.5 or more are considered to be interesting (Huang da et al., 2009). The enriched GO terms from the *biological processes* vocabulary were considered in our study. The significance of GO terms (and biological pathways) is estimated by DAVID tool on base of the number of genes from the list under study and the number of genes expected by chance. The significance of GO terms (or biological pathways) was estimated through the EASE score, a modified Fisher exact *p*-value (a built-in function of DAVID tool). The standard significance level $p < 0.05$ was applied. The count threshold value was 2 and the EASE threshold value was 0.1.

Another approach was based on the analysis of distribution of the SNP content in 500-bp long upstream regions of human genes from KEGG pathways (http://www.genome.jp/kegg/pathway.html). KEGG provides a large collection of manually derived schemes of metabolic and signaling pathways, as well as of a variety of related diseases and other processes. Namely, the pathways *Olfactory transduction* (Pathway_ID—hsa04740) and *Antigen processing and presentation* (Pathway_ID—hsa04612) were considered. In addition, the group of genes encoding ORs was considered. To estimate the promoter variability for genes encoding ORs, genes encoding ORs were extracted from HORDE (The Human Olfactory Data Explorer, http://genome.weizmann.ac.il/horde/) (Olender et al., 2013).

Final lists of transcripts for three groups were compiled according to criteria a, b, c, described above in this section for the whole-genome set of transcripts. The corrected numbers of transcripts/genes for all groups are given in **Table 1**.

The distributions of SNP contents for 500-bp long upstream regions for any k^{th} group ($k = 1, 2, 3$) of transcripts were compared to that for the whole-genome dataset. The statistical significance of differences was estimated by Welch's *t*-test for angular (arcsine square root) transformed proportions (Sokal and Rohlf, 1995). The first proportion $p_{1,n(k)}$ was computed as the ratio of the number of transcripts having at least *N* SNPs in upstream regions to the total number of transcripts in k^{th} group. The second proportion $p_{2,n}$ was calculated similarly for the whole genome dataset. For the range of thresholds *N* (from 1 to 20) the angular transformation $y(p_{i,n})$ was computed to apply the *t*-test as follows: $y_i = 2\arcsin\left(\sqrt{p_i}\right)$, where $i = 1, 2$. Additionally, in order to take into account missed annotations of 5′UTRs in some transcripts (**Table 1**), similarly to the aforementioned pipeline for analysis of 500-bp regions upstream TSSs we performed the corresponding analysis for: (a) 1000-bp regions upstream TSSs, (b) 500-bp regions upstream CRSs; in the next cases only transcripts with distinct annotated TSSs and CRSs were remained in analysis, (c) 500-bp regions upstream TSSs, and (d) 500/1000-bp regions upstream CRSs.

RESULTS

HUMAN PROMOTER VARIABILITY FOR THE WHOLE GENOME DATASET

Figure 1 shows the fractions of human transcripts (from the whole genome dataset of 23,372 transcripts, see Materials and Methods), possessing at least certain numbers of SNPs (SNP content) in 500-bp long regions upstream annotated TSSs. This number of SNPs is designated as the threshold for the SNP content in upstream region and is marked on the X-axis. The majority of transcripts have low or intermediate SNP contents in their 500-bp regions upstream annotated TSSs. For example, at least one SNP was found in the upstream regions of 81.5% of transcripts. This means that the other transcripts of the whole genome dataset (18.5%) do not contain SNP in their

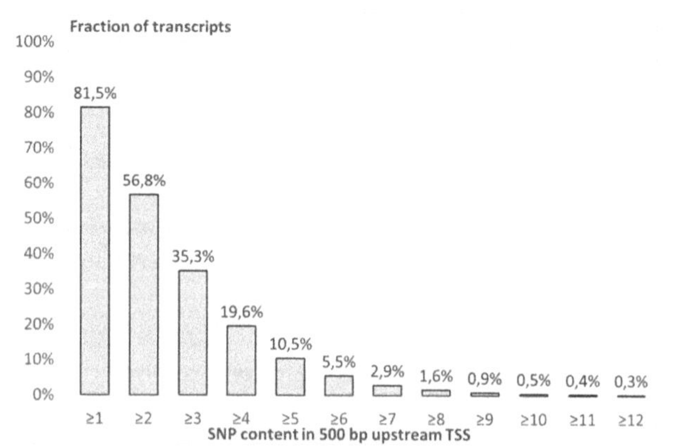

FIGURE 1 | The fraction of human transcripts from the whole genome dataset (Table 1), possessing at least certain number of SNPs in 500-bp long regions upstream annotated transcription start sites. X axis—SNP content in 500 bp upstream TSS. Y axis—fraction of the whole genome dataset of transcripts.

500-bp long upstream regions. At least two SNPs were observed in the upstream regions of 15,149 (56.8%) transcripts. However, at least six SNPs were found in 1,258 (5.5%) transcripts. As it was mentioned in Materials and Methods, this set of transcripts was designated as *SNP-rich*. The highest SNP content (53 SNPs) was found in the *HLA-DQA1* gene. Table S1 presents the list of all transcripts from the whole-genome dataset with the respective SNP contents in their 500-bp upstream regions.

BIOLOGICAL PROCESSES AND PATHWAYS OVERREPRESENTED AMONG GENES WHOSE TRANSCRIPTS WERE FOUND IN THE SNP-RICH DATASET

GO terms and biological pathways, which were overrepresented among genes whose transcripts were found to have at least six SNPs in their 500-bp long upstream regions (*SNP-rich dataset*) were selected by applying DAVID tool. As described in Materials and Methods DAVID annotation implies the classification of gene product function by relevant GO terms or KEGG pathway. Hence, in such a way, the gene sets could be functionally annotated and enriched GO terms and biologically relevant pathways could be identified. Inspection of GO categories overrepresented in the *SNP-rich dataset* revealed two biological processes among the top ones: *sensory perception of smell* and *antigen processing and presentation*. In both cases, fold enrichment exceeded 1.5, and *P*-Values were less than 0.01 (**Table 2**).

According to the DAVID report, the group of genes annotated by the GO term *sensory perception of smell* includes 45 genes encoding odorant receptors and three other genes: *OBP2A* (Odorant-binding protein 2a); *GNAL* (guanine nucleotide binding protein (G protein), alpha activating activity polypeptide, olfactory type); and *PDE1C* (phosphodiesterase 1C, calmodulin-dependent 70kDa). The upstream region of *OR9G1* (olfactory receptor, family 9, subfamily G, member 1 gene) was extremely variable, containing 15 SNPs per 500 bp.

Eighteen genes from *SNP-rich dataset* were annotated by the GO category antigen processing and presentation. Among them, 12 genes (*HLA-DQB1, HLA-DRB1, HLA-A, HLA-C, HLA-B, HLA-DQA2, HLA-G, HLA-DQA1, HLA-F, HLA-DRB5, HLA-DPA1, HLA-DRA*) belonged to the HLA gene family, and six genes (*MICB, MICA, LOC554223, TAP2, ULBP2, CTSE*) belonged to other families. This group contained two genes (*HLA-DQA1, HLA-B*) that had the highest promoter SNP contents (53 and 29, respectively) among all genes from the whole-genome dataset.

Inspection of KEGG pathways whose genes were overrepresented in the *SNP-rich dataset* identified two top pathways: *Olfactory transduction* (Pathway_ID—hsa04740) and *Antigen processing and presentation* (Pathway_ID—hsa04612). Since in both cases the fold enrichment exceeds 1.5 and *P*-Value is below 0.01 (**Table 3**), we conclude that genes from these two KEGG pathways are significantly overrepresented in the *SNP-rich dataset*. A substantial fraction of genes (96%, or 43 of 45) found to be involved in the olfactory transduction pathway were recognized as olfactory receptor genes. A half of genes (12 of 22) involved in antigen processing and presentation pathway belonged to the family of genes called the human leukocyte antigen (*HLA*) complex.

PROMOTER VARIABILITY FOR GENES CONTROLLING OLFACTORY TRANSDUCTION, ANTIGEN PROCESSING, AND PRESENTATION AND GENES ENCODING OLFACTORY RECEPTORS

Our second analysis was undertaken to compare promoter variability for genes controlling olfactory transduction or antigen processing and presentation to that for the whole-genome dataset. The lists of genes, belonging to these two pathways were extracted from the KEGG database. These lists are denoted below as *KEGG_Olf_Tr* and *KEGG_Ant_Pr_Pr*, respectively (**Table 1**).

Since olfactory receptor genes comprise a large fraction of genes detected in the *SNP-rich dataset* by GO and pathway analysis, it was interesting to analyze promoter variability for this genes. For this purpose, the gene list *HORDE_ORs* was compiled using data from HORDE (**Table 1**).

The comparison of distribution of the SNP content in 500-bp long regions upstream annotated TSSs in either group of transcripts and that for the whole-genome dataset shows that transcripts of all groups tend to have higher SNP contents

Table 2 | Biological processes overrepresented ($p < 0.05$) in the *SNP-rich dataset*, which includes transcripts with at least six SNPs in 500-bp upstream regions.

Biological process (GO category)	Number of genes from the *SNP-rich dataset* annotated by the category	Fold enrichment	*p*-Value	Genes
GO:0007608~sensory perception of smell	48	1.7	1.98E-04	*OR10A5, OR52H1, OR51B2, OR1L8, OR1A2, OR5D16, OR52J3, OR51F1, OR1N2, OR8S1, OR1L3, OR11G2, OR13C5, OR4C10, OR10G9, OR8I2, OR7C2, OR51L1, OR2C3, OR8G1, OR14C36, OR2AG1, OR2B11, OR8G5, OR11L1, OR4M2, OR6C74, OR9G1, OR6C75, OR6T1, OR2W3, OR51G2, OR10Z1, OR12D2, OR5H14, OR10AD1, OR52E6, OR11H6, OR4A15, OR5H15, OR10Q1, OR4C45, OR5H6, OR7D4, OR6K6, OBP2A, PDE1C, GNAL*
GO:0019882~antigen processing and presentation	18	3.32	3.95 E-05	*HLA-DQB1, HLA-DRB1, HLA-A, HLA-C, HLA-B, HLA-DQA2, HLA-G, HLA-DQA1, HLA-F, HLA-DRB5, HLA-DPA1, HLA-DRA, MICB, MICA, LOC554223, TAP2, ULBP2, CTSE*

Table 3 | Biological pathways overrepresented ($p < 0.05$) in the *SNP-rich dataset*, which includes transcripts with at least six SNPs in their 500-bp upstream regions.

KEGG pathway	Number of genes from the *SNP-rich dataset* belonging to the pathway	Fold enrichment	*p*-Value	Genes
Olfactory transduction (Pathway_ID—hsa04740)	45	1.68	6.37E-04	*OR10A5, OR52H1, OR51B2, OR1L8, OR1A2, OR5D16, OR52J3, OR51F1, OR1N2, OR8S1, OR1L3, OR11G2, OR13C5, OR4C16, OR10G9, OR8I2, OR51L1, OR7C2, OR2C3, OR8G1, OR14C36, OR2AG1, OR2B11, OR8G5, OR11L1, OR4M2, OR6C74, OR9G1, OR6C75, OR6T1, OR2W3, OR51G2, OR10Z1, OR12D2, OR10AD1, OR52E6, OR11H6, OR4A15, OR4C45, OR10Q1, OR5H6, OR7D4, OR6K6, GNAL, PDE1C*
Antigen processing and presentation (Pathway_ID—hsa04612)	24	4.0	2.11E-08	*HLA-DQB1, HLA-DRB1, HLA-A, HLA-C, HLA-B, HLA-DQA2, HLA-G, HLA-DQA1, HLA-F, HLA-DRB5, HLA-DPA1, HLA-DRA, HSP90AB1, IFNA21, KLRC3, IFNA10, KIR2DS4, HSPA2, TAP2, TAP1, HSPA6, IFNA16, IFNA17, CD4*

(**Figures 2A–C**). To confirm this conclusion, we applied the *t*-test for angular transformed proportions (see Materials and Methods). This test was applied for the range of thresholds of SNP content (**Figure 2D**). We concluded that for any threshold of SNP content from one to nine the significant enrichment of transcripts with SNPs was observed for all the three gene groups.

To ensure that missed annotation of 5′UTRs for transcripts of whole genome dataset, and especially for transcripts of *HORDE_ORs* and *KEGG_Olf_Tr* groups (**Table 1**) cannot substantially influence our conclusions, we performed additional analyses.

Below we will use the designations (−1 kb; TSS), (−500; TSS), (−1 kb; CRS), (−500; CRS) for 1000-bp or 500-bp regions upstream TSSs or CRSs. The prefixes 5′UTR ≥ 0 or 5′UTR > 0 mean that a 5′UTR may have any length, or only a positive value is allowed (i.e., the TSS and CRS positions are different). In these terms, a pipeline analysis in the case 5′UTR ≥ 0_(−500; TSS) is presented above in this section (**Figure 2**).

The results, similar to those depicted in **Figure 2D,** i.e., dependencies of the significance of the *t*-test on the threshold of SNP contents for the different combinations of upstream region lengths and locations and on 5′UTR's annotation availability are presented in Figure S2. We came to the following conclusions:

(a) 5′UTR ≥ 0_(−1 kb; TSS) case (Figure S2A). We observed the pattern similar to that in the 5′UTR > 0_(−500; TSS) case; however, the group of smallest size (*KEGG_Ant_Pr_Pr*) revealed very moderate significance of the *t*-test ($p < 0.02$ for at least eight SNPs).

(b) 5′UTR > 0_(−500; TSS) case. All groups show less significant results than in the 5′UTR ≥ 0_(−500; TSS) case described above (**Figure 2D**); nevertheless the significance $p < 0.05$ is observed for SNP content thresholds from two to six.

(c) 5′UTR ≥ 0_(−500; CRS) case. The overall results are similar to those described previously for the case 5′UTR ≥ 0_(−500; TSS).

(d) The 5′UTR > 0_(−500; CRS) and 5′UTR > 0_(−1 kb; CRS) cases show that only for the latter case an SNPs enrichment is observed for all three test groups (Figures S2D,E).

The 5′UTR ≥0 (−1 kb; TSS) case proves that the enrichment of upstream regions with SNPs hardly can strongly depend on region length. In the 5′UTR > 0_(−500; TSS) case, we are sure that the enrichment is related to the promoter region of a gene. The 5′UTR ≥ 0_(−500; CRS) case allows us to suppose that, as in case of promoter regions, 5′UTRs also have an enrichment of SNPs for transcripts of all three groups under study. However, the cases 5′UTR > 0_(−500; CRS) and 5′UTR > 0_(−1 kb; CRS) argue for the major impact of promoter region in the enrichment of SNPs in the upstream regions of transcripts classified into three groups.

DISCUSSION

INCREASED GENETIC VARIABILITY IN THE PROMOTER REGIONS OF GENES CONTROLLING SENSORY PERCEPTION OF SMELL AND ANTIGEN PROCESSING AND PRESENTATION

Our study revealed a broad variability of SNP contents in promoters of genes from the whole-genome dataset. Almost a one-fifth (18.5%) of the total number of promoters had no SNPs at all (**Figure 1**). However, a very interesting set of promoters characterized by high SNP contents (six or more SNPs) was found. Among the genes with high SNP content in promoters, three groups were overrepresented according to the DAVID tool (Huang da et al., 2007): (1) genes controlling the sensory perception of smell; (2) a specific subset of promoters of sensory perception genes encoding olfactory receptors (ORs), and (3) genes involved in antigen processing and presentation (**Tables 2, 3**). We compared the contents of SNPs in the upstream regions of genes of the aforementioned groups with that for the whole genome dataset by Welch's *t*-test for angular transformed proportions. It was shown that promoters of all three groups were characterized by increased genetic variability in comparison to that for the whole genome dataset. The detailed analysis showed that regions

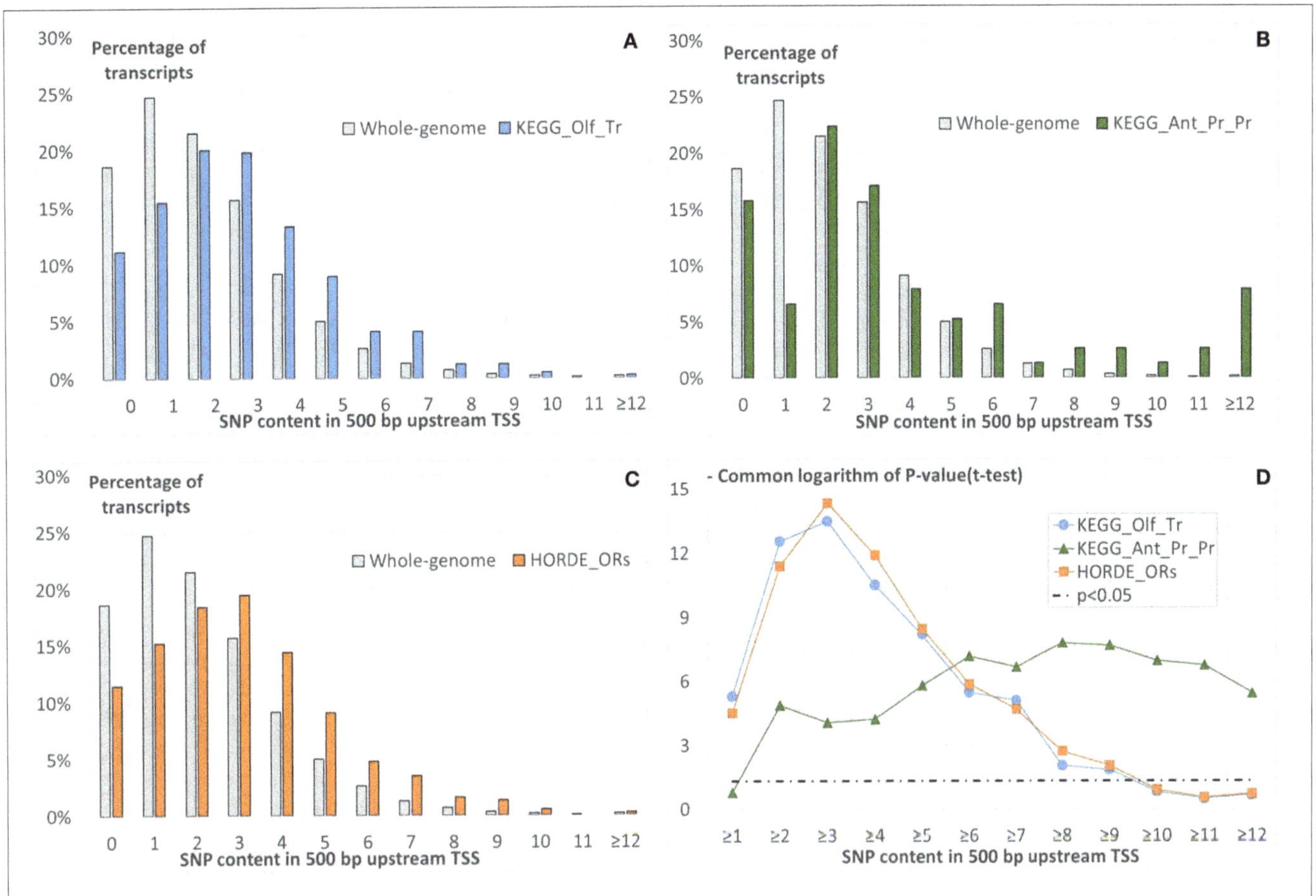

FIGURE 2 | The comparison of SNP content distributions in upstream regions of three groups of human transcripts with that for whole-genome dataset (Table 1). First 500-bp upstream annotated TSSs are analyzed. The groups are derived from KEGG pathways **(A)** *Olfactory transduction*, **(B)** *Antigen processing and presentation*, and **(C)** from HORDE. In panels from **(A** to **C)** the X axis denotes the SNP content; the Y axis, the count of transcripts with specific SNPs in the upstream regions. Panel **(D)** presents the significances of the *t*-test (Y axis), which compare the above-described SNP contents in three groups with that for the whole genome dataset as a function of the SNP content (X axis). The *t*-test was applied as described in Materials and Methods.

located both upstream and immediately downstream the transcription start, participated in SNPs enrichment (Figure S2). The clarification of this issue is still hampered by the scarce annotation of TSSs in genome. Nevertheless, the importance of 5′UTRs for transcription regulation is still underestimated (Omelina et al., 2011).

PARALLELISM BETWEEN OLFACTORY COGNITION AND FUNCTIONS OF THE IMMUNE SYSTEM (ABILITY TO DISTINGUISH BETWEEN SELF AND NON-SELF)

The whole-genome analysis of the SNP content in promoter DNA revealed two interesting groups of genes with the highest genetic variability: genes controlling sensory perception of smell and genes responsible for antigen processing and presentation. Actually, the biological functions of these two systems are similar. As far back as 1975, parallelism and even adaptive molecular convergence between olfactory cognition, on the one hand, and the heart of the immune system, its ability to distinguish between self and non-self, was found (Thomas, 1975). Both systems are targeted on the reception of extremely variable chemical compounds in the environment of living organisms and immune recognition of parasitic and commensal microbiotas, which evolve very rapidly. Therefore, it is not surprising that genes of both these systems have the highest promoter SNP contents among all genes in the human genome. Such extremely high variability may cause diversity in the expression levels of olfactory receptors and genes of the immune system as well. Recently, it has been suggested that OR diversity is maintained to an extent by balancing selection, similar to that acting upon the major histocompatibility complex alleles at the population level (Olender et al., 2012). Our results suggest that regulatory regions of OR genes and genes responsible for antigen processing and presentation may also be under such selection.

GENETIC DIVERSITY IN CODING REGIONS OF OR GENES AND VARIATIONS IN ODOR PERCEPTION

The ability to detect many odors varies among individuals; however, the contribution of genotype to this variation has been assessed for relatively few compounds. Several recent studies demonstrate that the genetic variation in the coding regions of human OR genes contributes to the variation in odor perception among individuals.

The human odorant receptor, *OR7D4*, is selectively activated *in vitro* by androstenone and the related odorous steroid androstadienone (androsta-4,16-dien-3-one), and it does not respond to a panel of other 64 odors and two solvents. Genotypic variation in *OR7D4* accounts for a significant proportion of the valence (pleasantness or unpleasantness) and intensity variance in perception of these steroidal odors. A common variant of this receptor contains two non-synonymous SNPs, resulting in two amino acid substitutions (R88W, T133M; hence 'RT') that severely impair its function *in vitro*. Human subjects with RT/WM or WM/WM genotypes were less sensitive to androstenone and androstadienone, and they found both odors less unpleasant than the RT/RT group did (Keller et al., 2007). Since androstenone is naturally present in meat derived from male pigs, the study evaluating the effect of two non-synonymous SNPs in *OR7D4* gene on food preferences was carried out. When pork containing varying levels of androstenone was cooked and tested by sniffing and tasting, subjects with two copies of the RT variant tended to rate the androstenone-containing meat as less favorable than subjects carrying the WM variant (Lunde et al., 2012). It was also found that the genetic variation in *OR7D4* (variant rs8109935) may influence odor perception (pleasantness/unpleasantness) between heterosexual partners (Sookoian et al., 2011).

The genetic basis of odorant-specific variations in human olfactory thresholds, and, in particular, of enhanced odorant sensitivity (hyperosmia) was explored. The association between olfactory detection threshold phenotypes for four odorants and segregating pseudogene genotypes of 43 ORs was examined (Menashe et al., 2007). A strong association signal was observed between the SNP variants in *OR11H7P* and sensitivity to the odorant isovaleric acid. This association was largely due to the low frequency of homozygous pseudogenized genotype in individuals with specific hyperosmia to this odorant, implying a possible functional role of *OR11H7P* in isovaleric acid detection.

Resting on the fact that smoking behavior has been associated in two independent European cohorts with the most common Caucasian human leukocyte antigen (HLA) haplotype (A1-B8-DR3), a study linking smoking to a distinct OR allele was carried out (Santos et al., 2008). The non-synonymous SNP within the *OR12D3* gene (rs3749971) was found to be associated with the HLA haplotype-dependent differential recognition of cigarette smoke components for the Hungarian cohort. This polymorphism leads to a Thr → Ile substitution that affects a putative ligand-binding region of the OR12D3 protein.

A genetic basis for the ability to detect the flavor compound cis-3-hexen-1-ol was determined recently (McRae et al., 2012). This compound is typically described as "green grassy" or the smell of "cut grass." One SNP variant (rs28757581), found in the coding region of the *OR2J3* gene, was strongly associated with cis-3-hexen-1-ol detection threshold concentrations. This polymorphism encodes a T113A substitution in OR2J3 protein. The *OR2J3* gene contained five predicted haplotypes in the 52 individuals from New Zealand. The majority of the individuals studied were Caucasians (73.6%), and other subjects were Indians (13.2%), Asians (11.3%), and Maoris (1.9%). All five haplotypes were tested *in vitro*. It was shown that two amino acid substitutions, T113A and R226Q, impaired the ability of OR2J3 to respond to *cis*-3-hexen-1-ol, and the presence of both effectively abolished the response to the compound. The haplotype of *OR2J3* containing both T113A and R226Q was responsible for 26.4% of the variation in cis-3-hexen-1-ol detection in the cohort under consideration.

THE BIOLOGICAL SIGNIFICANCE OF SNPs LOCATED IN UPSTREAM REGIONS OF GENES INVOLVED IN OLFACTORY TRANSDUCTION

Evidence for biological significant variation found in the upstream region of the olfactory receptor 2M7 (*OR2M7*) gene was obtained from two unrelated studies. Thirty-eight adult men and women from Philadelphia (Caucasian; African-American; Asian etc.) participated in the first study (Pelchat et al., 2011). One SNP within a cluster of fifty olfactory receptor genes was found to be associated with the inability to smell the asparagus odor, which is detected in urine of people who have recently eaten asparagus. The urine of these people has a sulfurous odor, which is distinct and similar to cooked cabbage. Asparagusic acid (1,2-dithiolane-4-carboxylic acid) is found in asparagus, and it may be the precursor to some of the sulfur metabolites found in asparagus urine. The most common odorant detected in asparagus urine is methanethiol. The inability to smell the asparagus odor in urine was associated with the variant rs4481887 located upstream the *OR2M7* gene. The A allele was associated with greater ability to detect the asparagus odorant than G. There were racial differences in rs4481887 allele frequency, with Caucasian subjects having a minor allele frequency of 0.35, whereas there was no observed genetic variation in subjects of African descent (all genotypes were GG) (Pelchat et al., 2011). The same allele was associated with the ability to smell the asparagus odor in the second study, which reported results for individuals having European ancestry (Eriksson et al., 2010). Since this SNP is located approximately 9 kb upstream of the *OR2M7* translation initiation codon, these two studies provide the first piece of evidence for significant biological variation found in the upstream region of an olfactory receptor gene. It is conceivable that the nucleotide substitution in this position changes the affinity of some transcription factor to the DNA region containing the SNP, affecting the *OR2M7* gene expression level.

The obvious demonstration that the nucleotide substitution in promoter region of gene from olfactory transduction pathway can alter the binding of a transcription factor and thus result in impaired gene transcription was obtained for the *ADRBK2* gene. *ADRBK2* encodes G-protein-coupled receptor kinase 3R (GRK3) which participates in termination of olfactory signaling, phosphorylating activated olfactory receptors and thus transforming them to the desensitized state (Boekhoff et al., 1997). It was demonstrated that the rare variant of SNP G-384A (rs41261045) disrupts Sp1 transcription factor binding to DNA *in vitro*, and increases *ADRBK2* promoter-driven expression in cell transfection models (Zhou et al., 2008). The rare variant of SNP G-384A was reported to be associated with bipolar disorder in two independent samples (Barrett et al., 2003). However, in this case the possible effect of the G→A nucleotide substitution on olfactory cognition has not been studied.

Two SNPs in the upstream region of *OR51B4* gene were found among genetic modifiers of Hb E/b0 thalassemia identified by a two-stage genome-wide association study (Sherva et al., 2010). Both SNPs were significantly associated with disease severity. One SNP (rs10837774) was less than 500 bp upstream from the start of *OR51B4* transcript. The other (rs3886223) located ~20 kb upstream from *OR51B4* was the most closely associated SNP in this group, with the common allele contributing to increased risk of severe disease in an additive fashion.

Thus, only few studies describe the effects of polymorphisms found in upstream regions of olfactory receptors genes. Nevertheless, investigations of SNPs in the upstream regions of the *OR2M7, OR51B4,* and *ADRBK2* genes involved in olfactory transduction (Zhou et al., 2008; Eriksson et al., 2010; Pelchat et al., 2011) as well as SNPs in the upstream regions of *ERβ, LPH, TBX21* and many other genes controlling a variety of cellular processes (Lewinsky et al., 2005; Li et al., 2011, 2012; Chen et al., 2013) show that such SNPs may have a great impact on phenotypic traits.

THE EXTREMELY HIGH GENETIC DIVERSITY OF HUMAN OLFACTORY RECEPTOR GENES ESTIMATED FROM THE 1000 GENOMES PROJECT DATASET

Olfactory receptor genes are the largest gene family in the human genome comprising ~400 genes and ~600 pseudogenes (Firestein, 2001; Hasin et al., 2008; Olender et al., 2012). Therefore, ORs may be a special challenge for high-throughput sequencing and genotyping due to the high level of homology observed in their coding regions. Nevertheless, we believe, that the high genetic diversity of upstream regions of OR genes observed in our study could not be explained, entirely or partially, by incorrect assemblage of the olfactory genome.

First, in both phase 1 and pilot stages of the 1000 Genomes project the special filter *depth threshold* was applied to remove miscalling of SNPs based on the mapping of paralogous sequences (1000 Genomes Project Consortium et al., 2010). The filters on coverage and fraction of reads with low mapping quality lead to the exclusion of a substantial fraction of sites in the genome. More details are presented in the Supplementary section (Part 3). We are sure that if the upstream regions of olfactory receptor genes had any assembly problems their SNPs would certainly be excluded from the final SNP set.

Second, an unusually high genetic diversity of genes of the olfactory transduction pathway was described in the 1000 Genomes Project report (1000 Genomes Project Consortium et al., 2012). According to table S13 presented in the Supplementary Information to this report, genes belonging to the KEGG pathway *Olfactory transduction* (of which 92% belong to the odorant receptor family) had the highest SNP content in coding regions (16.9 SNPs per 1000 bp) among examined KEGG pathways. As presented in Figure S11b in the Supplementary Information to 1000 Genomes Project report, the genes from the olfactory transduction pathway had an excessive number of rare non-synonymous SNPs and a high level of conservation in the American ancestry-based group.

Third, an unusually high genetic diversity was found previously in coding regions of human olfactory receptor genes. On average, two individuals have functional differences at over 30% of their odorant receptor alleles (Mainland et al., 2014). The degree of genomic variation for coding regions of OR genes was one SNP per 66 bases, 2.5 times larger than in coding exons of the control genes (Olender et al., 2012). In that study, a comprehensive catalog of genetic variability in the human olfactory receptor genes was compiled. A major resource for this work was the 1000 Genomes Projects whole genome sequence data, and to a lesser extent, dbSNP. The authors performed experimental validation of non-functional SNPs using a custom SNP array (Illumina GoldenGate Genotyping Assay). The final design included 285 non-functional OR variations, of which 268 were successfully genotyped in a cohort of 468 individuals of two ethnicities (validation rate 94%). The majority (65%) of the unsupported variations were mined from dbSNP (Olender et al., 2012). We believe that this high validation rate (94%) revealed for non-functional SNPs in coding regions of OR genes by Olender et al. (2012) confirms the validity of the 1000 Genomes Projects data for all olfactory receptor loci in whole.

FINAL CONCLUSIONS

The majority of investigations of OR genes demonstrate that genetic variability in coding regions of OR genes may be associated with differences in olfactory cognition and odor perception, confirming the idea of functional importance of coding SNPs. The impact of SNPs, located in the 5′regions of OR genes on gene function and phenotype is still defined very poorly. However, the examples considered above demonstrate that (a) some polymorphic alleles in upstream regions of genes involved in olfactory cognition may be associated with variations in odor perception; (b) genetic variation in the promoter region may considerably impair transcriptional regulation of a particular gene, changing morphological, behavioral, physical, and/or biochemical traits of an organism. We suggest that the extremely high SNP content in the promoters of OR genes revealed in our study causes variations in gene expression. In turn, the elevated variability in ORs expression may partly explain individual differences in odor perception.

The extremely high level of the SNP content in promoters of olfactory receptor genes revealed in our study raises the question about the functional significance of such SNPs for olfactory cognition as well as about their association with human diseases. The genome-wide view on human olfaction with the emphasis on regulatory SNPs may provide understanding of some aspects of personalized odor coding. Theoretical analysis of the potential functional role of nucleotide substitutions found in upstream regions of genes may outline possible molecular mechanisms of SNP effects at the gene expression level. These two approaches combined with subsequent experimental verification of theoretical assumptions and hypotheses may be helpful for understanding the molecular mechanism linking olfactory cognition with individual emotional and behavioral reactions to a broad variety of olfactory stimuli: air pollutants, human body odors (including body odors affected by anxiety or bacteria), odors in culinary etc.

AUTHOR CONTRIBUTIONS

Elena V. Ignatieva, Mikhail P. Moshkin and Nikolay A. Kolchanov designed the study. Elena V. Ignatieva, Victor G. Levitsky performed the study. Elena V. Ignatieva, Victor G. Levitsky, Nikolay S. Yudin were involved in data analysis. Elena V. Ignatieva drafted the manuscript. Victor G. Levitsky, Nikolay S. Yudin, Mikhail P. Moshkin and Nikolay A. Kolchanov corrected the manuscript. All authors read and approved the final manuscript.

ACKNOWLEDGMENTS

The authors are grateful to Victor V. Gulevich for editing the English translation. Nikolay A. Kolchanov was partly supported by Presidium of the Siberian Branch of the Russian Academy of Sciences (project No. VI.61.1.2 from nominate VI.61). Elena V. Ignatieva was partly supported by project No. 14.B25.31.0033 (of 28.07.2013) under Russian Federation government decree N 220 (of 09.04.2010). Nikolay S. Yudin was partly supported by Russian Foundation for Basic Research (grant no. 13-04-00968). Victor G. Levitsky was partly supported by Russian Foundation for Basic Research (grant no. 12-04-33112). Mikhail P. Moshkin was partly supported by the Interdisciplinary Integration Research grants from the Siberian Branch of the Russian Academy of Sciences (grants no. 57, 60, 61, 108, and 122).

REFERENCES

1000 Genomes Project Consortium, Abecasis, G. R., Altshuler, D., Auton, A., Brooks, L. D., Durbin, R. M., et al. (2010). A map of human genome variation from population-scale sequencing. *Nature* 467, 1061–1073. doi: 10.1038/nature09534

1000 Genomes Project Consortium, Abecasis, G. R., Auton, A., Brooks, L. D., DePristo, M. A., Durbin, R. M., et al. (2012). An integrated map of genetic variation from 1,092 human genomes. *Nature* 491, 56–65. doi: 10.1038/nature11632

Ayabe-Kanamura, S., Saito, S., Distel, H., Martínez-Gómez, M., and Hudson, R. (1998). Differences and similarities in the perception of everyday odors. A Japanese-German cross-cultural study. *Ann. N.Y. Acad. Sci.* 855, 694–700. doi: 10.1111/j.1749-6632.1998.tb10647.x

Barrett, T. B., Hauger, R. L., Kennedy, J. L., Sadovnick, A. D., Remick, R. A., Kec, P. E., et al. (2003). Evidence that a single nucleotide polymorphism in the promoter of the G protein receptor kinase 3 gene is associated with bipolar disorder. *Mol. Psychiatry* 8, 546–557. doi: 10.1038/sj.mp.4001268

Benson, C. C., Zhou, Q., Long, X., and Miano, J. M. (2011). Identifying functional single nucleotide polymorphisms in the human CArGome. *Physiol. Genomics* 43, 1038–1048. doi: 10.1152/physiolgenomics.00098.2011

Boekhoff, I., Touhara, K., Danner, S., Inglese, J., Lohse, M. J., Breer, H., et al. (1997). Phosducin, potential role in modulation of olfactory signaling. *J. Biol. Chem.* 272, 4606–4612. doi: 10.1074/jbc.272.7.4606

Buck, L., and Axel, R. (1991). A novel multigene family may encode odorant receptors: a molecular basis for odor recognition. *Cell* 65, 175–187. doi: 10.1016/0092-8674(91)90418-X

Chen, L., Liang, Y., Qiu, J., Zhang, L., Chen, X., Luo, X., et al. (2013). Significance of rs1271572 in the estrogen receptor beta gene promoter and its correlation with breast cancer in a southwestern Chinese population. *J. Biomed. Sci.* 20, 32. doi: 10.1186/1423-0127-20-32

Chorley, B. N., Wang, X., Campbell, M. R., Pittman, G. S., Noureddine, M. A., and Bell, D. A. (2008). Discovery and verification of functional single nucleotide polymorphisms in regulatory genomic regions: current and developing technologies. *Mutat. Res.* 659, 147–157. doi: 10.1016/j.mrrev.2008.05.001

De Palo, G., Boccaccio, A., Miri, A., Menini, A., and Altafini, C. (2012). A dynamical feedback model for adaptation in the olfactory transduction pathway. *Biophys. J.* 102, 2677–2686. doi: 10.1016/j.bpj.2012.04.040

Eriksson, N., Macpherson, J. M., Tung, J. Y., Hon, L. S., Naughton, B., Saxonov, S., et al. (2010). Web-based, participant-driven studies yield novel genetic associations for common traits. *PLoS Genet.* 6:e1000993. doi: 10.1371/journal.pgen.1000993

Firestein, S. (2001). How the olfactory system makes sense of scents. *Nature* 413, 211–218. doi: 10.1038/35093026

Gilad, Y., Bustamante, C. D., Lancet, D., and Pääbo, S. (2003). Natural selection on the olfactory receptor gene family in humans and chimpanzees. *Am. J. Hum. Genet.* 73, 489–501. doi: 10.1086/378132

Glusman, G., Yanai, I., Rubin, I., and Lancet, D. (2001). The complete human olfactory subgenome. *Genome Res.* 11, 685–702. doi: 10.1101/gr.171001

Greenberg, M. I., Curtis, J. A., and Vearrier, D. (2013). The perception of odor is not a surrogate marker for chemical exposure: a review of factors influencing human odor perception. *Clin. Toxicol. (Phila).* 51, 70–76. doi: 10.3109/15563650.2013.767908

Hasin, Y., Olender, T., Khen, M., Gonzaga-Jauregui, C., Kim, P. M., Urban, A. E., et al. (2008). High-resolution copy-number variation map reflects human olfactory receptor diversity and evolution. *PLoS Genet.* 4:e1000249. doi: 10.1371/journal.pgen.1000249

Hrdlicka, M., Vodicka, J., Havlovicova, M., Urbanek, T., Blatny, M., and Dudova, I. (2011). Brief report: significant differences in perceived odor pleasantness found in children with ASD. *J. Autism Dev. Disord.* 41, 524–527. doi: 10.1007/s10803-010-1084-x

Huang da, W., Sherman, B. T., and Lempicki, R. A. (2009). Systematic and integrative analysis of large gene lists using DAVID bioinformatics resources. *Nat. Protoc.* 4, 44–57. doi: 10.1038/nprot.2008.211

Huang da, W., Sherman, B. T., Tan, Q., Collins, J. R., Alvord, W. G., Roayaei, J., et al. (2007). The DAVID gene functional classification tool: a novel biological module-centric algorithm to functionally analyze large gene lists. *Genome Biol.* 8:R183. doi: 10.1186/gb-2007-8-9-r183

Jahromi, M. M. (2012). Haplotype specific alteration of diabetes MHC risk by olfactory receptor gene polymorphism. *Autoimmun. Rev.* 12, 270–274. doi: 10.1016/j.autrev.2012.05.001

Jia, P., and Zhao, Z. (2012). Personalized pathway enrichment map of putative cancer genes from next generation sequencing data. *PLoS ONE* 7:e37595. doi: 10.1371/journal.pone.003759

Keller, A., Hempstead, M., Gomez, I. A., Gilbert, A. N., and Vosshall, L. B. (2012). An olfactory demography of a diverse metropolitan population. *BMC Neurosci.* 13:122. doi: 10.1186/1471-2202-13-122

Keller, A., Zhuang, H., Chi, Q., Vosshall, L. B., and Matsunami, H. (2007). Genetic variation in a human odorant receptor alters odour perception. *Nature* 449, 468–472. doi: 10.1038/nature06162

Kim, B. C., Kim, W. Y., Park, D., Chung, W. H., Shin, K. S., and Bhak, J. (2008). SNP@Promoter: a database of human SNPs (single nucleotide polymorphisms) within the putative promoter regions. *BMC Bioinformatics* 9(Suppl. 1):S2. doi: 10.1186/1471-2105-9-S1-S2

Knaapila, A., Zhu, G., Medland, S. E., Wysocki, C. J., Montgomery, G. W., Martin, N. G., et al. (2012). A genome-wide study on the perception of the odorants androstenone and galaxolide. *Chem. Senses* 37, 541–552. doi: 10.1093/chemse/bjs008

Kolchanov, N. A., Ignatieva, E. V., Ananko, E. A., Podkolodnaya, O. A., Stepanenko, I. L., Merkulova, T. I., et al. (2002). Transcription regulatory regions database (TRRD): its status in 2002. *Nucleic Acids Res.* 30, 312–317. doi: 10.1093/nar/30.1.312

Kolchanov, N. A., Ignatieva, E. V., Podkolodnaya, O. A., Ananko, E. A., Khlebodarova, T. M., Stepanenko, I. L., et al. (2008). TRRD: technology for extraction, storage, and use of knowledge about the structural-functional organization of the transcriptional regulatory regions in the eukaryotic genes. *Intell. Data Anal.* 12, 443–461.

Kolchanov, N. A., Podkolodnaya, O. A., Ananko, E. A., Ignatieva, E. V., Stepanenko, I. L., Kel-Margoulis, O. V., et al. (2000). Transcription regulatory regions database (TRRD): its status in 2000. *Nucleic Acids Res.* 28, 298–301. doi: 10.1093/nar/28.1.298

Lewcock, J. W., and Reed, R. R. (2004). A feedback mechanism regulates monoallelic odorant receptor expression. *Proc. Natl. Acad. Sci. U.S.A.* 101, 1069–1074. doi: 10.1073/pnas.0307986100

Lewinsky, R. H., Jensen, T. G., Møller, J., Stensballe, A., Olsen, J., and Troelsen, J. T. (2005). T-13910 DNA variant associated with lactase persistence interacts with Oct-1 and stimulates lactase promoter activity *in vitro*. *Hum. Mol. Genet.* 14, 3945–3953. doi: 10.1093/hmg/ddi418

Li, J., Li, J., You, Y., and Chen, S. (2012). The role of upstream stimulatory factor 1 in the transcriptional regulation of the human TBX21 promoter mediated by the T-1514C polymorphism associated with systemic lupus erythematosus. *Immunogenetics* 64, 361–370. doi: 10.1007/s00251-011-0597-6

Li, J. R., Li, J. G., Deng, G. H., Zhao, W. L., Dan, Y. J., Wang, Y. M., et al. (2011). Common promoter variant of TBX21 is associated with allele specific binding to Yin-Yang 1 and reduced gene expression. *Scand. J. Immunol.* 73, 449–458. doi: 10.1111/j.1365-3083.2011.02520.x

Lunde, K., Egelandsdal, B., Skuterud, E., Mainland, J. D., Lea, T., Hersleth, M., et al. (2012). Genetic variation of an odorant receptor OR7D4 and sensory perception of cooked meat containing androstenone. *PLoS ONE* 7:e35259. doi: 10.1371/journal.pone.0035259

Mainland, J. D., Keller, A., Li, Y. R., Zhou, T., Trimmer, C., Snyder, L. L., et al. (2014). The missense of smell: functional variability in the human odorant receptor repertoire. *Nat. Neurosci.* 17, 114–120. doi: 10.1038/nn.3598

Malnic, B., Godfrey, P. A., and Buck, L. B. (2004). The human olfactory receptor gene family. *Proc. Natl. Acad. Sci. U.S.A.* 101, 2584–2589. doi: 10.1073/pnas.0307882100

Mashukova, A., Spehr, M., Hatt, H., and Neuhaus, E. M. (2006). Beta-arrestin2-mediated internalization of mammalian odorant receptors. *J. Neurosci.* 26, 9902–9912. doi: 10.1523/JNEUROSCI.2897-06.2006

McRae, J. F., Mainland, J. D., Jaeger, S. R., Adipietro, K. A., Matsunami, H., and Newcomb, R. D. (2012). Genetic variation in the odorant receptor OR2J3 is associated with the ability to detect the "grassy" smelling odor, cis-3-hexen-1-ol. *Chem. Senses* 37, 585–593. doi: 10.1093/chemse/bjs049

Menashe, I., Abaffy, T., Hasin, Y., Goshen, S., Yahalom, V., Luetje, C. W., et al. (2007). Genetic elucidation of human hyperosmia to isovaleric acid. *PLoS Biol.* 5:e284. doi: 10.1371/journal.pbio.0050284

Menashe, I., Aloni, R., and Lancet, D. (2006). A probabilistic classifier for olfactory receptor pseudogenes. *BMC Bioinformatics* 7, 393. doi: 10.1186/1471-2105-7-393

Merkulova, T. I., Ananko, E. A., Ignatieva, E. V., and Kolchanov, N. A. (2013). Transcription regulatory codes of eukaryotic genomes. *Russ. J. Genet.* 49, 29–45. doi: 10.1134/S1022795413010079

Mombaerts, P. (2001). The human repertoire of odorant receptor genes and pseudogenes. *Annu. Rev. Genomics Hum. Genet.* 2, 493–510. doi: 10.1146/annurev.genom.2.1.493

Moshkin, M. P., Litvinova, N. A., Bedareva, A. V., Bedarev, M. S., Litvinova, E. A., and Gerlinskaia, L. A. (2011). [Scent as an element of subjective assessment of young males and females] [Article in Russian]. *Zh. Evol. Biokhim. Fiziol.* 47, 62–72.

Nguyen, M. Q., Zhou, Z., Marks, C. A., Ryba, N. J., and Belluscio, L. (2007). Prominent roles for odorant receptor coding sequences in allelic exclusion. *Cell* 131, 1009–1017. doi: 10.1016/j.cell.2007.10.050

Olender, T., Lancet, D., and Nebert, D. W. (2008). Update on the olfactory receptor (OR) gene superfamily. *Hum. Genomics* 3, 87–97. doi: 10.1186/1479-7364-3-1-87

Olender, T., Nativ, N., and Lancet, D. (2013). HORDE: comprehensive resource for olfactory receptor genomics. *Methods Mol. Biol.* 1003, 23–38. doi: 10.1007/978-1-62703-377-0_2

Olender, T., Waszak, S. M., Viavant, M., Khen, M., Ben-Asher, E., Reyes, A., et al. (2012). Personal receptor repertoires: olfaction as a model. *BMC Genomics* 13, 414. doi: 10.1186/1471-2164-13-414

Omelina, E. S., Baricheva, E. M., Oshchepkov, D. Y., and Merkulova, T. I. (2011). Analysis and recognition of the GAGA transcription factor binding sites in Drosophila genes. *Comput. Biol. Chem.* 35, 363–370. doi: 10.1016/j.compbiolchem.2011.10.008

Pelchat, M. L., Bykowski, C., Duke, F. F., and Reed, D. R. (2011). Excretion and perception of a characteristic odor in urine after asparagus ingestion: a psychophysical and genetic study. *Chem. Senses* 36, 9–17. doi: 10.1093/chemse/bjq081

Plessy, C., Pascarella, G., Bertin, N., Akalin, A., Carrieri, C., Vassalli, A., et al. (2012). Promoter architecture of mouse olfactory receptor genes. *Genome Res.* 22, 486–497. doi: 10.1101/gr.126201.111

Saito, H., Chi, Q., Zhuang, H., Matsunami, H., and Mainland, J. D. (2009). Odor coding by a Mammalian receptor repertoire. *Sci. Signal.* 2, ra9. doi: 10.1126/scisignal.2000016

Santos, P. S., Füst, G., Prohászka, Z., Volz, A., Horton, R., Miretti, M., et al. (2008). Association of smoking behavior with an odorant receptor allele telomeric to the human major histocompatibility complex. *Genet. Test.* 12, 481–486. doi: 10.1089/gte.2008.0029

Seo, H. S., Guarneros, M., Hudson, R., Distel, H., Min, B. C., Kang, J. K., et al. (2011). Attitudes toward olfaction: a cross-regional study. *Chem. Senses* 36, 177–187. doi: 10.1093/chemse/bjq112

Seo, H. S., Lee, S., and Cho, S. (2013). Relationships between personality traits and attitudes toward the sense of smell. *Front. Psychol.* 4:901. doi: 10.3389/fpsyg.2013.00901

Sherva, R., Sripichai, O., Abel, K., Ma, Q., Whitacre, J., Angkachatchai, V., et al. (2010). Genetic modifiers of Hb E/beta0 thalassemia identified by a two-stage genome-wide association study. *BMC Med. Genet.* 11:51. doi: 10.1186/1471-2350-11-51

Sinnarajah, S., Dessauer, C. W., Srikumar, D., Chen, J., Yuen, J., Yilma, S., et al. (2001). RGS2 regulates signal transduction in olfactory neurons by attenuating activation of adenylyl cyclase III. *Nature* 409, 1051–1055. doi: 10.1038/35059104

Smirnova, N. P., Ptitsyn, A. A., Austin, K. J., Bielefeldt-Ohmann, H., Van Campen, H., Han, H., et al. (2009). Persistent fetal infection with bovine viral diarrhea virus differentially affects maternal blood cell signal transduction pathways. *Physiol. Genomics* 36, 129–139. doi: 10.1152/physiolgenomics.90276.2008

Sokal, R. R., and Rohlf, F. J. (1995). *Biometry: The Principles and Practice of Statistics in Biological Research, 3rd Edn.* New York, NY: W.H. Freeman.

Sookoian, S., Burgueño, A., Gianotti, T. F., Marillet, G., and Pirola, C. J. (2011). Odor perception between heterosexual partners: its association with depression, anxiety, and genetic variation in odorant receptor OR7D4. *Biol. Psychol.* 86, 153–157. doi: 10.1016/j.biopsycho.2010.11.003

Sosinsky, A., Glusman, G., and Lancet, D. (2000). The genomic structure of human olfactory receptor genes. *Genomics* 70, 49–61. doi: 10.1006/geno.2000.6363

Thomas, L. (1975). "Symbiosis as an immunologic problem," in *The Immune System and Infectious Diseases. 4th International Convocation on Immunology*, eds E. Neter and F. Milgrom (Buffalo, NY, Basel: Karger), 2–11.

Vaskin, Y. Y., Khomicheva, I. V., Ignatieva, E. V., and Vityaev, E. E. (2011–2012). ExpertDiscovery and UGENE integrated system for intelligent analysis of regulatory regions of genes. *In Silico Biol.* 11, 97–108. doi: 10.3233/ISB-2012-0448

Weiss, J., Pyrski, M., Jacobi, E., Bufe, B., Willnecker, V., Schick, B., et al. (2011). Loss-of-function mutations in sodium channel Nav1.7 cause anosmia. *Nature* 472, 186–190. doi: 10.1038/nature09975

Wingender, E., Schoeps, T., and Dönitz, J. (2013). TFClass: an expandable hierarchical classification of human transcription factors. *Nucleic Acids Res.* 41, Database issue, D165–D170. doi: 10.1093/nar/gks1123

Zhang, H. M., Chen, H., Liu, W., Liu, H., Gong, J., Wang, H., et al. (2012). AnimalTFDB: a comprehensive animal transcription factor database. *Nucleic Acids Res.* 40, D144–D149. doi: 10.1093/nar/gkr965

Zhou, X., Barrett, T. B., and Kelsoe, J. R. (2008). Promoter variant in the GRK3 gene associated with bipolar disorder alters gene expression. *Biol. Psychiatry* 64, 104–110. doi: 10.1016/j.biopsych.2007.12.017

8

Olfaction in alcohol-dependence: a neglected yet promising research field

Pierre Maurage[1]*, Philippe Rombaux[2] and Philippe de Timary[1,3]

[1] Laboratory for Experimental Psychopathology, Psychological Sciences Research Institute, Université catholique de Louvain, Louvain-la-Neuve, Belgium
[2] Department of Otorhinolaryngology, St Luc Hospital and Institute of Neuroscience, Université catholique de Louvain, Brussels, Belgium
[3] Department of Adult Psychiatry, St Luc Hospital and Institute of Neuroscience, Université catholique de Louvain, Brussels, Belgium

Correspondence:
Pierre Maurage, Laboratory for Experimental Psychopathology, Psychological Sciences Research Institute, Université catholique de Louvain, 10, Place C. Mercier, B-1348 Louvain-la-Neuve, Belgium
e-mail: pierre.maurage@uclouvain.be

Olfaction research deeply renewed the knowledge of the pathophysiological mechanisms involved in various psychopathological states and showed that olfactory deficits might constitute an onset or trait marker in psychiatry. However, while alcohol-dependence is the most wide spread psychiatric disorder and while olfaction might be involved in its development and maintenance, olfactory abilities have been little explored in this population. The central aim of this paper is thus to underline the usefulness of olfaction research in alcohol-dependence. After reviewing the few olfaction studies available, a research agenda will be proposed, identifying the major challenges for future research, and particularly: (1) the identification of the origin, extent and cerebral correlates of olfaction deficits; (2) the links between olfaction and emotional-cognitive deficits, and the use of olfaction to understand the pathomechanisms of alcohol-dependence; (3) the interactions between olfaction and other sensory modalities; (4) the use of olfaction to predict the appearance and intensity of cognitive impairments; (5) the impact of olfaction deficits on everyday life in alcohol-dependence.

Keywords: olfaction, cognition, emotion, alcohol-dependence, orbitofrontal cortex, executive functions

INTRODUCTION

Alcohol-dependence represents a major concern for public health, annually leading to more than two million deaths worldwide (World Health Organization [WHO], 2011). The excessive consumption of alcohol has deleterious physiological effects, notably on the central nervous system as alcohol-dependence is associated with cerebral impairments (see Bühler and Mann, 2011 for a review of more than 190 papers on brain correlates of alcohol-dependence). The consequences of these brain deficits on cognitive and emotional abilities have also been widely described: alcohol-dependent individuals present impaired performance in attentional, executive, or memory abilities (Stavro et al., 2013), but also in affective and interpersonal processing (Philippot et al., 1999; Maurage et al., 2012). This large amount of data now offers a nearly exhaustive view of the deleterious consequences of excessive alcohol consumption.

However, these numerous studies have nearly all be based on visual or auditory stimulations. This can be explained by the fact that vision and audition are the most frequently used sensorial modalities among humans and are also the easiest to implement in experimental settings. Nevertheless, the exclusive focus on two modalities led to the nearly total neglect of other senses, and particularly olfaction. This lack of data on olfactory abilities constitutes a major shortcoming for the understanding of alcohol-dependence, as odors might play a crucial role in the development and persistence of this addictive state. The main aim of the present paper will thus first be to underline this importance of olfactory processes in alcohol-related disorders. After reviewing the results of the few studies which explored olfaction in alcohol-dependent patients, we will then underline the usefulness of olfactory studies to offer a better understanding of the impairments presented in alcohol-dependence. Particularly, we will show how olfaction might deeply renew and improve the current knowledge about this pathology, at fundamental (e.g., by renewing the knowledge on the pathophysiological mechanisms involved) and clinical (e.g., by developing olfaction rehabilitation programs to improve quality of life) levels.

WHY SHOULD OLFACTION BE EXPLORED IN ALCOHOL-DEPENDENCE?

There are at least four main arguments promoting further exploration of olfaction in alcohol-dependence:

THE IMPACT OF OLFACTORY LOSS ON EVERYDAY LIFE

Olfactory impairments could influence the decreased quality of life observed in alcohol-dependence. Indeed, olfactory loss is deleterious for everyday activities (Shu et al., 2011) as it increases the risk of injury by hampering the identification of environmental hazards (Stevenson, 2010). It also lowers the richness of social life (Schiffman, 1997), as smells are involved in social choices (Li et al., 2007; Prehn-Kristensen et al., 2009). Olfaction impairments thus have major consequences on personal and social life. As odors are crucial for food enjoyment (Smeets et al., 2009) and regulation (Stevenson, 2010), altered olfaction might participate in abnormal feeding behaviors (Santolaria et al., 2000) and nutrition deficiencies reported in alcohol-dependence (Carey, 1989). Olfaction impairments might largely alter food choices or eating motivation in this population, which underlines the need to better understand these impairments.

THE INTERACTIONS BETWEEN OLFACTION AND EMOTIONAL-COGNITIVE ABILITIES

The olfactory system is connected with cognitive and emotional brain regions, and exploring olfaction might improve the understanding of emotional-cognitive deficits in alcohol-dependence (up to now explored with visuo–auditory stimulations). Olfaction is indeed directly connected with limbic (Soudry et al., 2011) and fronto-temporal regions (Rolls, 2004). The orbitofrontal cortex is a crucial area in this perspective, being simultaneously involved in emotional, executive, and olfactory processing (Rolls, 2008). Strong correlations between olfactory and cognitive abilities have been shown (Purdon, 1998; Schubert et al., 2008; Sohrabi et al., 2012), underlining their common cerebral basis. Olfaction testing is also used to explore cognitive impairments in neurodegenerative disorders (Velayudhan et al., 2013). Olfaction thus constitutes an interesting way to renew the exploration of emotional-executive deficits in alcohol-dependence.

THE PROMISING RESULTS OF OLFACTION STUDIES IN PSYCHIATRY

Odor-processing impairments have been described in schizophrenia (Strauss et al., 2010), autism (Wiggins et al., 2009), anorexia nervosa (Roessner et al., 2005), and depression (Clepce et al., 2010). Beyond the mere description of impaired olfactory abilities, olfaction research offered new fundamental insights on psychiatric states, notably on three aspects. First, it renewed the knowledge on the psychophysiological mechanisms involved [e.g., dopamine regulation in schizophrenia (Moberg et al., 2013; Schecklmann et al., 2013)]. Second, it proposed early diagnostic tool for neurodegenerative diseases [e.g., Alzheimer (Luzzi et al., 2007) or Parkinson disease (Kranick and Duda, 2008)] and schizophrenia (Brewer et al., 2003; Turetsky et al., 2008). Third, as the level of olfactory deficit varies across pathologies, olfaction might constitute a cognitive marker in psychiatry (Atanasova et al., 2008) and a reliable evaluator of disease severity (Rupp, 2010; Segalàs et al., 2011). However, while constituting a topic of rising importance in psychiatry, odor processing remains little investigated in alcohol-dependence.

THE POSSIBLE ROLE OF OLFACTION IN THE DEVELOPMENT AND MAINTENANCE OF ALCOHOL-DEPENDENCE

Alcohol beverages provoke massive orthonasal and retronasal stimulations (Bragulat et al., 2008) which constitute strong appetitive cues (Bienkowski et al., 2004) and might be involved in the arisen of alcohol-dependence as they rapidly lead to conditioned alcohol-seeking behaviors (Pautassi et al., 2009). Olfactory stimulations elicit strong drinking desires (Schneider et al., 2001), this olfactory craving being even stronger than those provoked by visual–auditory cues, particularly during withdrawal (Kareken et al., 2004; Little et al., 2005) and thus being potentially involved in relapse. These preliminary results suggest that olfactory cues might play a role in the appearance of alcohol-dependence, but further studies are needed to explore their role at different stages of dependence.

WHAT IS CURRENTLY KNOWN ABOUT OLFACTION DEFICITS IN ALCOHOL-DEPENDENCE?

Earlier studies used olfactory cues in alcohol-dependence to elicit a consumption urge, and showed that alcohol-related odors can provoke strong subjective and physiological craving responses (Stormark et al., 1995; Bordnick et al., 2008). Neuroimaging studies showed that odor-induced craving mostly relies on a limbic and reward network including nucleus accumbens (Kareken et al., 2004), amygdala–hippocampal (Schneider et al., 2001), and orbitofrontal (Bragulat et al., 2008) regions. Nevertheless, as they were designed to test whether odors elicit craving, these studies did not explore odor processing and brought no insight on olfaction impairments.

Few studies directly explored olfaction in alcohol-dependence. The initial explorations led to contradictory results, some showing impaired odor discrimination, identification, or recall (Potter and Butters, 1979; DiTraglia et al., 1991) while others described preserved olfaction (Jones et al., 1975, 1978; Mair et al., 1986; Kesslak et al., 1991). These discrepancies might be explained by large methodology and population variations, and by the lack of control for medication and comorbidities. More recently, the use of a validated battery separately exploring three olfaction abilities [odor detection threshold, discrimination, identification (Kobal et al., 2000)] allowed to show a generalized olfactory deficit in alcohol-dependence, independent of medication and smoking habits (Rupp et al., 2003), as well as impaired familiarity and edibility odor judgments (Rupp et al., 2004). As olfactory judgments largely rely on orbitofrontal cortex (Royet et al., 2001), these results support the involvement of this region in olfaction deficits. However, this hypothesis had to be confirmed by studies including neuroimaging exploration or other cognitive tasks testing orbitofrontal cortex.

To explore this orbitofrontal implication, a simultaneous exploration of odor processing and executive functions was subsequently proposed (Rupp et al., 2006). Results confirmed olfaction impairments and showed a strong correlation between odor discrimination and executive performance, suggesting that orbitofrontal cortex is involved in olfactory impairments. Nevertheless, these executive tasks did not specifically rely on orbitofrontal functioning but rather on a large frontal network. In line with these results, we recently explored these olfaction-executive links by simultaneously administrating a complete odor processing test, the confabulation task [a source memory test specifically involving the orbitofrontal cortex (Schnider et al., 1996)] and another executive task unrelated to orbitofrontal cortex. Alcohol-dependence was associated with impaired odor identification and source memory, but preserved non-orbitofrontal performance. Centrally, a strong correlation was found between olfaction and source memory performances, suggesting that both abilities rely on orbitofrontal cortex (Maurage et al., 2011a).

Finally, only two studies directly explored the cerebral correlates of olfaction in alcohol-dependence. A MRI study showed a correlation between olfaction deficits and decreased cerebral volumes in a large cortico-subcortical network (Shear et al., 1992).

More recently, we explored the electrophysiological consequences of alcohol-dependence on olfaction (Maurage et al., 2011b) using chemosensory event-related potentials. Results showed altered olfactory event-related potentials (related to smell and indexing olfactory nerve activation) in alcohol-dependence, with preserved trigeminal activity (related to nasal somatosensory feelings and indexing trigeminal nerve activation). This shows that the olfactory deficit is specific and not due to a general impairment also affecting trigeminal functioning. Moreover, the electrophysiological deficit was mostly present for the P2 wave (a high-level cognitive component related to endogenous cortical olfactory processing) with partial preservation of the N1 wave (indexing low-level sensory processing linked with the exogenous activity provoked by the odor). This suggests that olfaction deficits rely on impaired high-level cognition based on fronto-limbic network (including orbitofrontal cortex and amygdala) and not on low-level olfactory processing in primary olfactory cortex.

SEVEN CRUCIAL QUESTIONS FOR FUTURE RESEARCH

Earlier studies presented above suggest that odor processing modifications might influence the everyday life of alcohol-dependent patients and claim for further exploration of olfaction deficits. Seven of the central questions that should be addressed will now be described, drawing a potential research agenda:

WHAT ARE THE ORIGIN AND EXTENT OF OLFACTION DEFICITS?

The presence of olfaction impairments is established, but controversial results were obtained across earlier studies concerning the respective impairment of different olfactory abilities. Variations in alcohol-dependence's characteristics (e.g., duration/severity of alcohol-dependence, duration of abstinence) might explain this controversy, and future studies should evaluate olfactory sub-components on larger populations to determine which factors modulate the impairment. A second step is to further explore other olfactory functions and particularly high-level odor judgments, which appear impaired (Rupp et al., 2004). Future studies should determine the preserved/impaired abilities, notably by using more subtle tests (Delplanque et al., 2008). As earlier studies focused on recently detoxified patients, the evolution of olfactory impairments across the successive stages of alcohol-dependence should also be explored. Cognitive functions recover with abstinence (Pitel et al., 2009), and testing olfaction at several stages of abstinence would determine how this deficit evolves when alcohol consumption stops. Finally, olfactory impairments are supposed to be provoked by alcohol-dependence, but this causal link should be tested. Studies in populations at-risk for schizophrenia showed that olfactory deficit precedes the pathology (Turetsky et al., 2008). Accordingly, exploring olfaction in populations at-risk for alcohol-dependence would determine if olfaction impairments mostly precede or follow alcohol-dependence.

WHAT ARE THE CEREBRAL BASES OF THE DEFICIT?

While the brain correlates of olfactory impairments have been explored in clinical populations (Turetsky et al., 2003; Welge-Lüssen et al., 2009), underlining the key role of orbitofrontal cortex (Frasnelli et al., 2010; Li et al., 2010), only two studies investigated this question in alcohol-dependence (Shear et al., 1992; Maurage et al., 2011b). Behavioral explorations suggested an implication of the orbitofrontal cortex in olfactory dysfunctions but no neuroimaging data confirmed it. A combined neuroscience approach could identify these cerebral impairments and particularly the processing level at which olfactory deficits begins. Indeed, if the deficit is, as suggested (Maurage et al., 2011b), focused on high-level cognitive stages (limbic areas, orbitofrontal cortex) with preserved low-level sensory ones (olfactory bulb, primary olfactory cortex), therapeutic programs should focus on these high-level functions. More globally, neuroimaging studies of olfaction would complement the knowledge on the cerebral consequences of alcohol-dependence, currently based on visuo–auditory modalities. Another important issue is the contradiction between impaired processing (and reduced cerebral activations) for non-alcohol-related odors and increased cerebral activations for alcohol-related odors (Bragulat et al., 2008). Alcohol-dependence might lead to a double olfactory system modification: over-activation for alcohol-related cues, reduced activation for other stimuli. A better understanding of how motivational factors may persistently activate olfactive responses to some but not all olfactory stimuli would also give new insights on olfaction-motivation interactions.

WHAT ARE THE LINKS BETWEEN OLFACTION AND EMOTIONAL-COGNITIVE FUNCTIONS?

Large-scale cognitive and emotional impairments have been described in alcohol-dependence using visual and auditory stimuli. As olfaction is the only modality possessing straightforward connections (Price, 1987) with emotional (amygdala) and cognitive (orbitofrontal cortex) areas, olfaction studies could renew the exploration of these emotion–cognition deficits. At the cognitive level, results suggesting links between olfaction and executive dysfunctions (Rupp et al., 2006; Maurage et al., 2011a) and showing that olfaction impairments might predict cognitive decline (Killgore et al., 2010) should lead to further explore these mutual influences. This is reinforced by the strong connections observed between olfaction, executive functions and memory in psychiatry (Murphy et al., 2001; Good et al., 2002). At the emotional level, the simultaneous implication of limbic structures in odor and affective processing (Soudry et al., 2011) and the olfaction–emotion interactions in healthy populations (Retiveau et al., 2004; Chrea et al., 2009) encourage the use of olfaction to explore emotional alterations. Moreover, odors strongly influence affective states (Lehrner et al., 2005; Moss et al., 2008, 2010), and applying these paradigms in alcohol-dependence might open new perspectives. Finally, as connections between olfactory and social deficits have been suggested (Malaspina and Coleman, 2003; Lahera et al., 2013), olfaction might also offer original tools to explore interpersonal abilities in alcohol-dependence.

HOW DOES OLFACTION INTERACT WITH OTHER MODALITIES?

Crossmodal processing is the ability to construct a unified percept on the basis of distinct sensory inputs. This crucial capacity for everyday life has been explored among healthy and psychiatric populations (Campanella and Belin, 2007; De Jong et al., 2009), and is impaired in alcohol-dependence (Maurage et al., 2007, 2008, 2013). However, previous studies focused on audio-visual integration, and it is unclear whether the observed behavioral and cerebral correlates of integration reflect general crossmodal integration or are somehow specific to audio-visual processing. Exploring crossmodal integration between olfactory and visual–auditory stimulations would test the generalization of earlier results to other modalities. Preliminary results exist on olfactory–visual crossmodality, showing that olfactory cues influence emotional visual processing (Leppänen and Hietanen, 2003; Seubert et al., 2010a), while these olfactory–visual influences appear impaired in schizophrenia (Seubert et al., 2010b). Moreover, some cerebral regions (middle frontal gyrus) are activated in all crossmodal situations, while others (anterior insula) seem specifically involved in olfactory–visual interactions (Small, 2004). Applying these paradigms to alcohol-dependence would deepen the understanding of crossmodal processing.

IS THERE A GLOBAL IMPAIRMENT FOR CHEMICAL SENSES?

Olfaction and taste are intimately linked, notably by the retronasal stimulation (Hornung and Enns, 1987) which appears altered in alcohol-dependence (Maurage et al., 2011b) but has been little explored. Moreover, while links have been shown between gustatory characteristics and risk for alcohol-dependence (Sandstrom et al., 2003), tasting abilities remain surprisingly underexplored. Earlier studies exploring taste in alcohol-dependence indeed focused on sucrose detection, showing preserved (Tremblay et al., 2009) or increased (Kampov-Polevoy et al., 1998) sensitivity to sucrose. Other aspects of taste remain unexplored, despite their role in malnutrition problems. The recent development of validated taste evaluations should lead to the precise exploration of this sensorial modality, in order to complete the description of chemical senses deficits.

COULD OLFACTION TESTING DETECT COGNITIVE IMPAIRMENT IN ALCOHOL-DEPENDENCE?

Simple olfactory tests have been used to assess cognitive impairments in the early stages of neurological diseases (Moscovich et al., 2012; Conti et al., 2013; Stamps et al., 2013). As it is still currently difficult to detect individuals who are bound to develop alcohol-dependence, these tests might be used to rapidly assess the cognitive decline in alcohol-dependence, and hence serve as early detectors of brain impairments potentially facilitating the maintenance of alcohol abuse.

WHAT IS THE IMPACT OF OLFACTORY LOSS ON EVERYDAY LIFE IN ALCOHOL-DEPENDENCE?

While it is clearly established that olfaction impairments have a major impact on life satisfaction (Shu et al., 2011) and nutrition (Stevenson, 2010), the precise consequences of olfactory loss on alcohol-dependent individuals' everyday life remain unexplored. Future studies should thus directly determine how olfaction deficits modulate the quality of life and nutritional habits in alcohol-dependence.

CONCLUSION

This perspective paper underlined the usefulness of developing a structured and thorough exploration of olfaction in alcohol-dependence. Olfaction is deeply involved in a wide range of everyday life activities (Stevenson, 2010) but olfactory impairments remain largely under-diagnosed and under-treated in healthy and psychiatric populations. Recent findings have underlined the involvement of odor processing impairments in schizophrenia and their usefulness as an endophenotypic marker of vulnerability, which shows that olfaction studies constitute a promising research field to understand this pathology (Rupp, 2010). Accordingly, olfactory cues might be involved in the emergence of alcohol-dependence and in relapse after detoxification. However, data are currently lacking in this field, as earlier studies focused on visual and auditory stimulations.

We tried to show that this lack of data is detrimental for the understanding of alcohol-dependence and to propose several perspectives for the development of this research field. At the fundamental level, further exploring olfaction in alcohol-dependence could on the one hand enrich the knowledge concerning the behavioral and cerebral consequences of excessive alcohol consumption, and thus complement the current theoretical models of this pathology. Specifically, following what has been done in other psychiatric states (Moberg et al., 2013; Schecklmann et al., 2013), olfaction deficits might give crucial new insights on the pathophysiological mechanisms involved in the appearance and maintenance of alcohol-related disorders. On the other hand, these explorations could complement the understanding of the mutual influences between olfaction and cognitive-emotional processes. At the clinical level, circumscribing the extent of olfactory impairments in alcohol-dependence would help clinicians to take into account this deficit and its consequences on everyday life, as it is currently totally neglected in clinical settings. It might also allow the inclusion of olfactory stimulations in crossmodal retraining programs, or even the development of innovative olfaction training programs capitalizing on existing rehabilitation tools used in other populations with olfactory loss (Hummel et al., 2009; Konstantinidis et al., 2013). Actually, nearly everything remains to be done in the exploration of olfaction in alcohol-dependence, but we hope that the preliminary data and research perspectives described here will encourage the development of this research field.

ACKNOWLEDGMENTS

Pierre Maurage (Research Associate) and Philippe de Timary (Clinical Research Associate) are founded by the Belgian Fund for Scientific Research (F.N.R.S., Belgium), but this fund did not exert any editorial direction or censorship on any part of this article.

REFERENCES

Atanasova, B., Graux, J., El Hage, W., Hommet, C., Camus, V., and Belzung, C. (2008). Olfaction: a potential cognitive marker of psychiatric disorders. *Neurosci. Biobehav. Rev.* 32, 1315–1325. doi: 10.1016/j.neubiorev.2008.05.003

Bienkowski, P., Rogowski, A., Korkosz, A., Mierzejewski, P., Radwanska, K., Kaczmarek, L., et al. (2004). Time-dependent changes in alcohol-seeking behaviour during abstinence. *Eur. Neuropsychopharmacol.* 14, 355–360. doi: 10.1016/j.euroneuro.2003.10.005

Bordnick, P. S., Traylor, A., Copp, H. L., Graap, K. M., Carter, B., Ferrer, M., et al. (2008). Assessing reactivity to virtual reality alcohol based cues. *Addict. Behav.* 33, 743–756. doi: 10.1016/j.addbeh.2007.12.010

Bragulat, V., Dzemidzic, M., Talavage, T., Davidson, D., O'Connor, S. J., and Kareken, D. A. (2008). Alcohol sensitizes cerebral responses to the odors of alcoholic drinks: an fMRI study. *Alcohol. Clin. Exp. Res.* 32, 1124–1134. doi: 10.1111/j.1530-0277.2008.00693.x

Brewer, W. J., Wood, S. J., McGorry, P. D., Francey, S. M., Phillips, L. J., Yung, A. R., et al. (2003). Impairment of olfactory identification ability in individuals at ultrahigh risk for psychosis who later develop schizophrenia. *Am. J. Psychiatry* 160, 1790–1794. doi: 10.1176/appi.ajp.160.10.1790

Bühler, M., and Mann, K. (2011). Alcohol and the human brain: a systematic review of different neuroimaging methods. *Alcohol. Clin. Exp. Res.* 35, 1–23. doi: 10.1111/j.1530-0277.2011.01540.x

Campanella, S., and Belin, P. (2007). Integrating face and voice in person perception. *Trends Cogn. Sci.* 11, 535–543. doi: 10.1016/j.tics.2007.10.001

Carey, G. B. (1989). Nutrition and alcoholism: problems and therapies. *Occup. Med.* 4, 311–326.

Chrea, C., Grandjean, D., Delplanque, S., Cayeux, I., Le Calvé, B., Aymard, L., et al. (2009). Mapping the semantic space for the subjective experience of emotional responses to odors. *Chem. Senses* 34, 49–62. doi: 10.1093/chemse/bjn052

Clepce, M., Gossler, A., Reich, K., Kornhuber, J., and Thuerauf, N. (2010). The relation between depression, anhedonia and olfactory hedonic estimates – a pilot study in major depression. *Neurosci. Lett.* 47, 139–143. doi: 10.1016/j.neulet.2010.01.027

Conti, M. Z., Vicini-Chilovi, B., Riva, M., Zanetti, M., Liberini, P., Padovani, A., et al. (2013). Odor identification deficit predicts clinical conversion from mild cognitive impairment to dementia due to Alzheimer's disease. *Arch. Clin. Neuropsychol.* 28, 391–399. doi: 10.1093/arclin/act032

De Jong, J. J., Hodiamont, P. P., Van den Stock, J., and de Gelder, B. (2009). Audiovisual emotion recognition in schizophrenia: reduced integration of facial and vocal affect. *Schizophr. Res.* 107, 286–293. doi: 10.1016/j.schres.2008.10.001

Delplanque, S., Grandjean, D., Chrea, C., Aymard, L., Cayeux, I., Le Calvé, B., et al. (2008). Emotional processing of odors: evidence for a nonlinear relation between pleasantness and familiarity evaluations. *Chem. Senses* 33, 469–479. doi: 10.1093/chemse/bjn014

DiTraglia, G. M., Press, D. S., Butters, N., Jernigan, T. L., Cermak, L. S., Velin, R. A., et al. (1991). Assessment of olfactory deficits in detoxified alcoholics. *Alcohol* 8, 109–115. doi: 10.1016/0741-8329(91)91318-V

Frasnelli, J., Lundström, J. N., Boyle, J. A., Djordjevic, J., Zatorre, R. J., and Jones-Gotman, M. (2010). Neuroanatomical correlates of olfactory performance. *Exp. Brain Res.* 201, 1–11. doi: 10.1007/s00221-009-1999-7

Good, K. P., Martzke, J. S., Milliken, H. I., Honer, W. G., and Kopala, L. C. (2002). Unirhinal olfactory identification deficits in young male patients with schizophrenia and related disorders: association with impaired memory function. *Schizophr. Res.* 56, 211–223. doi: 10.1016/S0920-9964(01)00227-4

Hornung, D. E., and Enns, M. P. (1987). Odor-taste mixtures. *Ann. N. Y. Acad. Sci.* 510, 86–90. doi: 10.1111/j.1749-6632.1987.tb43471.x

Hummel, T., Rissom, K., Reden, J., Hahner, A., Weidenbecher, M., and Hüttenbrink, K. B. (2009). Effects of olfactory training in patients with olfactory loss. *Laryngoscope* 119, 496–499. doi: 10.1002/lary.20101

Jones, B. P., Butters, N., Moskowitz, H. R., and Montgomery, K. (1978). Olfactory and gustatory capacities of alcoholic Korsakoff patients. *Neuropsychologia* 16, 323–337. doi: 10.1016/0028-3932(78)90026-X

Jones, B. P., Moskowitz, H. R., and Butters, N. (1975). Olfactory discrimination in alcoholic Korsakoff patients. *Neuropsychologia* 13, 173–179. doi: 10.1016/0028-3932(75)90026-3

Kampov-Polevoy, A. B., Garbutt, J. C., Davis, C. E., and Janowsky, D. S. (1998). Preference for higher sugar concentrations and Tridimensional Personality Questionnaire scores in alcoholic and nonalcoholic men. *Alcohol. Clin. Exper. Res.* 22, 610–614. doi: 10.1111/j.1530-0277.1998.tb04300.x

Kareken, D. A., Claus, E. D., Sabri, M., Dzemidzic, M., Kosobud, A. E. K., Radnovich, A. J., et al. (2004). Alcohol-related olfactory cues activate the nucleus accumbens and the ventrotemental area in high-risk drinkers: preliminary findings. *Alcohol. Clin. Exp. Res.* 28, 550–557. doi: 10.1097/01.ALC.0000122764.60626.AF

Kesslak, J. P., Proffit, B. F., and Criswell, P. (1991). Olfactory function in chronic alcoholics. *Percept. Mot. Skills* 73, 551–554. doi: 10.2466/pms.1991.73.2.551

Killgore, W. D., Killgore, D. B., Grugle, N. L., and Balkin, T. J. (2010). Odor identification ability predicts executive function deficits following sleep deprivation. *Int. J. Neurosci.* 120, 328–334. doi: 10.3109/00207450903389396

Kobal, G., Klimek, L., Wolfensberger, M., Gudziol, H., Temmel, A., Owen, C. M., et al. (2000). Multicenter investigation of 1,036 subjects using a standardized method for the assessment of olfactory function combining tests of odor identification, odor discrimination, and olfactory thresholds. *Eur. Arch. Otorhinolaryngol.* 257, 205–211. doi: 10.1007/s004050050223

Konstantinidis, I., Tsakiropoulou, E., Bekiaridou, P., Kazantzidou, C., and Constantinidis, J. (2013). Use of olfactory training in post-traumatic and postinfectious olfactory dysfunction. *Laryngoscope* doi: 10.1002/lary.24390 [Epub ahead of print].

Kranick, S. M., and Duda, J. E. (2008). Olfactory dysfunction in Parkinson's disease. *Neurosignals* 16, 35–40. doi: 10.1159/000109757

Lahera, G., Ruiz-Murugarren, S., Fernández-Liria, A., Saiz-Ruiz, J., Buck, B. E., and Penn, D. L. (2013). Relationship between olfactory function and social cognition in euthymic bipolar patients. *CNS Spectr.* 12, 1–7. doi: 10.1017/S1092852913000382

Lehrner, J., Marwinski, G., Lehr, S., Johren, P., and Deecke, L. (2005). Ambient odors of orange and lavender reduce anxiety and improve mood in a dental office. *Physiol. Behav.* 86, 92–95. doi: 10.1016/j.physbeh.2005.06.031

Leppänen, J. M., and Hietanen, J. K. (2003). Affect and face perception: odors modulate the recognition advantage of happy faces. *Emotion* 3, 315–326. doi: 10.1037/1528-3542.3.4.315

Li, W., Lopez, L., Osher, J., Howard, J. D., Parrish, T. B., and Gottfried, J. A. (2010). Right orbitofrontal cortex mediates conscious olfactory perception. *Psychol. Sci.* 21, 1454–1463. doi: 10.1177/0956797610382121

Li, W., Moallem, I., Paller, K. A., and Gottfried, J. A. (2007). Subliminal smells can guide social preferences. *Psychol. Sci.* 18, 1044–1049. doi: 10.1111/j.1467-9280.2007.02023.x

Little, H. J., Stephens, D. N., Ripley, T. L., Borlikova, G., Duka, T., Schubert, M., et al. (2005). Alcohol withdrawal and conditioning. *Alcohol. Clin. Exp. Res.* 29, 453–464. doi: 10.1097/01.ALC.0000156737.56425.E3

Luzzi, S., Snowden, J. S., Neary, D., Coccia, M., Provinciali, L., and Lambon Ralph, M. A. (2007). Distinct patterns of olfactory impairment in Alzheimer's disease, semantic dementia, frontotemporal dementia, and corticobasal degeneration. *Neuropsychologia* 45, 1823–1831. doi: 10.1016/j.neuropsychologia.2006.12.008

Mair, R. G., Doty, R. L., Kelly, K. M., Wilson, C. S., Langlais, P. J., McEntee, W. J., et al. (1986). Multimodal sensory discrimination deficits in Korsakoff's psychosis. *Neuropsychologia* 24, 831–839. doi: 10.1016/0028-3932(86)90082-5

Malaspina, D., and Coleman, E. (2003). Olfaction and social drive in schizophrenia. *Arch. Gen. Psychiatry* 60, 578–584. doi: 10.1001/archpsyc.60.6.578

Maurage, P., Callot, C., Chang, B., Philippot, P., Rombaux, P., and de Timary, P. (2011a). Olfactory impairment is correlated with confabulation in alcoholism: towards a multimodal testing of orbitofrontal cortex. *PLoS ONE* 6:e23190. doi: 10.1371/journal.pone.0023190

Maurage, P., Callot, C., Philippot, P., Rombaux, P., and de Timary, P. (2011b). Chemosensory event-related potentials in alcoholism: a specific impairment for olfactory function. *Biol. Psychol.* 88, 28–36. doi: 10.1016/j.biopsycho.2011.06.004

Maurage, P., Campanella, S., Philippot, P., Pham, T., and Joassin, F. (2007). The crossmodal facilitation effect is disrupted in alcoholism: a study with emotional stimuli. *Alcohol Alcohol.* 42, 552–559. doi: 10.1093/alcalc/agm134

Maurage, P., Joassin, F., Pesenti, M., Grandin, C., Heeren, A., Philippot, P., et al. (2013). The neural network sustaining crossmodal integration is impaired in alcohol-dependence: an fMRI study. *Cortex* 49, 1610–1626. doi: 10.1016/j.cortex.2012.04.012

Maurage, P., Joassin, F., Philippot, P., Heeren, A., Vermeulen, N., Mahau, P., et al. (2012). Disrupted regulation of social exclusion in alcohol-dependence: an fMRI study. *Neuropsychopharmacology* 37, 2067–2075. doi: 10.1038/npp.2012.54

Maurage, P., Philippot, P., Joassin, F., Pauwels, L., Pham, T., Alonso Prieto, E. A., et al. (2008). The auditory-visual integration of anger is impaired in alcoholism: an ERP study. *J. Psychiatry Neurosci.* 33, 111–122.

Moberg, P. J., Kamath, V., Marchetto, D. M., Calkins, M. E., Doty, R. L., Hahn, C. G., et al. (2013). Meta-analysis of olfactory function in schizophrenia, first-degree family members, and youths at-risk for psychosis. *Shizophr. Bull.* doi: 10.1093/schbul/sbt049 [Epub ahead of print].

Moscovich, M., Munhoz, R. P., Teive, H. A., Raskin, S., Carvalho, M., Barbosa, E. R., et al. (2012). Olfactory impairment in familial ataxias. *J. Neurol. Neurosurg. Psychiatry* 83, 970–974. doi: 10.1136/jnnp-2012-302770

Moss, L., Rouse, M., Wesnes, K. A., and Moss, M. (2010). Differential effects of the aromas of *Salvia* species on memory and mood. *Hum. Psychopharmacol. Clin. Exp.* 25, 388–396. doi: 10.1002/hup.1129

Moss, M., Hewitt, S., Moss, L., and Wesnes, K. (2008). Modulation of cognitive performance and mood by aromas of peppermint and ylang-ylang. *Int. J. Neurosci.* 118, 59 doi: 10.1080/00207450601042094

Murphy, K. R., Barkley, R. A., and Bush, T. (2001). Executive functioning and olfactory identification in young adults with attention deficit-hyperactivity disorder. *Neuropsychology* 15, 211–220. doi: 10.1037/0894-4105.15.2.211

Pautassi, R. M., Nishnikov, M. E., and Spear, N. E. (2009). Assessing appetitive, aversive, and negative ethanol-mediated reinforcement through an immature rat model. *Neurosci. Biobehav. Rev.* 33, 953–974. doi: 10.1016/j.neubiorev.2009.03.008

Philippot, P., Kornreich, C., Blairy, S., Baerts, I., Den Dulk, A., Le Bon, O., et al. (1999). Alcoholics' deficits in the decoding of emotional facial expression. *Alcohol. Clin. Exp. Res.* 23, 1031–1038.

Pitel, A. L., Rivier, J., Beaunieux, H., Vabret, F., Desgranges, B., and Eustache, F. (2009). Changes in the episodic memory and executive functions of abstinent and relapsed alcoholics over a 6-month period. *Alcohol. Clin. Exp. Res.* 33, 490–498. doi: 10.1111/j.1530-0277.2008.00859.x

Potter, H., and Butters, N. (1979). Continuities in the olfactory deficits of chronic alcoholics and alcoholics with the Korsakoff syndrome. *Curr. Alcohol* 7, 261–271.

Prehn-Kristensen, A., Wiesner, C., Bergmann, T. O., Wolff, S., Jansen, O., Mehdorn, H. M., et al. (2009). Induction of empathy by the smell of anxiety. *PLoS ONE* 4:e101371. doi:10.1371/journal.pone.0005987

Price, J. L. (1987). "The central olfactory and accessory olfactory systems," in *Neurobiology of Taste and Smell*, eds T. E. Finger and W. L. Silver (New York, NY: John Wiley), 179–203.

Purdon, S. E. (1998). Olfactory identification and stroop interference converge in schizophrenia. *J. Psychiatry Neurosci.* 23, 163–171.

Retiveau, A. N., Chambers, I. V. E., and Milliken, G. A. (2004). Common and specific effects of fine fragrances on the mood of women. *J. Sens. Stud.* 19, 373–394. doi: 10.1111/j.1745-459x.2004.102803.x

Roessner, V., Bleich, S., Banaschewski, T., and Rothenberger, A. (2005). Olfactory deficits in anorexia nervosa. *Eur. Arch. Psychiatry Clin. Neurosci.* 255, 6–9. doi: 10.1007/s00406-004-0525-y

Rolls, E. T. (2004). The functions of the orbitofrontal cortex. *Brain. Cogn.* 55, 11–29. doi: 10.1016/S0278-2626(03)00277-X

Rolls, E. T. (2008). Functions of the orbitofrontal and pregenual cingulate cortex in taste, olfaction, appetite and emotion. *Acta Physiol. Hung.* 95, 131–164. doi: 10.1556/APhysiol.95.2008.2.1

Royet, J. P., Hudry, J., Zald, D. H., Godinot, D., Gregoire, M. C., Lavenne, F., et al. (2001). Functional neuroanatomy of different olfactory judgments. *Neuroimage* 13, 506–519. doi: 10.1006/nimg.2000.0704

Rupp, C. I. (2010). Olfactory function and schizophrenia: an update. *Curr. Opin. Psychiatry* 23, 97–102. doi: 10.1097/YCO.0b013e328336643f

Rupp, C. I., Fleischhacker, W., Drexler, A., Hausmann, A., Hinterhuber, H., and Kurz, M. (2006). Executive function and memory in relation to olfactory deficits in alcoholdependent patients. *Alcohol. Clin. Exp. Res.* 30, 1355–1362. doi: 10.1111/j.1530-0277.2006.00162.x

Rupp, C. I., Fleischhacker, W., Hausmann, H., Mair, D., Hinterhubern, H., and Kurz, M. (2004). Olfactory functioning in patients with alcohol dependence: impairments in odor judgments. *Alcohol Alcohol.* 39, 514–519. doi: 10.1093/alcalc/agh100

Rupp, C. I., Kurz, M., Kemmler, G., Mair, D., Hausmann, A., Hinterhuber, H., et al. (2003). Reduced olfactory sensitivity, discrimination, and identification in patients with alcohol dependence. *Alcohol. Clin. Exp. Res.* 27, 432–439. doi: 10.1097/01.ALC.0000057945.57330.2C

Sandstrom, K. A., Rajan, T. M., Feinn, R., and Kranzler, H. R. (2003). Salty and sour taste characteristics and risk of alcoholism. *Alcohol. Clin. Exp. Res.* 27, 955–961. doi: 10.1111/j.1530-0277.2003.tb04420.x

Santolaria, F., González-Reimers, E., Pérez-Manzano, J. L., Milena, A., Gómez-Rodríguez, M. A., González-Díaz, A., et al. (2000). Osteopenia assessed by body composition analysis is related to malnutrition in alcoholic patients. *Alcohol* 22, 147–157. doi: 10.1016/S0741-8329(00)00115-4

Schecklmann, M., Schwenck, C., Taurines, R., Freitag, C., Warnke, A., Gerlach, M., et al. (2013). A systematic review on olfaction in child and adolescent psychiatric disorders. *J. Neural. Transm.* 120, 121–130. doi: 10.1007/s00702-012-0855-2

Schiffman, M. (1997). Taste and smell losses in normal aging and disease. *JAMA* 278, 1357–1362. doi: 10.1001/jama.1997.0355010077042

Schneider, F., Habel, U., Wagner, M., Franke, P., Salloum, J. B., Jon Shah, N., et al. (2001). Subcortical correlates of craving in recently abstinent alcoholic patients. *Am. J. Psychiatry* 158, 1075–1083. doi: 10.1176/appi.ajp.158.7.1075

Schnider, A., von Daniken, C., and Gutbrod, K. (1996). The mechanisms of spontaneous and provoked confabulations. *Brain* 119, 1365–1375. doi: 10.1093/brain/119.4.1365

Schubert, C. R., Carmichael, L. L., Murphy, C., Klein, B. E., Klein, R., and Cruickshanks, K. J. (2008). Olfaction and the 5-year incidence of cognitive impairment in an epidemiological study of older adults. *J. Am. Geriatrics Soc.* 56, 1517–1521. doi: 10.1111/j.1532-5415.2008.01826.x

Segalàs, C., Labad, J., Alonso, P., Real, E., Subirà, M., Bueno, B., et al. (2011). Olfactory identification and discrimination in obsessive-compulsive disorder. *Depress. Anxiety* 28, 932–940. doi: 10.1002/da.20836

Seubert, J., Kellermann, T., Loughead, J., Boers, F., Brensinger, C., Schneider, F., et al. (2010a). Processing of disgusted faces is facilitated by odour primes: a functional MRI study. *Neuroimage* 53, 746–756. doi: 10.1016/j.neuroimage.2010.07.012

Seubert, J., Loughead, J., Kellermann, T., Boers, F., Brensinger, C. M., and Habel, U. (2010b). Multisensory integration of emotionally valenced olfactory-visual information in patients with schizophrenia and healthy controls. *J. Psychiatry Neurosci.* 35, 185–194. doi: 10.1503/jpn.090094

Shear, P. K., Butters, N., Jernigan, T. L., DiTraglia, G. M., and Irwin, M. (1992). Olfactory loss in alcoholics: correlations with cortical and subcortical MRI indices. *Alcohol* 9, 247–255. doi: 10.1016/0741-8329(92)90061-E

Shu, C. H., Lee, P. O., Lan, M. Y., and Lee, Y. L. (2011). Factors affecting the impact of olfactory loss on the quality of life and emotional coping ability. *Rhinology* 49, 337–341. doi: 10.4193/Rhino10.130

Small, D. A. (2004). Crossmodal integration – insights from the chemical senses. *Trends Neurosci.* 27, 123–124. doi: 10.1016/j.tins.2004.01.003

Smeets, M. A., Veldhuizen, M. G., Galle, S., Gouweloos, J., de Haan, A. M., Vernooij, J., et al. (2009). Sense of smell disorder and health-related quality of life. *Rehabil. Psychol.* 54, 404–412. doi: 10.1037/a0017502

Sohrabi, H. R., Bates, K. A., Weinborn, M. G., Johnston, A. N. B., Bahramian, A., Taddei, K., et al. (2012). Olfactory discrimination predicts cognitive decline among community-dwelling older adults. *Transl. Psychiatry* 2:e118. doi: 10.1038/tp.2012.43

Soudry, Y., Lemogne, C., Malinvaud, D., Consoli, S. M., and Bonfils, P. (2011). Olfactory system and emotion: common substrates. *Eur. Ann. Otorhinolaryngol. Head Neck Dis.* 128, 18–23. doi: 10.1016/j.anorl.2010.09.007

Stamps, J. J., Bartoshuk, L. M., and Heilman, K. M. (2013). A brief olfactory test for Alzheimer's disease. *J. Neurol. Sci.* 333, 19–24. doi: 10.1016/j.jns.2013.06.033

Stavro, K., Pelletier, J., and Potvin, S. (2013). Widespread and sustained cognitive deficits in alcoholism: a meta-analysis. *Addict. Biol.* 18, 203–213. doi: 10.1111/j.1369-1600.2011.00418.x

Stevenson, R. J. (2010). An initial evaluation of the functions of human olfaction. *Chem. Senses* 35, 3–20. doi: 10.1093/chemse/bjp083

Stormark, K. M., Laberg, J. C., Bjerland, T., Nordby, H., and Hugdahl, K. (1995). Autonomic cued reactivity in alcoholics: the effect of olfactory stimuli. *Addict. Behav.* 20, 571–584. doi: 10.1016/0306-4603(95)00017-7

Strauss, G. P., Allen, D. N., Ross, S. A., Duke, L. A., and Schwartz, J. (2010). Olfactory hedonic judgment in patients with deficit syndrome schizophrenia. *Schizophr. Bull.* 36, 860–868. doi: 10.1093/schbul/sbn178

Tremblay, K. A., Bona, J. M., and Kranzler, H. R. (2009). Effects of a diagnosis or family history of alcoholism on the taste intensity and hedonic value of sucrose. *Am. J. Addict.* 18, 494–499. doi: 10.3109/10550490903206023

Turetsky, B. I., Kohler, C. G., Gur, R. E., and Moberg, P. J. (2008). Olfactory physiological impairment in first-degree relatives of schizophrenia patients. *Schizophr. Res.* 102, 220–229. doi: 10.1016/j.schres.2008.03.013

Turetsky, B. I., Moberg, P. J., Owzar, K., Johnson, S. C., Doty, R. L., and Gur, R. E. (2003). Physiologic impairment of olfactory stimulus processing in schizophrenia. *Biol. Psychiatry* 53, 403–411. doi: 10.1016/S0006-3223(02)01865-6

Velayudhan, L., Pritchard, M., Powell, J. F., Proitsi, P., and Lovestone, S. (2013). Smell identification function as a severity and progression marker in Alzheimer's disease. *Int. Psychogeriatr.* 25, 1157–1166. doi: 10.1017/S1041610213000446

Welge-Lüssen, A., Wattendorf, E., Schwerdtfeger, U., Fuhr, P., Bilecen, D., Hummel, T., et al. (2009). Olfactory-induced brain activity in Parkinson's disease relates to the expression of event-related potentials: a functional magnetic resonance imaging study. *Neuroscience* 162, 537–543. doi: 10.1016/j.neuroscience.2009.04.050

Wiggins, L. D., Robins, D. L., Bakeman, R., and Adamson, L. B. (2009). Brief report: sensory abnormalities as distinguishing symptoms of autism spectrum disorders in young children. *J. Autism Dev. Disord.* 39, 1087–1091. doi: 10.1007/s10803-009-0711-x

World Health Organization [WHO]. (2011). *Global Status Report on Alcohol and Health.* Geneva: World Health Organization. Available at: http://www.who.int/substance_abuse/publications/global_alcohol_report [accessed July 27, 2013].

9

Hedonic appreciation and verbal description of pleasant and unpleasant odors in untrained, trainee cooks, flavorists and perfumers

Caroline Sezille[1]*, Arnaud Fournel[1], Catherine Rouby[1], Fanny Rinck[2†] and Moustafa Bensafi[1†]*

[1] CNRS, UMR5292, INSERM1028, Lyon Neuroscience Research Center, University of Lyon, Lyon, France
[2] Lidilem Laboratory, University of Grenoble, Grenoble, France

***Correspondence:**
Caroline Sezille and Moustafa Bensafi, CNRS, UMR5292, INSERM1028, Lyon Neuroscience Research Center, University of Lyon, 50 Avenue Tony Garnier, 69366 Lyon, France
e-mail: csezille@olfac.univ-lyon1.fr, bensafi@olfac.univ-lyon1.fr

Olfaction is characterized by a salient hedonic dimension. Previous studies have shown that these affective responses to odors are modulated by physicochemical, physiological, and cognitive factors. The present study examined expertise influenced processing of pleasant and unpleasant odors on both perceptual and verbal levels. For this, performance on two olfactory tasks was compared between novices, trainee cooks, and experts (perfumers and flavorists): Members of all groups rated the intensity and pleasantness of pleasant and unpleasant odors (perceptual tasks). They were also asked to describe each of the 20 odorants as precisely as possible (verbal description task). On a perceptual level, results revealed that there were no group-related differences in hedonic ratings for unpleasant and pleasant odors. On a verbal level, descriptions of smells were richer (e.g., chemical, olfactory qualities, and olfactory sources terms) and did not refer to pleasantness in experts compared to untrained subjects who used terms referring to odor sources (e.g., candy) accompanied by terms referring to odor hedonics. In conclusion, the present study suggests that as novices, experts are able to perceptually discriminate odors on the basis of their pleasantness. However, on a semantic level, they conceptualize odors differently, being inclined to avoid any reference to odor hedonics.

Keywords: olfaction, expertise, hedonic, emotion, perfumery

INTRODUCTION

Hedonic treatment is a crucial level of processing sensory information. The sense of smell is of particular interest in this regard: in humans, odors induce attractive or repulsive reactions and may influence cognition and behavior in various contexts (Alaoui-Ismaili et al., 1997a,b; Yeshurun and Sobel, 2010; Croy et al., 2011). From a cognitive point of view, odor-grouping experiments showed that hedonics is the most salient dimension of olfaction (Harper, 1966; Berglund et al., 1973; Schiffman, 1977). In these studies, subjects were exposed to various pairs of olfactory stimuli and asked to judge their similarity. It was usually observed that two main clusters were formed: one grouping together pleasant and the other unpleasant odors (Schiffman, 1974; Godinot et al., 1995).

Whereas psychophysical investigations have shown that such hedonic processing of smells is influenced by physicochemical properties (Khan et al., 2007; Mandairon et al., 2009; Poncelet et al., 2010; Joussain et al., 2011; Kermen et al., 2011; Zarzo, 2011), many other experiments, however, showed that odor pleasantness can be modulated by physiological (Fernandez et al., 2013; Joussain et al., 2013a,b) or cognitive factors (Herz, 2003; Rolls, 2004; de Araujo et al., 2005; Barkat et al., 2008; Rinck et al., 2011). For example, it has been shown that pleasantness judgments are enhanced when subjects are able to identify the odorant source (Ayabe-Kanamura et al., 1998). When verbal information about an odor is available, subjects shift their pleasantness judgment in line with the affective connotation of the label (Herz, 2003). Such top-down modulation by verbal association has been found even in children (Bensafi et al., 2007; Rinck et al., 2011). In summary, it would seem that both bottom-up (molecular feature coding) and top-down (training and language) processes contribute to build our hedonic responses to smells, which may be thus very variable across individuals.

Another factor that may explain olfactory individual differences is expertise. Training and verbal associations are crucial in professional situations in which odorants have to be associated systematically to label in order to ensure a common vocabulary to enhance perceptual agreement between individuals. Past and more recent studies showed that experts in olfaction used more consistent, rich, and precise language to describe smells (Bende and Nordin, 1997; Valentin and Chollet, 2000; Parr et al., 2002). Moreover, it has been shown that wine experts use more specific and relevant wine descriptors (Zucco et al., 2011). Although experts are known not only to acquire a systematic knowledge of the chemistry of odorants but also to learn to describe olfactory qualities of odorants and odor sources in a shared language, very little is known about the importance of hedonic processing in both the ways: (i) they describe but also (ii) they perceive smells. On a descriptive level, the literature in the field suggests that whereas pleasantness is a prominent attribute that drives odor verbalizations (Dubois and Rouby, 1997; Dubois, 2000), experts may be inclined to avoid any reference to pleasantness (Yoshida, 1964; Ehrlichman and Bastone, 1992; Holley, 2002). In the present study, we aim to test experimentally this hypothesis on a verbal level and to further assess how expertise modulates hedonic perception of odors. To this end, experts and non-experts in olfaction were compared during two olfactory tasks: (i) a verbal description task whereby participants were asked to freely describe odors and (ii) a perceptual rating task whereby participants were asked to judge the pleasantness of odors. Practically, four groups of subjects, differing in their levels of expertise, were tested: (i) an untrained group, (ii) a group of apprentice cooks, who had no specific course on olfaction but were daily exposed to odors, (iii) a group of experts in aroma formulation, and (iv) a group of experts in perfume formulation.

Moreover, because there is evidence of the existence of two different systems dedicated to treating aversive and appetitive smells [unpleasant odors are processed faster than pleasant ones (Bensafi et al., 2002d; Jacob et al., 2003), induced specific patterns of autonomic (Miltner et al., 1994; Brauchli et al., 1995; Ehrlichman et al., 1995; Alaoui-Ismaili et al., 1997a,b; Ehrlichman et al., 1997; Bensafi et al., 2002a,c) and olfactomotor responses (Bensafi et al., 2003a; Rouby et al., 2009) and specific neural activations (Zald and Pardo, 1997; Gottfried et al., 2002b; Anderson et al., 2003; Rolls et al., 2003; Royet et al., 2003; Bensafi et al., 2012)], odor hedonic valence *per se* was included as a factor in the analysis. Here, all participants were thus presented with unpleasant and pleasant odorant molecules. Specific hypotheses were: (i) on a verbal and descriptive level, experts (flavorists and perfumers) should use precise terminology without reference to pleasantness, whereas non-experts (novices and trainee cooks) should use less precise terminology accompanied by references to pleasantness; (ii) on a perceptual level, experts should not consider pleasantness and thus should rate pleasant odors as less pleasant and unpleasant odors as less unpleasant than non-experts.

MATERIALS AND METHODS

SUBJECTS

Sixty-four subjects without neurological disease or olfactory disorder were tested. Participants were divided into four groups according to their level of expertise: (i) a group of untrained individuals ("novices": $n = 16$; mean age, 23.5 ± 0.423 years; six male), composed of subjects who had no specific training on olfaction; (ii) a group of trainee cooks ("trainee cooks": $n = 16$; mean age, 21.313 ± 0.285 years; nine male), composed of subjects in their second year of training in a cookery institute where they received no specific training in olfaction, but were exposed daily to odors; (iii) a group of flavorists ("flavorists": $n = 16$; mean age, 31.063 ± 2.765 years; three male; with 9.065 ± 2.497 years expertise), who had previous knowledge of artificial and natural flavors through intensive learning in school and/or at work; and (iv) a group of perfumers ("perfumers": $n = 16$; mean age, 34.063 ± 1.296 years; five male; with 9.933 ± 1.487 years expertise), who had previous knowledge of olfactory compounds for designing new fragrances through intensive learning in school and/or at work.

ODORANTS

Twenty odorants covering a wide range of hedonic valence were used. [Odor code: compound ID; *v/v* concentration in mineral oil, as used by Kermen et al. (2011)]: 3-hexanol (3HEX: 12178; 0.076), heptanol (HEP: 8129; 0.911), butyric acid (BUA: 6590; 0.098), heptanal (HEPa: 8130; 0.075), ethyl butyrate (ETB: 7762; 0.012), caproic acid (CAP: 8892; 3.631), 2′3-butane-di-one (23BD: 650; 0.003), benzaldehyde (BZ: 240; 0.154), guaiacol (GUA: 460; 2.087), isoamylacetate (IAA: 31276; 0.032), diphenyl oxide (DPO: 7583; 13.552), allyl caproate (ACA: 31266; 0.553), benzyl acetate (BZA: 8785; 1.467), citronellal (CITa: 7794; 1.271), eugenol (EUG: 3314; 13.122), methyl anthranilate (MA: 8635; 12.653), linalol (LIN: 6549; 2.164), alpha-pinene (aPIN: 6654; 0.099), D-carvone (CAR: 16724; 1.924), and beta-ionone (ION: 638014; 30.604). To further examine the hedonic assessment of each of these odors, a pilot experiment was conducted in healthy subjects ($n = 19$; mean age, 19.47 ± 0.207 years; 13 male) who rated the pleasantness of each stimulus on a scale from 1 (not at all pleasant) to 9 (very pleasant). Results revealed that the stimuli did indeed cover a wide range of affective evaluation, from the most unpleasant to the most pleasant (**Figure 1A**). Moreover, it was also ensured that the odorants covered the entire physicochemical olfactory space by including molecules with a full range of molecular weight and structural complexity (**Figure 1B**). All odorants were diluted in mineral oil so as to achieve an approximate gas-phase partial pressure of 1 Pa.

EXPERIMENTAL PROCEDURE

The experimental procedure was explained in great detail to the subjects, who provided written consent prior to participation. The study was conducted according to the Declaration of Helsinki and was approved by the local ethics committee of Lyon.

After providing written informed consent, subjects started the experiment. Odorants were presented in 15-ml flasks (opening diameter, 1.7 cm; height, 5.8 cm; filled with 5 ml), absorbed on a scentless polypropylene fabric (3 × 7 cm; 3M, Valley, NE, USA) to optimize evaporation and air/oil partitioning.

The experimenter presented the odorant vial 1 cm below the subject's nose and subjects were instructed to sniff at each presentation of a vial then rate odor intensity and pleasantness on a scale from 1 (not at all intense/ pleasant) to 9 (very intense/ pleasant). Although the two ratings were performed in the same perceptual task, participants were asked to first complete the intensity judgment that refers more to the stimulus itself (i.e., concentration).

Once odor ratings were completed, participants were asked to verbalize on each odor by describing it as precisely as possible. The instructions given to the subjects were as follows: "You are going to smell several odors one after the other. Your task will be to sniff each vial and then to rate how intense and pleasant the smell was. To give your estimates, you will rate each odorant on a scale from 1 (not at all intense/ pleasant) to 9 (very intense/ pleasant). Then, after rating each odor, you will have to describe the smell as precisely as possible." Odorants were presented every 45 s. In order to habituate the subjects to the experimental setting, a training session was carried out with a sequence of 1–3 empty flasks.

DATA ANALYSIS

Partitioning the odorant data set into two groups of pleasant and unpleasant odors

A cluster analysis (using k-means partitioning) was used to separate the odorant sample into two groups of pleasant and

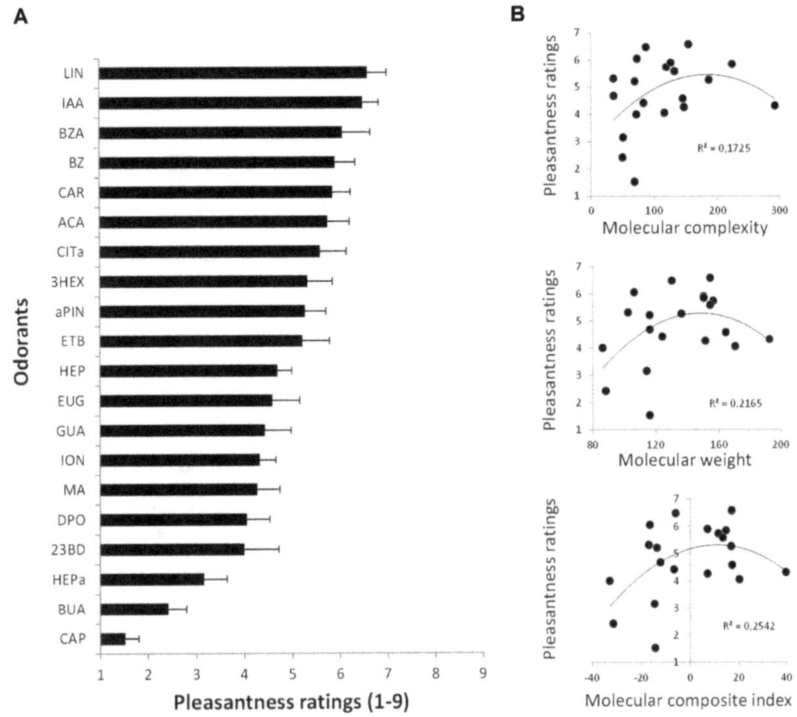

FIGURE 1 | Pilot study. (A) The tested odorants cover a large range of pleasantness ratings. **(B)** Odorant molecules covered a full range of structural complexity (complexity index was collected from PubChem, one of the largest databases of chemical molecules – http://pubchem.ncbi.nlm.nih.gov/; see also Kermen et al., 2011 for details), of molecular weight and of physicochemical properties (molecular composite index based on a principal component analysis with physicochemical data obtained from Dragon® software).

unpleasant odors. Here, all pleasantness ratings data from all odorants and all subjects (from the four groups) were considered. This analysis revealed that the ten most unpleasant were CAP, BUA, HEPa, DPO, 23BD, HEP, MA, GUA, EUG, and ETB and the ten most pleasant odors were CITa, 3HEX, ION, aPIN, ACA, CAR, IAA, BZ, BZA, and LIN. It is noteworthy that the pleasantness scores of the 20 odorants in the main study correlated positively with those obtained in the pilot study ($r = 0.92$, $p < 0.0001$).

Verbal description of pleasant and unpleasant odors

To illustrate the verbal descriptions provided by the four groups, we considered the descriptions of each individual (in a given group) by counting the number of times a word was used. Thus, for each group, a table including all words and their occurrences was set. These four tables were then expressed graphically (https://github.com/amueller/word_cloud; **Figure 2A**). Afterward, to analyze each subject's olfactory description, the 20 verbalizations produced by each subject (for the 20 odorants) were processed by exploratory lexical analysis, first counting references to pleasantness (e.g., "pleasant," "unpleasant"). Here, a mark of "-1" was attributed for unpleasant labels, and a mark "$+1$" was used for pleasant labels. Second, three types of references were considered: (1) references to an odor source (e.g., "flower"), (2) references to an olfactory quality [e.g., "woody," Chastrette et al. (1988) being used to determine whether a term was an olfactory quality], and (3) references to chemical terminology (e.g., "beta ionone").

Statistical analyses

Perceptual ratings and verbal data were analyzed using a 4 × 2 ANOVA using "group" (novices, trainee cooks, flavorists, perfumers) as a between-subjects factor and "hedonic valence" (unpleasant, pleasant) as a within-subject factor. If significant effects of "group" or "hedonic valence" or a significant "group"*"hedonic valence" interaction were observed, the analysis was followed by Bonferroni tests to allow for multiple statistical comparisons.

RESULTS

PERCEPTUAL RATING TASK

Because the four groups had heterogeneous distributions in terms of age and gender, as a control analysis, we first explored whether age correlated with hedonic appreciation in each pleasantness category (independent of learning group). Results revealed no significant relationship between hedonic appreciation of (i) pleasant odors and age ($r = 0.007$, $p > 0.05$) and, (ii) unpleasant odors and age ($r = 0.056$, $p > 0.05$). Moreover, gender did not influence hedonic appreciation of pleasant odors [$F(1,62) = 0.049$, $p > 0.05$] and unpleasant odors [$F(1,62) = 0.175$, $p > 0.05$].

Statistical analysis of pleasantness ratings revealed a significant effect of hedonic valence [$F(1,60) = 267.171$, $p < 0.0001$; pleasant odors being rated as more pleasant than unpleasant odors; mean ± SEM: unpleasant odors, 3.86 ± 0.10; pleasant odors,

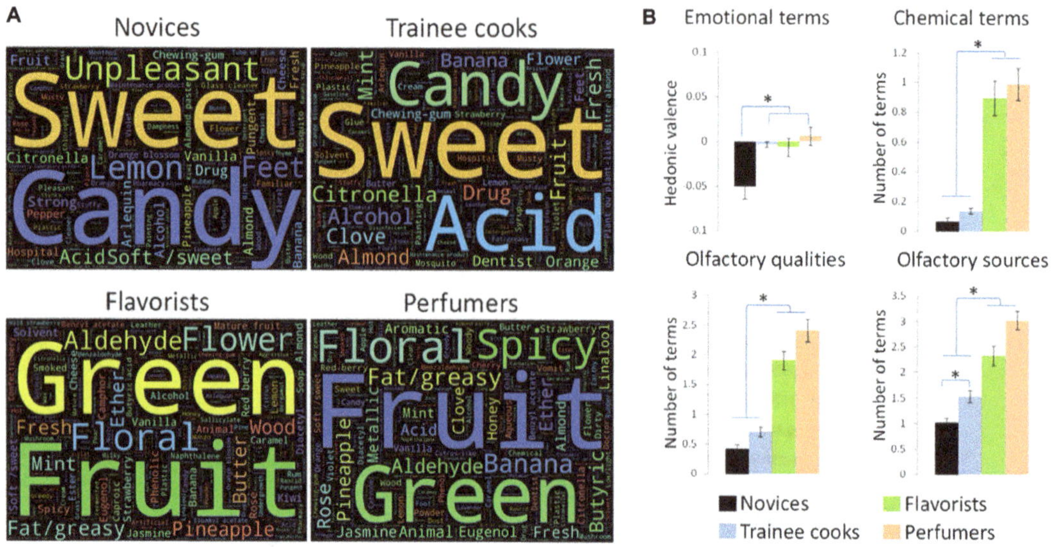

FIGURE 2 | Verbal descriptions of odors in untrained subjects, trainee cooks, flavorists, and perfumers. (A) Whereas novice (untrained) subjects used more often sources and negative emotional terms to describe smells, experts used more technical terms when asked to verbalize about odors. **(B)** Novices used more emotional terms than trainee cooks, flavorists and perfumers and these terms are more often negatives. The number of chemical terms and olfactory qualities to describe odors is significantly higher in flavorists and perfumers than in novices and trainee cooks. Further, novices used less odor source references than trainee cooks, flavorists and perfumers and trainee cooks used less odor source references than flavorists and perfumers. $^{*}p < 0.05$ (corrected for multiple comparisons).

5.54 ± 0.09]. In addition, a significant effect of groups was noted [$F(3,60) = 3.416$, $p < 0.03$], but paired comparisons revealed no significant difference between the four groups ($p > 0.05$ in all cases; **Table 1**).

Regarding intensity ratings, a significant effect of hedonic valence was observed [$F(2,120) = 17.008$, $p < 0.0001$; pleasant odors being rated as less intense than unpleasant odors; mean ± SEM: unpleasant odors, 6.59 ± 0.10; pleasant odors, 5.75 ± 0.10].

This effect was accompanied by a significant effect of groups [$F(3,60) = 4.045$, $p < 0.02$] and a significant groups*hedonic valence interaction [$F(3,60) = 6.108$, $p < 0.002$]. The effect of groups reflected that odors were rated as significantly more intense by perfumers than novices ($p < 0.03$) (**Table 2**). The significant group*hedonic valence interaction reflected that unpleasant odors were rated more intense than pleasant odors in novices ($p < 0.006$), trainee cooks ($p < 0.0001$), flavorists ($p < 0.005$), and perfumers ($p < 0.0001$).

Table 1 | Pleasantness ratings of pleasant and unpleasant odors in novice (untrained) subjects, trainee cooks, flavorists, and perfumers.

	Unpleasant odors		Pleasant odors	
	Mean	**SEM**	**Mean**	**SEM**
Novices	3.63	0.13	5.58	0.17
Trainee cooks	3.66	0.18	5.41	0.19
Flavorists	4.55	0.24	5.76	0.21
Perfumers	3.62	0.19	5.45	0.22

Table 2 | Intensity ratings of pleasant and unpleasant odors in novice (untrained) subjects, trainee cooks, flavorists, and perfumers.

	Unpleasant odors		Pleasant odors	
	Mean	**SEM**	**Mean**	**SEM**
Novices	6.21	0.19	5.44	0.23
Trainee cooks	6.19	0.23	5.64	0.22
Flavorists	6.73	0.16	6.09	0.20
Perfumers	7.25	0.13	5.83	0.18

VERBAL DESCRIPTION TASK

A descriptive analysis performed on the verbal data revealed differences between groups regarding their odor description. Whereas novices seems to use specific sources (e.g., "feet," "candy") and "emotional" words (e.g., "unpleasant"), flavorists and perfumers describe smells using more technical terms (chemical terminology and references to olfactory qualities and sources; **Figure 2A**).

Specifically, regarding emotional terms, a significant effect of hedonic valence was observed reflecting that unpleasant odors were described using more negative emotional words than pleasant odors [mean ± SEM: unpleasant odors, -0.033 ± 0.011; pleasant odors, 0.006 ± 0.009; $F(3,60) = 5.958$, $p < 0.002$]. Moreover, a significant effect of group was observed [$F(1,60) = 5.306$, $p < 0.03$], reflecting that novices used more negative emotional words to describe odors than trainee cooks ($p < 0.03$) and perfumers ($p < 0.02$; **Figure 2B**). It is worth noting that the difference between novices and flavorists was significant ($p = 0.0187$) but did not survive multiple comparisons.

For chemical terms, a significant effect of group was observed [$F(3,60) = 36.353$, $p < 0.0001$], reflecting the fact that perfumers and flavorists used more chemical terms than novices and trainee cooks ($p < 0.0001$). No significant differences were observed between perfumers and flavorists ($p > 0.05$) or between novices and trainee cooks ($p > 0.05$; **Figure 2B**).

With regard to olfactory qualities, a significant effect of group was likewise observed [$F(3,60) = 48.818$, $p < 0.0001$]: perfumers and flavorists used more olfactory quality terms than novices and trainee cooks ($p < 0.005$). No significant differences were observed between perfumers and flavorists ($p > 0.05$) or between novices and trainee cooks ($p > 0.05$; **Figure 2B**). In addition, a significant effect of hedonic valence was observed [mean ± SEM: unpleasant odors, 1.30 ± 0.11; pleasant odors, 1.41 ± 0.13; $F(1,60) = 5.877$, $p < 0.02$] reflecting that pleasant odors were described using more olfactory qualities than unpleasant odors.

Finally, regarding references to odor sources, a significant effect of group was also observed [$F(2,60) = 34.622$, $p < 0.0001$]: (i) novices used fewer odor source references than trainee cooks, flavorists and perfumers ($p < 0.05$); and (ii) trainee cooks used fewer odor source references than flavorists and perfumers. No significant differences were observed between perfumers and flavorists ($p > 0.05$; **Figure 2B**). Apart from main effect of group, a significant effect of hedonic valence was observed reflecting the fact that pleasant odors were described using more odor source references than unpleasant odors [mean ± SEM: unpleasant odors, 1.84 ± 0.11; pleasant odors, 2.1 ± 0.13; $F(1,60) = 20.610$, $p < 0.0001$].This latter finding corroborates previous results in the field showing a negative correlation between the number of olfactory qualities and odor unpleasantness: odorants that evoked few sources and qualities were also perceived as more unpleasant (Kermen et al., 2011).

DISCUSSION

The main question addressed by the present investigation concerned the effect of expertise on verbal descriptions and perceptual assessments of pleasant and unpleasant odors. It was assumed that flavorists and perfumers should rate pleasant odors as less pleasant, and unpleasant odors as less unpleasant than non-experts. Moreover, on a descriptive level, whereas flavorists and perfumers were expected to use chemical and odor terminology without referring to odor hedonics, novices were expected to accompany their odor descriptions by references to pleasantness.

An important finding of the present study is that, in contrast to our expectations, hedonic perceptual ratings of unpleasant and pleasant odors was not affected by expertise: novices, trainee cooks, flavorists and perfumers rated similarly unpleasant odors on the one hand and pleasant odors on the other hand. As was shown in wine tasting (Valentin and Chollet, 2000) where experts and naïve subjects do not significantly differ in perceptual similarity judgment, the present study suggests that experts in olfaction are able to discriminate and/or categorize odors on the basis of their hedonic valence. However, although this is true at an evaluative or perceptual level (pleasantness ratings), verbal data suggest that experts describe and conceptualize odors with few references to pleasantness: a result of interest of our study was the low number of references to pleasantness in the verbal descriptions of experts, whereas novices used hedonic terms to describe odors (especially words with negative connotation). These results are in line with the literature in the field suggesting that experts in olfaction avoid references to odor hedonic valence (Yoshida, 1964; Ehrlichman and Bastone, 1992; Holley, 2002).

An interpretation of the discrepancy between an expert's ability to use less references to unpleasantness than controls vs. his actual perceptual hedonic appreciation of unpleasant (and pleasant) odors which remains the same, could be that on a perceptual level, hedonic valence and especially its negative side, represents the basic level of odor categorization for any perceiver, independent of his/her expertise. This affective perception would occur quickly and unwittingly. In accordance with the above, autonomic responses to unpleasant odors occur implicitly when subjects are not given any particular instruction (Bensafi et al., 2002b), and response times are significantly shorter for unpleasant than for pleasant odors (Bensafi et al., 2003b). These results seem to indicate a “quick and dirty” pathway, fast-tracking decision for bad odors. Brain imaging studies also show that pleasant and unpleasant odors activate different neural networks (Zald and Pardo, 1997; Gottfried et al., 2002a; Anderson et al., 2003; Rolls et al., 2003; Royet et al., 2003; de Araujo et al., 2005; Bensafi et al., 2008). Taken together, these results support the hypothesis that only a rudimentary level of processing is necessary to hedonically pre-process odors, and that this pre-processing takes place when perceivers do not attend to any other specific feature of the odorant stimulus, whatever the expertise level. However, when experts are engaged in a verbal task requiring subtle discrimination and description, they process the same odors more deeply on a lexico-semantic level, with few hedonic references.

On a lexical level, verbal descriptions in relation to smells were significantly longer in experts than untrained subjects, confirming expectations regarding experts' explicit knowledge. Previous studies described the language of experts (perfumers and flavorists) as richer, more proficient, precise, expressive and/or consistent (Bende and Nordin, 1997; Parr et al., 2002). In line with this, the linguistic-based criteria used here showed that experts' verbal skills were characterized by the use of chemical names and terms referring to odor qualities and sources. Moreover, trainee cooks used more odor source references than novices, suggesting that daily exposure to odor sources (food sources in this case, without explicit olfactory associative learning) can increase the verbal ability to describe smells.

Lack of verbal resources in odor processing is a characteristic of untrained subjects. Indeed, it is a common experience to like (or dislike) a specific odor, and to be quite sure of recognizing it even if no name can be put on it: this so-called ‘tip of the nose phenomenon’ highlights implicit knowledge of odors, despite failure to name them. This interaction between language and olfaction can be seen in the development of olfactory function: whereas a 3-year-old child learns to name colors, odor naming is mostly developed through autonomous learning (Rouby and Sicard, 1997) and expressed in terms of idiosyncratic experience (Engen, 1987). On the contrary, expert verbal skills in our study were characterized by the use of domain-specific terminology, with very few references to pleasantness. These differences between experts and novices reflect the effect of learning for flavorists and perfumers since their olfactory education includes learning of chemical names and olfactory qualities with adjectives (see the "the field of odors," Jaubert et al., 1987; Jaubert, 1995). For example, in perfumers and flavorists particularly, the creation of fragrances and flavors involves recognizing hundreds of odorants and memorizing the effects of their combinations. Reports indicate that perfumers are better able to imagine odors (Gilbert et al., 1998; see also Rinck et al., 2009) and can routinely group odors in classes, from 18 (Rimmel, 1895) to 88 (Arctander, 1969; Chastrette et al., 1988). For perfumers, these classes usually contain further sub-classes (Roudnitska, 1991; Ellena, 2007). Moreover, notions such as "notes," "faces," and "sub-tones" are used in perfumery to represent odors (Ellena, 2007). Experts, through such continuous repetitive olfactory training, can communicate their perception using verbal supports which is of upmost importance in their professional practice.

Although the present study provides evidence for an influence of expertise on odor verbalization, some of the findings warrant discussion. Indeed, another particular feature of the present findings was the increased perceived intensity in perfumers. One potential explanation may be that perfumers have lower odor threshold leading to higher perceived intensity due to their past training. Unfortunately, very little information is available to confirm this hypothesis and one of the few studies that compared experts and novices on a sensory level was that of (Bende and Nordin, 1997) who showed no expertise effect on olfactory detection, rendering less likely this possibility. Another explanation may be that perceived intensity is higher for identified odors (Distel and Hudson, 2001). In this psychophysical study, the authors tested human participants with a large set of everyday odorants, and asked their subjects to rate odor pleasantness, familiarity and intensity. Results showed that all these ratings (including odor intensity) were enhanced when participants either were given the name by the experimenter or could identify the odorant source themselves. In the same line, the increase in odor intensity seen in experts of our study may be related to their better ability to describe, name and identified the odors used.

In conclusion, we showed here that expertise does not influence odor hedonic perception *per se* when the subject's attention is focused on pleasantness: experts and novices appreciated similarly pleasant and unpleasant odors. On a verbal level, in contrast to experts, novices do not have rich lexical representations of smells, and they often use words referring to environmental odor sources accompanied by perceptually hedonic terms, often referring to unpleasantness. However, when attention is directed toward the lexical component of odor representations, experts seem to avoid references to pleasantness. These findings offer new insights into odor hedonic perception in untrained and expert populations, highlighting for the first time an influence of expertise at the verbal but not at the perceptual level of processing, providing new understanding on perceptual processing of pleasant and unpleasant odors.

ACKNOWLEDGMENTS

This study was supported a grant from the ANR to Moustafa Bensafi (EMCO program, ICEO Project) and by the Region Rhone-Alpes (CIBLE 2011 program).

REFERENCES

Alaoui-Ismaili, O., Robin, O., Rada, H., Dittmar, A., and Vernet-Maury, E. (1997a). Basic emotions evoked by odorants: comparison between autonomic responses and self-evaluation. *Physiol. Behav.* 62, 713–720. doi: 10.1016/S0031-9384(97)90016-0

Alaoui-Ismaili, O., Vernet-Maury, E., Dittmar, A., Delhomme, G., and Chanel, J. (1997b). Odor hedonics: connection with emotional response estimated by autonomic parameters. *Chem. Senses* 22, 237–248. doi: 10.1093/chemse/22.3.237

Anderson, A. K., Christoff, K., Stappen, I., Panitz, D., Ghahremani, D. G., Glover, G., et al. (2003). Dissociated neural representations of intensity and valence in human olfaction. *Nat. Neurosci.* 6, 196–202. doi: 10.1038/nn1001

Arctander, S. (1969). *Perfume and Flavor Chemicals (Aroma Chemicals)*. Montclair, NJ: Allured Publishing Corporation.

Ayabe-Kanamura, S., Schicker, I., Laska, M., Hudson, R., Distel, H., Kobayakawa, T., et al. (1998). Differences in perception of everyday odors: a Japanese-German cross-cultural study. *Chem. Senses* 23, 31–38. doi: 10.1093/chemse/23.1.31

Barkat, S., Poncelet, J., Landis, B. N., Rouby, C., and Bensafi, M. (2008). Improved smell pleasantness after odor-taste associative learning in humans. *Neurosci. Lett.* 434, 108–112. doi: 10.1016/j.neulet.2008.01.037

Bende, M., and Nordin, S. (1997). Perceptual learning in olfaction: professional wine tasters versus controls. *Physiol. Behav.* 62, 1065–1070. doi: 10.1016/S0031-9384(97)00251-5

Bensafi, M., Iannilli, E., Gerber, J., and Hummel, T. (2008). Neural coding of stimulus concentration in the human olfactory and intranasal trigeminal systems. *Neuroscience* 154, 832–838. doi: 10.1016/j.neuroscience.2008.03.079

Bensafi, M., Iannilli, E., Poncelet, J., Seo, H. S., Gerber, J., Rouby, C., et al. (2012). Dissociated representations of pleasant and unpleasant olfacto-trigeminal mixtures: an FMRI study. *PLoS ONE* 7:e38358. doi: 10.1371/journal.pone.0038358

Bensafi, M., Rinck, F., Schaal, B., and Rouby, C. (2007). Verbal cues modulate hedonic perception of odors in 5-year-old children as well as in adults. *Chem. Senses* 32, 855–862. doi: 10.1093/chemse/bjm055

Bensafi, M., Rouby, C., Farget, V., Bertrand, B., Vigouroux, M., and Holley, A. (2002a). Autonomic nervous system responses to odours: the role of pleasantness and arousal. *Chem. Senses* 27, 703–709. doi: 10.1093/chemse/27.8.703

Bensafi, M., Rouby, C., Farget, V., Bertrand, B., Vigouroux, M., and Holley, A. (2002b). Influence of affective and cognitive judgments on autonomic parameters during inhalation of pleasant and unpleasant odors in humans. *Neurosci. Lett.* 319, 162–166. doi: 10.1016/S0304-3940(01)02572-1

Bensafi, M., Rouby, C., Farget, V., Bertrand, B., Vigouroux, M., and Holley, A. (2002c). Psychophysiological correlates of affects in human olfaction. *Neurophysiol. Clin.* 32, 326–332. doi: 10.1016/S0987-7053(02)00339-8

Bensafi, M., Rouby, C., Farget, V., Vigouroux, M., and Holley, A. (2002d). Asymmetry of pleasant vs. unpleasant odor processing during affective judgment in humans. *Neurosci. Lett.* 328, 309–313. doi: 10.1016/S0304-3940(02)00548-7

Bensafi, M., Porter, J., Pouliot, S., Mainland, J., Johnson, B., Zelano, C., et al. (2003a). Olfactomotor activity during imagery mimics that during perception. *Nat. Neurosci.* 6, 1142–1144. doi: 10.1038/nn1145

Bensafi, M., Rouby, C., Farget, V., Bertrand, B., Vigouroux, M., and Holley, A. (2003b). Perceptual, affective, and cognitive judgments of odors: pleasantness and handedness effects. *Brain Cogn.* 51, 270–275. doi: 10.1016/S0278-2626(03)00019-8

Berglund, B., Berglund, U., Engen, T., and Ekman, G. (1973). Multidimensional analysis of twenty-one odors. *Scand. J. Psychol.* 14, 131–137. doi: 10.1111/j.1467-9450.1973.tb00104.x

Brauchli, P., Ruegg, P. B., Etzweiler, F., and Zeier, H. (1995). Electrocortical and autonomic alteration by administration of a pleasant and an unpleasant odor. *Chem. Senses* 20, 505–515. doi: 10.1093/chemse/20.5.505

Chastrette, M., Elmouaffek, A., and Sauvegrain, P. (1988). A multidimensional statistical study of similarities between 74 notes used in perfumery. *Chem. Senses* 13, 295–305. doi: 10.1093/chemse/13.2.295

Croy, I., Olgun, S., and Joraschky, P. (2011). Basic emotions elicited by odors and pictures. *Emotion* 11, 1331–1335. doi: 10.1037/a0024437 de Araujo, I. E., Rolls, E. T., Velazco, M. I., Margot, C., and Cayeux, I. (2005). Cognitive modulation of olfactory processing. *Neuron* 46, 671–679. doi: 10.1016/j.neuron.2005.04.021

Distel, H., and Hudson, R. (2001). Judgement of odor intensity is influenced by subjects' knowledge of the odor source. *Chem. Senses* 26, 247–251. doi: 10.1093/chemse/26.3.247

Dubois, D. (2000). Categories as acts of meaning: the case of categories in olfaction and audition. *Cogn. Sci. Q.* 1, 35–68.

Dubois, D., and Rouby, C. (1997). Une approche de l'olfaction: du linguistique au neuronal. *Intellectica* 24, 9–20.

Ehrlichman, H., and Bastone, L. (1992). "Olfaction and emotion," in *Science of Olfaction*, M. Serby and K. Chobor (New York: Springer), 410–438. doi: 10.1007/978-1-4612-2836-3_15

Ehrlichman, H., Brown, S., Zhu, J., and Warrenburg, S. (1995). Startle reflex modulation during exposure to pleasant and unpleasant odors. *Psychophysiology* 32, 150–154. doi: 10.1111/j.1469-8986.1995.tb03306.x

Ehrlichman, H., Kuhl, S. B., Zhu, J., and Warrenburg, S. (1997). Startle reflex modulation by pleasant and unpleasant odors in a between-subjects design. *Psychophysiology* 34, 726–729. doi: 10.1111/j.1469-8986.1997.tb02149.x

Ellena, J. (2007). *La Note Verte.* Paris: Sabine Wespieser Editeur.

Engen, T. (1987). Remembering odors and their names. *Am. Sci.* 75, 497–503.

Fernandez, P., Bensafi, M., Rouby, C., and Giboreau, A. (2013). Does olfactory specific satiety take place in a natural setting? *Appetite* 60, 1–4. doi: 10.1016/j.appet.2012.10.006

Gilbert, A. N., Crouch, M., and Kemp, S. E. (1998). Olfactory and visual mental imagery. *J. Ment. Imagery* 22, 137–146.

Godinot, N., Sicard, G., and Dubois, D. (1995). Categories, familiarity and unpleasantness of odours. *Odours VOC's J.* 3, 202–208.

Gottfried, J. A., Deichmann, R., Winston, J. S., and Dolan, R. J. (2002a). Functional heterogeneity in human olfactory cortex: an event-related functional magnetic resonance imaging study. *J. Neurosci.* 22, 10819–10828.

Gottfried, J. A., O'Doherty, J., and Dolan, R. J. (2002b). Appetitive and aversive olfactory learning in humans studied using event-related functional magnetic resonance imaging. *J. Neurosci.* 22, 10829–10837.

Harper, R. (1966). On odour classification. *Int. J. Food Sci. Technol.* 1, 167–176. doi: 10.1111/j.1365-2621.1966.tb01803.x

Herz, R. S. (2003). The effect of verbal context on olfactory perception. *J. Exp. Psychol. Gen.* 132, 595–606. doi: 10.1037/0096-3445.132.4.595

Holley, A. (2002). "Cognitive aspects of olfaction in perfumer practice," in *Olfaction, Taste and Cognition*, eds C. Rouby, B. Schaal, D. Dubois, R. Gervais, and A. Holley. (Cambridge, NY: Cambridge University Press), 16–26. doi: 10.1017/CBO9780511546389.006

Jacob, T. J., Fraser, C., Wang, L., Walker, V., and O'Connor, S. (2003). Psychophysical evaluation of responses to pleasant and mal-odour stimulation in human subjects; adaptation, dose response and gender differences. *Int. J. Psychophysiol.* 48, 67–80. doi: 10.1016/S0167-8760(03)00020-5

Jaubert, J. N. (1995). The field of odors: toward a universal language for odor relationships. *Perfumer and flavorist* 20, 1–15.

Jaubert, J. N., Gordon, G., and Dore, J.-C. (1987). Une organisation du champ des odeurs. *Parfums, cosmétiques, arômes* 77, 53–56.

Joussain, P., Chakirian, A., Kermen, F., Rouby, C., and Bensafi, M. (2011). Physicochemical influence on odor hedonics: where does it occur first? *Commun. Integr. Biol.* 4, 563–565. doi: 10.4161/cib.4.5.15811

Joussain, P., Giboreau, A., Fontas, M., Laville, M., Hummel, T., Souquet, P. J., et al. (2013a). Cisplatin chemotherapy induces odor perception changes in bronchial cancer patients. *Lung Cancer* 82, 168–170. doi: 10.1016/j.lungcan.2013.06.009

Joussain, P., Thevenet, M., Rouby, C., and Bensafi, M. (2013b). Effect of aging on hedonic appreciation of pleasant and unpleasant odors. *PLoS ONE* 8:e61376. doi: 10.1371/journal.pone.0061376

Kermen, F., Chakirian, A., Sezille, C., Joussain, P., Le Goff, G., Ziessel, A., et al. (2011). Molecular complexity determines the number of olfactory notes and the pleasantness of smells. *Sci. Rep.* 1, 206. doi: 10.1038/srep00206

Khan, R. M., Luk, C. H., Flinker, A., Aggarwal, A., Lapid, H., Haddad, R., et al. (2007). Predicting odor pleasantness from odorant structure: pleasantness as a reflection of the physical world. *J. Neurosci.* 27, 10015–10023. doi: 10.1523/JNEUROSCI.1158-07.2007

Mandairon, N., Poncelet, J., Bensafi, M., and Didier, A. (2009). Humans and mice express similar olfactory preferences. *PLoS ONE* 4:e4209. doi: 10.1371/journal.pone.0004209

Miltner, W., Matjak, M., Braun, C., Diekmann, H., and Brody, S. (1994). Emotional qualities of odors and their influence on the startle reflex in humans. *Psychophysiology* 31, 107–110. doi: 10.1111/j.1469-8986.1994.tb01030.x

Parr, W. V., Heatherbell, D., and White, K. G. (2002). Demystifying wine expertise: olfactory threshold, perceptual skill and semantic memory in expert and novice wine judges. *Chem. Senses* 27, 747–755. doi: 10.1093/chemse/27.8.747

Poncelet, J., Rinck, F., Ziessel, A., Joussain, P., Thevenet, M., Rouby, C., et al. (2010). Semantic knowledge influences prewired hedonic responses to odors. *PLoS ONE* 5:e13878. doi: 10.1371/journal.pone.0013878

Rimmel, E. (1895). *The Base of Perfumes.* London (French translation 1990, Le livre des parfums. Paris: les éditions 1900).

Rinck, F., Barkat-Defradas, M., Chakirian, A., Joussain, P., Bourgeat, F., Thevenet, M., et al. (2011). Ontogeny of odor liking during childhood and its relation to language development. *Chem. Senses* 36, 83–91. doi: 10.1093/chemse/bjq101

Rinck, F., Rouby, C., and Bensafi, M. (2009). Which format for odor images? *Chem. Senses* 34, 11–13. doi: 10.1093/chemse/bjn060

Rolls, E. T. (2004). The functions of the orbitofrontal cortex. *Brain Cogn.* 55, 11–29. doi: 10.1016/S0278-2626(03)00277-X

Rolls, E. T., Kringelbach, M. L., and De Araujo, I. E. (2003). Different representations of pleasant and unpleasant odours in the human brain. *Eur. J. Neurosci.* 18, 695–703. doi: 10.1046/j.1460-9568.2003.02779.x

Rouby, C., Bourgeat, F., Rinck, F., Poncelet, J., and Bensafi, M. (2009). Perceptual and sensorimotor differences between "good" and "poor" olfactory mental imagers. *Ann. N. Y. Acad. Sci.* 1170, 333–337. doi: 10.1111/j.1749-6632.2009.03915.x

Rouby, C., and Sicard, G. (1997). "Des catégories d'odeurs," in *Catégorisation et cognition : de la perception au discours,* ed. D. Dubois (Paris: Edition Kimé), 59–81.

Roudnitska, E. (1991). "The art of perfumery," in *Perfumes Art, Science and Technology,* eds P. M. Müller and D. Lamparsky (London: Elsevier), 3–48.

Royet, J. P., Plailly, J., Delon-Martin, C., Kareken, D. A., and Segebarth, C. (2003). fMRI of emotional responses to odors: influence of hedonic valence and judgment, handedness, and gender. *Neuroimage* 20, 713–728. doi: 10.1016/S1053-8119(03)00388-4

Schiffman, S. (1977). Food recognition by the elderly. *J. Gerontol.* 32, 586–592. doi: 10.1093/geronj/32.5.586

Schiffman, S. S. (1974). Physicochemical correlates of olfactory quality. *Science* 185, 112–117. doi: 10.1126/science.185.4146.112

Valentin, D., and Chollet, S. (2000). Le degré d'expertise a-t-il une influence sur la perception olfactive? Quelques éléments de réponse dans le domaine du vin. *L'année psychologique* 100, 11–36. doi: 10.3406/psy.2000.28625

Yeshurun, Y., and Sobel, N. (2010). An odor is not worth a thousand words: from multidimensional odors to unidimensional odor objects. *Annu. Rev. Psychol.* 61, 219–241, C211–215. doi: 10.1146/annurev.psych.60.110707.163639

Yoshida, M. (1964). Studies in psychometric classification of odors. *Jpn. Psychol. Res.* 6, 115–124.

Zald, D. H., and Pardo, J. V. (1997). Emotion, olfaction, and the human amygdala: amygdala activation during aversive olfactory stimulation. *Proc. Natl. Acad. Sci. U.S.A.* 94, 4119–4124. doi: 10.1073/pnas.94.8.4119

Zarzo, M. (2011). Hedonic judgments of chemical compounds are correlated with molecular size. *Sensors (Basel)* 11, 3667–3686. doi: 10.3390/s110403667

Zucco, G. M., Carassai, A., Baroni, M. R., and Stevenson, R. J. (2011). Labeling, identification, and recognition of wine-relevant odorants in expert sommeliers, intermediates, and untrained wine drinkers. *Perception* 40, 598–607. doi: 10.1068/p6972

10

Sadness might isolate you in a non-smelling world: olfactory perception and depression

Sylvia Schablitzky and Bettina M. Pause*

Department of Experimental Psychology, Heinrich-Heine-University, Düsseldorf, Germany

***Correspondence:**
Bettina M. Pause, Department of Experimental Psychology, Heinrich-Heine-University, Universitaetsstraße 1, 40225 Duesseldorf, Germany
e-mail: bettina.pause@hhu.de

Major depressive disorder (MDD) occurs with a high prevalence among mental illnesses. MDD patients experience sadness and hopelessness, with blunted affective reactivity. However, such depressive episodes are also key symptoms in other depressive disorders, like Bipolar Disorder (BPD) or Seasonal Affective Disorder (SAD). Moreover, depressive symptoms can also be found in healthy individuals, but are experienced as less severe or for a shorter duration than in patients. Here, it is aimed to summarize studies investigating odor perception in depression, including depressive states in healthy individuals and patient populations. Odor perception in depression has been assessed with psychophysical methods (olfactory sensitivity, odor identification, and discrimination), and odor ratings (intensity, emotional valence, familiarity). In addition, some studies investigated affective reactions to odors, and physiological and anatomical correlates of odor perception in depression. The summary reveals that MDD is associated with reduced olfactory sensitivity. However, odor identification and discrimination scores seem to be unaffected by depression. The reduced olfactory sensitivity might be associated with a reduced ability to encode olfactory information and a reduced volume of the olfactory bulb. While similar processes seem to occur in healthy individuals experiencing depressive states, they have not been observed in BPD or SAD patients. However, in order to conclude that the reduced olfactory sensitivity is directly linked to depression, it is suggested that studies should implement control measures of cognitive performances or perceptual abilities in other stimulus modalities. It is concluded that the reduced olfactory performance in MDD patients seems to be disorder-, modality-, and test-specific, and that the application of an appropriate olfactory and cognitive test-battery might be highly useful in the differential diagnosis of MDD.

Keywords: major depression, sadness, odor perception, olfactory sensitivity, bipolar disorder, emotion

INTRODUCTION

Everybody knows the feeling of sadness as a transient mood state. Sadness is considered to be one of six basic emotions, all of which being experienced in healthy humans independent of culture (anger, disgust, fear, happiness, sadness, and surprise; Ekman and Davidson, 1994). Several brain areas involved in cerebral processing of these emotions are described (Panksepp, 2011; LeDoux, 2012), with sad states being regulated most prominently by the anterior cingulate cortex and the dorsomedial prefrontal cortex (Murphy et al., 2003). But what kind of feelings and behavior differentiate the normal experience of transient sadness from an affective state of depression? The clinical categories and diagnostic criteria for mood and other mental disorders can be assessed via the diagnostic and statistical manual of mental disorders (DSM-5, American Psychiatric Association, APA, 2013).

Whereas in former times (DSM IV; APA, 2000) depression belonged to the category of affective disorders that included unipolar and bipolar depressive disorders, in the present view both disorders are clearly separated from each other (DSM-5, APA, 2013). Among the unipolar depressive disorders, the two most prevalent disorders are Major Depressive Disorder (MDD) and Dysthymia. Both of them share the key symptoms of a depressed mood and a loss of interest or pleasure. However, MDD patients strongly suffer from the depressive mood during at least a 2-weeks period, while in Dysthymia patients, the depressive mood is less severe but lasts at least for 2 years. Bipolar disorders (BPDs) on the other hand, differ from unipolar depressive disorders in the experience of manic (Bipolar Disorder I, BPD I) or hypomanic episodes (Bipolar Disorder II, BPD II), states of abnormally elevated physical or mental activity, usually accompanied by an inflated self-esteem. In BPD patients, the manic phases often alternate with depressive episodes. Both, BPD and MDD, can occur with a seasonal pattern, with depressive episodes regularly reoccurring during fall or winter time.

MDD as well as BPD are described to include one or more major depressive episodes. Therefore, the occurrence of an episode of major depression is not a diagnostic category by itself. The criteria of a major depressive episode are as follows: during 2 weeks nearly the whole time, at least five of the following symptoms have to be present: depressive mood like sadness or hopelessness, reduced interest in activities, significant loss of appetite or increased appetite as well as weight loss or weight-gain without going on a diet, insomnia or hypersomnia, increased psychomotor agitation or retardation, fatigue, feelings of worthlessness, diminished ability to concentrate, and thoughts of suicide. Regarding these symptoms, MDD and BPD are mood disorders affecting functions of motor behavior, perception, memory, cognition, and motivation.

Among all mental disorders, MDD occurs with a high prevalence. The 12-month prevalence in the United States is approximately 7%, with females experiencing 1.5–3-fold higher rates than males. With a 12-month prevalence of 0.6%, BPD has a lower prevalence than MDD (USA, APA, 2013).

There are several theories explaining different aspects of MDD. Cognitive approaches focus on biased information processing and dysfunctional beliefs about the self, the outside world and the future (Beck, 1979). Studies using neuroimaging techniques show alterations of cerebral blood flow and metabolic differences between depressed patients and healthy controls in the amygdala and anatomically related areas of the prefrontal cortex (see Drevets, 2003). Moreover, it is suggested that dysfunctions in the serotonin receptor and other monoaminergic systems could lead to MDD (see Savitz et al., 2009; Savitz and Drevets, 2013). Recently, it has been shown that the deviant serotonergic neurotransmission seems to be responsible for a decoupled cingulated-amygdala-interaction (Pezawas et al., 2005).

Depressive episodes occurring predominately during a particular time of the year (e.g., in the fall or winter) have been termed Seasonal Affective Disorder (SAD). The underlying mechanisms of SAD, MDD, or BPD are supposed to be different, considering the improvement of SAD symptoms, but not MDD or BPD symptoms, through light therapy (exposure to a standard regimen of 10,000 lux cool-white fluorescent light, e.g., Eastman et al., 1998). In SAD, functional deviations within the suprachiasmatic nucleus of the hypothalamus are described (Krout et al., 2002). The suprachiasmatic nucleus is a central structure that mediates behavioral responses induced by the change in the length of daylight.

As mentioned before, alterations of cerebral blood flow and metabolism in the limbic cingulated cortex and prefrontal cortex are consistently observed in MDD patients. Within these brain areas, the amygdala and the ventromedial (orbitofrontal) prefrontal cortex seem to be the most affected in MDD patients (Murray et al., 2011). As well as in emotional processing (LeDoux, 2007), the amygdala is inherently involved in the processing of odor perception (Soudry et al., 2011) and is part of the primary olfactory cortex (Carmichael et al., 1994). From the amygdala olfactory information can be directly transmitted to the orbitofrontal cortex, which is the main neocortical relay for olfactory information (Carmichael et al., 1994; Gottfried, 2006). According to this overlap in odor and emotion processing structures, affective disorders like MDD should accompany alterations of olfactory perception.

Human olfaction has been divided into hierarchical organized levels that are characterized as either primary or secondary. As described by Martzke et al. (1997), olfactory sensitivity is a part of a primary and sensory level of stimulus processing in the olfactory system. However, abilities like olfactory identification, discrimination or odor recognition and odor ratings belong to the secondary and evaluative level of olfaction. The various functions of the olfactory system are to be assessed by suitable methods (Weierstall and Pause, 2012). Most tests for the assessment of olfactory functions fall into three main classes: threshold (absolute sensitivity), identification, and discrimination. Olfactory sensitivity is understood as a measure of the lowest concentration of a particular olfactory stimulus required to activate the receptor neurons resulting in the detection of that odor (Martzke et al., 1997). For the assessment of the odor threshold, a staircase threshold procedure (Bekesy, 1947; Doty, 1991) has been developed that can be used with several odors (Doty and Laing, 2003). This threshold test has been adopted by numerous laboratories (e.g., Pause et al., 2001; Lötsch et al., 2008).

Odor identification is a measure of an individual's ability to perceive and name an odor. Three types are common: first, a simple naming task, prompting the individual to supply a name for a given odor; second, a yes-no odor identification test, in which the participant has to decide whether the odor presented matches a given verbal label or not; or third, a multiple choice odor identification test, with a list of odor names provided for each stimulus. The 40-item, multiple choice University of Pennsylvania Smell Identification Test (UPSIT) is widely used to assess identification performance (Doty et al., 1984b). In the UPSIT, the participant has to choose the odor quality of a given odor out of four verbal descriptors. An odor identification test is also included in the Sniffin' Sticks test battery (Hummel et al., 2007), which is constructed similar to the UPSIT but contains 16 items only.

Odor discrimination is defined as a measure of an individual's ability to differentiate between a set of odors. The most simple form is to state whether two odors are the same or different. However, common tasks involve participants picking out the odd odor out of a series of odors, all of which identical except for one. The only commercially available odor discrimination test is included in the Sniffin' Sticks (Hummel et al., 2007). It comprises 16 items, of which participants are required to choose the odd stimulus out of three given odors.

Psychological attributes of odors are assessed mainly with regard to their intensity, hedonic aspects (pleasantness and unpleasantness) or familiarity. Rating scales can be used to estimate the relative amount of a psychological attribute perceived by an individual. According to Doty and Laing (2003) in chemosensory assessment, two types are popular: category scales, and analog scales. Using category scales, the relative amount of a sensation is signified by indicating which of a series of discrete categories best describes the sensation. Using visual analog scales, the strength of the sensation is indicated by placing a mark along a line that might have descriptors (termed anchors) located at its extremes (e.g., very weak—very strong). Contrary to olfactory sensitivity, odor evaluations are suprathreshold procedures mostly and therefore part of the secondary cognitive evaluative level of the olfactory processing system. For some odors, pleasantness and intensity are closely related psychological dimensions and negatively correlated (Doty, 1975).

In the following review, psychophysical and neurophysiological findings of olfactory performances (sensitivity, identification, discrimination, and odor ratings) in depressed patients (MDD, BPD, SAD) and in healthy individuals experiencing only some depressive symptoms or a transient state of sad mood will be summarized. By expanding this review to healthy people and including the recent literature, this review will add on existing summaries on olfaction and depression (Settle and Amsterdam, 1991; Serby et al., 1992; Atanasova et al., 2008; Burón and Bulbena, 2013).

METHODS

Literature research was based on PubMed (National Center for Biotechnology Information, Bethesda, MDUSA). Only studies investigating distinct groups of MDD, BPD, or SAD patients were included. Mixed samples consisting of BPD and MDD patients in one group or different psychiatric patients in one group were excluded. Further, only publications on chemical perception of standard odors were taken into account. Publications regarding the perception of body odors were not considered, because body odors might be processed by different systems than the olfactory system (Pause, 2012). As it was aimed to focus on the distinct emotional experience of sadness, studies examining olfaction in personality disorders were excluded from the literature search. Finally, effects of odors on mood or therapeutic effect of odors were not considered.

FINDINGS ON OLFACTORY FUNCTION IN DEPRESSION

Research on olfactory dysfunction in patients with depressive disorders mainly focused on psychophysical assessment of olfactory perception. Particularly, olfactory sensitivity, identification and odor ratings including evaluations of odor characteristics like pleasantness, unpleasantness, intensity or familiarity were investigated. To a lesser extent, patients with depressive disorders have been examined with reference to psychophysiological and neuroanatomical aspects of odor perception, like chemosensory event-related potentials (CSERPs, Pause et al., 2003) or the volume of the olfactory bulb (Negoias et al., 2010). In the following sections, we will review the psychophysics, psychophysiology, and neuroanatomy of olfactory perception in patients with depressive disorders.

OLFACTORY SENSITIVITY IN DEPRESSIVE DISORDERS

Almost all studies regarding olfactory acuity in MDD indicate that olfactory sensitivity is reduced (corresponding to elevated detection thresholds) in patients, as compared to healthy controls (**Table 1**). Pause et al. (2001) examined olfactory sensitivity in medicated patients with acute MDD. The Beck's depression score (BDI; Beck et al., 1961) was 28.5 ± 11.4 in the patient group. Olfactory thresholds for eugenol (clove-like odor) and phenyl-ethylalcohol (PEA, rose-like odor) were determined using a two-alternative staircase detection procedure (Bekesy, 1947; Doty, 1991). The study showed reduced olfactory sensitivity in MDD patients compared to healthy controls. Similarly, Thomas et al. (2002) reported slightly ($p < 0.10$) elevated thresholds in a sample of 16 unselected depressives without comorbidity and with a mean BDI-Score of 23.8 ± 9.5. In line with these studies, Lombion-Pouthier et al. (2006) reported sensitivity impairments in patients with severe depression (without any comorbidity) and a BDI-Score of 23.8 ± 5.7. Olfactory perception was assessed by means of the Test Olfactif. The Test Olfactif evaluates olfactory sensitivity using L-carvone and tetrahydrothiopene (forced choice procedure for 5 successive concentrations). Odor detection and identification performance are examined with a panel of 16 odors. Participants have to choose the odor bottle out of four bottles (detection task) and they are asked to choose the correct odor label among a list of four labels (indentification task). Negoias et al. (2010) also showed sensitivity impairments in MDD patients [comorbidities (somatoform disorders, posttraumatic stress disorder and anxiety disorders) were accepted for inclusion] with a mean BDI-Score of 29.7 ± 10.8. All participants were screened for possible cognitive impairments by the mini mental state examination (MMSE, Folstein et al., 1975) and olfactory thresholds were assessed by the Sniffin' Sticks (Hummel et al., 2007) with PEA in 16 dilutions.

Two studies investigated whether the reduced olfactory sensitivity is directly related to the depressive disorder or secondary to the effects of antidepressant drugs. Serby et al. (1990, 1992) examined a sample of 9 MDD patients with a mean Hamilton-Depression-Score (HAM-D; Hamilton, 1960) of 19.9 ± 1.6 under no antidepressant medication. They found a slightly ($p < 0.10$) reduced olfactory sensitivity (elevated olfactory thresholds) to geraniol in patients with MDD compared to healthy controls. Pause et al. (2005) investigated 11 antidepressant drug-free MDD patients. They found significantly elevated olfactory thresholds (PEA and menthol) in patients with moderate MDD (BDI-Score = 17.7 ± 6.9). These results support the conclusion that the decline in olfactory sensitivity in MDD is directly related to the disorder and not mediated by psychiatric treatment.

Gross-Isseroff et al. (1994) investigated olfactory thresholds (androstenone and isoamylacetate) in 9 MDD patients, three times during the course of their psychiatric treatment (HAM-D-Score: Day 0: 24.1 ± 1.2, Day 21: 11.7 ± 1.1 and Day 42: 6.4 ± 0.6). They observed a significant increase in olfactory sensitivity (only isoamylacetate) in MDD patients 6 weeks after initiation of antidepressant drug treatment. This finding is in line with the results from Pause et al. (2001) who showed that after successful medical treatment, sensitivity impairments in MDD patients were reduced. Further, Pause et al. (2001, 2005) and Negoias et al. (2010) reported a significant negative correlation between olfactory sensitivity and the severity of depression.

To our knowledge, only one study did not find any alterations of olfactory thresholds in MDD patients (Swiecicki et al., 2009). In this patient group, the mean HAM-D-Score was 15.2 ± 1.6 and the mean BDI-Score was 27.2 ± 2.8; olfactory thresholds were assessed using the Sniffin' Sticks (n-butanol). Only non-demented (MMSE-score > 24) patients without another psychiatric disorder were included. However, according to the authors, in many of the depressed patients, pharmacotherapy had led to improvement in depressive symptomatology before inclusion to the study. Hence, in line with the findings of Gross-Isseroff et al. (1994) and Pause et al. (2001) successful psychiatric treatment in MDD seems to renormalize olfactory performance.

While the vast majority of studies have investigated odor perception in MDD patients, few studies have examined olfactory sensitivity in related depressive disorders. Swiecicki et al. (2009) reported no differences of olfactory thresholds in patients with BPD, suggesting that sensory aspects of olfactory function cannot

Table 1 | Summary of studies of olfactory sensitivity in affective disorders.

Study	Number of participants (f/m) and diagnosis	Mean age ± *SD*	Severity-scores	Odorants and test method	Olfactory sensitivity
Gross-Isseroff et al., 1994	C: 9 (8/1) P: 9 (8/1); MDD	C: 49,11 ± 4.82 P: 49.00 ± 4.56	P: 24.11 ± 1.17 (Day 0), 11.67 ± 1.13 (Day 21), 6.44 ± 0.58 (Day 42, HAM-D)	Androstenone, isoamyl acetate, three way forced choice ascending method	Day 0 and Day 21: P = C, Day 42: P > C (isoamyl acetate)
Krüger et al., 2006	BPD + ETE: 7 (1/6) BPD – ETE: 9 (5/4)	BPD + ETE: 33.9 ± 10.7 BPD – ETE: 46.1 ± 11.6	BPD + ETE: 0.8 ± 1 (HAM-D) 0.8 ± 1.2 (SRMI) BPD – ETE: 0.4 ± 0.7 (HAM-D) 1.4 ± 1 (SRMI)	PEA, Sniffin' Sticks	BPD + ETE > BPD – ETE
Lombion-Pouthier et al., 2006	C: 58 (36/22) P: 49 (35/14); MDD	C: 38.4 ± 13.96 P: 43.4 ± 17.54	P: 23.75 ± 5.74 (BDI)	L-carvone, tetrahydrothiopene, Test Olfactif	P < C
Negoias et al., 2010	C: 21 (15/6) P: 21 (17/4); MDD	C: 39.62 ± 11.39 P: 36.86 ± 10.13	P: 29.67 ± 10.84 (BDI)	PEA, Sniffin' Sticks, laterized	P < C
Pause et al., 2001	1. Session: C: 24 (15/9) P: 24 (15/9); MDD 2. Session: C: 18 (13/5) P: 18 (13/5); MDD in remission	C: 44.2 ± 12.6 P: 48.4 ± 13.2 C: 46.6 ± 12.8 P: 47.9 ± 13.4	C: 4.8 ± 2.5 (BDI) P: 28.5 ± 11.4 (BDI) C: 4.6 ± 3.4 (BDI) P: 11.5 ± 7.1 (BDI)	PEA, eugenol, 2alt.-staircase PEA, eugenol, 2alt.-staircase	P < C P = C
Pause et al., 2005	C: 11 (6/5) P: 11 (7/4); MDD (drug-free)	C: 33.0 ± 8.6 P: 32.7 ± 5.5	C: 2.1 ± 2.3 (BDI) P: 17.7 ± 6.9 (BDI)	PEA, menthol, 2alt.-staircase	P < C
Postolache et al., 1999	C: 24 (17/7) P: 24 (17/7); SAD	C: 42.1 ± 11.8 P: 42.8 ± 9.7	/	PEA, 2alt.-staircase	P (SAD) = C
Postolache et al., 2002	C: 16 (9/7) P: 14(7/7); SAD	C: 39.0 ± 10.8 P: 42.3 ± 11.5	/	PEA, 2alt.-staircase	P (SAD) > C
Serby et al., 1990, 1992	C: 9 (/) P: 9 (0/9); MDD (drug free)	C: 50 – 59 P: 50 – 59	P: 19.9 ± 1.6 (HAM-D)	Geraniol, forced-choice ascending method	P < C ($p < 0.1$)
Swiecicki et al., 2009	C: 30 (20/10) P: 46 (RDD: 20, BPD: 21)	C: 35.4 ± 2.1 RDD: 35.7 ± 2.3 BPD: 39.6 ± 2.5	C: 0.5 ± 0.3 (HAM-D), 1.9 ± 0.5 (BDI) RDD: 15.2 ± 1.6 (HAM-D), 27.2 ± 2.8 (BDI); BPD: 14.1 ± 1.0 (HAM-D), 23.2 ± 1.8 (BDI)	n-butanol, Sniffin' Sticks	RDD = BP = C
Thomas et al., 2002	C: 24 P: 16 (unselected depressed with major depressive episode)	/	23.8 ± 9.5 (BDI)	/	P < C ($p < 0.1$)

f, female; m, male; C, controls; P, patients; MDD, major depressive disorder; HAM-D, Hamilton Depression Rating-Scale; =, no difference between groups; P > C, patients performed better than controls; P < C, patients performed worse than controls; BPD + ETE, bipolar disorder with event triggered episodes; BPD – ETE, bipolar disorder without event triggered episodes; SRMI, Self-Report Manic Inventory; PEA, phenyl-ethylalcohol; BDI, Beck's Depression Inventory; 2alt.-staircase, two-alternative staircase detection procedure; SAD, Seasonal affective disorder; RDD, unipolar recurrent depressive disorder; BPD, bipolar disorder; /, no information available.

serve as a reliable indicator of patients' polarity. Contrasting BPD patients with and without a history of event-triggered episodes, Krüger et al. (2006) showed in a pilot study that olfactory sensitivity (as assessed by the Sniffin' Sticks) was higher in patients vulnerable to emotional stress (with event-triggered episodes, $n = 7$) than in patients without event-triggered episodes ($n = 9$). A healthy control group did not exist in this study.

To our knowledge, there are only two studies on olfactory performance and SAD, however, with conflicting results. In one study, Postolache et al. (1999) found no differences in olfactory thresholds between patients (SAD without comorbidity) and healthy controls or between patients before and after light treatment (exposure to a standard regimen of 10,000 lux cool-white fluorescent light therapy for 45 min twice daily). In the other study, Postolache et al. (2002) observed lower olfactory detection thresholds (a higher olfactory acuity) in SAD patients compared to controls regardless of season.

In summary, the presented evidence shows that olfactory sensitivity is reduced in MDD. The olfactory impairment is directly related to the affective state and is not affected by anti-depressive medication. Furthermore, the decline in sensitivity is related to the severity of MDD. After successful treatment the olfactory dysfunction in MDD patients disappears. Importantly, the decline in olfactory sensitivity seems to be specifically related to MDD, and has not been observed in other depressive disorders like BPD or SAD. The disorder specificity indicates that the reduced olfactory sensitivity is not caused by a general cognitive decline in depressive disorders. However, only one study controlled cognitive performances in MDD patients (Negoias et al., 2010). Therefore, olfactory threshold measurements seem to serve as a differential diagnostic tool and a reduced olfactory sensitivity might play a role as a marker of MDD.

OLFACTORY IDENTIFICATION AND DISCRIMINATION ABILITIES IN DEPRESSIVE DISORDERS

Odor identification

Most studies examining olfactory identification abilities in depressive patients have not found differences compared to healthy controls (**Table 2**). Using the UPSIT, Amsterdam et al. (1987) found no impairments of odor identification ability in a sample of MDD patients with HAM-D-Scores ranging from 18 to 37. Kopala et al. (1994) and Warner et al. (1990) replicated these results, also measuring olfactory identification ability by the UPSIT in MDD patients (Warner et al., 1990), or patients experiencing a major depressive episode (Kopala et al., 1994). They gave no information about the severity of depression. Pause et al. (2003) asked 20 MDD patients (mean BDI-Score $= 26.4 \pm 9.3$) and 20 healthy controls (mean BDI-Score $= 3.2 \pm 3.2$) to identify the odors of PEA and isobutyraldehyde, presented via an olfactometer. It was shown that the identification rates were similar in patients and controls. Assessing patients with severe depression (mean BDI-Score $= 23.8 \pm 5.7$), Lombion-Pouthier et al. (2006) found identification scores, as indicated by the Test Olfactif, to be similar to those in the control group. In line with these results, Swiecicki et al. (2009) reported no alteration of olfactory identification ability, measured by the Sniffin' Sticks in MDD patients. The mean HAM-D-Score was 15.2 ± 1.6 and the mean BDI-Score was 27.2 ± 2.8 in the patient group. Using the Sniffin Sticks as well, Negoias et al. (2010) showed no differences in olfactory identification ability between healthy controls and MDD patients (mean BDI-Score $= 29.7 \pm 10.8$, ranging from 11 to 51). Another study (Naudin et al., 2012) evaluated psychiatric patients during acute episodes of depression and 6 weeks after antidepressant treatment against healthy controls. On the identification task, participants had to identify single odors ($n = 8$) from a list of four descriptors. Regarding the participants' odor identification performances, there was no significant difference among the three groups, considering all odors or each odor independently.

In three studies MDD patients' identification performance was compared to the identification performance in patients with Alzheimer's dementia (AD). Solomon et al. (1998) and McCaffrey et al. (2000) applied the Pocket Smell Test, a three-item short version of the UPSIT to 20 MDD and 20 AD patients. In the latter study the patients' cognitive status was assessed by the MMSE, revealing cognitive impairments in AD patients but not in MDD patients. The authors found that depressive patients scored significantly better on the identification test than AD patients, thereby, resembling the performance of healthy controls. Pentzek et al. (2007) investigated odor identification performance by means of the Sniffin' Sticks in 20 AD patients, 20 MDD patients and 30 healthy controls. Whereas MDD patients did not differ from healthy participants in their cognitive status (evaluated by the German version of the Alzheimer's disease assessment scale; Ihl and Weyer, 1993), AD patients showed a significant cognitive decline compared to the two other groups. With respect to the odor identification test, AD patients performed significantly worse than MDD patients and the control group, whereas MDD patients and healthy controls did not differ in their odor identification ability.

Few studies have shown reduced olfactory identification ability in depressed patients. First, Serby et al. (1990, 1992) reported odor identification deficits in patients with MDD (mean HAM-D-Score of 19.9 ± 1.6) using the UPSIT. However, the same authors employed the yes-no identification task and did not show differences between MDD patients and controls. In the yes-no identification task, odors were presented in similar quality pairs (e.g., lemon and orange) and participants were asked to decide, whether the presented odor matched a given verbal label. As compared to the UPSIT, the yes-no identification task might be easier to perform, requiring less cognitive resources. The authors hypothesized that the differences between UPSIT and yes-no performance in depressive patients may be a function of task-specific difficulty, suggesting that the reduced identification performance in MDD might be due to general deficits in cognitive demanding tasks. Assessing odor identification performance by the Sniffin' Sticks in a sample of MDD patients during a depressive episode and in a remitted state, Clepce et al. (2010) showed a significant reduced odor identification score only during the depressive state. In line with Serby et al. (1992), Clepce et al. (2010) attributed the poor identification performance in MDD patients to strong general cognitive impairments. Zucco and Bollini (2011) investigated olfactory identification and olfactory recognition performance in patients with mild MDD and in patients with severe MDD as well as in healthy controls. On the identification task, participants had

Table 2 | Summary of studies of olfactory identification in affective disorders.

Study	Number of participants (f/m) and diagnosis	Mean age ± *SD*	Severity-scores	Odors and test method	Olfactory identification
Amsterdam et al., 1987	C: 51 (34/17) P: 51 (34/17); MDD/BPD II	C: / P: m: 49 ± 14 f: 43 ± 13	P: 18 – 37 (HAM-D)	UPSIT	P = C
Clepce et al., 2010	C: 37 (21/16) P: 37 (21/16); MDD	C: / P: m: 48.31 ± 11.95 f: 47.52 ± 11.33	/ (BDI and SHAPS)	Sniffin' sticks	P < C (acute MDD) P = C (in remission)
Cumming et al., 2011	C: 22 (11/11) P: 20 (10/10); BPD	C: 35.5 ± 9.8 P: 34.6 ± 11.3	P: 16.3 ± 9.5 (BPRS) 9.9 ± 8.0 (YMRS) 12.0 ± 8.2 (HAM-D)	UPSIT	BPD < C
Kopala et al., 1994	C: 77 (47/30) P: 21 (13/8); MDD	C: 32.5 ± 11.1 P: 37.0 ± 9.6	/	UPSIT	P = C
Krüger et al., 2006	BPD + ETE: 7 (1/6) BPD – ETE: 9 (5/4)	BPD + ETE: 33.9 ± 10.7 BPD – ETE: 46.1 ± 11.6	BPD + ETE: 0.8 ± 1 (HAM-D) 0.8 ± 1.2 (SRMI) BPD – ETE: 0.4 ± 0.7 (HAM-D) 1.4 ± 1 (SRMI)	Sniffin' sticks	BPD + ETE = BPD – ETE
Lombion-Pouthier et al., 2006	C: 58 (36/22) P: 49 (35/14); MDD	C: 38.4 ± 13.96 P: 43.4 ± 17.54	P: 23.75 ± 5.74 (BDI)	Test olfactif	P = C
McCaffrey et al., 2000	AD: 20 (13/7) MDD: 20 (11/9)	AD: 74.15 ± 7.86 MDD: 67.55 ± 7.29	AD: 20.85 ± 5.22 (MMSE) MDD: 28.6 ± 1.54 (MMSE)	Pocket smell test	MDD > AD
Naudin et al., 2012	C: 54 (36/18) P: 18 (12/16); MDD	C: 49.5 ± 12.5 P: 50.1 ± 13.3	C: 2.33 ± 2.3 (MADRS) P (acute MDD): 35.1 ± 4.5 (MADRS) P (clinically improved): 9.1 ± 5.6 (MADRS)	Identification of odors (*n* = 8) from a list of four descriptors	P(acute MDD) = P(clinically improved) = C
Negoias et al., 2010	C: 21 (15/6) P: 21 (17/4); MDD	C: 39.62 ± 11.39 P: 36.86 ± 10.13	P: 29.67 ± 10.84 (BDI)	Sniffin' sticks	P = C
Oren et al., 1995	C: 21 (16/5) P: 21 (16/5); SAD	C: 38 ± 9 P: 38 ± 9	P: 29 ± 6 (HAM-D,SAD-Version)	UPSIT	P (SAD) = C
Pause et al., 2003	C: 22 (14/8) P: 22 (14/8); MDD	C: 48.4 ± 11.9 P: 47.2 ± 10	C: 3.6 ± 3.2 (BDI); 2.6 ± 3.5 (HAM-D) P: 25.7 ± 9.4 (BDI), 21.8 ±8.9 (HAM-D)	PEA, isobutyraldehyde, identification of odors from a set of three odors	P = C
Pentzek et al., 2007	C: 30 (24/6) P: AD: 20 (15/5) MDD 20 (15/5)	C: 77.07 ± 6.81 AD: 75.95 ± 9.09 MDD: 73.45 ± 5.61	C: 4.5 ± 3.34 (HAM-D), 8.83 ± 3.02 (ADAS-cog); AD: 5.1 ± 4.72 (HAM-D), 25.05 ± 7.57 (ADAS-cog); MDD: 19.05 ± 7.57 (HAM-D), 9.4 ± 3.22 (ADAS-cog)	Sniffin' sticks	A < C A < MDD MDD = C

(Continued)

Table 2 | Continued

Study	Number of participants (f/m) and diagnosis	Mean age ± *SD*	Severity-scores	Odors and test method	Olfactory identification
Postolache et al., 1999	C: 24 (17/7) P: 24 (17/7); SAD	C: 42.1 ± 11.8 P: 42.8 ± 9.7	/	UPSIT	P = C
Serby et al., 1990, 1992	C: 9 (/) P: 9 (0/9) MDD	C: 50 – 59 P: 50 – 59	P: 19.9 ± 1.6 (HAM-D)	UPSIT; Yes/No task	UPSIT: P < C Yes/No task: P = C
Solomon et al., 1998	AD: 20 (12/8) MDD: 20 (13/7)	AD: 74.5 ± 7.77 MDD: 69.4 ± 7.69	/	Pocket smell test	MDD > AD
Swiecicki et al., 2009	C: 30 (20/10) P: 46 (RDD: 20, BPD: 21)	C: 35.4 ± 2.1 RDD: 35.7 ± 2.3 BPD: 39.6 ± 2.5	C: 0.5 ± 0.3 (HAM-D), 1.9 ± 0.5 (BDI) RDD: 15.2 ± 1.6 (HAM-D), 27.2 ± 2.8 (BDI); BPD: 14.1 ± 1.0 (HAM-D), 23.2 ± 1.8 (BDI)	Sniffin' sticks	RDD = BPD = C
Warner et al., 1990	C: 8 P: 6; MDD	C: 32 (20 – 44) P: 37 (28 – 50)	/	UPSIT	P = C
Zucco and Bollini, 2011	C: 12 (6/6) P: 12 (6/6) Mild MDD; 12 (6/6) Severe MDD	C: 39.8 ± 7.1 P: Mild MDD: 41.3 ± 6.4 Severe MDD: 41.9 ± 6.2	/	Identification of odors (*n* = 10) from a list of four descriptors	Severe MDD < Mild MDD = C

f, female; m, male; C, controls; P, patients; MDD, major depressive disorder; BPD II, bipolar disorder II; HAM-D, Hamilton Depression Rating-Scale; UPSIT, University of Pennsylvania Smell Identification Test; =, no difference between groups; P < C: patients performed worse than controls; P > C patients performed better than controls; BDI, Beck's Depression Inventory; SHAPS, Snaith-Hamilton-pleasure-scale; BPRS, Brief Psychiatric Rating Scale; YMRS, Young Mania Rating Scale; BPD + ETE, bipolar disorder with event triggered episodes; BPD – ETE, bipolar disorder without event triggered episodes; SRMI, Self-Report Manic Inventory; AD, Alzheimer's dementia; MMSE, Mini-Mental State Exam; PEA, Phenyl-ethylalcohol; MADRS, Montgomery-Asberg Depression Rating Scale; SAD, seasonal Affective Disorder;ADAS-cog, Alzheimer's disease Assessment Scale; RDD, unipolar recurrent depressive disorder; BPD, bipolar disorder; /, no information available.

to smell an odor randomly selected from a set of 10 (aniseed, cinnamon, coffee, garlic, ink, lavender, marsala liquor, mint, petrol, and shoe-polish cream) and had to identify the correct label for each odor (four-alternative-forced choice). The study revealed significantly worse identification performance in the severe MDD group compared to both the mild MDD group and the healthy control group. In addition, olfactory identification performance was significantly correlated with olfactory recognition performance. The authors concluded that the results indicate the suitability of olfactory identification tasks for the assessment of cognitive decline in MDD.

Few studies have examined olfactory identification performance in other depressive disorders than MDD. Oren et al. (1995) examined the odor identification performance (UPSIT) in 21 medication-free patients with SAD, and found that the patients scored as high as the 21 healthy controls. Postolache et al. (1999) applied the UPSIT to 24 SAD patients and 24 matched controls. Even though the UPSIT score did not significantly differ between patients and controls, a negative correlation between the UPSIT score and the score for typical depressive syndromes emerged in depressed patients. This correlation was only observed for right nostril stimulation, but not for left nostril stimulation.

Krüger et al. (2006) examined BPD patients with ($n = 7$) and without ($n = 9$) event triggered episodes. Odor identification performance was assessed by the Sniffin' Sticks and no differences between groups were observed. Swiecicki et al. (2009) investigated olfactory identification performance in 21 BPD patients, using the Sniffin' Sticks, and found no olfactory alterations in the patient group, as compared to healthy controls. A more recent study with 20 BPD patients (without comorbidity; Cumming et al., 2011) observed lower odor identification scores (UPSIT) in BPD patients than in healthy controls. However, the olfactory deficit in the BPD group was significantly less pronounced than in a group of Schizophrenia patients. In this study, participants with IQs < 75 were excluded (evaluated by the Wechsler abbreviated scale of intelligence; Wechsler, 1999).

Summarizing odor identification performances in MDD patients, most studies indicate that patients do not differ from healthy controls. In line with this conclusion, MDD patients have been found to perform significantly better on olfactory identification tasks than AD patients. Few studies reporting reduced olfactory identification scores in MDD point to the possibility that a general cognitive decline in severe depression affects higher order odor processing, such as odor identification. As in MDD, odor identification deficits seem neither to be pronounced in SAD nor in BPD.

Odor discrimination

To our knowledge, so far, only one study has investigated odor discrimination ability in MDD patients (**Table 3**). Using the Sniffin' Sticks Negoias et al. (2010) reported no differences in olfactory discrimination performance between MDD patients and healthy controls. The mean BDI-Score was 29.7 ± 10.8. Odor discrimination performance in BPD was investigated by Krüger et al. (2006). They reported that 7 BPD patients with an event-triggered episode did not differ from 9 BPD patients without event-triggered episodes in their ability to discriminate odors.

ODOR RATINGS IN DEPRESSIVE DISORDERS

In the following, studies assessing the intensity, emotionality (hedonic profile), and familiarity of odors in depressive disorders will be reviewed.

Intensity ratings

Most studies observed intensity ratings of odors not to be altered with MDD (**Table 4**). In a study by Pause et al. (2001) medicated MDD patients (mean BDI-Score: 28.5 ± 11.4) gave intensity ratings of ten odors using a 7-point scale ranging from 0 to 6. Compared to 24 healthy controls (mean BDI-Score: 4.8 ± 2.5), there were no differences of odor intensity ratings. After successful treatment, 18 MDD patients (mean BDI-Score: 11.5 ± 7.1) and 18 healthy controls were tested again and also showed no differences in intensity ratings. In an unselected sample of 16 patients with an MDD-episode (no diagnosis of the disorder, the episode was related to), Thomas et al. (2002) did not show any differences of odor intensity evaluations compared to a control sample of 24 participants. To obtain ratings of six odors an analog scale was used, grading from 1 (minimal intensity) to 5 (maximal intensity). Testing 5 patients with a MDD-episode in stable remission and 5 controls a second time, Thomas et al. (2002) also reported no group differences. In a study by Pause et al. (2003) 20 MDD patients (mean BDI-Score = 26.4 ± 9.3) and 20 healthy controls (mean BDI-Score = 3.2 ± 3.2) were asked to judge the intensity of PEA and isobutyraldehyde (7-point scale ranging from 0 to 6). No differences between patients and controls were observed. Pause et al. (2005) examined odor intensity ratings in 11 psychotropic non-medicated MDD patients (mean BDI-Score: 17.7 ± 6.9) and 11 control participants. They used a 20 cm analog scale, ranging from not intense at all to extremely intense, to observe the ratings of two odors (PEA and menthol). Groups did not differ with respect to their odor intensity ratings. In a sample of 49 MDD patients (mean BDI-Score: 23.8 ± 5.7), Lombion-Pouthier et al. (2006) also observed similar intensity ratings compared to 58 healthy individuals. Intensity analog scales grading from 0 (low intensity) to 10 (high intensity) were used in order to investigate ratings of 16 odors. Clepce et al. (2010) also reported no differences of odor intensity estimations in 37 MDD patients and 37 healthy controls either in an acute MDD or a remission state of MDD. By means of a 200 mm visual analog scale ranging from 0 (very low intensity) and 200 (very high intensity) participants were asked to rate the intensity of the 16 Sniffin Sticks odors.

In studies by Atanasova et al. (2010) and Naudin et al. (2012) participants' task was to evaluate the intensity of a pleasant odor and an unpleasant odor that were presented in three different concentrations. Vanillin and butyric acid (Atanasova et al., 2010) as well as PEA and isovaleric acid (Naudin et al., 2012) were used to evaluate the odor intensity, either by means of a magnitude estimate method (Atanasova et al., 2010) or by a 10 cm analog scale, labeled at each end (very low intensity/very high intensity; Naudin et al., 2012). Both studies revealed that MDD patients perceived the unpleasant odor as significantly more intense than the control group. Furthermore, Atanasova et al. (2010) reported the perception of the pleasant odor by the MDD patients as less intense compared to the healthy individuals. After 6 weeks of treatment, Naudin et al. (2012) observed similar odor intensity ratings between MDD patients and healthy controls. It was suggested that presented results might indicate an olfactory anhedonia for pleasant odors and an olfactory alliesthesia for unpleasant odors.

In one study, odor intensity ratings of MDD patients (mean BDI score = 22.9 ± 9.0) were compared to odor intensity ratings

Table 3 | Summary of studies of olfactory discrimination in affective disorders.

Study	Number of participants (f/m) and diagnosis	Mean age ± *SD*	Severity-scores	Odors and test method	Olfactory discrimination
Krüger et al., 2006	BPD + ETE: 7 (1/6) BPD – ETE: 9 (5/4)	BPD + ETE: 33.9 ± 10.7 BPD – ETE: 46.1 ± 11.6	BPD + ETE: 0.8 ± 1 (HAM-D) 0.8 + 1.2 (SRMI) BPD – ETE: 0.4 ± 0.7 (HAM-D) 1.4 ± 1 (SRMI)	Sniffin' Sticks	BPD + ETE = BPD – ETE
Negoias et al., 2010	C: 21 (15/6) P: 21 (17/4); MDD	C: 39.62 ± 11.39 P: 36.86 ± 10.13	P: 29.67 ± 10.84 (BDI)	Sniffin' Sticks	P = C

f, female; m, male; C, controls; P, patients; BPD + ETE, bipolar disorder with event triggered episodes; BPD – ETE, bipolar disorder without event triggered episodes; HAM-D, Hamilton Depression Rating-Scale; SRMI: Self-Report Manic Inventory; =, no difference between groups; MDD, major depressive disorder; BDI, Beck's Depression Inventory.

Table 4 | Summary of studies of odor intensity ratings in affective disorders.

Study	Number of participants (f/m) and diagnosis	Mean age ± *SD*	Severity-scores	Odors and test method	Olfactory intensity rating
Atanasova et al., 2010	C: 30 (12/18) P: 30 (12/18); MDD	C: 33.4 ± 9.9 P: 34.6 ±11.1	C: 2 ± 2.1 (MADRS) P: 36.3 ± 6.3 (MADRS)	6 olfactory stimuli, prepared from vanillin (pleasant) and butyric acid (unpleasant) in different concentrations magnitude estimate method	Vanillin (three concentrations)/pleasant: P < C Butyric acid (three concentrations)/unpleasant: P > C
Clepce et al., 2010	C: 37 (21/16) P: 37 (21/16); MDD	C: / P: m: 48.31 ± 11.95 f: 47.52 ± 11.33	/: (BDI and SHAPS)	16 odors of the sniffin' sticks, visual analog scale	P = C (in acute MDD and in remission)
Lombion-Pouthier et al., 2006	C: 58 (36/22) P: 49 (35/14); MDD	C: 38.4 ± 13.96 P: 43.4 ± 17.54	P: 23.75 ± 5.74 (BDI)	Test olfactif; rating scale	P = C
Naudin et al., 2012	C: 54 (36/18) P: 18 (12/16); MDD	C: 49.5 ± 12.5 P: 50.1 ± 13.3	C: 2.33 ± 2.3 (MADRS) P (acute MDD): 35.1 ± 4.5 (MADRS) P (clinically improved): 9.1 ± 5.6 (MADRS)	Isovaleric acid, PEA; rating scale	2-phenylethanol: acute MDD = clinically improved = C Isovaleric acid: acute MDD > C; clinically improved = C
Pause et al., 2001	1. Session: C: 24 (15/9) P: 24 (15/9); MDD	C: 44.2 ± 12.6 P: 48.4 ± 13.2	C: 4.8 ± 2.5 (BDI) P: 28.5 ± 11.4 (BDI)	10 odors; rating scale	P = C
	2. Session: C: 18 (13/5) P: 18 (13/5); MDD in remission	C: 46.6 ± 12.8 P: 47.9 ± 13.4	C: 4.6 ± 3.4 (BDI) P: 11.5 ± 7.1 (BDI)	10 odors; rating scale	P = C
Pause et al., 2003	C: 22 (14/8) P: 22 (14/8); MDD	C: 48.4 ± 11.9 P: 47.2 ± 10	C: 3.6 ± 3.2 (BDI), 2.6 ± 3.5 (HAM-D) P: 25.7 ± 9.4 (BDI), 21.8 ±8.9 (HAM-D)	PEA, isobutyraldehyde, linear scale	P = C
Pause et al., 2005	C: 11 (6/5) P: 11 (7/4); MDD (drug-free)	C: 33.0 ± 8.6 P: 32.7 ± 5.5	C: 2.1 ± 2.3 (BDI) P: 17.7 ± 6.9 (BDI)	PEA, menthol; visual analog scale	P = C
Pause et al., 2008	MDD: 9 (0/9) SZ: 9 (0/9)	MDD: 55.1 ± 4.5 SZ: 33.4 ± 7.9	SZ: 31.9 ± 7.1 (BPRS) MDD: 22.9 ± 9 (BDI); 40.3 ± 16.4 (HAM-D)	PEA, isobutyraldehyde, linear scale	SZ = MDD
Thomas et al., 2002	C: 24 P: 16 (unselected depressed with major depressive episode)	/	23.8 ± 9.5 (BDI)	8 odors, rating scale	P = C

f, female; m, male; C, controls; P, patients; MDD, major depressive disorder; MADRS, Montgomery-Asberg Depression Rating Scale; SHAPS, Snaith-Hamilton-pleasure-scale; PEA, phenyl-ethylalcohol; P < C, patients rated odors less intense; P > C patients rated odors more intense; =, no difference between groups; BDI, Beck's Depression Inventory; SZ, Schizophrenia patients; BPRS, Brief Psychiatric Rating Scale; /, no information available.

of schizophrenia patients (range of intensity ratings: 0 to 6; Pause et al., 2008). Intensity ratings did not differ between patient groups.

In summary, the results of most studies regarding odor intensity ratings in MDD showed evaluations of odor intensity to be unaffected by MDD. However, intensity ratings for highly pleasant or unpleasant odors might be changed in patients experiencing major depressive episodes.

Hedonic ratings

In a study by Pause et al. (2001) valence ratings of ten odors were investigated in MDD patients in an acute state of MDD (mean BDI score: 28.5 ± 11.4) and in a remission state after successful medical treatment (mean BDI score: 11.5 ± 7.1; see **Table 5** for a summary of results regarding hedonic ratings). To assess ratings of odor pleasantness a 7-point scale ranging from −3 to +3 was used. Valence ratings of nine out of the ten odors were similar in acute state MDD patients and healthy controls. However, citral was perceived as significantly more pleasant by depressive patients. After medical treatment, MDD patients and healthy controls gave similar ratings to all odors. As citral has been discussed to have relaxing and anti-depressant properties, the authors suggested that citral might be perceived as more distinct by depressed patients than by healthy controls. The finding that MDD patients rated the hedonic tone of odors similarly to healthy controls was confirmed in three other studies: Assessing perceived odor pleasantness of seven odors in a sample of unselected MDD patients in an acute state and in a stable remission state, Thomas et al. (2002) also reported no differences between the patients' group and the control group. In order to assess hedonic evaluations analog scales were used ranging from −5 (maximal unpleasant) to +5 (maximal pleasant). Pause et al. (2003) asked 20 MDD patients (mean BDI-Score = 26.4 ± 9.3) and 20 healthy controls (mean BDI-Score = 3.2 ± 3.2) to judge the emotional valence of PEA and isobutyraldehyde (7-point scale: −3 to +3). It was shown that the hedonic judgments were similar in patients and controls. Swiecicki et al. (2009) reported that MDD patients (mean BDI score: 27.2 ± 2.8, mean HAM-D score: 15.2 ± 1.5) evaluated the pleasantness of 16 odors similar to healthy participants. The participants' task was to rate each odor of the Sniffin' Sticks identification test as pleasant, unpleasant or neutral.

Similiar to the finding that certain odors (like citral; Pause et al., 2001) may be perceived as more pleasant in MDD patients, Lombion-Pouthier et al. (2006) observed that MDD patients (mean BDI score: 23.75 ± 5.7) evaluated pleasant odors as more pleasant than healthy individuals. Participants gave ratings of 13 pleasant odors using analog scales graduated from 0 (displeasure) to 10 (pleasure). Another study by Pause et al. (2005) found that drug free MDD patients (mean BDI score: 17.7 ± 6.9) were inclined ($p < 0.10$) to rate odors (PEA and menthol) as less unpleasant than healthy controls (mean BDI score: 2.1 ± 2.3).

However, other studies found depressive patients to rather evaluate odors as more unpleasantness than more pleasant, suggesting that the occurrence of anhedonia in MDD might affect hedonic ratings. Clepce et al. (2010) assessed BDI-Scores as well as Snaith-Hamilton-Pleasure-Scale (SHAPS; Franz et al., 2005) scores. MDD patients (acute and remitted state) and healthy controls rated the pleasantness of the 16 odors of the Sniffin' Sticks using 200 mm visual analog scales ranging from −100 (unpleasantness) to +100 (pleasantness). The study revealed a significant correlation between anhedonia and hedonic estimates during the acute episode of MDD, demonstrating that high depression scores are related to low hedonic estimates of odors.

Atanasova et al. (2010) examined hedonic odor ratings in MDD patients with a mean score of 36.3 ± 6.3 on the Montgomery-Asberg Depression rating scale (MADRS; Montgomery and Asberg, 1979). On a 10 cm analog scale (highly unpleasant/highly pleasant) participants were asked to rate the perceived pleasantness of vanillin (representing a pleasant odor), and butyric acid (representing an unpleasant odor), and binary mixtures of both odors, all in three different concentrations. The study revealed that depressed patients perceived unpleasant odors as significantly more unpleasant than controls. Atanasova et al. interpreted this result as an indicator for olfactory negative alliesthesia in MDD.

Naudin et al. (2012) aimed at determining whether olfactory impairments are state or trait markers of a major depressive episode. They evaluated depressed patients during acute episodes of depression (mean MADRS = 35.1 ± 4.5) and 6 weeks after antidepressant treatment (mean MADRS = 9.1 ± 5.6) against healthy controls (mean MADRS = 2.3 ± 2.3). Hedonic ratings of eight odors (four unpleasant odors, four pleasant odors) were assessed using a 10 cm analog scale (highly unpleasant/highly pleasant). During their acute phase, MDD patients rated five out of the eight odors as less pleasant as controls. The deviant pleasantness ratings were rather observed for pleasant and unpleasant odors than for neutral odors. However, after initiation of psychiatric treatment, only two out of eight odors were still judged as less pleasant by depressive patients.

There are only a few studies available that contrast odor hedonics in MDD patients to another psychiatric population. Pause et al. (2008) found no differences in odor valence ratings between MDD patients (mean BDI score: 22.9 ± 9.0; mean HAM-D score: 40.3 ± 16.4) and schizophrenia patients. In this study, valence ratings (7-point scale: −3 to +3) were obtained for PEA and isobutyraldehyde. Swiecicki et al. (2009) reported that MDD patients (mean BDI score: 27.2 ± 2.8, mean HAM-D score: 15.2 ± 1.5) rated fewer olfactory stimuli as pleasant compared to a BPD group (mean BDI score: 23.2 ± 1.8, mean HAM-D score: 14.1 ± 1.0). Participants were to rate each of the 16 odors of the Sniffin' Sticks identification test as pleasant, unpleasant or neutral. Similar to the outcome that BPD patients seem to judge odors as more pleasant than a comparable patient group, Cumming et al. (2011) found that patients with BPD rated odors (40 odors corresponding to the UPSIT items) as significantly more pleasant than healthy controls. The ratings were judged on a five-point scale (−2 to +2).

In conclusion, odor hedonics are not consistently changed in depressive patients (**Table 5**). Two studies point to the possibility that MDD patients judge certain odors to be more pleasant than healthy controls (Pause et al., 2001; Lombion-Pouthier et al., 2006). However, the majority of studies found MDD patients to judge the emotional valence of odors either in a normal range or as less positive than healthy controls. This effect has

Table 5 | Summary of studies of hedonic odor ratings in affective disorders.

Study	Number of participants (f/m) and diagnosis	Mean age ± *SD*	Severity-scores	Odors and test method	Hedonic odor rating
Atanasova et al., 2010	C: 30 (12/18) P: 30 (12/18); MDD	C: 33.4 ± 9.9 P: 34.6 ±11.1	C: 2 ± 2.1 (MADRS) P: 36.3 ± 6.3 (MADRS)	15 olfactory stimuli, prepared from vanillin (pleasant) and butyric acid (unpleasant) in different concentrations and their mixtures; linear scale	Patients rated unpleasant odors as significantly more unpleasant than controls; 9 out of 15 stimuli were rated as less pleasant by patients
Clepce et al., 2010	C: 37 (21/16) P: 37 (21/16); MDD	C: / P: m: 48.31 ± 11.95 f: 47.52 ± 11.33	/: (BDI and SHAPS)	16 odors of the sniffin' sticks, visual analog scale	P = C (in acute MDD and in remission); significant interrelation between anhedonia and hedonic estimates during an acute MDD episode
Cumming et al., 2011	C: 22 (11/11) P: 20 (10/10) BPD	C: 35.5 ± 9.8 P: 34.6 ± 11.3	C: / P: 16.3 ± 9.5 (BPRS) 9.9 ± 8.0 (YMRS) 12.0 ± 8.2 (HAM-D)	Odors of the UPSIT; likert like scale	BPD patients rated odors as more pleasant than controls
Lombion-Pouthier et al., 2006	C: 58 (36/22) P: 49 (35/14); MDD	C: 38.4 ± 13.96 P: 43.4 ± 17.54	P: 23.75 ± 5.74 (BDI)	Test olfactif; rating scale	Patients over-evaluate the pleasantness of pleasant odors
Naudin et al., 2012	C: 54 (36/18) P: 18 (12/16); MDD	C: 49.5 ± 12.5 P: 50.1 ± 13.3	C: 2.33 ± 2.3 (MADRS) P (acute MDD): 35.1 ± 4.5 (MADRS) P (clinically improved): 9.1 ± 5.6 (MADRS)	8 odors, linear scale	Acute MDD: P rated 5 odors as less pleasant, Clinically improved: two odors were rated to be less pleasant by the patients
Pause et al., 2001	1. Session: C: 24 (15/9) P: 24 (15/9); MDD 2. Session: C: 18 (13/5) P: 18 (13/5); MDD in remission	C: 44.2 ± 12.6 P: 48.4 ± 13.2 C: 46.6 ± 12.8 P: 47.9 ± 13.4	C: 4.8 ± 2.5 (BDI) P: 28.5 ± 11.4 (BDI) C: 4.6 ± 3.4 (BDI) P: 11.5 ± 7.1 (BDI)	10 odors; rating scale 10 odors; rating scale	9 odors:P = C; citral was rated to be more pleasant by the patients P = C
Pause et al., 2003	C: 22 (14/8) P: 22 (14/8); MDD	C: 48.4 ± 11.9 P: 47.2 ± 10	C: 3.6 ± 3.2 (BDI); 2.6 ± 3.5 (HAM-D) P: 25.7 ± 9.4 (BDI), 21.8 ± 8.9 (HAM-D)	PEA, isobutyraldehyde, linear scale	P = C
Pause et al., 2005	C: 11 (6/5) P: 11 (7/4); MDD (drug-free)	C: 33.0 ± 8.6 P: 32.7 ± 5.5	C: 2.1 ± 2.3 (BDI) P: 17.7 ± 6.9 (BDI)	PEA, menthol; visual analog scale	Patients tended ($p < 0.1$) to rate odors as less unpleasant than controls

(Continued)

Table 5 | Continued

Study	Number of participants (f/m) and diagnosis	Mean age ± *SD*	Severity-scores	Odors and test method	Hedonic odor rating
Pause et al., 2008	MDD: 9 (0/9) SZ: 9 (0/9)	MDD: 55.1 ± 4.5 SZ: 33.4 ± 7.9	SZ: 31.9 ± 7.1 (BPRS) MDD: 22.9 ± 9 (BDI); 40.3 ± 16.4 (HAM-D)	PEA, isobutyraldehyde, linear scale	SZ = MDD
Swiecicki et al., 2009	C: 30 (20/10) P: 46 (RDD: 20, BPD: 21)	C: 35.4 ± 2.1 RDD: 35.7 ± 2.3, BPD: 39.6 ± 2.5	C: 0.5 ± 0.3 (HAM-D), 1.9 ± 0.5 (BDI); RDD: 15.2 ± 1.6 (HAM-D), 27.2 ± 2.8 (BDI); BPD: 14.1 ± 1.0 (HAM-D), 23.2 ± 1.8 (BDI)	Odors of the sniffin' sticks	RDD and BPD = C; RDD patients rated less olfactory stimuli as pleasant as compared to BPD patients
Thomas et al., 2002	C: 24 P: 16 (unselected depressed with major depressive episode)	/	23.8 ± 9.5 (BDI)	8 odors, rating scale	P = C

f, female; m, male; C, controls; P, patients; MDD, major depressive disorder; MADRS: Montgomery asberg depression rating scale; BDI: Beck's depression inventory; SHAPS, Snaith-Hamilton-pleasure-scale; BPD: bipolar disorder; BPRS, Brief Psychiatric Rating Scale; YMRS, Young Mania Rating Scale; HAM-D: Hamilton depression scale; =, no difference between groups; UPSIT, University of Pennsylvania Smell Identification Test; PEA, phenyl-ethylalcohol; SZ, Schizophrenia; RDD, recurrent depressive disorder; /, no information available.

been observed for standard test odors and especially for emotionally negative odors (Atanasova et al., 2010). The hypothesis that depressive patients perceive the hedonic profile of emotionally negative odors as more intense than healthy individuals is supported by the finding that MDD patients report a higher physiological arousal in response to emotionally negative odors than healthy controls (Pause et al., 2000). The findings in MDD patients cannot be generalized to BPD patients, who seem to perceive odors as more pleasant than healthy controls.

Familiarity ratings

To our knowledge, there are only four studies concerning ratings of odor familiarity in MDD patients (**Table 6**). There are no studies with respect to familiarity ratings in BPD or SAD. Thomas et al. (2002) found slight differences between a sample of 16 unselected patients suffering from an acute MDD-episode without comorbidity and 24 healthy controls. Familiarity ratings of odors (dried fish, parmesan cheese, gyran, alpha-methylnaphtylketone, coffee, and vanilla) were assessed by means of visual analog scales ranging from −5 (most unfamiliar) to +5 (most familiar). Depressed patients tended to rate vanilla ($p = 0.051$) and dried fish ($p = 0.099$) to be less common than healthy controls. Five MDD patients in a stable remission state of MDD were retested. Compared to 5 retested controls, patients rated odor familiarity in a similar way. Pause et al. (2005) examined 11 antidepressant drug-free MDD patients (mean BDI-Score: 17.7 ± 6.9) and 11 controls (mean-BDI-Score: 2.1 ± 2.3). To assess odor familiarity ratings, they used visual analog scales (anchor: familiar—unfamiliar) and presented PEA and menthol as odors. Groups did not differ in familiarity ratings of either PEA or menthol. Atanasova et al. (2010) assessed odor familiarity ratings in 30 MDD patients (mean MADRS-Score: 36.3 ± 6.3) and 30 healthy controls. They used a 10 cm analog scale, labeled at each end (unfamiliar odor and very unfamiliar odor), for ratings of vanillin and butyric acid. They found no differences between groups for either odor in familiarity evaluations. Naudin et al. (2012) examined odor familiarity ratings in 18 MDD patients and a control group ($n = 54$). They used analog scales for the ratings and assessed ratings again after MDD patients in remission. For all odors, except vanillin, the authors reported no group differences in odor familiarity ratings. Vanillin was evaluated as less familiar by MDD patients and patients in remission as compared to healthy controls.

In sum, ratings of odor familiarity do not seem to be strongly altered in MDD.

AFFECTIVE REACTIONS TO OLFACTORY STIMULI IN MDD

Only two studies investigated emotional reactivity or affective states after odor exposure. Steiner et al. (1993) investigated valence ratings and facial expressive features (assessed by observer ratings with regard to the quality, strength and duration of facial expressions) in 21 MDD patients as an indicator for affective reactions to olfactory stimuli (rose oil and amyl acetate representing pleasant odors and butyric acid and methyl mercaptan representing unpleasant stimuli). The patient sample was found to display reduced facial expressions while presenting pleasant odors and to show reduced durations of facial expressions in response to either pleasant or unpleasant odors. That was contrary to the valence ratings that did not differ between patients and healthy controls.

In another study by Pause et al. (2000), affective reactions to olfactory and visual stimuli (emotional scenes) were assessed in 26 MDD patients (mean BDI-Score: 29.4 ± 11.4) and 26 healthy controls (mean BDI-Score: 4.7 ± 2.5). Participants were to describe their emotional reaction to 10 odors (pleasant, unpleasant and neutral) and 20 pictures on three dimensions (valence, arousal, and dominance) by means of the self-assessment-manikin (Bradley and Lang, 1994). The study revealed higher arousal in MDD patients while presenting negative stimuli for all stimulus modalities.

In sum, both studies indicate that emotional reactions to odors are altered in MDD patients, irrespective of odor evaluation strategies. However, elevated affective reactions to emotionally negative odors do not seem to be modality-specific.

PSYCHOPHYSIOLOGY AND NEUROANATOMY OF OLFACTION IN MDD

The data presented in the previous section indicate that olfactory sensitivity is reduced in depressed patients. Therefore, and following the annotations by Martzke et al. (1997), odor perception in depression seems to be altered on an early sensory processing level. Other perceptual performances, like odor identification and discrimination, do not seem to be strongly altered in MDD patients, indicating that the cognitive-evaluative level of olfactory processing is not impaired in depression.

By means of event-related potential (ERP) analysis, Pause et al. (2003) investigated olfactory, visual, and emotional stimulus processing in MDD patients and in healthy controls. Patients were examined at the beginning of their therapy and after successful medical treatment. Pause and colleagues focused on whether olfactory function in depression is disturbed in a modality-specific manner. Within the ERP, early and late potentials were analyzed. While early potentials, such as the P2, are related to early pre-attentive stimulus encoding, late potentials, such as the P3 and the late positive Slow Wave (pSW), are rather related to late evaluative stimulus processing. The study revealed that MDD patients responded to odors with reduced early (P2) and late (P3-1) potential amplitudes. In response to colors, and emotional slides they showed reduced late potential amplitudes only (colors: P3 and pSW; emotional slides: pSW). After successful psychiatric treatment, the event-related potentials to either stimuli did not differ between groups. The authors discuss the reduction of the early potential amplitudes of the chemosensory ERP in

Table 6 | Summary of studies of odor familiarity ratings in affective disorders.

Study	Number of participants (f/m) and diagnosis	Mean age ± *SD*	Severity-scores	Odors and test method	Odor familiarity rating
Atanasova et al., 2010	C: 30 (12/18) P: 30 (12/18); MDD	C: 33.4 ± 9.9 P: 34.6 ±11.1	C: 2 ± 2.1 (MADRS) P: 36.3 ± 6.3 (MADRS)	15 olfactory stimuli, prepared from vanillin (pleasant) and butyric acid (unpleasant) in different concentrations and their mixtures; linear scale	Vanillin and butyric acid: P = C
Naudin et al., 2012	C: 54 (36/18) P: 18 (12/16); MDD	C: 49.5 ± 12.5 P: 50.1 ± 13.3	C: 2.33 ± 2.3 (MADRS) P (acute MDD): 35.1 ± 4.5 (MADRS) P (clinically improved): 9.1 ± 5.6 (MADRS)	8 odors	7 odors: P = C; vanillin: P < C
Pause et al., 2005	C: 11 (6/5) P: 11 (7/4); MDD (drug-free)	C: 33.0 ± 8.6 P: 32.7 ± 5.5	C: 2.1 ± 2.3 (BDI); P: 17.7 ± 6.9 (BDI)	PEA, menthol; visual analog scale	P = C
Thomas et al., 2002	C: 24 P: 16 (unselected depressed with major depressive episode) and 5 retested patients in stable remission	/	23.8 ± 9.5 (BDI)	8 odors, rating scale	Vanilla: P < C, (*p* = 0.051); dried fish: P < C (*p* = 0.099); patients in stable remission = C

f, female; m, male; C, controls; P, patients; MDD, major depressive disorder; MADRS, Montgomery-Asberg Depression Rating Scale; PEA, phenyl-ethylalcohol; =, no difference between groups; P < C, patients rated odors less intense; BDI, Beck's Depression Inventory; /, no information available.

MDD patients to reflect a modality-specific reduction in the ability to encode basic olfactory information on an early level of sensory processing. This interpretation is in line with the data demonstrating a reduced olfactory sensitivity in MDD patients. However, the reduction of the late positive potentials in response to colored and emotional slides might have been related to the non-modality specific effect of a reduced late evaluative stimulus processing in MDD patients.

In another ERP study, Pause et al. (2008) contrasted olfactory and visual stimulus (colored slides) processing in 9 MDD patients and 9 Schizophrenia patients (all males). In response to odors (PEA and isobutyraldahyde), MDD patients showed longer latencies of all ERP components than Schizophrenia patients. Additionally, the amplitude of the pSW in response to colors was larger in MDD patients than in Schizophrenia patients. These results indicate that the reduced olfactory processing capacities (as shown in longer latencies or reduced amplitudes) in MDD patients are modality-specific and prominent in comparison to healthy individuals and also in comparison to other psychiatric patient groups.

Negoias et al. (2010) assessed olfactory function and the volume of the olfactory bulb (OB) in patients with acute MDD. Participants underwent measures of odor threshold, discrimination and identification using the Sniffin' Sticks test battery in a lateralized fashion. OB volumes were calculated by manual segmentation of acquired T2-weighted coronal slices according to a standardized protocol. The study revealed that MDD patients had a significantly lower olfactory sensitivity and smaller OB volumes as compared to healthy controls. There were no group differences for olfactory discrimination and identification scores. A significant correlation between OB volumes and odor thresholds was observed for the left nostril: the lower the olfactory sensitivity, the smaller the OB volume. Additionally, Negoias et al. (2010) found a significant negative correlation between olfactory bulb volume and depression scores (BDI).

In sum, the data indicate that olfactory stimulus processing is altered on an early sensory processing level in patients with acute severe MDD. This olfactory dysfunction seems to be modality- and disorder-specific. Furthermore, the reduced capacity to encode olfactory information in MDD seems to be accompanied by higher olfactory thresholds and smaller OB volumes. Whether or not olfaction is impaired on the later cognitive-evaluative level seems to depend on the progress of general cognitive decline during depressive episodes, but seems not to be depend on the stimulus modality.

OLFACTORY PERFORMANCE IN HEALTHY INDIVIDUALS WITH DEPRESSIVE SYMPTOMS

In the following section, studies will be outlined, which investigated healthy individuals scoring high on some depressive symptoms but not fulfilling the diagnostic criteria for MDD or any other psychiatric disorder.

Satoh et al. (1996) examined odor ratings in Japanese elderly participants (mean age in men: 73.2 ± 6.0; in women: 72.4 ± 5.9). Odor ratings were obtained for the 40 odor items of the UPSIT. As a main result, it was found that elderly men with increased depression scores (assessed by the self-rating depression scale; Zung, 1965) rated odors to be weaker than their non-depressive counterparts.

In another study (Economou, 2003) smell identification performance (UPSIT) was investigated in elderly Greek people, ranging in age from 49 to 88 years. Correlations between the UPSIT and the BDI-II score were not significant, suggesting that in elderly healthy individuals, a small number of depressive symptoms does not affect odor identification.

Olfactory discrimination scores were assessed in young adults (mean age: 19.3 ± 1.6) by Goel and Grasso (2004). The olfactory discrimination test included 7 items and was based on five different blends of commercially available lavender oil. Participants were to indicate, whether a certain blend was the same, stronger, or weaker than another blend, briefly presented before. All participants rated their depressive symptoms on the BDI manual. Whereas overall olfactory performance was not related to the BDI score, participants with higher BDI scores solved two out of the seven items better than participants with a lower BDI score.

Pollatos et al. (2007a) examined 48 participants who reported a small number of depressive symptoms (BDI score < 10). Olfactory sensitivity and discrimination performance were assessed by means of Sniffin' Sticks (odor for the threshold test: n-butanol). Concerning olfactory sensitivity, the degree of depressive symptoms was inversely correlated to the olfactory threshold score: The higher the number of depressive symptoms the lower the olfactory sensitivity. However, olfactory discrimination performance was not related to the degree of depressive symptoms. These results correspond to data of studies concerning olfactory sensitivity in patients with MDD that reported elevated thresholds in MDD patients.

Pouliot et al. (2008) investigated the relation between olfactory perception (odor detection, identification and ratings of odor pleasantness and intensity) in 32 healthy menopausal women. Anhedonia, one symptom frequently occurring in MDD, was assessed by the Physical Anhedonia Scale (Chapman et al., 1976). Women below or equaling the median anhedonia score of 14 were classified as low-anhedonic and women with a higher anhedonia score than 14 were assigned to the high-anhedonia group. Participants underwent the European test of olfactory capabilities (ETOC; Thomas-Danguin et al., 2003). The test consists of an odor detection task and an odor identification task using a panel of 16 odors. Firstly, Participants are asked to detect the odor bottle out of four bottles (three bottles that are not holding any odor) and, secondly, to identify the detected odor by choosing a label out of four given labels. Olfactory performances of detection (an indicator of olfactory sensitivity) and identification are integrated in one olfactory performance score. Additionally, in the study by Pouliot et al. (2008) pleasantness and intensity of the ETOC-odors were rated by the participants on a 9 point scale. Pouliot et al. (2008) reported that high-anhedonic menopausal women had a worse olfactory function than women with a lower anhedonia score. Women in the low anhedonia group rated more odors as pleasant and as neutral than as unpleasant. Moreover, it was observed that the anhedonia score correlated negatively with the perceived odor pleasantness.

Conflicting results were obtained in a study conducted by Scinska et al. (2008). In a sample of non-clinical older adults (mean age: 63.0 ± 1.1), the relation between depressive symptoms and olfactory performance (odor detection thresholds and odor identification ability) was investigated. Depression scores were assessed by the Geriatric Depression Scale (GDS; Yesavage, 1988). Depending on the GDS-Score, participants were classified as depressed (GDS-Score > 5) or as non-depressed (GDS-Score < 5). In order to assess olfactory performance, Sniffin' Sticks were used and the odor for the threshold test was n-butanol. The study revealed that depressive symptoms were not related to any measurement of olfactory performance. However, the authors found that age was significantly correlated with both olfactory measures; as expected older participants performed worse on the olfactory tests.

In sum, three out of six studies (Satoh et al., 1996; Pollatos et al., 2007a; Pouliot et al., 2008) reveal that the experience of depressive symptoms in healthy individuals affects olfactory performances. All of these studies found scores of odor sensitivity (as assessed by intensity ratings, odor detection performances and threshold tests) to be reduced in individuals with depressive symptoms. However, two studies investigated odor perception (identification and sensitivity) in older adults and failed to establish a relation between olfaction and depression scores (Economou, 2003; Scinska et al., 2008). As olfactory functions have been repeatedly reported to decline with age (e.g., Doty et al., 1984a; Hummel et al., 2007), in these two studies, effects of age might have overshadowed effects of depression, resulting in overall low olfactory performances, which are unlikely to be further reduced by psychiatric symptoms. In addition, one study (Goel and Grasso, 2004) indicated that olfactory discrimination performance for certain odors might even be increased during depressive mood states.

OLFACTORY PERFORMANCE IN HEALTHY INDIVIDUALS WITH TRANSIENTLY EXPERIENCED DEPRESSION-LIKE FEELINGS

To our knowledge, there are only two studies investigating odor perception in healthy participants who transiently experience depression-like feelings.

Laudien et al. (2006) considered symptoms of learned helplessness as a mood state similar to symptoms occurring in depression. The term "helplessness" has been adopted to denote a negative emotion, which is characterized by lack of control, significant negative expectancies for the future and deterioration of cognitive performance (e.g., Hiroto and Seligman, 1975). By means of ERP analysis, olfactory and auditory stimulus processing was investigated in healthy individuals who transiently experienced helplessness or were in a neutral mood state. In order to induce helplessness, participants were exposed to uncontrollable failure in an unsolvable face-classification task. Odors (PEA and menthol) were presented by an olfactometer. While experiencing helplessness, participants' responses to odorous stimuli were attenuated at an early processing stage: the amplitudes of P2 and P3-1 were smaller and the latencies of N1, P2 and P3-1 were longer. Effects were only shown for the olfactory modality and not for the auditory modality. Results indicate that the CSERP displays transient mood effects, resembling the CSERP effects in MDD patients (Pause et al., 2003).

Pollatos et al. (2007b) investigated olfactory sensitivity and olfactory discrimination ability by Sniffin' Sticks (odor for the threshold test: n-butanol) as well as perceived pleasantness and intensity of n-butanol by a 9 point scale in 32 healthy participants. Prior to the olfactory testing, participants underwent a procedure of emotion induction by presenting pleasant, unpleasant and neutral pictures from the IAPS (International Affective Picture System; the center for the study of emotion and attention). Results show that olfactory sensitivity was decreased after presentation of unpleasant pictures, and only in male participants were olfactory thresholds increased after viewing pleasant pictures as well. Olfactory discrimination ability did not show any alterations in dependence of the emotional state condition. The authors concluded that negative emotional experience is accompanied by a reduced olfactory sensitivity. They suggested that, in addition, odor perception in men is strongly interfered with arousing states.

The studies by Laudien et al. (2006) and Pollatos et al. (2007b) show that even transient experiences of negative mood or helplessness affect odor perception at a sensory level. As in depressive patients, threshold values are increased during negative mood states, but tests involving cognitive performance, like odor discrimination, are not affected by a transient mood decline (Pollatos et al., 2007b). Moreover, as in depressive patients, central nervous processing of odors in helpless individuals is attenuated at an early processing stage, related to stimulus encoding, but unchanged at a late processing stage, related to cognitive odor evaluation.

DISCUSSION

METHODOLOGICAL CONSIDERATIONS ON OLFACTORY ASSESSMENT AND THEIR IMPLICATIONS FOR STUDY DIFFERENCES

Obviously, measuring olfaction in patients with depressive disorders needs to be reliable and valid. Thus, olfaction as well as depression should be assessed with unambiguous measurements.

Measuring olfaction requires the standardization of context variables inherently linked to the chemical senses. Temperature and air humidity are factors that can alter the evaporation rate of odors (Mozell et al., 1986) and should thus be controlled in tests on olfactory performance. Most volatile chemicals stimulate the olfactory as well as the trigeminal nerve. Stimulating the trigeminal nerve produces stinging, burning, tickling, warm, or cold sensations. Regarding olfactory acuity, odors that only stimulate the olfactory nerve (nervus olfactorius) should be used in olfactory testing. Odors, for example n-butanol, which do not exclusively stimulate the first cranial nerve (nervus olfactorius), can also produce sensations in anosmic individuals. PEA or vanillin may be more suitable in olfactory acuity assessment because they seem to be nearly pure olfactory stimulants (Doty et al., 1978). Further, it should be considered whether participants should take a natural sniff in the olfactory test procedure. Berglund et al. (1986) and Laing (1983) showed that olfactory threshold assessment using an external constant airflow produced more elevated thresholds than olfactory assessment with natural sniffing. In addition, sniffing seems to be necessary for the neuronal priming of odor processing within the olfactory bulb (Gerkin et al., 2013). Several procedures have been published which have been used in the measurement of olfactory performance (e.g., number of items, ascending or descending stimulus presentation in threshold tests). These test characteristics have been reviewed elsewhere (Doty, 2006, 2007). In general, implementing a standard test procedure, comparable between different studies, seems to be advantageous. Besides olfaction-specific requirements, performance testing relies on general test characteristics. For example, in olfactory testing the item difficulty is rarely considered. However, in olfaction, easy items (tasks, which are easy to solve in the general population) may be useful in testing relatively strong deficits in elderly individuals or neurologic or psychiatric patients, while difficult items (tasks, which are difficult to solve in the general population) seem to be more suitable in measuring performance differences in healthy young individuals (Weierstall and Pause, 2012).

As already mentioned, functions of human olfaction can be characterized as either primary (olfactory sensitivity) or secondary (olfactory identification, discrimination or recognition). The distinction of human olfaction as either primary or secondary indicates that one single test of olfactory performance might not be a sufficient marker of olfactory functioning (Martzke et al., 1997). However, olfactory sensitivity performance can be altered by centrally mediated events known as top-down processing, and furthermore, the interpretation of secondary olfactory functions (e.g., identification or discrimination) is contingent upon available data about the intactness of the primary sensory systems (e.g., intact olfactory acuity). Many studies of olfactory performance do not regard the necessity to obtain measures on primary and secondary olfactory functions in order to judge olfactory abilities in patients.

Besides psychophysical test procedures, electrophysiological measures, like CSERPs, are promising tools aiding to differentiate primary from secondary odor processing. Research on the relation between olfaction and depression, has demonstrated that early sensory odor processing is attenuated in MDD patients and in healthy individuals experiencing helplessness, while late evaluative odor processing is not affected (or only affected in a modality non-specific manner). These findings correspond to studies showing that olfactory sensitivity is reduced in MDD patients, while odor discrimination and odor identification often remains unaffected.

Similar to the considerations on the tests of olfaction, also the tests of depression need to be appropriate. Thus, in patient studies, it is required to assess the distinct type of depressive disorder and the severity of the depressive symptoms. While most studies include measures of symptom severity (e.g., HAM-D, or BDI), some studies lack a precise diagnosis of the depressive symptoms. Major depressive episodes might occur in MDD, in BPD, in SAD or mood disorders, which are due to other medical conditions (e.g., multiple sclerosis, stroke, hypothyroidism). However, the foregone summary reveals that there are disorder specific alterations of olfactory perception. Therefore, in depression research, it is a prerequisite to specify the differential diagnosis.

A general cognitive decline that occurs during a depressive episode has been suggested to be the underlying process of impaired olfactory identification ability showed by some studies that examined MDD patients. However, cognitive impairments should be considered in olfactory testing in general. For example, memory, attention, executive functions, or language deficits can affect olfactory identification or discrimination performance. The amount of influence by these factors is partly task-dependent: whereas olfactory discrimination tests vary with the amount of attentional resources and working memory performance, olfactory identification tasks, vary with language skills, semantic memory, and executive functions (Doty and Laing, 2003; Schubert et al., 2013; Zucco et al., 2014). Furthermore, the familiarity of an odor can lead to increased discrimination performance (Rabin, 1988). However, olfactory sensitivity seems to be rather unaffected by cognitive factors. According to Hedner et al. (2010) cognitive factors like executive functioning, semantic memory, and episodic memory are unrelated to odor threshold scores. Thus, in order to make sure that alterations in olfactory perception are directly related to the disorder (and it's specific neurological underpinnings) and not secondary to cognitive or motivational deficits, appropriate control conditions need to be implemented. Such control conditions should consist of cognitive tests (most importantly assessing short-term memory, and attentional capacities) or control tests which assess perceptional performances in other modalities than olfaction (Pause et al., 2003).

In summary, there are some methodological considerations which should be taken into account in investigating olfactory performance in depressive disorders. The considerations refer to the kind of olfactory test, which might be most suitable and to the precise measurement of the kind of depressive disorder. To control influences of cognitive or motivational factors on olfactory performance (especially odor identification and odor discrimination), cognitive functioning should be evaluated. As summarized above, the alterations in olfactory performances are specific to the depressive disorder (e.g., MDD or BPD), therefore, direct comparisons of sensory performances between and within psychiatric populations are recommended (see e.g., Pentzek et al., 2007; Pause et al., 2008).

GENERAL IMPLICATIONS

The literature on olfaction in depressive disorders and healthy people experiencing a negative mood state has been summarized. Regarding olfactory sensitivity in MDD, almost all studies show elevated olfactory thresholds in patients as compared to healthy controls. The olfactory impairments can be observed whether or not patients are treated with antidepressants, indicating that the reduced odor sensitivity is directly related to the depressive disorder. Furthermore, the sensitivity impairments disappear with successful treatment of MDD. Accordingly, two studies reveal that severity of MDD and reduced olfactory sensitivity are significantly correlated. The decline in olfactory sensitivity seems to be specific for MDD and has not been observed in BPD or SAD.

Olfactory identification ability in MDD was found to be unaffected in most of the studies. However, some studies found reduced odor identification performances in patients with severe MDD. It is likely that the worse odor identification performance in these MDD patients is due to a general cognitive deficit, which accompanies severe depressive symptoms. Due to the limited evidence, the degree of olfactory identification performance in BPD and SAD remains unclear. There is only one study (Negoias et al., 2010) investigating discrimination ability in MDD, revealing no differences between patients and control group.

Evaluations of odor characteristics are assessed with regard to intensity, hedonic aspects or familiarity. Odor intensity ratings seem to be unaffected by MDD. However, intensity ratings for highly pleasant or unpleasant odors might be changed in MDD patients. Most studies reveal the emotional valence of odors to be rated in a normal range or as less positive in MDD patients as compared to healthy participants. This is in line with the findings that MDD patients report a higher arousal in response to emotionally negative odors than healthy participants. In contrast to MDD patients, BPD patients seem to judge odors as emotionally more positive than healthy controls. Familiarity ratings seem not to be altered in MDD.

Regarding the psychophysiology of olfaction, early potential amplitudes of the CSERP in MDD patients are reduced in a modality-specific manner. Further, regarding the neuroanatomy of olfaction in MDD, patients showed smaller OB volumes compared to healthy controls and reduced olfactory sensitivity was negatively correlated with the OB volume. Both findings indicate that odor perception in MDD is altered at an early sensory processing level.

Similar to depressive patients, healthy individuals with depressive symptoms as well as individuals experiencing a transient negative mood seem to show a reduced olfactory sensitivity, whereas odor identification or discrimination appears to be unchanged. In addition, early sensory odor processing, as indexed by CSERP analysis is attenuated in MDD patients as well as in healthy individuals experiencing helplessness. These findings indicate that similar neurophysiological processes appear to modulate the effects of negative mood or depression on the olfactory system.

Altogether, reviewed data show that odor perception in MDD and healthy but sad individuals is altered on an early sensory processing level. Alterations of olfaction on a later cognitive-evaluative level seem to vary with the magnitude of a general cognitive impairment during depressive episodes. These findings have practical and theoretical implications: First, as even healthy individuals experiencing sad mood show reduced olfactory performances it is highly probable that alterations in odor perception precede the manifestation of a depressive disorder. Therefore, olfactory tests could be useful to be added to the early diagnosis of depressive symptoms during the development of a depressive disorder. Furthermore, as the reduced olfactory performance in MDD patients seems to be disorder-, modality-, and test-specific, the application of an appropriate olfactory and cognitive test-battery might be highly useful in the differential diagnosis of MDD (as compared to other disorders which also include the manifestation of depressive episodes).

Second, it is likely that structures of the primary olfactory cortex are affected during depressive experiences. Primary cortical processing structures of the olfactory system are the OB and its direct project areas (the anterior olfactory nucleus, the piriform cortex, the anterior cortical nucleus of the amygdala, the periamygdaloid cortex and the anteromediate part of the entorhinal cortex). The amygdala, especially the anterior cortical nucleus, receives direct information from the OB (see Carmichael and Price, 1994; Cleland and Linster, 2003).

Rats with excised OBs (OB rats) are proposed to be an animal model of depression. It is observed that OB rats show behavioral, neurotransmitter, immune and endocrine changes similar to patients with depression. Additionally, behavioral changes in the OB rat can be treated by antidepressants given chronically (Richardson, 1991). Regarding behavioral changes, OB rats show increased locomotor activity in a novel environment, impaired spatial learning and taste aversion learning. In addition, they show increased reactivity to stressors, which is related to higher levels of adrenocorticotrophic hormone (see Kelly et al., 1997; Harkin et al., 2003). The alterations of the physiology and behavior after bulbectomy are not caused by the loss of smell, as peripherally induced anosmia does not generate depression like symptoms (Song and Leonard, 2005). It is suggested that the bulbectomy disrupts the limbic circuit responsible for flexible modulating of behavior. Probably most important, after bulbectomy the tonic inhibition of amygdala activity through the OB is reduced, resulting in a dysinhibition of the amygdala (McNish and Davis, 1997; Harkin et al., 2003). The amygdala is basically involved in the processing of emotional signals of threat and fear (LeDoux, 2007), and further plays a central role in the physiopathology of depressive disorders (Hamilton et al., 2012). Processing negative stimuli is accompanied by hyperactivity of the amygdala (see Soudry et al., 2011). Following these considerations, reduced olfactory sensitivity might be due to dysfunctions of the OB in depressive patients (Lu and Slotnick, 1998) and additionally, an impaired OB can cause an intensified experience of sadness and fear via disinhibition of the amygdala (Pause et al., 2001).

Individuals experiencing depression show a loss of interest or pleasure in nearly all activities and describe their mood to be sad, hopeless or discouraged. Their emotional experience is generally blunted, involving reduced experiences of positive as well as of negative emotions. Here, we conclude that the reduced emotionality during depressive states is accompanied by a reduced olfactory experience. It is hypothesized that similar neuronal networks are responsible for the attenuated olfactory and emotional experience. The olfactory environment is usually low in distinctiveness and in general only few smells reach our awareness. Therefore, it has been postulated that, in everyday life, olfaction is a rather implicit sense (Köster, 2002). Considering, that a reduced olfactory sensitivity contributes to a still lesser experience of environmental smells, leads to the assumption that sadness might not only to isolate individuals in terms of their emotional belongingness, but also might isolate them with regard to reduced sensory (olfactory) experiences.

ACKNOWLEDGMENTS

The authors thank Sabine Schlösser for proof-reading the manuscript.

REFERENCES

American Psychiatric Association. (2000). *Diagnostic and Statistical Manual of Mental Disorders, 4th Edn.* Arlington, VA: American Psychiatric Association. doi: 10.1176/appi.books.9780890423349

American Psychiatric Association. (2013). *Diagnostic and Statistical Manual of Mental Disorders, 4th Edn.* Arlington, VA: American Psychiatric Association.

Amsterdam, J. D., Settle, R. G., Doty, R. L., Abelman, E., and Winokur, A. (1987). Taste and smell perception in depression. *Biol. Psychiatry* 22, 1481–1485. doi: 10.1016/0006-3223(87)90108-9

Atanasova, B., El-Hage, W., Chabanet, C., Gaillard, P., Belzung, C., and Camus, V. (2010). Olfactory anhedonia and negative olfactory alliesthesia in depressed patients. *Psychiatry Res.* 176, 190–196. doi: 10.1016/j.psychres.2008.11.016

Atanasova, B., Graux, J., El Hage, W., Hommet, C., Camus, V., and Belzung, C. (2008). Olfaction: a potential cognitive marker of psychiatric disorders. *Neurosci Biobehav. Rev.* 32, 1315–1325. doi: 10.1016/j.neubiorev.2008.05.003

Beck, A. T. (1979). *Cognitive Therapy of Depression.* New York, NY: Guilford Press.

Beck, A. T., Ward, C. M., Mendelson, M., Mock, J. E., and Erbaugh, J. K. (1961). An inventory for measuring depression. *Arch. Gen. Psychiatry* 4, 561–571. doi: 10.1001/archpsyc.1961.01710120031004

Bekesy, G. V. (1947). A new audiometer. *Acta Otolaryngol.* 35, 411–422. doi: 10.3109/00016484709123756

Berglund, B., Berglund, U., and Linvall, T. (1986). Theory and methods for odor evaluation. *Experientia* 42, 280–187. doi: 10.1007/BF01942508

Bradley, M. M., and Lang, P. J. (1994). Measuring emotion: the self-assessment manikin and the semantic differential. *J. Behav. Ther. Exp. Psychiatry* 25, 49–59. doi: 10.1016/0005-7916(94)90063-9

Burón, E., and Bulbena, A. (2013). Olfaction in affective and anxiety disorders: a review of the literature. *Psychopathology* 46, 63–74. doi: 10.1159/000338717

Carmichael, S. T., Clugnet, M. C., and Price, J. L. (1994). Central olfactory connections in the macaque monkey. *J. Comp. Neurol.* 346, 403–434. doi: 10.1002/cne.903460306

Carmichael, S. T., and Price, J. L. (1994). Architectonic subdivision of the orbital and medial prefrontal cortex in the macaque monkey. *J. Comp. Neurol.* 346, 366–402. doi: 10.1002/cne.903460305

Chapman, L. J., Chapman, J. P., and Raulin, M. L. (1976). Scales for physical and social anhedonia. *J. Abnorm. Psychol.* 85, 374–382. doi: 10.1037/0021-843X.85.4.374

Cleland, T. A., and Linster, C. (2003). "Central olfactory structures," in *Handbook of Olfaction and Gustation 2nd Edn* ed R. L. Doty (New York, NY: Marcel Dekker), 165–180.

Clepce, M., Gossler, A., Reich, K., Kornhuber, J., and Thuerauf, N. (2010). The relation between depression, anhedonia and olfactory hedonic estimates – A pilot study in major depression. *Neurosci. Lett.* 471, 139–143. doi: 10.1016/j.neulet.2010.01.027

Cumming, A. G., Matthews, N. L., and Park, S. (2011). Olfactory identification and preference in bipolar disorder and schizophrenia. *Eur. Arch. Psychiatry Clin. Neurosci.* 261, 251–259. doi: 10.1007/s00406-010-0145-7

Doty, R. L. (1975). An examination of relationships between the pleasantness, intensity, and concentration of 10 odorous stimuli. *Percept. Psychophys.* 17, 492–496. doi: 10.3758/BF03203300

Doty, R. L. (1991). "Olfactory system," in *Smell and Taste in Health and Disease*, eds T. V. Getchell, R. L. Doty, L. M. Bartoshuk, and J. B. Snow (New York, NY: Raven Press), 735–751.

Doty, R. L. (2006). Olfactory dysfunction and its measurement in the clinic and workplace. *Int. Arch. Occup. Environ. Health* 79, 268–282. doi: 10.1007/s00420-005-0055-6

Doty, R. L. (2007). Office procedures for quantitative assessment of olfactory function. *Am. J. Rhinol.* 21, 460–473. doi: 10.2500/ajr.2007.21.3043

Doty, R. L., Brugger, W. E., Jurs, P. C., Orndorff, M. A., Snyder, P. J., and Lowry, L. D. (1978). Intranasal trigeminal stimulation from odorous volatiles: psychometric responses from anosmic and normal humans. *Physiol. Behav.* 20, 175–185. doi: 10.1016/0031-9384(78)90070-7

Doty, R. L., and Laing, D. G. (2003). "Psychophysical measurement of human olfactory function, including odorant mixture assessment," in *Handbook of Olfaction and Gustation 2nd Edn,* ed R. L. Doty (New York, NY: Marcel Dekker), 203–228.

Doty, R. L., Shaman, P., Applebaum, S. L., Giberson, R., Siksorski, L., and Rosenberg, L. (1984a) Smell identification ability: changes with age. *Science* 226, 1441–1443. doi: 10.1126/science.6505700

Doty, R. L., Shaman, P., and Dann, M. (1984b). Development of the university of pennsylvania smell identification test: a standardized microencapsulated test of olfactory function. *Physiol. Behav.* 32, 489–502. doi: 10.1016/0031-9384(84)90269-5

Drevets, W. C. (2003). Neuroimaging abnormalities in the amygdala in mood disorders. *Ann. N.Y. Acad. Sci.* 985, 420–44. doi: 10.1111/j.1749-6632.2003.tb07098.x

Eastman, C. I., Young, M. A., Fogg, L. F., Liu, L., and Meaden, P. M. (1998). Bright light treatment of winter depression: a placebo-controlled trial. *Arch. Gen. Psychiatry* 55, 883–889. doi: 10.1001/archpsyc.55.10.883

Economou, A. (2003). Olfactory identification in elderly Greek people in relation to memory and attention measures. *Arch. Gerontol. Geriatr.* 37, 119–130. doi: 10.1016/S0167-4943(03)00025-6

Ekman, P. E., and Davidson, R. J. (1994). *The Nature of Emotion: Fundamental Questions.* New York, NY: Oxford University Press.

Folstein, M. F., Folstein, F. E., and McHugh, P. R. (1975). Mini mental state. A practical methodfor grading the cognitive state of patients for the clinician. *J. Psychiatr. Res.* 12, 189–198. doi: 10.1016/0022-3956(75)90026-6

Franz, M., Lemke, M. R., Meyer, T., Ulferts, J., Puhl, P., and Snaith, R. P. (2005). *Snaith-Hamilton Pleasure Scale (SHAPS-D).* Göttingen: Hogrefe.

Gerkin, R. C., Tripathy, S. J., and Urban, N. N. (2013). Origins of correlated spiking in the mammalian olfactory bulb. *Proc. Natl. Acad. Sci. U.S.A.* 110, 17083–17088. doi: 10.1073/pnas.1303830110

Goel, N., and Grasso, D. J. (2004). Olfactory discrimination and transient mood change in young men and women: variation by season, mood state, and time of day. *Chronobiol. Int.* 21, 691–719. doi: 10.1081/CBI-200025989

Gottfried, J. (2006). Smell: central nervous processing. *Adv. Otorhinolaryngol.* 63, 44–69. doi: 10.1159/000093750

Gross-Isseroff, R., Luca-Haimovici, K., Sasson, Y., Kindler, S., Kotler, M., and Zohar, J. (1994). Olfactory sensitivity in major depressive disorder and obsessive compulsive disorder. *Biol. Psychiatry* 35, 798–802. doi: 10.1016/0006-3223(94)91142-8

Hamilton, J. P., Etkin, A., Furman, D. J., Lemus, M. G., Johnson, R. F., and Gotlib, I. H. (2012). Functional neuroimaging of major depressive disorder: a meta-analysis and new integration of baseline activation and neural response data. *Am. J. Psychiatry* 169, 693–703. doi: 10.1176/appi.ajp.2012.11071105

Hamilton, M. (1960). A rating scale for depression. *J. Neurol. Neurosurg. Psychiatry* 23, 56–62. doi: 10.1136/jnnp.23.1.56

Harkin, A., Kelly, J. P., and Leonard; B. E. (2003). A review of the relevance and validity of olfactory bulbectomy as a model of depression. *Clin. Neurosci. Res.* 3, 253–262. doi: 10.1016/S1566-2772(03)00087-2

Hedner, M., Larsson, M., Arnold, N., Zucco, G. M., and Hummel, T. (2010). Cognitive factors in odor detection, odor discrimination, and odor identification tasks. *J. Clin. Exp. Neuropsychol.* 10, 1062–1067. doi: 10.1080/13803391003683070

Hiroto, D. S., and Seligman, M. E. (1975). Generality of learned helplessness in man. *J. Pers. Soc. Psychol.* 31, 311–327. doi: 10.1037/h0076270

Hummel, T., Kobal, G., Gudziol, H., and Mackay-Sim, A. (2007). Normative data for the "Sniffin'Sticks" including tests of odor identification, odor discrimination, and olfactory thresholds: an upgrade based on a group of more than 3,000 subjects. *Eur. Arch. Otolaryngol.* 264, 237–243. doi: 10.1007/s00405-006-0173-0

Ihl, P., and Weyer, G. (1993). *Alzheimer's Disease Assessment Scale (ADAS), German Version.* Weinheim: Beltz.

Kelly, J. P., Wrynn, A. S., and Leonard, B. E. (1997). The olfactory bulbectomized rat as a model of depression: an update. *Pharmacol. Ther.* 74, 299–316. doi: 10.1016/S0163-7258(97)00004-1

Kopala, L. C., Good, K. P., and Honer, W. G. (1994). Olfactory hallucinations and olfactory identification ability in patients with schizophrenia and other psychiatric disorders. *Schizophr. Res.* 12, 205–211. doi: 10.1016/0920-9964(94)90030-2

Köster, E. P. (2002). "The specific characteristics of the sense of smell," in *Olfaction, Taste, and Cognition*, eds C. Rouby, B. Schaal, D. Dubois, R. Gervais, and A. Holley (New York, NY: Cambridge University Press), 27–43. doi: 10.1017/CBO9780511546389.007

Krout, K. E., Kawano, J., Mettenleiter, T. C., and Loewy, A. D. (2002). CNS inputs to the suprachiasmatic nucleus of the rat. *Neuroscience* 110, 73–92. doi: 10.1016/S0306-4522(01)00551-6

Krüger, S., Frasnelli, J., Braunig, P., and Hummel, T. (2006). Increased olfactory sensitivity in euthymic patients with bipolar disorder with event-related episodes compared with patients with bipolar disorder without such episodes. *J. Psychiatry Neurosci.* 31, 263–270.

Laing, D. G. (1983). Natural sniffing gives optimum odour perception for humans. *Perception* 12, 99–107. doi: 10.1068/p120099

Laudien, J. H., Küster, D., Sojka, B., Ferstl, R., and Pause, B. M. (2006). Central odor processing in subjects experiencing helplessness. *Brain Res.* 1120, 141–150. doi: 10.1016/j.brainres.2006.08.090

LeDoux, J. (2007). The amygdala. *Curr. Biol.* 17, 868–874. doi: 10.1016/j.cub.2007.08.005

LeDoux, J. (2012). Rethinking the emotional brain. *Neuron* 73, 653–676. doi: 10.1016/j.neuron.2012.02.004

Lombion-Pouthier, S., Vandel, P., Nezelof, S., Haffen, E., and Millot, J.-L. (2006). Odor perception in patients with mood disorders. *J. Affect. Disord.* 90, 187–191. doi: 10.1016/j.jad.2005.11.012

Lötsch, J., Reichmann, H., and Hummel, T. (2008). Different odor tests contribute differently to the evaluation of olfactory loss. *Chem. Senses* 33, 17–21. doi: 10.1093/chemse/bjm058

Lu, X. C., and Slotnick, B. M. (1998). Olfaction in rats with extensive lesions of the olfactory bulbs: implications for odor coding. *Neuroscience* 84, 849–866. doi: 10.1016/S0306-4522(97)00520-4

Martzke, J. S., Kopala, L. C., and Good, K. P. (1997). Olfactory dysfunction in neuropsychiatric disorders: review and methodological considerations. *Biol. Psychiatry* 42, 721–732. doi: 10.1016/S0006-3223(96)00442-8

McCaffrey, R. J., Duff, K., and Solomon, G. S. (2000). Olfactory dysfunction discriminates probable Alzheimer's dementia from major depression: a cross-validation and extension. *J. Neuropsychiatry Clin. Neurosci.* 12, 29–33.

McNish, K. A., and Davis, M. (1997). Olfactory bulbectomy enhances sensitization of the acoustic startle reflex produced by acute or repeated stress. *Behav. Neurosci.* 111, 80–91. doi: 10.1037/0735-7044.111.1.80

Montgomery, S. A., and Asberg, M. (1979). A new depression scale designed to be sensitive to change. *Brit. J. Psychiat.* 134, 382–389. doi: 10.1192/bjp.134.4.382

Mozell, M. M., Hornung, D. E., Sheehe, P. R., and Kurtz, D. B. (1986). "What should be controlled in studies of smell?," in *Clinical Measurement of Taste and Smell*, eds H. L. Meiselmann and R. S. Rivlin (New York, NY: Macmillian Publishing Company), 154–169.

Murphy, F. C., Nimmo-Smith, I., and Lawrence, A. D. (2003). Functional neuroanatomy of emotions: a meta-analysis. *Cogn. Affect. Behav. Neurosci.* 3, 207–233. doi: 10.3758/CABN.3.3.207

Murray, E. A., Wise, S. P., and Drevets, W. C. (2011). Localization of dysfunction in major depressive disorder: prefrontal cortex and amygdala. *Biol. Psychiatry* 69, e43–e54. doi: 10.1016/j.biopsych.2010.09.041

Naudin, M., El-Hage, W., Gomes, M., Gaillard, P., Belzung, C., Atanasova, B., et al. (2012). State and trait olfactory markers of major depression. *PLoS ONE* 7:e46938. doi: 10.1371/journal.pone.0046938

Negoias, S., Croy, I., Gerber, J., Puschmann, S., Petrowski, K., Joraschky, P., et al. (2010). Reduced olfactory bulb volume and olfactory sensitivity in patients with acute major depression. *Neuroscience* 169, 415–421. doi: 10.1016/j.neuroscience.2010.05.012

Oren, D. A., Schwartz, P. J., Turner, E. H., and Rosenthal, N. E. (1995). Olfactory function in winter seasonal affective disorder. *Am. J. Psychiatry* 152, 1531–1532.

Panksepp, J. (2011). The basic emotional circuits of mammalian brains: do animals have affective lives? *Neurosci. Biobehav. Rev.* 35, 1791–1804. doi: 10.1016/j.neubiorev.2011.08.003

Pause, B. M. (2012). Processing of body odor signals by the human brain. *Chem. Percept.* 5, 55–63. doi: 10.1007/s12078-011-9108-2

Pause, B. M., Hellmann, G., Göder, R., Aldenhoff, J. B., and Ferstl, R. (2008). Increased processing speed for emotionally negative odors in schizophrenia. *Int. J. Psychophysiol.* 70, 16–22. doi: 10.1016/j.ijpsycho.2008.04.003

Pause, B. M., Lembcke, J., Reese, I., Hinze-Selch, D., Aldenhoff, J. B., and Ferstl, R. (2005). Reduced olfactory sensitivity in antidepressant drug-free patients with major depression. *Z. Klin. Psychol. Psychother.* 34, 79–85. doi: 10.1026/1616-3443.34.2.79

Pause, B. M., Miranda, A., Göder, R., Aldenhoff, J. B., and Ferstl, R. (2001). Reduced olfactory performance in patients with major depression. *J. Psychiatr. Res.* 35, 271–277. doi: 10.1016/S0022-3956(01)00029-2

Pause, B. M., Miranda, A., Nysterud, M., and Ferstl, R. (2000). Geruchs- und emotionale Reizbewertung bei Patienten mit Major Depression. *Z. Klin. Psychol. Psychother.* 29, 16–23. doi: 10.1026//0084-5345.29.1.16

Pause, B. M., Raack, N., Sojka, B., Göder, R., Aldenhoff, J. B., and Ferstl, R. (2003). Convergent and divergent effects of odors and emotions in depression. *Psychophysiology* 40, 209–225. doi: 10.1111/1469-8986.00023

Pentzek, M., Grass-Kapanke, B., and Ihl, R. (2007). Odor identification in Alzheimer's disease and depression. *Aging Clin. Exp. Res.* 19, 255–258. doi: 10.1007/BF03324698

Pezawas, L., Meyer-Lindenberg, A., Drabant, E. M., Verchinski, B. A., Munoz, K. E., Kolachana, B. S., et al. (2005). 5-HTTLPR polymorphism impacts human cingulate-amygdala interactions: a genetic susceptibility mechanism for depression. *Nat. Neurosci.* 8, 828–834. doi: 10.1038/nn1463

Pollatos, O., Albrecht, J., Kopietz, R., Linn, J., Schoepf, V., Kleemann, A. M., et al. (2007a). Reduced olfactory sensitivity in subjects with depressive symptoms. *J. Affect. Disord.* 102, 101–108. doi: 10.1016/j.jad.2006.12.012

Pollatos, O., Kopietz, R., Linn, J., Albrecht, J., Sakar, V., Anzinger, A., et al. (2007b). Emotional stimulation alters olfactory sensitivity and odor judgment. *Chem. Senses* 32, 583–589. doi: 10.1093/chemse/bjm027

Postolache, T. T., Doty, R. L., Wehr, T. A., Jimma, L. A., Han, L., Turner, E. H., et al. (1999). Monorhinal odor identification and depression scores in patients with seasonal affective disorder. *J. Affect. Disord.* 56, 27–35. doi: 10.1016/S0165-0327(99)00027-0

Postolache, T. T., Wehr, T. A., Doty, R. L., Sher, L., Turner, E. H., Bartko, J. J., et al. (2002). Patients with seasonal affective disorder have lower odor detection thresholds than control subjects. *Arch. Gen. Psychiatry* 59, 1119–1122. doi: 10.1001/archpsyc.59.12.1119

Pouliot, S., Bourgeat, F., Barkat, S., Rouby, C., and Bensafi, M. (2008). Increase in anhedonia level in menopausal women is accompanied by a shift in olfactory function. *Chem. Percept.* 1, 43–47. doi: 10.1007/s12078-007-9001-1

Rabin, M. D. (1988). Experience facilitates odor quality discrimination. *Percept. Psychophys.* 44, 185–192. doi: 10.3758/BF03207487

Richardson, J. S. (1991). Animal models of depression reflect changing views on the essence and etiology of depressive disorders in humans. *Prog. Neuro-Psychopharmacol. Biol. Psychiat.* 15, 199–204. doi: 10.1016/0278-5846(91)90081-B

Satoh, S., Morita, N., Matsuzaki, I., Konishi, T., Nakano, T., Minoshita, S., et al. (1996). Relationship between odor perception and depression in the Japanese elderly. *Psychiatry Clin. Neurosci.* 50, 271–275. doi: 10.1111/j.1440-1819.1996.tb00563.x

Savitz, J., and Drevets, W. C. (2013). Neuroreceptor imaging in depression. *Neurobiol. Dis.* 52, 49–65. doi: 10.1016/j.nbd.2012.06.001

Savitz, J., Lucki, I., and Drevets, W. C. (2009). 5-HT1A receptor function in major depressive disorder. *Prog. Neurobiol.* 88, 17–31. doi: 10.1016/j.pneurobio.2009.01.009

Schubert, C. R., Cruickshanks, K. J., Fischer, M. E., Huang, G. H., Klein, R., Pankratz, N., et al. (2013). Odor identification and cognitive function in the Beaver Dam Offspring Study. *J. Clin. Exp. Neuropsychol.* 35, 669–676. doi: 10.1080/13803395.2013.809701

Scinska, A., Wrobel, E., Korkosz, A., Zatorski, P., Sienkiewicz–Jarosz, H., Lojkowska, W., et al. (2008). Depressive symptoms and olfactory function in older adults. *Psychiatry Clin. Neurosci.* 62, 450–456. doi: 10.1111/j.1440-1819.2008.01824.x

Serby, M., Larson, P., and Kalkstein, D. (1990). Olfactory sense in psychoses. *Biol. Psychiatry* 28, 830. doi: 10.1016/0006-3223(90)90520-C

Serby, M., Larson, P., and Kalkstein, D. (1992). "Olfaction and neuropsychiatry," in *Science of olfaction*, eds M. J. Serby and K. L. Chobor (New York, NY: Springer), 559–584. doi: 10.1007/978-1-4612-2836-3_21

Settle, R. G., and Amsterdam, J. D. (1991). "Depression and chemical senses," in *Smell and Taste in Health and Disease*, eds T. V. Getchell, R. L. Doty, L. M. Bartoshuk, and J. B. Snow Jr (New York, NY: Raven Press), 851–862.

Solomon, G. S., Petrie, W. M., Hart, J. R., and Brackin, H. B. Jr. (1998). Olfactory dysfunction discriminates Alzheimer's dementia from major depression. *J. Neuropsychiatry Clin. Neurosci.* 10, 64–67.

Song, C., and Leonard, B. E. (2005). The olfactory bulbectomised rat as a model of depression. *Neurosci. Biobehav. Rev.* 29, 627–647. doi: 10.1016/j.neubiorev.2005.03.010

Soudry, Y., Lemogne, C., Malinvaud, D., Consoli, S. M., and Bonfils, P. (2011). Olfactory system and emotion: common substrates. *Eur. Ann. Otorhinolaryngol. Head. Neck. Dis.* 128, 18–23. doi: 10.1016/j.anorl.2010.09.007

Steiner, J. E., Lidar-Lifschitz, D., and Perl, E. (1993). Taste and odor: reactivity in depressive disorders, a multidisciplinary approach. *Percept. Mot. Skills* 77, 1331–1346. doi: 10.2466/pms.1993.77.3f.1331

Swiecicki, L., Zatorski, P., Bzinkowska, D., Sienkiewicz-Jarosz, H., Szyndler, J., and Scinska, A. (2009). Gustatory and olfactory function in patients with unipolar and bipolar depression. *Prog. Neuro-Psychopharmacol. Biol. Psychiatry* 33, 827–834. doi: 10.1016/j.pnpbp.2009.03.030

Thomas, H. J., Fries, W., and Distel, H. (2002). Bewertung von Geruchsreizen bei depressiv Erkrankten. *Nervenarzt* 73, 71–77. doi: 10.1007/s115-002-8150-9

Thomas-Danguin, T., Rouby, C., Sicard, G., Vigouroux, M., Farget, V., Johanson, A., et al. (2003). Development of the ETOC: a European test of olfactory capabilities. *Rhinology* 41, 134–151.

Warner, M. D., Peabody, C. A., and Csernansky, J. G. (1990). Olfactory functioning in schizophrenia and depression. *Biol. Psychiatry* 27, 457–458. doi: 10.1016/0006-3223(90)90557-I

Wechsler, D. (1999). *Wechsler Abbreviated Scale of Intelligence*. San Antonio, TX: Psychological Corporation.

Weierstall, R., and Pause, B. M. (2012). Development of a 15-item odour discrimination test (Düsseldorf Odour Discrimination Test). *Perception* 41, 193–203. doi: 10.1068/p7113

Yesavage, J. A. (1988). Geriatric depression scale. *Psychopharmacol. Bull.* 82, 899–904.

Zucco, G. M., and Bollini, F. (2011). Odour recognition memory and odour identification in patients with mild and severe major depressive disorders. *Psychiatry Res.* 190, 217–220. doi: 10.1016/j.psychres.2011.08.025

Zucco, G. M., Hummel, T., Tomaiuolo, F., and Stevenson, R. J. (2014). The influence of short-term memory on standard discrimination and cued indentification olfactory tasks. *J. Neurosci. Methods* 222, 138–141.

Zung, W. W. K. (1965). A self-rating depression scale. *Arch. Gen. Psychiatry* 12, 63–70. doi: 10.1001/archpsyc.1965.01720310065008

11

The impact of expertise in olfaction

Jean-Pierre Royet[1]*, Jane Plailly[1], Anne-Lise Saive[1], Alexandra Veyrac[1] and Chantal Delon-Martin[2,3]

[1] Olfaction: From Coding to Memory Team, Centre de Recherche en Neurosciences de Lyon, CNRS UMR 5292, INSERM U1028, Université Lyon 1, Lyon, France
[2] INSERM, U836, NeuroImagerie Fonctionnelle et Perfusion Cerebrale, Grenoble, France
[3] Université Joseph Fourier, Grenoble Institut des Neurosciences, Grenoble, France

***Correspondence:**
Jean-Pierre Royet, Olfaction: From Coding to Memory Team, Centre de Recherche en Neurosciences de Lyon, CNRS UMR 5292, INSERM U1028, Université Lyon 1, 50 Avenue Tony Garnier, 69366 Lyon Cedex 07, France
e-mail: royet@olfac.univ-lyon1.fr

Olfactory expertise remains poorly understood, most likely because experts in odor, such as perfumers, sommeliers, and oenologists, are much rarer than experts in other modalities, such as musicians or sportsmen. In this review, we address the specificities of odor expertise in both odor experts and in *a priori* untrained individuals who have undergone specific olfactory training in the frame of an experiment, such as repeated exposure to odors or associative learning. Until the 21st century, only the behavioral effects of olfactory training of untrained control individuals had been reported, revealing an improvement of olfactory performance in terms of sensitivity, discrimination, memory, and identification. Behavioral studies of odor experts have been scarce, with inconsistent or inconclusive results. Recently, the development of cerebral imaging techniques has enabled the identification of brain areas and neural networks involved in odor processing, revealing functional and structural modifications as a function of experience. The behavioral approach to odor expertise has also evolved. Researchers have particularly focused on odor mental imagery, which is characteristic of odor experts, because this ability is absent in the average person but is part of a perfumer's professional practice. This review summarizes behavioral, functional, and structural findings on odor expertise. These data are compared with those obtained using animals subjected to prolonged olfactory exposure or to olfactory-enriched environments and are discussed in the context of functional and structural plasticity.

Keywords: odor expert, perfumer, oenologist, mental imagery, perceptual learning, functional and structural reorganization, brain plasticity, neurogenesis

INTRODUCTION

Grenouille, who had phenomenal olfactory ability, was able to remember the olfactory imprint of a person and to instantly discern his mood. As a perfumer's apprentice in 18th-century France, Grenouille attempted to create the ultimate, love-inspiring perfume. However, Grenouille was only a fictional character in a story written by the German writer Süskind (1986). Other testimonies of individuals with a noteworthy sense of smell have been reported in the literature. Bedichek (1960, p. 57), who was a writer, teacher, and naturalist, reported in a posthumously published book that there are "notable noses," people who are exceptionally sensitive to odors. For instance, he explained that Helen Keller (1908a,b), who described her experience in The Century Magazine, was able to "*recognize an old-fashioned country house because it has several layers of odors, left by a succession of families, of plants, perfumes and draperies.*" Bedichek (1960, p. 57) further highlighted that "*She disentangles and identifies odors by their respective ages, a discrimination I have not found claimed by any nose except that of the bee which one observer declares identifies passage of time by displacement of antennae in flight.*" More recently, Engen (1982), an eminent scientific authority in sensory perception, described an example of experienced noses used in the Vietnam War to detect the whereabouts of machinery and other items. In his famous book, Sachs (1985), a British-American neurologist, also reported the clinical case of a young student, D. Stephen, who experimented with drugs (cocaine, amphetamine). One night, Stephen vividly dreamt that he was a dog, experiencing a world unimaginably rich and significant in smells. On waking, he found that he actually retained this amazingly acute olfactory ability. As emphasized by Engen (1982), one problem with notable noses is that information about them is always anecdotal and is obtained from indirect testimonies, which are not experimentally verifiable. What can we say about the olfactory performances of these noses?

OLFACTORY PERFORMANCE IN TRAINED INDIVIDUALS AND ODOR EXPERTS

The concept of perceptual learning refers to a phenomenon whereby sensory experience induces changes in behavior and brain function (Gibson, 1991; Goldstone, 1998; Gilbert et al., 2001; Fahle and Poggio, 2002). However, Gawel (1997, p. 268) indicated that the literature does not always clearly delineate what constitutes training and what is experience: "*following training, a panelist can be said to be more experienced, but he can also obtain experience without any formal training.*" Gawel (1997) suggested that, in the first case, better performances result from a uniform and directed program of instruction, whereas in the second case, experience relates to passive exposure to a wide variety of stimuli, which makes them more familiar. He specifies (p. 268) that "*thought may be molded by discussion with others with more or less experience, but always in an unstructured way.*"

In this review, we shall focus on two aspects of perceptual learning by examining data from *a priori* untrained subjects who improved their performance by specific olfactory training (in the frame of an experiment) and from odor experts whose performance is the result of both learning and experience. These experts are mainly perfumers, oenologists, and sommeliers. Surprisingly, most behavioral studies dedicated to evaluating the performance of odor experts have examined wine experts[1]. To the best of our knowledge, only three studies have been devoted to perfumers (Livermore and Laing, 1996; Gilbert et al., 1998; Zarzo and Stanton, 2009). Therefore, when we present expert performances, most of the studies described will concern wine professionals (oenologists and sommeliers). Interestingly, wine discrimination has been used as an example of perceptual learning since the end of the 19th century (James, 1890; Gibson, 1953; Gibson and Gibson, 1955). It is further important to emphasize that wine experts use not only their olfactory system but also their gustatory and trigeminal functions to form a unitary perceptual experience (Small and Prescott, 2005). Wine experts also employ visual perception when identifying a wine (Panghorn et al., 1963; Morrot et al., 2001).

ODOR SENSITIVITY

In the olfactory domain, the repeated presentation of an odor (within the perithreshold concentration range) in untrained subjects results in the lowering of thresholds and the enhancement of signal detection sensitivity measures (Engen, 1960; Doty et al., 1981; Rabin and Cain, 1986; Dalton et al., 2002). Similar results are observed for volatile substances such as androstenone[2], for which an individual is conspicuously anosmic but is able to detect with training (Wysocki et al., 1989; Mainland et al., 2002). These data suggest that odor experts who are trained daily can acquire better olfactory sensitivity. However, surprisingly, when the performances of wine experts were compared with those of wine novices or controls, no difference in olfactory sensitivity was revealed for either wine-related components such as tannin or alcohol or non-wine-related components such as *n*-butyl-alcohol (Berg et al., 1955; Bende and Nordin, 1997; Parr et al., 2002; Brand and Brisson, 2012). Bende and Nordin (1997) explained that the non-superiority in detection of wine tasters was due to their professional inexperience with a detection task *per se*. It is also possible that these results were due to the inadequacy of the experimental procedures used in studies.

Several authors state that the plasticity that underpins the emergence of better detection following repeated exposure to odors originates in the central components of the olfactory system, although they do not rule a contribution from peripheral components (Rabin and Cain, 1986; Mainland et al., 2002). In this context, repeated exposure to an odorant (e.g., androstenone, amyl acetate, isovaleric acid, or phenyl ethyl alcohol) can increase olfactory sensitivity to the odorant in mice (Yee and Wysocki, 2001) and rats (Doty and Ferguson-Segall, 1989) and can also increase the sensitivity of the olfactory receptor cells to that odorant in genetically anosmic mice (Wang et al., 1993) and in salmon (Nevitt et al., 1994). Thus, these data provide evidence for stimulus-induced plasticity in sensory receptor cells and suggest that the ability of olfactory cells to exhibit plasticity may be related to their continual turnover (Wang et al., 1993; Huart et al., 2013).

ODOR DISCRIMINATION

Stimulus "differentiation" also represents an important mechanism of perceptual learning in which experience refines sensory perception through the differentiation of stimulus features, dimensions, or categories (Gibson, 1991; Goldstone, 1998; Schyns et al., 1998). In olfaction, the discrimination task usually consists of comparing two odors in order to determine if they are identical or not[3]. Since it has been claimed that an expert can distinguish as many as 10,000 or even 15,000 odors, not including mixtures (Wright, 1964, 1972), the ability to discriminate between odors could be considered as an area of competence of odor experts. Several studies have shown that wine or beer experts have better discrimination or memory abilities than novices (Walk, 1966; Owen and Machamer, 1979; Peron and Allen, 1988; Solomon, 1990; Bende and Nordin, 1997; Parr et al., 2002; Hughson and Boakes, 2009; Zucco et al., 2011). For instance, Bende and Nordin (1997) reported that sommeliers have greater abilities to discriminate odors of eugenol and citral in a mixture than untrained subjects, although they reported only occasionally experiencing these two odors in their profession. The authors claimed that perceptual learning in odor discrimination can be generalized to other odors as well. Peron and Allen (1988) also demonstrated that novice drinkers of beer improve their ability to discriminate beer flavors with experience.

Rather than evaluating discrimination abilities between two odors, some studies have aimed to determine the maximum number of components that an individual can distinguish within a mixture. Untrained subjects can distinguish only three or four components within a mixture (Laing and Francis, 1989; Schab and Cain, 1992). Using a trained panel of 10 women and an expert panel of 8 male professional perfumers and flavorists, Livermore and Laing (1996) observed that the number of components that experts can discriminate and identify is not higher than that of untrained subjects. Nevertheless, when mixtures of two and three components only were used, experts recorded significantly more hits and fewer false alarms[4] than did trained non-experts. Livermore and Laing (1996) suggested that the inability

[1]We identified approximately 50 studies devoted to wine expertise (without taking into account expertise of other types of alcohol such as beer or brandy). This number is not huge but is much higher than the three behavioral studies that have been devoted to perfumers. Whereas the number of perfumers in the world is approximately 500 (120 in France and Switzerland), the number of oenologists (without sommeliers) can be estimated at more than 150,000 (of which 9,500 live in France) in 44 wine-producing countries.

[2]Androstenone is a pheromone that has been identified in pigs. Although this steroid is also found in sweat and urine of both human male and female, and that gender-specific differences in olfactory sensitivity to this odor have been demonstrated (see, e.g., Dalton et al., 2002), it has not yet been recognized as being a human pheromone. Androstadienone, that is a compound closely-related to androstenone, has also been suggested to be a human pheromonal substance.

[3]Other types of discrimination tasks are used, such as the triangle test, in which three samples, two of which are identical, are presented to participants. The task consists of determining which stimulus is different (Amerine et al., 1965). Another task asks subjects to rank samples along a sensory dimension. In the case of wine, the sensory dimension can be attributes of odor (e.g., alcohol, fruit) or taste such as sugared or astringency (produced by tannin; Solomon, 1990).

[4]In such a discrimination task, a hit is defined when the subject correctly identifies a component that is present; a false alarm is defined when the subject incorrectly identifies a component as being present.

of participants to discriminate more than three of four stimuli is a physiologically imposed limit that could be related to the overlap of the odorants' perceptual or cognitive representations. Thus, when odors are not sufficiently separated in multidimensional perceptual space, the addition of other odorants to the mixture can increase the chance of their representations overlapping, increasing the possibility of perceptual confusion and reducing the ability of the subjects to identify odors. Nevertheless, given that descriptions of wine by sommeliers are usually rich in vocabulary, Hughson and Boakes (2001) suggested that these experts might distinguish more components in a mixture than perfumers or flavorists.

ODOR MEMORY

A wide variety of tests are used to evaluate odor recognition memory (Doty, 1991). One test assesses short-term recognition memory and is similar to the discrimination procedure described above, except that a delay of a few seconds to several tens of seconds separates the two odors of a pair (Engen et al., 1973; Jehl et al., 1994). To our knowledge, only a single study with naïve subjects has investigated the impact of training on odor memory by passive exposure to stimuli (Jehl et al., 1995). The authors demonstrated that familiarization by repeated presentation of target or distractor odors improved discrimination performance by reducing the number of false alarms[5], that is, incorrect recognition (**Figure 1**). More recently, Hughson and Boakes (2009) evaluated wine drinkers using a different procedure and demonstrated that experience can improve short-term wine recognition (4 min) by passive perceptual learning.

[5]In the short-term recognition task, the subject must indicate whether the two odors of a pair are identical or different. A hit is defined when the two odors are identical and are so declared by the subject. A false alarm is defined when the two odors are different but are declared as identical by the subject.

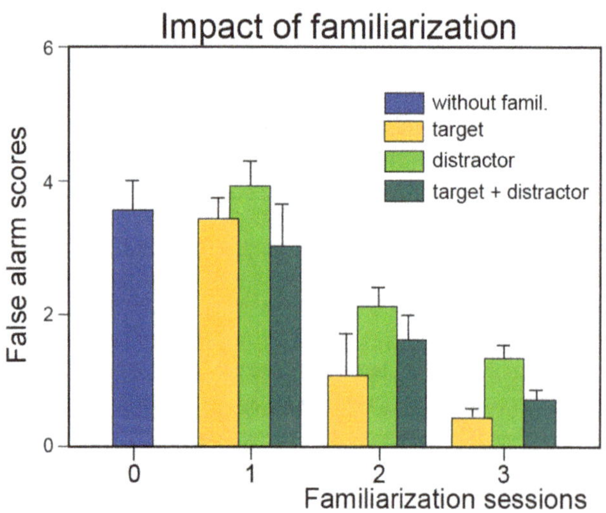

FIGURE 1 | Effect of familiarization. Number of incorrect recognitions (false alarm scores) as a function of the number of familiarization sessions (0, 1, 2, and 3) and of the type of odor (target, distractor, or both target and distractor) to which subjects were familiarized. Vertical bars, standard errors of the mean (modified from Jehl et al., 1995).

To investigate long-term odor recognition memory, the procedure typically consists of using a set of odors for inspection, followed by the presentation of a second set of odors, including equal numbers of previously presented odors (old) and new odors, in a later testing session (Walk and Johns, 1984). For each item, subjects then indicate whether they have previously smelt the odor or not. Using such a memory test, Rabin and Cain (1984) observed that recognition performances increased with odor familiarity rated at inspection, but they did not specifically examine the influence of repeated presentation of stimuli.

ODOR IDENTIFICATION

Smell is likely the most difficult sensory modality to verbalize (Wippich et al., 1989). Human beings possess an excellent odor detection and discrimination abilities but typically have great difficulty in identifying specific odorants (Richardson and Zucco, 1989). The fact that there are no specific terms to describe odor and that odors are identified in terms of idiosyncratic personal experience can explain this difficulty. It has been hypothesized that odor information processing shares some of the cortical resources used in language processing and that these two types of processing can interfere with each other (Lorig, 1999).

Correlating with these observations, the human ability to identify and to name[6] odors is extremely limited (Engen, 1987; Richardson and Zucco, 1989). Estimates vary from approximately 6 to 22 odors when subjects are tested for the first time (Engen, 1960; Sumner, 1962; Desor and Beauchamp, 1974; Lawless and Engen, 1977; Cain, 1979). However, all investigations in naïve subjects have consistently shown that identification performance improves with practice (Desor and Beauchamp, 1974; Cain and Krause, 1979; Cain, 1982). This result is observed as well when subjects must use only labels generated during the first exposure as when they have the option to change labels (Cain, 1979).

IMPACT OF VERBALIZATION ON OLFACTORY PERFORMANCE

Cain (1979) suggested that experts such as perfumers, flavor chemists, food technologists, and wine tasters must verbalize their olfactory experiences and thus identify odors better than untrained persons. To facilitate the description of complex mixtures of stimuli and the classification of sensations, experts are trained to use descriptors of odors, aromas, and flavors. Accordingly, specific terminologies are employed to describe and classify perfumes (**Figure 2**; Zarzo and Stanton, 2009), wines (Noble et al., 1987), Brandies (Jolly and Hattingh, 2001), or certain alimentary products such as cereals or Cheddar cheese (Chambers and Smith, 1993; Roberts and Vickers, 1994; Drake et al., 2001). Correlatively, it is natural to observe that experts (e.g., trained panelists) better characterize or describe wines (Lawless, 1984; Solomon, 1990; Gawel, 1997; Solomon, 1997;

[6]In a typical multiple-choice identification test, the subject has a list of labels when the olfactory stimulus is presented. One of the labels is veridical (e.g., strawberry). A second label is an alternative name and evokes a similar odor (a near miss, such as raspberry). Other names are more distinct alternatives (far misses, such as tar). The number of names can vary from three to four to several dozen. In a naming test, only the odor is presented to the subject. This test is therefore more difficult than the multiple-choice test. The results can be analyzed in terms of response accuracy (veridical label, near and far misses; see, e.g., Rabin and Cain, 1984; Lyman and McDaniel, 1986).

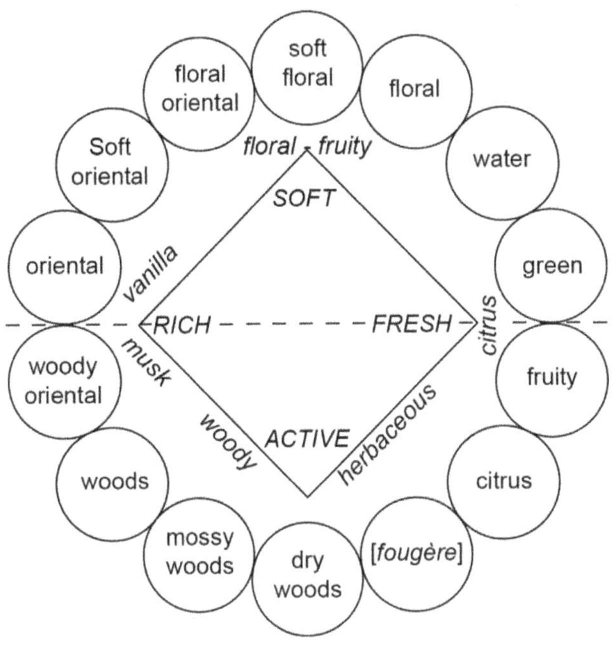

FIGURE 2 | Fragrance wheel. Fourteen perfume categories (within circles) are depicted. For the purposes of comparison, the odor effects diagram (inner square, letters in italics) proposed by Calkin and Jellinek (1994) is also illustrated (with permission from Zarzo and Stanton, 2009).

Chollet and Valentin, 2000; Hughson and Boakes, 2001), beers (Clapperton and Piggott, 1979), fishes (Cardello et al., 1982), and perfumes (Lawless, 1988) than non-experts. Consistent with these data, perfumers (or wine professionals) are less prone to classify odors in terms of their hedonic quality than non-experts, suggesting that they are able to discern (or label) perceptual qualities not available to untrained individuals (Yoshida, 1964; Ballester et al., 2008). Chollet and Valentin (2000) suggested that the perceptual representation of wine is similar in experts and novices but the verbalization of this representation varies with the level of expertise. Experts use analytical terms, whereas non-experts use holistic terms (Schab, 1991; Chollet and Valentin, 2000). Gawel (1997) even hypothesized that superior sensorial knowledge in trained panelists not only leads to the search for descriptors but also facilitates the expectation of prototypical characters, which can result in a higher probability of the detection of components.

Discrimination and recognition memory performances of odors and aromas, as described above (see Odor Discrimination and Odor Memory), were evaluated in perceptual terms only. However, except for two studies in which the authors knowingly used unfamiliar odors (Jehl et al., 1994, 1995), semantic impact was likely largely present but not considered in these studies. In addition, it was demonstrated, in an experimental frame, that discrimination and memory performances can partly be improved by verbalization of the stimuli or the knowledge of their names. Such results have been observed in wine experts (Solomon, 1990; Melcher and Schooler, 1996) and in naïve subjects (Lawless and Engen, 1977; Rabin, 1988; Jehl et al., 1997). For instance, Rabin (1988) reported that naïve subjects trained to label specific odors significantly enhanced their ability to discriminate them one day later. According to Rabin (1988, p. 539), "*endowing a layperson with a perfumer's experience would make subtle mixture components more salient stimuli.*"

In short, it emerges from these data that perceptual (via passive exposure) and cognitive (label learning, development of classification schemas) changes accompany the development of wine expertise (Solomon, 1997; Hughson and Boakes, 2001, 2002; Zucco et al., 2011). However, if perceptual learning of wine, which depends on the frequency and diversity of exposure to stimuli, is rapid and passive, cognitive expertise (semantic) is slower and difficult to develop and requires many years of practice (Zucco et al., 2011). Similar changes are likely associated with the development of expertise in perfumers or flavorists (Jones, 1968; Schab and Cain, 1992). With time, the expert can then acquire perceptual abilities incredibly superior to that of an untrained person (Schab and Cain, 1992).

ODOR MENTAL IMAGERY

The review of the literature described above shows that it is difficult to propose a test to reveal the higher sensory capacities of odor experts compared to naïve subjects. Data are often conflicting, and it is difficult to decide what is sensory and what is semantic in these tasks. The mental imagery task can satisfy these requirements.

With regards to olfaction, the widespread assertion is that it is very difficult for the average person to mentally imagine odors, in contrast to our ability to mentally imagine images, sounds, or music (Stevenson and Case, 2005; Stevenson et al., 2007). Despite behavioral and psychophysical studies demonstrating the existence of odor imagery (Lyman and McDaniel, 1990; Algom and Cain, 1991; Algom et al., 1993; Carrasco and Ridout, 1993; Ahsen, 1995; Djordjevic et al., 2004a,b, 2005), several authors have even claimed that recalling physically absent odors is not possible (Engen, 1991; Crowder and Schab, 1995; Herz, 2000). However, odor experts do not appear to have difficulty in mentally smelling odors. When perfumers are questioned, they claim that they are quite able to do this and that these images provide the same sensations as the olfactory experiences evoked by odorous stimuli themselves. Gilbert et al. (1998) were the first to investigate olfactory imagery abilities in fragrance experts and to provide evidence that they are better than in non-expert controls. Importantly, they did not observe a difference between the visual mental imagery abilities of the expert and non-expert groups.

BRAIN REORGANIZATION WITH OLFACTORY PERFORMANCE

The Polish neuroscientist Jerzy Konorski (1948) is regarded as being the first to introduce the term neuroplasticity (also referred to as brain plasticity, cortical plasticity, or cortical re-mapping) to the scientific literature (Jancke, 2009). Konorski presented one of the earliest comprehensive theories of associative learning as a result of long-term neuronal plasticity and also proposed the idea that synapses strengthen with use. The advent of modern brain imaging methods has boosted the study of cortical plasticity in healthy human subjects in the last 20 years (Jancke, 2009). These techniques have enabled the investigation of functional as well as structural plasticity[7] in experts such as musicians or sportsmen. What about olfactory expertise?

FUNCTIONAL AND STRUCTURAL DATA IN NON-EXPERTS

A few recent studies suggest that, even in the absence of specific learning, everyday olfactory experience improves olfactory performance and simultaneously shapes olfactory bran regions in the average person (Buschhuter et al., 2008; Frasnelli et al., 2010; Seubert et al., 2013). For instance, the volumes of the olfactory bulb, orbitofrontal cortex (OFC), and insula are positively correlated with the composite measure of olfactory threshold, discrimination, and identification scores (Frasnelli et al., 2010). Moreover, to compensate for their lack of vision, it is well established that blind subjects develop enhanced abilities in the use of their remaining senses. Accordingly, Rombaux et al. (2010) observed that blind subjects have better olfactory performance than sighted control subjects and correlatively have higher olfactory bulb volumes. Congenital or early blind subjects also activate olfactory areas (amygdala, OFC, hippocampus) and occipital areas more strongly than sighted control subjects during an olfactory task (Kupers et al., 2011; Renier et al., 2013), providing evidence that blind individuals undergo adaptive neuroplastic changes.

Other studies demonstrate that changes in brain activity can be observed in healthy control subjects after training. Li et al. (2008) demonstrated that odor aversive learning enhances the perceptual discrimination of initially indistinguishable odor enantiomers and that these results parallel the spatial divergence of ensemble activity patterns in the primary olfactory cortex (piriform cortex). These results indicate that aversive learning updates odor quality representations in the piriform cortex or, in other terms, emphasizes a spatial reorganization of odor coding. The same team also demonstrated that prolonged exposure (3.5 min) to a floral-smelling odorant is sufficient to enhance perceptual differentiation of novel odorants that are related in odor quality or functional groups (**Figure 3**; Li et al., 2006). This finding indicates that subjects become floral "experts." This effect is paralleled by increased responses in both the posterior piriform cortex and the medial OFC. The authors of this older work speculated that this learning-induced plasticity could reflect two neuronal mechanisms: an enlargement of cortical receptive fields that results in the recruitment of more neurons (spatial summation), or, alternatively, a synchronization of neuronal activity (temporal summation; Gilbert et al., 2001).

The results of Li et al. (2006) are echoed by electrophysiological data reported by Wilson (2000, 2003) using anesthetized rats. The authors suggested that perceptual learning via prolonged odorant exposure (habituation) can modify odor-evoked activity in the piriform cortex independently of the responses in the olfactory bulb. These data suggest that adequate sensory experience favors the formation of novel odor representations in the piriform cortex, which could promote olfactory differentiation at both the behavioral (Cleland et al., 2002; Fletcher and Wilson, 2002; Johnson et al., 2002) and neural (Wilson, 2000, 2003) levels.

FUNCTIONAL AND STRUCTURAL DATA IN ODOR EXPERTS

The first study to investigate brain changes related to odor-taste expertise was reported in 2005. Castriota-Scanderbeg et al. (2005) found that, in contrast to naïve drinkers of wine, who activate the primary gustatory cortex and brain areas implicated in emotional processing (e.g., the amygdala), sommeliers activate more brain regions involved in high-level cognitive processes such as working memory and selection of behavioral strategies (the dorsolateral prefrontal cortex) when they taste wine than when they taste glucose.

The second study was performed in perfumers (Plailly et al., 2012). The authors postulated that, in contrast to laymen, perfumers learn to form olfactory sensory representations through daily practice and extensive training. Because they claim to have the ability to produce perceptual images of smells in the total absence of odorants, we estimated that the ability to form odor mental images is a crucial component of a perfumer's

[7] The concept of "functional brain plasticity" refers to modifications of brain activity, whereas "structural brain plasticity" refers to changes at the anatomical level.

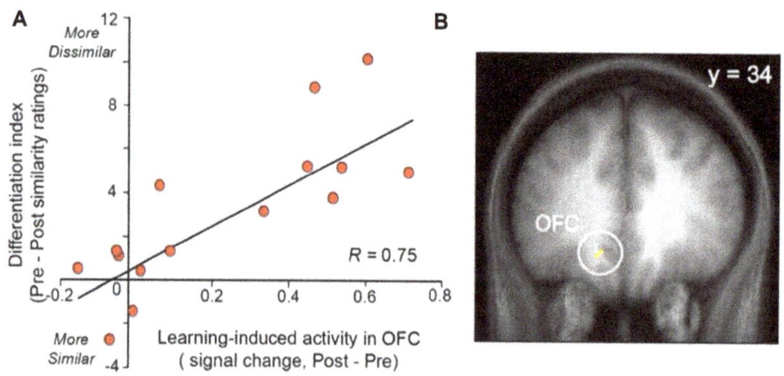

FIGURE 3 | Experience-induced neural plasticity in the OFC predicts olfactory perceptual learning. (A) The scatterplot demonstrates a strong correlation between the level of learning-induced OFC signal and the behavioral magnitude of perceptual learning. **(B)** Activation is superimposed on a mean T1-weighted coronal section and displays the area in OFC exhibiting this correlation. OFC, orbitofrontal cortex (modified with permission from Li et al., 2006).

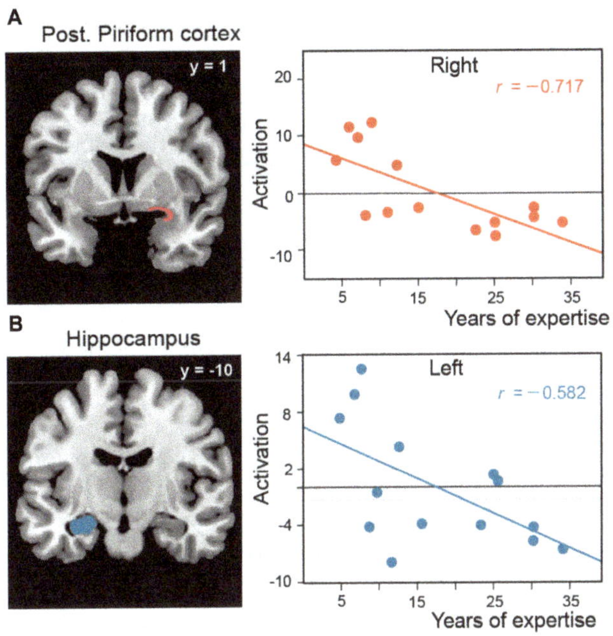

FIGURE 4 | Functional reorganization in perfumers. Significant negative correlations between the length of expertise in professional experts and the level of activation (amplitude) in **(A)** the posterior piriform cortices and **(B)** the left hippocampus (modified from Plailly et al., 2012).

expertise (Royet et al., 2013). Finally, as for other sensory modalities (Kosslyn et al., 2001), we hypothesized that similar neural networks are activated during mental imagery and the actual perception of odorous sensory stimuli.

As in two studies performed in untrained subjects (Djordjevic et al., 2005; Bensafi et al., 2007), we observed that the piriform cortex is activated when perfumers mentally imagine odors. We further revealed that, during the creation of mental images of odors, expertise influences not only this primary olfactory area but also the OFC and the hippocampus, regions that are involved in memory and the formation of complex sensory associations, respectively. In these areas, the magnitude of activation was negatively correlated with experience: the greater the level of expertise, the lower the activation of these key regions (**Figure 4**). We explained these results in terms of improvements of perceptual capacity and, consequently, gains in performance. Perfumers require less effort to mentally imagine odors than novices. The evocation of mental images is more spontaneous, almost instantaneous, and do not need to rely on high-level cognitive processes to gather information. These abilities, acquired with time and experience, are essential for perfumers because they allow them to devote all of their cognitive resources to the artistic activity that is the creation of novel fragrances.

Many studies have shown brain anatomical modifications as a result of learning and training. In experts with enhanced visual, auditory, or motor skills, such as musicians and athletes, greater performances are associated with structural brain changes in modality-specific brain areas. In olfaction, studies indicating structural modifications have only been performed in patients suffering from anosmia, hyposmia, or neurological disease (e.g., Abolmaali et al., 2002; Mueller et al., 2005; Rupp et al., 2005; Rombaux et al., 2006, 2009a,b; Wattendorf et al., 2009; Bitter et al., 2010). Therefore, these studies focus on alterations of olfactory processes associated with atrophy in olfactory-related areas. Recently, we studied structural modifications in the brains of perfumers (Delon-Martin et al., 2013). Using voxel-based morphometry and all possible methodological improvements to reduce false positives, we detected an increase in gray-matter volume in the bilateral gyrus rectus/medial orbital gyrus (GR/MOG), an orbitofrontal area that surrounds the olfactory sulcus, in perfumers. In addition, the gray-matter volumes in the anterior piriform cortex and left GR/MOG were positively correlated with experience in professional perfumers but negatively correlated with age in control subjects (**Figure 5**), suggesting that training counteracts the effects of aging.

Our data are the first to demonstrate the functional and structural impact of long-term odor training. What characterizes odor experts compared with other types of experts? Professional musicians practice several hours a day; their practice begins early in life and continues intensively throughout their lives. Sportsmen such as gymnasts or swimmers also begin early in life, but their careers end more rapidly than those of musicians, at approximately 30–35 years of age, when their physical performance does not allow them to be competitive. In contrast to musicians and sportsmen, odor experts such as perfumers and flavorists begin their training only in early adulthood, at the beginning of their

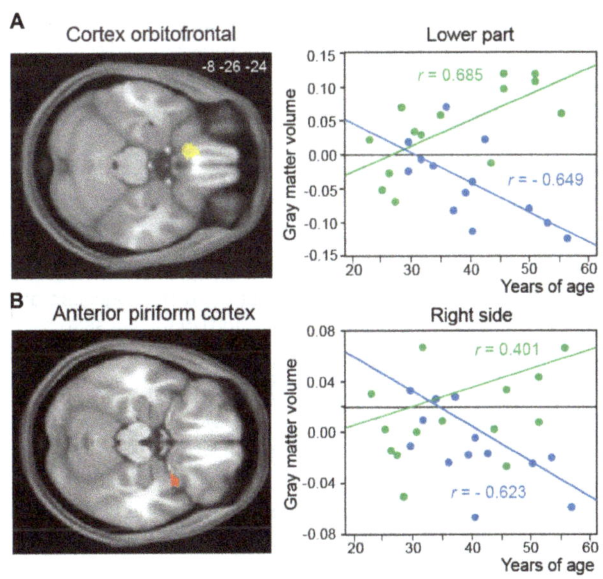

FIGURE 5 | Structural reorganization in perfumers. Relationship between structural modifications and years of age. The regression lines between the gray-matter volume and years of age (from 20 to 60 years old) show a positive slope in older experts (OE, green) and a negative slope in older controls (OC, blue) for **(A)** the left GR/MOG and **(B)** the right anterior piriform cortex. GR/MOG, gyrus rectus/medial orbital gyrus (modified from Delon-Martin et al., 2013).

working life or when they join a specialized school. They then live in an enriched olfactory environment in which they learn to characterize and recognize numerous stimuli daily and to learn to discriminate minute differences between odors. They can continue their training into old age. Olfactory performance is usually reported to decrease with age in the layman (e.g., Doty et al., 1984; Stevens et al., 1990; Murphy et al., 1991), and these deficits are partly due to both degenerative processes within the olfactory epithelium (Doty et al., 1984; Welge-Lussen, 2009) and changes in central olfactory structures (e.g., Tomlinson and Henderson, 1976). However, our functional and structural data demonstrate that perfumers can improve their performance throughout their lives and that intensive olfactory training can also counteract the effects of age. The volume of several brain regions involved in odor processing increases in perfumers but decreases in laymen. Thus, the metaphor "*use it or lose it*" used by Jancke (2009, p. 535) in reference to brain plasticity can also be applied to the olfactory modality. Furthermore, even if a peripheral dysfunction is observed in elderly odor experts, our findings further suggest that elderly perfumers would still be able to mentally imagine perfumes, just as deaf professional musicians are still able to continue to compose and conduct by mentally imagining music.

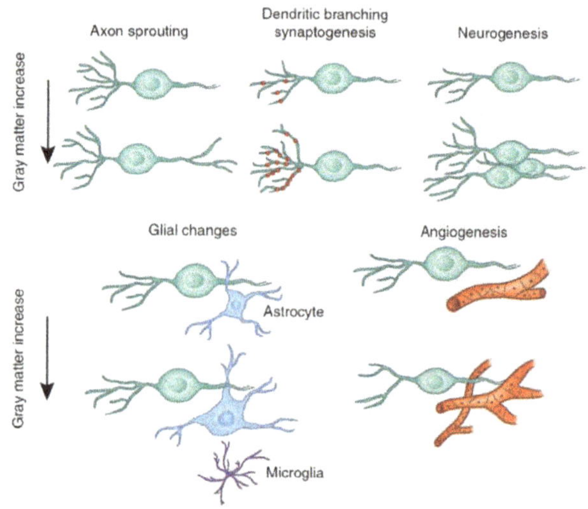

FIGURE 6 | Candidate cellular mechanisms for gray matter plasticity. Cellular events in gray matter regions underlying changes detected by magnetic resonance imaging during learning include axon sprouting, dendritic branching, and synaptogenesis, neurogenesis, changes in glial number and morphology, and angiogenesis (image courtesy of Marina Corral; modified with permission from Zatorre et al., 2012).

NEURONAL AND CELLULAR MECHANISMS RELATED TO OLFACTORY LEARNING

In the frame of our functional study in which perfumers were asked to generate mental images of odors (Plailly et al., 2012), a decrease in the amplitude of brain activation with the level of expertise could be due to greater selectivity of neurons resulting from the decorrelation of neuronal activity (Gilbert et al., 2001). Similar mechanisms have been observed in the antennal lobe of honeybees that are trained on one odorant. The sensorial representation of that odorant becomes smaller, more compact, and non-overlapping with representations of other odorants (Faber et al., 1999). This effect has also been observed in rats that are trained to discriminate highly overlapping odorous mixtures (Chapuis and Wilson, 2012).

The nature of the cellular events that underlie structural changes in the human brain is still unknown (May, 2011), although it is widely assumed that gray matter loss in neurodegeneration corresponds to neural loss (Baron et al., 2001; Thieben et al., 2002). Several mechanisms have been proposed to explain increases in gray matter: neurogenesis, gliogenesis, synaptogenesis, and vascular changes (**Figure 6**; Zatorre et al., 2012). We will discuss only the two main mechanisms related to neuronal activity-dependent changes in gray matter.

First, gray matter increases can be explained by fast morphological changes in the intracortical axonal architecture, including the formation of new connections by dendritic spine growth (i.e., synaptogenesis) and changes in the strength of existing connections (Trachtenberg et al., 2002). These changes have been implicated in experience-related morphological modifications in the rat hippocampus (Moser et al., 1994; Geinisman et al., 2000; O'Malley et al., 2000) and have been suggested as a mechanism (long-term potentiation) underlying long-term memory (Bliss and Collingridge, 1993; Luscher et al., 2000). A 3-day olfactory learning in rats is accompanied by a dendritic spine density increase (15%) along apical dendrites of pyramidal neurons in the piriform cortex, suggesting an increased number of excitatory synapses (Knafo et al., 2001). As activity-induced dendritic morphogenesis in the hippocampus can occur within tens of minutes (Maletic-Savatic et al., 1999), the perceptual learning observed by Li et al. (2006) could be associated with such modifications.

Second, gray matter increases can be related to slow mechanisms, such as adult neurogenesis, which has been reported in the olfactory bulbs of rodents and primates, including humans (Bonfanti and Peretto, 2011; Curtis et al., 2011; Ming and Song, 2011; Huart et al., 2013; Lazarov and Marr, 2013). Although the functional impact of the addition of new olfactory neurons to mature circuits remains an outstanding question, many recent investigations have highlighted the role of network activity in shaping ongoing neurogenesis and, in turn, how the integration of new neurons refines pre-existing network functions and, consequently, olfactory behavior. To date, olfactory adult neurogenesis was associated with an improvement in short-term olfactory memory when mice were exposed daily to a novel but not familiar enriched olfactory environment (Rochefort et al., 2002; Bovetti et al., 2009; Veyrac et al., 2009). It was also demonstrated that olfactory perceptual learning both increases and requires adult neurogenesis (Moreno et al., 2009). Interestingly, constitutive neurogenesis has been described in the adult piriform cortex in several mammalian species (Bernier et al., 2002; Shapiro et al., 2007). Here, we suggest that the gray matter volume increase in the piriform cortex of perfumers could result from a fast remodeling of the intracortical neuronal network, but genesis of new neurons in this brain area cannot be excluded.

CONCLUSION

This review of the literature presents the findings of studies in which odor experts were subjects. In contrast to other domains of expertise, odor expertise has been rarely studied (Ericsson and Lehmann, 1996; Vicente and Wang, 1998; De Beni et al., 2007). In 1998, Vicente and Wang wrote that there were at least 51 studies of the effects of expertise in at least 19 different domains, including music (e.g., piano), sport (e.g., skating, baseball), games (e.g., bridge, go, chess), computer programming, medical diagnosis, maps, algebra, and circuit diagrams. The model of expertise research is the chess player because experts can reach very high levels of competence and the ability of participants is measurable and can be rated in a laboratory (De Beni et al., 2007). In all cases, studies of expertise emphasize the role of long-term working memory on performance (Ericsson and Kintsch, 1995) and highlight that "*memory recall performance on meaningful stimuli has almost always been found to be correlated with domain expertise*" (Vicente, 1988; Vicente and Wang, 1998, p. 33).

The extremely high performance of experts begs the fundamental question of whether their faculties are innate or acquired with training. In 1869, Francis Galton claimed that, because the limits on height and body size are genetically determined, innate mechanisms must also determine mental capacities (see Galton, 1979). Ericsson and Lehmann (1996) suggested that the influence of innate, domain-specific basic capacities (talent) on expert performance is small, possibly even negligible. However, more recent studies indicate that characteristics that distinguish experts from naïve subjects are mainly the result of adaptation. High expertise is typically associated with prolonged and maintained practice lasting many years and involving daily exercises (De Beni et al., 2007). The apparent emergence of early talent then depends on factors "*such as motivation, parental support, and access to the best training environments and teachers*" (Ericsson et al., 2009, p. 199).

In the context of odor experts, it is likely that expertise is acquired with training and experience rather than acquired innately, thus confirming a previous report that the notable nose is bred rather than born (Bedichek, 1960, p. 61; Engen, 1982, p. 5). Our work in cerebral imaging has led us to the same conclusions. Olfactory mental imagery capacities develop with practice and do not result from innate skill (Plailly et al., 2012). The structural modifications observed in the brain after intensive practice of an activity are not stable and rapidly disappear when this activity stops (Jancke, 2009). However, an exception that deserves to be noted is the case of synesthetes, who possess faculties to perceive a given sensory stimulus via another or several other sensory modalities. Synesthesia is a rare phenomenon that can have a genetic origin, which could explain the exceptional performances of experts such as mental calculators. Although relatively less frequent, examples of synesthesia involving olfactory sensation have been described in the literature (Day, 2005).

ACKNOWLEDGMENTS

This work was supported by the Centre National de la Recherche Scientifique (CNRS) and the LABEX Cortex (NR-11-LABX-0042) of Université de Lyon within the program "*Investissements d'Avenir*" (ANR-11-IDEX-0007) operated by the French National Research Agency (ANR). Alexandra Veyrac was funded by LABEX Cortex.

REFERENCES

Abolmaali, N. D., Hietschold, V., Vogl, T. J., Huttenbrink, K. B., and Hummel, T. (2002). MR evaluation in patients with isolated anosmia since birth or early childhood. *Am. J. Neuroradiol.* 23, 157–164.

Ahsen, A. (1995). Self-report questionnaires: new directions for imagery research. *J. Ment. Imag.* 19, 107–123.

Algom, D., and Cain, W. S. (1991). Remembered odors and mental mixtures: tapping reservoirs of olfactory knowledge. *J. Exp. Psychol. Hum. Percept. Perform.* 17, 1104–1119. doi: 10.1037/0096-1523.17.4.1104

Algom, D., Marks, L. E., and Cain, W. S. (1993). Memory psychophysics for chemosensation: perceptual and mental mixtures of odor and taste. *Chem. Senses* 18, 151–160. doi: 10.1093/chemse/18.2.151

Amerine, M., Panghorn, R., and Roessler, E. (1965). *Principles of Sensory Evaluation of Food.* New York: Academy Press.

Ballester, J., Patris, B., Symonaux, R., and Valentin, D. (2008). Conceptual vs. perceptual wine spaces: does expertise matter? *Food Qual. Pref.* 19, 267–276. doi: 10.1016/j.foodqual.2007.08.001

Baron, J. C., Chetelat, G., Desgranges, B., Perchey, G., Landeau, B., De La Sayette, V., et al. (2001). In vivo mapping of gray matter loss with voxel-based morphometry in mild Alzheimer's disease. *Neuroimage* 14, 298–309. doi: 10.1006/nimg.2001.0848

Bedichek, R. (1960). *The Sense of Smell.* New York: Doubleday.

Bende, M., and Nordin, S. (1997). Perceptual learning in olfaction: professional wine tasters versus controls. *Physiol. Behav.* 62, 1065–1070. doi: 10.1016/S0031-9384(97)00251-5

Bensafi, M., Sobel, N., and Khan, R. M. (2007). Hedonic-specific activity in piriform cortex during odor imagery mimics that during odor perception. *J. Neurophysiol.* 98, 3254–3262. doi: 10.1152/jn.00349.2007

Berg, H., Filipello, F., Hinreiner, E., and Webb, A. (1955). Evaluation of thresholds and minimum difference concentrations for various constituents of wine. *Food Technol.* 9, 23–26.

Bernier, P. J., Bedard, A., Vinet, J., Levesque, M., and Parent, A. (2002). Newly generated neurons in the amygdala and adjoining cortex of adult primates. *Proc. Natl. Acad. Sci. U.S.A.* 99, 11464–11469. doi: 10.1073/pnas.172403999

Bitter, T., Bruderle, J., Gudziol, H., Burmeister, H. P., Gaser, C., and Guntinas-Lichius, O. (2010). Gray and white matter reduction in hyposmic subjects – a voxel-based morphometry study. *Brain Res.* 1347, 42–47. doi: 10.1016/j.brainres.2010.06.003

Bliss, T. V., and Collingridge, G. L. (1993). A synaptic model of memory: long-term potentiation in the hippocampus. *Nature* 361, 31–39. doi: 10.1038/361031a0

Bonfanti, L., and Peretto, P. (2011). Adult neurogenesis in mammals – a theme with many variations. *Eur. J. Neurosci.* 34, 930–950. doi: 10.1111/j.1460-9568.2011.07832.x

Bovetti, S., Veyrac, A., Peretto, P., Fasolo, A., and De Marchis, S. (2009). Olfactory enrichment influences adult neurogenesis modulating GAD67 and plasticity-related molecules expression in newborn cells of the olfactory bulb. *PLoS ONE* 4:e6359. doi: 10.1371/journal.pone.0006359

Brand, G., and Brisson, R. (2012). Lateralisation in wine olfactory threshold detection: comparison between experts and novices. *Laterality* 17, 583–596. doi: 10.1080/1357650X.2011.595955

Buschhuter, D., Smitka, M., Puschmann, S., Gerber, J. C., Witt, M., Abolmaali, N. D., et al. (2008). Correlation between olfactory bulb volume and olfactory function. *Neuroimage* 42, 498–502. doi: 10.1016/j.neuroimage.2008.05.004

Cain, W. S. (1979). To know with the nose: keys to odor identification. *Science* 203, 467–470. doi: 10.1126/science.760202

Cain, W. S. (1982). Odor identification by males and females:predictions vs. performance. *Chem. Senses* 7, 129–142. doi: 10.1093/chemse/7.2.129

Cain, W. S., and Krause, R. J. (1979). Olfactory testing: rules for odor identification. *Neurol. Res.* 1, 1–9.

Calkin, R. R., and Jellinek, J. S. (1994). *Perfumery: Practice and Principles*, 1st Edn. New York: Wiley.

Cardello, A. V., Mealler, O., Kapsalis, J. G., Segars, R. A., Sawyer, F. M., Murphy, C., et al. (1982). Perception of texture by trained and consumer panels. *J. Food Sci.* 47, 1186–1197. doi: 10.1111/j.1365-2621.1982.tb07646.x

Carrasco, M., and Ridout, J. B. (1993). Olfactory perception and olfactory imagery: a multidimensional analysis. *J. Exp. Psychol. Hum. Percept. Perform.* 19, 287–301. doi: 10.1037/0096-1523.19.2.287

Castriota-Scanderbeg, A., Hagberg, G. E., Cerasa, A., Committeri, G., Galati, G., Patria, F., et al. (2005). The appreciation of wine by sommeliers: a functional magnetic resonance study of sensory integration. *Neuroimage* 25, 570–578. doi: 10.1016/j.neuroimage.2004.11.045

Chambers, E., and Smith, E. A. (1993). Effects of testing experience on performance of trained sensory panelists. *J. Sens. Stud.* 8, 155–166. doi: 10.1111/j.1745-459X.1993.tb00210.x

Chapuis, J., and Wilson, D. A. (2012). Bidirectional plasticity of cortical pattern recognition and behavioral sensory acuity. *Nat. Neurosci.* 15, 155–161. doi: 10.1038/nn.2966

Chollet, S., and Valentin, D. (2000). Le degré d'expertise a-t-il une influence sur la perception olfactive? Quelques éléments de réponse dans le domaine du vin. *Ann. Psychol.* 100, 11–36. doi: 10.3406/psy.2000.28625

Clapperton, J. F., and Piggott, J. R. (1979). Flavour characterization by trained and untrained assessors. *J. Inst. Brew.* 85, 275–277. doi: 10.1002/j.2050-0416.1979.tb03922.x

Cleland, T. A., Morse, A., Yue, E. L., and Linster, C. (2002). Behavioral models of odor similarity. *Behav. Neurosci.* 116, 222–231. doi: 10.1037/0735-7044.116.2.222

Crowder, R. G., and Schab, F. R. (1995). "Imagery for odors," in *Memory for Odors*, eds R. G. Crowder and F. R. Schab (Hilsdale, NJ: Erlbaum), 93–107.

Curtis, M. A., Kam, M., and Faull, R. L. (2011). Neurogenesis in humans. *Eur. J. Neurosci.* 33, 1170–1174. doi: 10.1111/j.1460-9568.2011.07616.x

Dalton, P., Doolittle, N., and Breslin, P. A. (2002). Gender-specific induction of enhanced sensitivity to odors. *Nat. Neurosci.* 5, 199–200. doi: 10.1038/nn803

Day, S. (2005). "Some demographic and socio-cultural aspects of synesthesia," in *Synesthesia*, eds L. C. Robertson and N. Sagiv (Oxford: University Press), 11–33.

De Beni, R., Cornoldi, C., Larsson, M., Magnussen, S., and Rönnberg, J. (2007). "Memory experts: visual learning, wine tasting, orienteering and speech-reading," in *Everydday Memory*, eds T. Helstrup and S. Magnussen (Hove: Psychological Press), 201–227.

Delon-Martin, C., Plailly, J., Fonlupt, P., Veyrac, A., and Royet, J. P. (2013). Perfumers' expertise induces structural reorganization in olfactory brain regions. *Neuroimage* 68C, 55–62. doi: 10.1016/j.neuroimage.2012.11.044

Desor, J. A., and Beauchamp, G. K. (1974). The human capacity to transmit olfactory information. *Percept. Psychophys.* 16, 551–556. doi: 10.3758/BF03198586

Djordjevic, J., Zatorre, R. J., and Jones-Gotman, M. (2004a). Effects of perceived and imagined odors on taste detection. *Chem. Senses* 29, 199–208. doi: 10.1093/chemse/bjh022

Djordjevic, J., Zatorre, R. J., Petrides, M., and Jones-Gotman, M. (2004b). The mind's nose: effects of odor and visual imagery on odor detection. *Psychol. Sci.* 15, 143–148. doi: 10.1111/j.0956-7976.2004.01503001.x

Djordjevic, J., Zatorre, R. J., Petrides, M., Boyle, J. A., and Jones-Gotman, M. (2005). Functional neuroimaging of odor imagery. *Neuroimage* 24, 791–801. doi: 10.1016/j.neuroimage.2004.09.035

Doty, R. L. (1991). "Psychophysical measurement of odor perception in humans," in *The Human Sense of Smell*, eds D. G. Laing, R. L. Doty, and W. Breipohl. (Berlin: Springer-Verlag), 95–134.

Doty, R. L., and Ferguson-Segall, M. (1989). Influence of adult castration on the olfactory sensitivity of the male rat: a signal detection analysis. *Behav. Neurosci.* 103, 691–694. doi: 10.1037/0735-7044.103.3.691

Doty, R. L., Shaman, P., Applebaum, S. L., Giberson, R., Siksorski, L., and Rosenberg, L. (1984). Smell identification ability: changes with age. *Science* 226, 1441–1443. doi: 10.1126/science.6505700

Doty, R. L., Snyder, P. J., Huggins, G. R., and Lowry, L. D. (1981). Endocrine, cardiovascular, and psychological correlated of olfactory sensitivity changes during the human menstrual cycle. *J. Comp. Physiol. Psychol.* 95, 45–60. doi: 10.1037/h0077755

Drake, M. A., McIngvale, S. C., Cadwallader, K. R., and Civille, G. V. (2001). Development of a descriptive language for Cheddar cheese. *J. Food Sci.* 66, 1422–1427. doi: 10.1111/j.1365-2621.2001.tb15225.x

Engen, T. (1960). Effect of practice and instruction on olfactory thresholds. *Percept. Motor Skills* 10, 195–198. doi: 10.2466/pms.1960.10.3.195

Engen, T. (1982). *The Perception of Odors*. New York: Academic Press.

Engen, T. (1987). Remembering odors and their names. *Am. Scientist* 75, 497–503.

Engen, T. (1991). *Odor Sensation and Memory*. New York: Praeger.

Engen, T., Kuisma, J. E., and Eimas, P. D. (1973). Short-term memory of odors. *J. Exp. Psychol.* 99, 222–225. doi: 10.1037/h0034645

Ericsson, K. A., and Kintsch, W. (1995). Long-term working memory. *Psychol. Rev.* 102, 211–245. doi: 10.1037/0033-295X.102.2.211

Ericsson, K. A., and Lehmann, A. C. (1996). Expert and exceptional performance: evidence of maximal adaptation to task constraints. *Annu. Rev. Psychol.* 47, 273–305. doi: 10.1146/annurev.psych.47.1.273

Ericsson, K. A., Nandagopal, K., and Roring, R. W. (2009). Toward a science of exceptional achievement: attaining superior performance through deliberate practice. *Ann. N. Y. Acad. Sci.* 1172, 199–217. doi: 10.1196/annals.1393.001

Faber, T., Joerges, J., and Menzel, R. (1999). Associative learning modifies neural representations of odors in the insect brain. *Nat. Neurosci.* 2, 74–78. doi: 10.1038/4576

Fahle, M., and Poggio, T. (2002). *Perceptual Learning*. Cambridge MA: MIT Press.

Fletcher, M. L., and Wilson, D. A. (2002). Experience modifies olfactory acuity: acetylcholine-dependent learning decreases behavioral generalization between similar odorants. *J. Neurosci.* 22, RC201.

Frasnelli, J., Lundstrom, J. N., Boyle, J. A., Djordjevic, J., Zatorre, R. J., and Jones-Gotman, M. (2010). Neuroanatomical correlates of olfactory performance. *Exp. Brain Res.* 201, 1–11. doi: 10.1007/s00221-009-1999-7

Galton, F. (1979). *Hereditary Genius: An Inquiry into its Laws and Consequences (First published in 1869)*. London: Friedman.

Gawel, R. (1997). The use of language by trained and untrained experienced wine tasters. *J. Sens. Stud.* 12, 267–284. doi: 10.1111/j.1745-459X.1997.tb00067.x

Geinisman, Y., Disterhoft, J. F., Gundersen, H. J., McEchron, M. D., Persina, I. S., Power, J. M., et al. (2000). Remodeling of hippocampal synapses after hippocampus-dependent associative learning. *J. Comp. Neurol.* 417, 49–59. doi: 10.1002/(SICI)1096-9861(20000131)417:1<49::AID-CNE4>3.0.CO;2-3

Gibson, E. J. (1953). Improvement in perceptual judgments as a function of controlled pratice or training. *Psychol. Bull.* 50, 401–431. doi: 10.1037/h0055517

Gibson, E. J. (1991). *An Odyssey in Learning and Perception*. Cambridge, MA: MIT Press.

Gibson, J. J., and Gibson, E. J. (1955). Perceptual learning: differentiation or enrichment? *Psychol. Rev.* 62, 32–41. doi: 10.1037/h0048826

Gilbert, A. N., Crouch, M., and Kemp, S. E. (1998). Olfactory and visual mental imagery. *J. Ment. Imag.* 22, 137–146.

Gilbert, C. D., Sigman, M., and Crist, R. E. (2001). The neural basis of perceptual learning. *Neuron* 31, 681–697. doi: 10.1016/S0896-6273(01)00424-X

Goldstone, R. L. (1998). Perceptual learning. *Annu. Rev. Psychol.* 49, 585–612. doi: 10.1146/annurev.psych.49.1.585

Herz, R. S. (2000). Verbal coding in olfactory versus nonolfactory cognition. *Mem. Cogn.* 28, 957–964. doi: 10.3758/BF03209343

Huart, C., Rombaux, P., and Hummel, T. (2013). Plasticity of the human olfactory system: the olfactory bulb. *Molecules* 18, 11586–11600. doi: 10.3390/molecules180911586

Hughson, A. L., and Boakes, R. A. (2001). Perceptual and cognitive aspects of wine expertise. *Aust. J. Psychol.* 53, 103–108. doi: 10.1080/00049530108255130

Hughson, A. L., and Boakes, R. A. (2002). The knowing nose: the role of knowledge in wine expertise. *Food Qual. Pref.* 13, 463–472. doi: 10.1016/S0950-3293(02)00051-4

Hughson, A. L., and Boakes, R. A. (2009). Passive perceptual learning in relation to wine: short-term recognition and verbal description. *Q. J. Exp. Psychol. (Hove)* 62, 1–8. doi: 10.1080/17470210802214890

James, W. (1890). *The Principles of Psychology*. New York: Holt.

Jancke, L. (2009). The plastic human brain. *Restor. Neurol. Neurosci.* 27, 521–538. doi: 10.3233/RNN-2009-0519

Jehl, C., Royet, J. P., and Holley, A. (1994). Very short term recognition memory for odors. *Percept. Psychophys.* 56, 658–668. doi: 10.3758/BF03208359

Jehl, C., Royet, J. P., and Holley, A. (1995). Odor discrimination and recognition memory as a function of familiarization. *Percept. Psychophys.* 57, 1002–1011. doi: 10.3758/BF03205459

Jehl, C., Royet, J. P., and Holley, A. (1997). Role of verbal encoding in short- and long-term odor recognition. *Percept. Psychophys.* 59, 100–110. doi: 10.3758/BF03206852

Johnson, B. A., Ho, S. L., Xu, Z., Yihan, J. S., Yip, S., Hingco, E. E., et al. (2002). Functional mapping of the rat olfactory bulb using diverse odorants reveals modular responses to functional groups and hydrocarbon structural features. *J. Comp. Neurol.* 449, 180–194. doi: 10.1002/cne.10284

Jolly, N. P., and Hattingh, S. (2001). A Brandy Aroma Wheel for South African brandy. *S. Afr. J. Enol. Vitic.* 22, 1–6.

Jones, F. N. (1968). "Information content of olfactory quality," in *Theories of Odors and Odor Measurement*, ed. N. Tanoyloac (Bebek: Robert College Center), 297.

Keller, H. (1908a). "Sense and Sensibility," in *The Century Magazine*, New York: The Century Company.

Keller, H. (1908b). "Sense of Sensibility," in *The Century Magazine*, New York: The Century Company.

Knafo, S., Grossman, Y., Barkai, E., and Benshalom, G. (2001). Olfactory learning is associated with increased spine density along apical dendrites of pyramidal neurons in the rat piriform cortex. *Eur. J. Neurosci.* 13, 633–638. doi: 10.1046/j.1460-9568.2001.01422.x

Konorski, J. (1948). *Conditioned reflexes and neuron organization.* Cambridge, MA: Cambridge University Press.

Kosslyn, S. M., Ganis, G., and Thompson, W. L. (2001). Neural foundations of imagery. *Nat. Rev. Neurosci.* 2, 635–642. doi: 10.1038/35090055

Kupers, R., Beaulieu-Lefebvre, M., Schneider, F. C., Kassuba, T., Paulson, O. B., Siebner, H. R., et al. (2011). Neural correlates of olfactory processing in congenital blindness. *Neuropsychologia* 49, 2037–2044. doi: 10.1016/j.neuropsychologia.2011.03.033

Laing, D. G., and Francis, G. W. (1989). The capacity of humans to identify odors in mixtures. *Physiol. Behav.* 46, 809–814. doi: 10.1016/0031-9384(89)90041-3

Lawless, H., and Engen, T. (1977). Associations to odors: interference, mnemonics, and verbal labeling. *J. Exp. Psychol. Hum. Learn.* 3, 52–59. doi: 10.1037/0278-7393.3.1.52

Lawless, H. T. (1984). Flavor description of white wine by "expert" and nonexpert wine consumers. *J. Food Sci.* 49, 120–123. doi: 10.1111/j.1365-2621.1984.tb13686.x

Lawless, H. T. (1988). "Odour description and odour classification revisited," in *Food Acceptability*, ed. D. M. H. Thompson (London: Elsevier Applied Science), 27–40.

Lazarov, O., and Marr, R. A. (2013). Of mice and men: neurogenesis, cognition and Alzheimer's disease. *Front. Aging Neurosci.* 5:43. doi: 10.3389/fnagi.2013.00043

Li, W., Howard, J. D., Parrish, T. B., and Gottfried, J. A. (2008). Aversive learning enhances perceptual and cortical discrimination of indiscriminable odor cues. *Science* 319, 1842–1845. doi: 10.1126/science.1152837

Li, W., Luxenberg, E., Parrish, T., and Gottfried, J. A. (2006). Learning to smell the roses: experience-dependent neural plasticity in human piriform and orbitofrontal cortices. *Neuron* 52, 1097–1108. doi: 10.1016/j.neuron.2006.10.026

Livermore, A., and Laing, D. G. (1996). Influence of training and experience on the perception of multicomponent odor mixtures. *J. Exp. Psychol. Hum. Percept. Perform.* 22, 267–277. doi: 10.1037/0096-1523.22.2.267

Lorig, T. S. (1999). On the similarity of odor and language perception. *Neurosci. Biobehav. Rev.* 23, 391–408. doi: 10.1016/S0149-7634(98)00041-4

Luscher, C., Nicoll, R. A., Malenka, R. C., and Muller, D. (2000). Synaptic plasticity and dynamic modulation of the postsynaptic membrane. *Nat. Neurosci.* 3, 545–550. doi: 10.1038/75714

Lyman, B. J., and McDaniel, M. A. (1986). Effects of encoding strategy on long-term memory for odours. *Q. J. Exp. Psychol.* 38, 753–765. doi: 10.1080/14640748608401624

Lyman, B. J., and McDaniel, M. A. (1990). Memory for odors and odor names: modalities of elaborating and imagery. *J. Exp. Psychol. Learn. Mem. Cogn.* 16, 656–664. doi: 10.1037/0278-7393.16.4.656

Mainland, J. D., Bremner, E. A., Young, N., Johnson, B. N., Khan, R. M., Bensafi, M., et al. (2002). Olfactory plasticity: one nostril knows what the other learns. *Nature* 419, 802. doi: 10.1038/419802a

Maletic-Savatic, M., Malinow, R., and Svoboda, K. (1999). Rapid dendritic morphogenesis in CA1 hippocampal dendrites induced by synaptic activity. *Science* 283, 1923–1927. doi: 10.1126/science.283.5409.1923

May, A. (2011). Experience-dependent structural plasticity in the adult human brain. *Trends Cogn. Sci. (Regul. Ed.)* 15, 475–482. doi: 10.1016/j.tics.2011.08.002

Melcher, J. M., and Schooler, J. W. (1996). The misrembrance of wines past: verbal and perceptual expertise differentially mediate verbal overshadowing of taste memory. *J. Mem. Lang.* 35, 231–245. doi: 10.1006/jmla.1996.0013

Ming, G. L., and Song, H. (2011). Adult neurogenesis in the mammalian brain: significant answers and significant questions. *Neuron* 70, 687–702. doi: 10.1016/j.neuron.2011.05.001

Moreno, M. M., Linster, C., Escanilla, O., Sacquet, J., Didier, A., and Mandairon, N. (2009). Olfactory perceptual learning requires adult neurogenesis. *Proc. Natl. Acad. Sci. U.S.A.* 106, 17980–17985. doi: 10.1073/pnas.0907063106

Morrot, G., Brochet, F., and Dubourdieu, D. (2001). The color of odors. *Brain Lang.* 79, 309–320. doi: 10.1006/brln.2001.2493

Moser, M. B., Trommald, M., and Andersen, P. (1994). An increase in dendritic spine density on hippocampal CA1 pyramidal cells following spatial learning in adult rats suggests the formation of new synapses. *Proc. Natl. Acad. Sci. U.S.A.* 91, 12673–12675. doi: 10.1073/pnas.91.26.12673

Mueller, A., Rodewald, A., Reden, J., Gerber, J., Von Kummer, R., and Hummel, T. (2005). Reduced olfactory bulb volume in post-traumatic and post-infectious olfactory dysfunction. *Neuroreport* 16, 475–478. doi: 10.1097/00001756-200504040-00011

Murphy, C., Cain, W. S., Gilmore, M. M., and Skinner, R. B. (1991). Sensory and semantic factors in recognition memory for odors and graphic stimuli: elderly versus young persons. *Am. J. Psychol.* 104, 161–192. doi: 10.2307/1423153

Nevitt, G. A., Dittman, A. H., Quinn, T. P., and Moody, W. J. Jr. (1994). Evidence for a peripheral olfactory memory in imprinted salmon. *Proc. Natl. Acad. Sci. U.S.A.* 91, 4288–4292. doi: 10.1073/pnas.91.10.4288

Noble, A. C., Arnold, R. A., Buechsenstein, J., Leach, E. J., Schmidt, J. O., and Stern, P. M. (1987). Modification of a standardized system of wine aroma terminology. *Am. J. Enol. Vitic.* 38, 143–146.

O'Malley, A., O'Connell, C., Murphy, K. J., and Regan, C. M. (2000). Transient spine density increases in the mid-molecular layer of hippocampal dentate gyrus accompany consolidation of a spatial learning task in the rodent. *Neuroscience* 99, 229–232. doi: 10.1016/S0306-4522(00)00182-2

Owen, D. H., and Machamer, P. K. (1979). Bias-free improvement in wine discrimination. *Perception* 8, 199–209. doi: 10.1068/p080199

Panghorn, R., Berg, H., and Hansen, B. (1963). The influence of color on discrimination of sweetness in dry table-wine. *Am. J. Psychol.* 76, 492–495. doi: 10.2307/1419795

Parr, W. V., Heatherbell, D., and White, K. G. (2002). Demystifying wine expertise: olfactory threshold, perceptual skill and semantic memory in expert and novice wine judges. *Chem. Senses* 27, 747–755. doi: 10.1093/chemse/27.8.747

Peron, R. M., and Allen, G. L. (1988). Attempts to train novices for beer flavor discrimination: a matter of taste. *J. Gen. Psychol.* 115, 403–418. doi: 10.1080/00221309.1988.9710577

Plailly, J., Delon-Martin, C., and Royet, J. P. (2012). Experience induces functional reorganization in brain regions involved in odor imagery in perfumers. *Hum. Brain Mapp.* 33, 224–234. doi: 10.1002/hbm.21207

Rabin, M. D. (1988). Experience facilitates olfactory quality discrimination. *Percept. Psychophys.* 44, 532–540. doi: 10.3758/BF03207487

Rabin, M. D., and Cain, W. S. (1984). Odor recognition: familiarity, identifiability, and encoding consistency. *J. Exp. Psychol. Learn. Mem. Cogn.* 10, 316–325. doi: 10.1037/0278-7393.10.2.316

Rabin, M. D., and Cain, W. S. (1986). Determinants of measured olfactory sensitivity. *Percept. Psychophys.* 39, 281–286. doi: 10.3758/BF03204936

Renier, L., Cuevas, I., Grandin, C. B., Dricot, L., Plaza, P., Lerens, E., et al. (2013). Right occipital cortex activation correlates with superior odor processing performance in the early blind. *PLoS ONE* 8:e71907. doi: 10.1371/journal.pone.0071907

Richardson, J. T., and Zucco, G. M. (1989). Cognition and olfaction: a review. *Psychol. Bull.* 105, 352–360. doi: 10.1037/0033-2909.105.3.352

Roberts, A. K., and Vickers, Z. M. (1994). A comparison of trained and untrained judges' evaluation of sensory attribute intensities and liking of cheddar cheeses. *J. Sens. Stud.* 9, 1–20. doi: 10.1111/j.1745-459X.1994.tb00226.x

Rochefort, C., Gheusi, G., Vincent, J. D., and Lledo, P. M. (2002). Enriched odor exposure increases the number of newborn neurons in the adult olfactory bulb and improves odor memory. *J. Neurosci.* 22, 2679–2689.

Rombaux, P., Grandin, C., and Duprez, T. (2009a). How to measure olfactory bulb volume and olfactory sulcus depth? *B-ENT* 5(Suppl. 13), 53–60.

Rombaux, P., Martinage, S., Huart, C., and Collet, S. (2009b). Post-infectious olfactory loss: a cohort study and update. *B-ENT* 5(Suppl. 13), 89–95.

Rombaux, P., Huart, C., De Volder, A. G., Cuevas, I., Renier, L., Duprez, T., et al. (2010). Increased olfactory bulb volume and olfactory function in early blind subjects. *Neuroreport* 21, 1069–1073. doi: 10.1097/WNR.0b013e32833fcb8a

Rombaux, P., Weitz, H., Mouraux, A., Nicolas, G., Bertrand, B., Duprez, T., et al. (2006). Olfactory function assessed with orthonasal and retronasal testing, olfactory bulb volume, and chemosensory event-related potentials. *Arch. Otolaryngol. Head Neck Surg.* 132, 1346–1351. doi: 10.1001/archotol.132.12.1346

Royet, J. P., Delon-Martin, C., and Plailly, J. (2013). Odor mental imagery in non-experts in odors: a paradox? *Front. Hum. Neurosci.* 7:87. doi: 10.3389/fnhum.2013.00087

Rupp, C. I., Fleischhacker, W. W., Kemmler, G., Oberbauer, H., Scholtz, A. W., Wanko, C., et al. (2005). Various bilateral olfactory deficits in male patients with schizophrenia. *Schizophr. Bull.* 31, 155–165. doi: 10.1093/schbul/sbi018

Sachs, O. (1985). *The Man Who Mistook His Wife for a Hat.* London: Gerald Duckworth & Co.

Schab, F. R. (1991). Odor memory – taking stock. *Psychol. Bull.* 109, 242–251. doi: 10.1037/0033-2909.109.2.242

Schab, F. R., and Cain, W. S. (1992). "Memory for odors," in *The Human Sense of Smell*, eds D. G. Laing, R. L. Doty, and W. Breipohl (Berlin: Springer-Verlag), 217–240.

Schyns, P. G., Goldstone, R. L., and Thibaut, J. P. (1998). The development of features in object concepts. *Behav. Brain Sci.* 21, 1–17; discussion 17–54. doi: 10.1017/S0140525X98000107

Seubert, J., Freiherr, J., Frasnelli, J., Hummel, T., and Lundstrom, J. N. (2013). Orbitofrontal cortex and olfactory bulb volume predict distinct aspects of olfactory performance in healthy subjects. *Cereb. Cortex* 23, 2448–2456. doi: 10.1093/cercor/bhs230

Shapiro, L. A., Ng, K. L., Kinyamu, R., Whitaker-Azmitia, P., Geisert, E. E., Blurton-Jones, M., et al. (2007). Origin, migration and fate of newly generated neurons in the adult rodent piriform cortex. *Brain Struct. Funct.* 212, 133–148. doi: 10.1007/s00429-007-0151-3

Small, D. M., and Prescott, J. (2005). Odor/taste integration and the perception of flavor. *Exp. Brain Res.* 166, 345–357. doi: 10.1007/s00221-005-2376-9

Solomon, G. E. A. (1990). Psychology of novice and expert wine talk. *Am. J. Psychol.* 103, 495–517. doi: 10.2307/1423321

Solomon, G. E. A. (1997). Conceptual change and wine expertise. *J. Learn. Sci.* 6, 41–60. doi: 10.1207/s15327809jls0601_3

Stevens, J. C., Cain, W. C., and Demarque, A. (1990). Memory and identification of simulated odors in elderly and young persons. *Bull. Psychon. Soc.* 28, 293–296. doi: 10.3758/BF03334025

Stevenson, R. J., and Case, T. I. (2005). Olfactory imagery: a review. *Psychon. Bull. Rev.* 12, 244–264. doi: 10.3758/BF03196369

Stevenson, R. J., Case, T. I., and Mahmut, M. (2007). Difficulty in evoking odor images: the role of odor naming. *Mem. Cognit.* 35, 578–589. doi: 10.3758/BF03193296

Sumner, D. (1962). On testing the sense of smell. *Lancet* 2, 895–897. doi: 10.1016/S0140-6736(62)90679-7

Süskind, P. (1986). *Le Parfum.* Paris: Editions Fayard.

Thieben, M. J., Duggins, A. J., Good, C. D., Gomes, L., Mahant, N., Richards, F., et al. (2002). The distribution of structural neuropathology in pre-clinical Huntington's disease. *Brain* 125, 1815–1828. doi: 10.1093/brain/awf179

Tomlinson, B. E., and Henderson, G. (1976). "Observations on the brains of demented old people," in *Neurobiology of Aging*, eds R. D. Terry and S. Gershon (New York: Raven), 88–94.

Trachtenberg, J. T., Chen, B. E., Knott, G. W., Feng, G., Sanes, J. R., Welker, E., et al. (2002). Long-term in vivo imaging of experience-dependent synaptic plasticity in adult cortex. *Nature* 420, 788–794. doi: 10.1038/nature01273

Veyrac, A., Sacquet, J., Nguyen, V., Marien, M., Jourdan, F., and Didier, A. (2009). Novelty determines the effects of olfactory enrichment on memory and neurogenesis through noradrenergic mechanisms. *Neuropsychopharmacology* 34, 786–795. doi: 10.1038/npp.2008.191

Vicente, K. J. (1988). Adapting the memory recall paradigm to evaluate interfaces. *Acta Psychol.* 69, 249–278. doi: 10.1016/0001-6918(88)90035-2

Vicente, K. J., and Wang, J. H. (1998). An ecological theory of expertise effects in memory recall. *Psychol. Rev.* 105, 33–57. doi: 10.1037/0033-295X.105.1.33

Walk, H. A., and Johns, E. E. (1984). Interference and facilitation in short-term memory for odors. *Percept. Psychophys.* 36, 508–514. doi: 10.3758/BF03207510

Walk, R. D. (1966). Perceptual learning and discrimination of wine. *Psychon. Sci.* 5, 57–58. doi: 10.3758/BF03328278

Wang, H. W., Wysocki, C. J., and Gold, G. H. (1993). Induction of olfactory receptor sensitivity in mice. *Science* 260, 998–1000. doi: 10.1126/science.8493539

Wattendorf, E., Welge-Lussen, A., Fiedler, K., Bilecen, D., Wolfensberger, M., Fuhr, P., et al. (2009). Olfactory impairment predicts brain atrophy in Parkinson's disease. *J. Neurosci.* 29, 15410–15413. doi: 10.1523/JNEUROSCI.1909-09.2009

Welge-Lussen, A. (2009). Ageing, neurodegeneration, and olfactory and gustatory loss. *B-ENT* 5(Suppl. 13), 129–132.

Wilson, D. A. (2000). Comparison of odor receptive field plasticity in the rat olfactory bulb and anterior piriform cortex. *J. Neurophysiol.* 84, 3036–3042.

Wilson, D. A. (2003). Rapid, experience-induced enhancement in odorant discrimination by anterior piriform cortex neurons. *J. Neurophysiol.* 90, 65–72. doi: 10.1152/jn.00133.2003

Wippich, W., Mecklenbrauker, S., and Trouet, J. (1989). Implicit and explicit memories of odors. *Arch. Psychol. (Frankf.)* 141, 195–211.

Wright, R. H. (1964). Odor and molecular vibration: the far infrared spectra of some perfume chemicals. *Ann. N. Y. Acad. Sci.* 116, 552–558. doi: 10.1111/j.1749-6632.1964.tb45084.x

Wright, R. H. (1972). Stereochemical and vibrational theories of odour. *Nature* 239, 226. doi: 10.1038/239226a0

Wysocki, C. J., Dorries, K. M., and Beauchamp, G. K. (1989). Ability to perceive androstenone can be acquired by ostensibly anosmic people. *Proc. Natl. Acad. Sci. U.S.A.* 86, 7976–7978. doi: 10.1073/pnas.86.20.7976

Yee, K. K., and Wysocki, C. J. (2001). Odorant exposure increases olfactory sensitivity: olfactory epithelium is implicated. *Physiol. Behav.* 72, 705–711. doi: 10.1016/S0031-9384(01)00428-0

Yoshida, M. (1964). Studies of psychometric classification of odors. *Jpn. Psychol. Res.* 6, 145–154.

Zarzo, M., and Stanton, D. T. (2009). Understanding the underlying dimensions in perfumers' odor perception space as a basis for developing meaningful odor maps. *Atten. Percept. Psychophys.* 71, 225–247. doi: 10.3758/APP.71.2.225

Zatorre, R. J., Fields, R. D., and Johansen-Berg, H. (2012). Plasticity in gray and white: neuroimaging changes in brain structure during learning. *Nat. Neurosci.* 15, 528–536. doi: 10.1038/nn.3045

Zucco, G. M., Carassai, A., Baroni, M. R., and Stevenson, R. J. (2011). Labeling, identification, and recognition of wine-relevant odorants in expert sommeliers, intermediates, and untrained wine drinkers. *Perception* 40, 598–607. doi: 10.1068/p6972

12

Do ambient urban odors evoke basic emotions?

Sandra T. Glass[1,2], Elisabeth Lingg[1] and Eva Heuberger[1,3,4]*

[1] *Division of Clinical Pharmacy and Diagnostics, Department of Pharmaceutical Chemistry, University of Vienna, Vienna, Austria*
[2] *Department of Health Sciences and Technology, Institute for Human Movement Sciences and Sport, ETH Zurich, Zurich, Switzerland*
[3] *Division of Clinical Psychology and Psychotherapy, Department of Psychology, Saarland University, Saarbruecken, Germany*
[4] *Pharmaceutical Biology, Department of Pharmacy, Saarland University, Saarbruecken, Germany*

***Correspondence:**
Eva Heuberger, Division of Clinical Psychology and Psychotherapy, Department of Psychology, Saarland University, Campus A1 3, 66123 Saarbruecken, Germany
e-mail: e.heuberger@mx.uni-saarland.de

Fragrances, such as plant odors, have been shown to evoke autonomic response patterns associated with Ekman's (Ekman et al., 1983) basic emotions happiness, surprise, anger, fear, sadness, and disgust. Inducing positive emotions by odors in highly frequented public spaces could serve to improve the quality of life in urban environments. Thus, the present study evaluated the potency of ambient odors connoted with an urban environment to evoke basic emotions on an autonomic and cognitive response level. Synthetic mixtures representing the odors of disinfectant, candles/bees wax, summer air, burnt smell, vomit and musty smell as well as odorless water as a control were presented five times in random order to 30 healthy, non-smoking human subjects with intact sense of smell. Skin temperature, skin conductance, breathing rate, forearm muscle activity, blink rate, and heart rate were recorded simultaneously. Subjects rated the odors in terms of pleasantness, intensity and familiarity and gave verbal labels to each odor as well as cognitive associations with the basic emotions. The results showed that the amplitude of the skin conductance response (SCR) varied as a function of odor presentation. Burnt smell and vomit elicited significantly higher electrodermal responses than summer air. Also, a negative correlation was revealed between the amplitude of the SCR and hedonic odor valence indicating that the magnitude of the electrodermal response increased with odor unpleasantness. The analysis of the cognitive associations between odors and basic emotions showed that candles/bees wax and summer air were specifically associated with happiness whereas burnt smell and vomit were uniquely associated with disgust. Our findings suggest that city odors may evoke specific cognitive associations of basic emotions and that autonomic activity elicited by such odors is related to odor hedonics.

Keywords: city odors, basic emotions, autonomic nervous system, hedonic valence, odor intensity

INTRODUCTION

In urban environments both residents and visitors are surrounded by a multitude of odors which, along with visual, acoustic and haptic sensations, accompany and shape their individual perceptual experiences. These contextual stimuli are believed to be encoded in episodic memory along with an event and with the emotions experienced at that event and can serve as triggers for the retrieval of event details, such as the experienced emotions, on subsequent encounters (Jellinek, 1997; Chu and Downes, 2000). A number of laboratory studies have shown that highly emotional stimuli are more efficient triggers of episodic memory than emotionally neutral ones (Koenig and Mecklinger, 2008) and that odors are such highly emotional cues (Chu and Downes, 2002; Goddard et al., 2005; Willander and Larsson, 2007). Particularly in big cities the olfactory environment might have great impact on the experience of public spaces of both inhabitants and visitors. For instance, feelings of pleasure might be experienced in the vicinity of a bakery emitting the smell of freshly baked bread or in a public garden with fragrant flowers (Weber and Heuberger, 2008). By contrast, negative emotions might be elicited in places where people crowd together in confined spaces, such as public transport, or in other places that are experienced as constricted, smelly, and unpleasant. To counteract such possible negative experiences efforts are being made to increase the pleasantness of the urban olfactory environment (Hosey, 2013). Although inducing positive emotions in highly frequented public spaces could be a simple and efficient means to improve the quality of life in urban environments no research exists to date that addresses this question.

One way to assess the potency of sensory stimuli to induce affective reactions is to measure self-reported emotions together with associated changes in autonomic nervous system (ANS) activity. Although the debate is still ongoing as to whether or not emotion-specific autonomic activity exists (see Kreibig, 2010 for an up-to-date review) and many studies have failed to reveal such specificity (Aue and Scherer, 2008), a considerable number of reports exists in favor of the hypothesis of emotion-specific physiological activity (Friedman, 2010; Stephens et al., 2010). The issue of specific physiological patterns is intrinsically linked with the concept of basic emotions, i.e., a limited number of primary affective states which are generated universally and prototypically in response to environmental demands and may be regarded as discrete points in dimensional affective space (Christie and Friedman, 2004). The discussion about unique autonomic response patterns allowing to distinguish between these basic emotions has received great support by the studies of Ekman et al. (1983) in which six basic emotions, i.e., happiness, surprise, anger, fear, sadness and disgust, were evoked by generating directed emotion-prototypical facial expressions, and by reliving an emotional experience. The authors reported that they were able to differentiate between positive and negative emotions as well as among negative emotions based on a decision tree that took into account changes in heart rate and skin temperature. More recent investigations have demonstrated that viewing these emotion-prototypic facial expressions (Collet et al., 1997) as well as viewing emotional film clips and listening to emotional music (Christie and Friedman, 2004; Etzel et al., 2006) may induce emotion specific autonomic response patterns. Also, stimuli from the gustatory domain (Rousmans et al., 2000) have been found to induce emotional states with distinguishable autonomic patterns.

In regard to olfaction, several investigations have revealed emotion-specific ANS response patterns (Alaoui-Ismaili et al., 1997a,b; Robin et al., 1999; Vernet-Maury et al., 1999; Bensafi et al., 2002b; Moller and Dijksterhuis, 2003). However, comparisons between verbal reports and physiological activity of the elicited emotions often showed a mismatch between these two response systems and the valence of the odor evoked affective reaction seems to be associated with the hedonic valence of the odor (Brauchli et al., 1995; Bensafi et al., 2002a; Delplanque et al., 2008; Weber and Heuberger, 2008). Alaoui-Ismaili et al. (1997a) were able to link both verbal responses and psychophysiological correlates of Ekman's basic emotions to a number of odors that differed in hedonic quality. In this study, they presented vanillin and menthol which were rated as pleasant and methyl methacrylate and propionic acid which were rated as unpleasant to 44 healthy students and recorded several electrodermal and cardio-respiratory parameters. In addition, subjects had to indicate which of the six basic emotions was evoked by each of these odors. The authors reported that the pleasant odors evoked happiness and surprise regarding both verbal reports and autonomic response patterns. The unpleasant odors, however, evoked disgust as the verbal response but anger as the autonomic response. Another study by the same group with a different set of odorants confirmed the association between the hedonic valence of the odors and the emotion specific autonomic response patterns (Alaoui-Ismaili et al., 1997b). In regard to the relationship between hedonic odor rating and the valence of the evoked emotion, an interesting finding was reported by Robin et al. (1999). Based on the observation that eugenol is contained in many materials used in restorative dental treatments (Sarrami et al., 2002), these authors compared basic emotions elicited by eugenol odor in fearful and non-fearful dental care subjects and reported that such prior experience with the odor modulated both the hedonic evaluation of the odor and the emotional response, i.e., in non-fearful subjects eugenol odor was rated as pleasant and evoked positive emotions, i.e., happiness and surprise, while in fearful participants the odor was rated as unpleasant and evoked negative emotions, i.e., fear, anger, and disgust.

In regard to verbal reports of odor induced affective reactions, a study by Bensafi et al. (2002b) in 12 healthy participants with 12 different food odors ranging from very pleasant to very unpleasant showed that from seven emotional terms "joy" and "disgust" were chosen more often than the other emotion terms. In addition, facial EMG activity differentiated between these two emotions. An explanation for these findings can be found in the results of Chrea et al. (2009) who argued that the small number of basic emotions may be insufficient and inappropriate to describe the multitude of emotional states which can be elicited by olfactory stimuli and that olfaction-specific dimensions were better suited to account for verbal descriptions of odor induced feelings (Delplanque et al., 2012). These authors presented a 6 to 7-factorial model that describes the semantic space of affective verbal responses to odors and showed that four of these dimensions which were related to disgust, happiness/well-being, sensuality/desire, and energy were shared by different cultures (Ferdenzi et al., 2011, 2013).

Concentrating on verbal reports of basic emotions triggered by olfactory cues Croy et al. (2011) took a different approach and came to slightly different conclusions. Instead of presenting preselected odors, they interviewed 119 healthy subjects about free associations between odors and each of the six basic emotions. As a control they asked another 97 participants about their associations of the basic emotions with pictures. The results of this study showed that the vast majority of subjects were able to report an odor that elicited happiness or disgust. Olfactory cues associated with anxiety were reported by 75% of the participants. In contrast, only 50% of the subjects were able to identify an olfactory elicitor for sadness and anger (Croy et al., 2011). The authors concluded that only a limited number of emotions, i.e., happiness, anxiety, and disgust, can be elicited verbally by olfactory cues.

The present study aimed to evaluate whether affective responses are evoked by ambient odors connoted with the City of Vienna. Specifically, we tested whether such odors elicit emotion specific autonomic response patterns and verbal associations with the basic emotions. Notwithstanding the above mentioned findings on the olfactory semantic space (Ferdenzi et al., 2011, 2013) we favored a discrete (basic) emotions model over a two-dimensional (valence-by-arousal) approach as a theoretical framework for our study. According to Levenson (2003) the former allows for more finely tuned responses than the latter not only at the physiological but also at the endocrine, cognitive, and behavioral level. In our view, this constitutes a functional advantage in the case of olfactory triggered emotions. For example, consider disgust and fear. Both emotions possess high negative valence, are highly arousing, and are associated with withdrawal behavior (Christie and Friedman, 2004). However, while disgust is associated with objects that are potentially harmful after ingestion (such as spoiled food because it may be toxic), or direct skin contact (such as excrement because it may carry germs), fearful stimuli, such as fire or an aggressor, are threatening because they may inflict severe injuries. Thus, one could generalize that disgusting stimuli convey a threat to the body interior while fearful stimuli impose a threat to the outside of the body. In regard to the responses, disgust eliciting stimuli require bodily reactions that help to remove the threat from the organism, such as vomiting (Croy et al., 2013). Fearful stimuli, on the other hand, should initiate behavior that mobilizes enough energy to remove oneself from the source of danger. Responding in the one or the other way of course requires a completely different sort of preparation, also in the ANS (Levenson, 2003). Olfaction is a proximal sense, and once an odor can be perceived its source is quite close. Consequently, the appropriate response, disgust and regurgitation or fear and flight in this example, must be induced quickly. Therefore, in response to odors we think that unique physiological patterns as predicted by the basic emotions model have greater adaptive value than adopting mere approach-avoidance behavior as the dimensional model would predict.

In order to increase the emotional valence of the odorous stimuli we combined the experimental approach reported by Croy et al. (2011) with that of other studies, i.e., rather than selecting odors on a random basis we first conducted semi-structured interviews in a larger sample of Viennese residents ($N = 50$) (Weber and Heuberger, 2011). Specifically, we asked them to think of and narrate to the experimenter an experience in the City of Vienna which involved one of the six basic emotions. Subjects were free to decide in how much detail they wanted to describe the experience. Then, they had to name at least one odor that was associated with this memory. In addition, the participants rated how emotional and how vivid the memory was, how brought back in time they felt when they thought of the odor, and how specific the odor was for the memory. For each basic emotion the same questions were asked. To identify olfactory stimuli that were specific for a given basic emotion the count of each nominated odor was assessed for each basic emotion. While in this study odor associated memories were reported for each of the basic emotions, the interviews demonstrated that only a very small number of the reported odors were specific for a particular basic emotion, such as "vomit" for disgust. Thus, to obtain the (potentially) full range of odor evoked basic emotions we decided to select odors that were specific in regard to their emotional impact even though they were reported by only a small number of participants in the preceding interviews. The next task in the stimulus selection process consisted of "translating" the odor names into "perfumes" that involved a manageable number of chemical constituents but would still be clearly recognizable by the tested sample. Thus, we identified the character impact compounds of the selected odors and created synthetic mixtures that best represented their olfactory properties. We limited the number of constituents to three. Several challenges had to be met during this step. For instance, in the case of "burnt smell" and "candles" a character impact compound (prop-2-enal, also known as acrolein) could not be used due to its toxicity. To circumvent this issue, we decided to use other non-toxic chemicals with appropriate olfactory properties (see **Table 1**). In the case of "summer air" the search for suitable character impact compounds did not yield satisfactory results due to the ambiguity of the odor concept so that we decided to choose a green note reminiscent of leaves and grass. We considered this to be the best choice because one of the most frequented places in Vienna during summer time is the so-called "Donauinsel," a man-made island at the Danube River that is vegetated with meadows and trees. Ultimately, we were interested in the question whether the emotional valence of the selected odors would transfer to another sample of subjects, i.e., whether the chosen odor representations would elicit the same basic emotions in a different sample of subjects. In our view this would constitute a basic prerequisite for the creation of olfactory environments which elicit distinct emotional states.

MATERIALS AND METHODS

ETHICS STATEMENT

The study was performed in accordance with the Declaration of Helsinki on Biomedical Research Involving Human Subjects and with the guidelines of the Institutional Review Board at the University of Vienna. All participants provided written informed consent, received financial compensation for their time commitment, and were free to withdraw from the study at any time.

OLFACTORY SCREENING

In a first step, the olfactory acuity of the subjects who enrolled for the study was determined using the odor discrimination and identification tests from the Sniffing Sticks olfactory test battery (Hummel et al., 1997). The discrimination test consisted of odor triplets, of which two fragrances were identical distractors and one was the target that smelled different from the distractors. Each subject was required to identify the target odor. The criterion for inclusion in the subsequent psychophysiological study was the correct identification of 11 (out of 16) triplets. In the odor identification test, each subject had to sample a target odor and pick the correct odor name among four written alternatives. The criterion for inclusion in the subsequent psychophysiological study was the correct identification of at least 13 (out of 16) odors. Only participants who successfully identified and discriminated the presented odors were tested in the main study, i.e., the psychophysiological measurements, which was conducted on a different day than the olfactory screening.

SUBJECTS

In total, 30 healthy and neurologically inconspicuous individuals (15 males) between the age of 18 and 34 (mean age 24 ± 4 years) participated in the main study. All participants had normal blood pressure, no history of olfactory deficits, allergies to fragrances, or neurological diseases. None of the women were pregnant and all participants were non-smokers. All subjects were Viennese residents and recruited by advertisement at the University of Vienna. They received financial compensation for their time commitment.

OLFACTORY STIMULI

The olfactory stimuli used in the main study were synthetic mixtures representing the odors of warm summer air, candles/bees wax, disinfectant, burnt smell, musty smell, and vomit. The number of components in each mixture was limited to three. Odorless water was used as a control. For each odor, the chemical composition and association with the basic emotions is given in **Table 1**.

EXPERIMENTAL DESIGN AND PROCEDURES

The psychophysiological study took place in a temperature controlled and well ventilated room at the Department of Clinical Pharmacy and Diagnostics at the University of Vienna. The

Table 1 | Chemical composition, concentration of constituents, and association with the basic emotions for all olfactory stimuli.

Odor	Components	Basic emotion
Summer air	Leaf alcohol (Z-hex-3-en-1-ol) (0.1% v/v in PG)	Happiness
Candles (bees wax)	Methyl 2-phenylacetate (0.5% v/v in PG)	Surprise
Disinfectant	Isopropyl alcohol (propan-2-ol) (50% v/v in PG)	Fear
Burnt smell	Guaiacol (2-methoxyphenol) (10% v/v in PG)	Anger
Musty smell	(±)-geosmin [(4R,4aR,8aS)-4,8a-dimethyl-1,2,3,4,5,6,7,8-octahydronaphthalen-4a-ol] (0.01% m/V in MeOH/EtOH 96%, 9 pt), green pea pyrazine [2-methoxy-3,5 or 6-(propan-2-yl)pyrazine] (0.1% v/v in EtOH 96%, 1 pt)	Sadness
Vomit	Butanoic acid (10% v/v in PG, 2 pt), isovaleric acid (3-methylbutanoic acid) (10% v/v in PG, 7 pt), hydrochloric acid (36% v/v, 1 pt)	Disgust

EtOH, ethanol; MeOH, methanol; PG, propylene glycol (propane-1,2-diol); m/v, mass per volume; v/v, volume per volume; pt, parts.

participants were seated in a comfortable chair and their non-dominant hand was placed on a soft pillow.

Skin conductance, forearm muscle activity, eye-blink rate, skin temperature, as well as breathing and heart rate were measured simultaneously and in real-time via MP100WSW hardware (Biopac Systems, Inc., Santa Barbara, California, USA) and AcqKnowledge® software (V 3.9.0.17, © 1992–2007, BIOPAC Systems, Inc., Santa Barbara, California, USA) with a sampling rate of 1000 Hz. All signals were filtered by means of hardware-based filters included in the amplifiers. Skin conductance was recorded using a GSR100B amplifier and 6 mm inner diameter Ag/AgCl finger electrodes (TSD203) via the constant voltage (0.5 V) technique. Electrodes were filled with conductive gel and placed on the second phalanx of the middle and the index finger of the non-dominant hand with non-caustic adhesive tape. Electrode positioning was in compliance with traditional recommendations (Fowles et al., 1981). The signal was low pass filtered at 1 Hz. Surface electromyogram (EMG) was recorded with a EMG100B amplifier, Ag/AgCl surface electrodes (EL208S), and adhesive disks (ADD208). Electromyographic activity was recorded by placing two electrodes, which were filled with conductive gel, over the forearm flexors of the non-dominant hand as suggested by Cacioppo et al. (1990). The raw EMG signal was band pass filtered (1–500 Hz), with a notch filter centered at 50 Hz, and converted to an average root-mean-square (rms) signal (time constant 500 ms, baseline removal). Eye-blinks were recorded by means of a EOG100B amplifier, Ag/AgCl surface electrodes (EL208S), and adhesive disks (ADD204). Two electrodes, which were filled with conductive gel, were placed over the left orbicularis oculi muscle on a vertical line (Stern et al., 2001). The signal was low pass filtered at 35 Hz and a 50 Hz notch filter was employed. ST was measured using a SKT100B amplifier and a fast response thermistor (TSD202A). The sensor was placed on the middle of the back of the non-dominant hand with non-caustic adhesive tape. The signal was low pass filtered at 1 Hz. Heart rate was measured via a ECG100C amplifier and Ag/AgCl surface electrodes (Skintact®, T601, Leonard Lang GmbH, Austria). The ECG signal was band pass filtered (0.05–35 Hz), with a 50 Hz notch filter. Heart rate was detected from the ECG via an integrated rate detector (peak interval window 40–180 bpm, noise rejection 5% of peak) and sampled at 250 Hz. Breathing was recorded via a RSP100C amplifier and a breathing belt (BIOPACTSD201) with an integrated electrical sensor. The belt was placed below the sternum and above the ECG electrodes. Any change in the belt's length was recorded by the electric sensor. The signal was low pass filtered at 10 Hz.

To each subject, the six olfactory stimuli and odorless water as a control stimulus were presented on sniffing stripes (Primavera Life GmbH, Germany) by one of two experimenters. 5 ml of each liquid stimulus were filled into 20 ml screw-cap brown glass vials coded by a number from 1 to 7. Stimulus concentration was kept constant by dipping the sniffing stripe into the vial until it reached the ground. To prevent the adulteration of the experimental stimuli with odors stemming from the hand of the experimenter, the experimenter wore cotton gloves. The stimuli were presented in randomized order. Each stimulus was presented 5 times. Stimulus presentation was synchronized with inspiration via the observation of the respiration channel and was marked in the recording by means of a hand switch. At the onset of inspiration the experimenter held a sniffing stripe soaked with the appropriate stimulus approximately 2 cm under the nostrils of the subject. Each stimulus presentation lasted for one breathing cycle. Subjects were instructed to breathe normally whether or not a stimulus was presented. The interstimulus interval was 2 min. Each stripe was used only once and discarded into a sealed container after use. The average duration of the experiment was 80 min. There was a 10 min baseline phase before the first odor presentation to ensure that all ANS parameters returned to their baseline levels before the first odor presentation took place.

After the psychophysiological measurements were finished, all participants completed a set of different questions. They had the opportunity to smell each of the odors again before giving their answers to the questions. The participants were asked to produce a verbal label for each odor. Using Likert scales they were then required to indicate the strength (1 = "very weak" and 10 = "very strong") of the association with each of the six basic emotions (i.e., happiness, surprise, anger, fear, sadness, and disgust). For a given odor, the emotion that received the highest rating was given one point, whereas all other emotions received zero points. If for a given odor two or more emotions received equal ratings, then one point was assigned to the category "no or unspecific association." Likert scales were also used to acquire data about the intensity of the odors (1 = "very weak" and 10 = "very strong"), the valence of the odors (1 = "very unpleasant" and 10 = "very pleasant") and the familiarity of the odors (1 = "very unfamiliar" and 10 = "very familiar").

DATA ANALYSIS

All recordings were edited offline for movement, breathing or electronic artefacts. No additional offline filtering was applied to the data. Since emotional reactions are quickly unfolding phasic events, a time window of 10 s post-stimulus was chosen (Ekman, 1992). The mean for each parameter was calculated across trials for each of the seven odor conditions. Only the first four blocks were included in the data analysis, since the participants showed signs of fatigue in the last (fifth) block due to the overall length of the experiment. Changes in muscle tension (rms EMG), number of eye-blinks, ST, number of breaths and heart rate were expressed as the difference between the respective mean of the prestimulus (10 s) and the post-stimulus (10 s) time interval. The change in heart rate variability (HRV) was calculated as the difference between the standard deviation (SD) of the heart rate before (10 s) and after (10 s) stimulus onset. The amplitude as well as the latency and the recovery time of the skin conductance response (SCR) were analyzed separately. The time window for the latency response was 1–4 s after stimulus onset. The criterion for a SCR to be included in the analysis was 0.05 $\mu S/cm^2$ (Boucsein, 1988). In order to be able to compare the SCR amplitudes (SCR-a) across subjects, each amplitude value in a given odor condition was divided by the corresponding maximum value across all trials (Schandry, 1989).

STATISTICAL ANALYSIS

To evaluate the impact of the different odor stimuli One-Way repeated measures ANOVAs with the within-subjects factor "odor" were conducted for each of the psychophysiological parameters and for each of the odor ratings (i.e., intensity, valence, and familiarity). Degrees of freedom were adjusted via the Greenhouse-Geisser method. *Post-hoc* pairwise comparisons were calculated using Bonferroni corrected *P*-values to control for alpha inflation. Two-sided Pearson product-moment correlations were calculated to identify potential relationships between the ANS parameters and the different odor ratings as well as between the odor ratings themselves. These analyses were conducted with the data of 16 subjects. For 14 subjects the data was not sufficient (in most cases due to SCRs that did not meet the amplitude or temporal criteria) to allow for further analyses.

The association between each odor and the six basic emotions was analyzed using a Pearson's χ^2 test ($N = 30$). The observed associations were compared to hypothetical associations based on our previous findings (Weber and Heuberger, 2011).

RESULTS

AUTONOMIC NERVOUS SYSTEM PARAMETERS

The *amplitude of the skin conductance responses* (SCR-a) varied significantly with the presented olfactory stimulus. A One-Way repeated measures ANOVA with the within-subjects factor "odor" revealed a significant main effect for the factor "odor" [$F_{(6, 90)} = 7.579, P = 0.000$]. Mean values of SCR-a are depicted in **Figure 1**. *Post-hoc* pairwise comparisons showed that the unpleasant odor "vomit" elicited significantly larger responses than all other odors

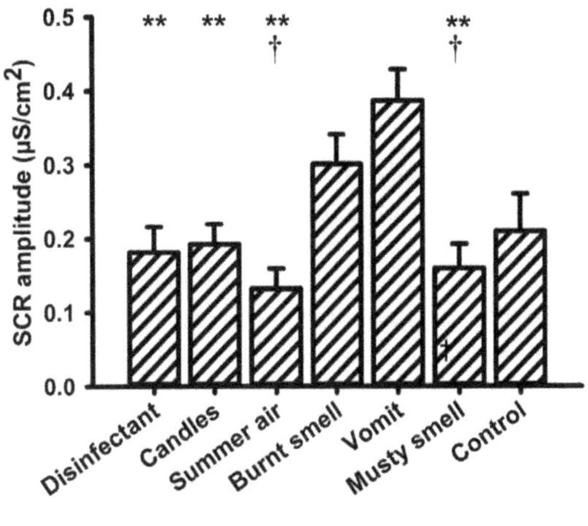

FIGURE 1 | Mean values (and s.e.m.) of the amplitude of the skin conductance response (SCR) to all olfactory stimuli. **Differs significantly ($P < 0.005$) from "vomit," †differs significantly ($P < 0.05$) from "burnt smell."

("disinfectant": $P = 0.002$, "candles": $P = 0.004$, "summer air": $P = 0.001$, and "musty smell": $P = 0.002$) except "burnt smell" and odorless water (i.e., the control stimulus). We also found a significant difference between "summer air" and "burnt smell" ($P = 0.022$) and between "burnt smell and "musty smell" ($P = 0.031$). In addition, there was a significant negative correlation between SCR-a and the odor valence ratings ($N = 7, r = -0.927, P = 0.003$; **Figure 2**), i.e., the amplitude of the SCR decreased with the perceived pleasantness of a fragrance. This correlation was unaffected by either intensity ($N = 7, r = -0.962, P = 0.002$) or familiarity ratings ($N = 7, r = -0.951, P = 0.003$) as revealed by partial correlation analyses. The correlation between SCR-a and perceived intensity was marginally significant only after controlling for the perceived pleasantness of the odors ($N = 7, r = -0.768, P = 0.074$) and significant after controlling for ratings of familiarity ($N = 7, r = -0.823, P = 0.044$) indicating that SCR-a increased with the perceived intensity of an odor. There was no significant correlation between SCR-a and familiarity ($P > 0.1$).

The *latency* and *the half recovery time of the skin conductance response* were analyzed using One-Way repeated measures ANOVAs with the within-subjects factor "odor" but no significant main effects were found (all $P > 0.1$; mean values and s.e.m. of the latency and half recovery time of the SCR are given in Table S1 in the supplementary material). Neither the correlation analyses between the subjective odor ratings (i.e., perceived odor pleasantness, intensity, and familiarity) and the latency of the SCR nor those between the subjective odor ratings and the half recovery time of the SCR revealed any significant relationships (all $P > 0.1$).

Changes in *heart rate variability (HRV)* in response to the different olfactory stimuli were analyzed using a One-Way repeated measures ANOVA with the within-subjects factor "odor." The analysis revealed no significant effects ($P > 0.1$; mean values and s.e.m. of the HRV changes are given in Table S1 in the supplementary material). The correlation analysis, however, showed a significant negative correlation between HRV changes and the odor intensity ratings ($N = 7$, $r = -0.763$, $P = 0.046$; **Figure 3A**). This correlation remained significant after controlling for the ratings of familiarity ($N = 7$, $r = -0.905$, $P = 0.013$) but disappeared after controlling for their perceived pleasantness ($P > 0.1$). The correlation between HRV changes and the odor valence ratings was also significant ($N = 7$, $r = 0.843$, $P = 0.017$; **Figure 3B**). This correlation remained significant after controlling for the perceived familiarity of the odors ($N = 7$, $r = 0.846$, $P = 0.034$), but disappeared after controlling for their perceived intensity ($P > 0.1$). The correlation between HRV changes and the familiarity ratings revealed no significant relationship ($P > 0.1$).

Skin temperature (ST) responses to the olfactory stimuli did not change depending on the different olfactory stimuli. A One-Way repeated measures ANOVA with the within-subjects factor "odor" did not yield a significant main effect for this factor [$F_{(6, 90)} = 2.664$, $P = 0.068$; mean values and s.e.m. of the ST changes are given in Table S1 in the supplementary material]. A significant negative correlation was revealed between the ST responses and the odor familiarity ratings ($N = 7$, $r = -0.697$, $P = 0.041$; **Figure 4**).

Number of breaths, heart rate, number of eye-blinks and *forearm muscle activity* did not vary dependent on the presented olfactory stimuli. Neither the One-Way repeated measures ANOVAs with the within-subjects factor "odor" nor the correlation analyses (with the valence, intensity, and familiarity ratings) revealed a significant result (all $P > 0.1$; mean values and s.e.m. of the changes of number of breaths, heart rate, number of eye-blinks, and forearm muscle activity are given in Table S1 in the supplementary material).

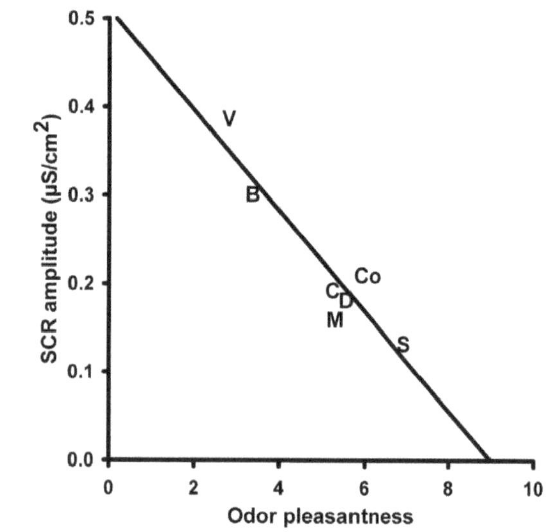

FIGURE 2 | Correlation between the amplitude of the skin conductance response (SCR) to the olfactory stimuli and perceived odor pleasantness. S, Summer air; C, Candles; D, Disinfectant; B, Burnt smell; M, Musty smell; V, Vomit; Co, Control.

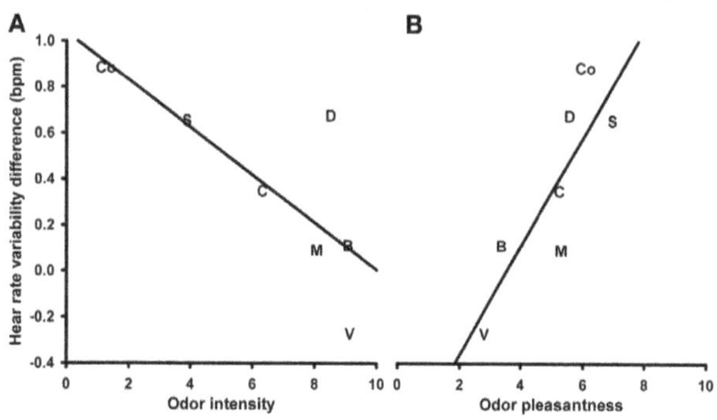

FIGURE 3 | Correlation between heart rate variability in response to the olfactory stimuli and perceived odor intensity (A) and pleasantness (B), respectively. S, Summer air; C, Candles; D, Disinfectant; B, Burnt smell; M, Musty smell; V, Vomit; Co, Control.

VALENCE, INTENSITY, AND FAMILIARITY RATINGS

Figures 5–7 show the mean values of the valence, intensity, and familiarity ratings, respectively. With respect to the valence ratings, a One-Way repeated measures ANOVA revealed a significant main effect for the within-subjects factor "odor" [$F_{(6, 90)} = 6.440$, $P < 0.001$]. The highest valence rating was observed for "summer air," whereas the lowest rating was recorded for "vomit." *Post-hoc* pairwise comparisons revealed significant differences between "burnt smell" and "summer air" ($P = 0.012$), "burnt smell" and "musty smell" ($P = 0.016$) and "burnt smell" and odorless water ($P = 0.019$) as well as between "vomit" and "disinfectant" ($P = 0.032$), "vomit" and "summer air" ($P = 0.004$) and "vomit" and odorless water ($P = 0.008$).

For the intensity ratings the One-Way ANOVA showed a significant main effect for the within-subjects factor "odor" [$F_{(6, 90)} = 66.308$, $P < 0.001$]. The lowest intensity rating was

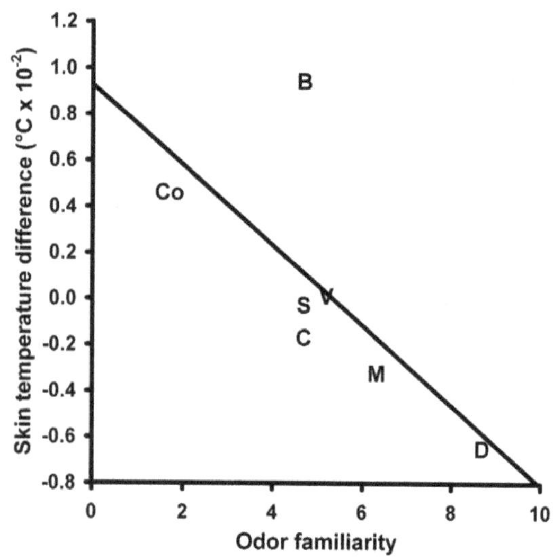

FIGURE 4 | Correlation between the skin temperature response to the olfactory stimuli and perceived odor familiarity. S, Summer air; C, Candles; D, Disinfectant; B, Burnt smell; M, Musty smell; V, Vomit; Co, Control.

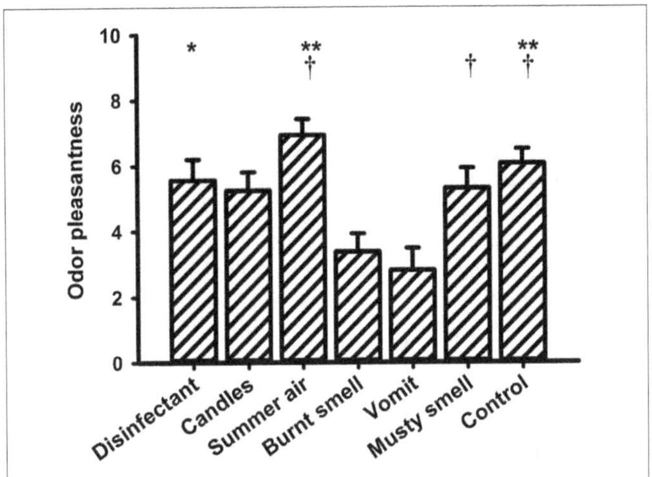

FIGURE 5 | Mean values (and s.e.m.) of the ratings of odor valence. **Differs significantly ($P < 0.01$) from "vomit," *differs significantly ($P < 0.05$) from "vomit," †differs significantly ($P < 0.05$) from "burnt smell."

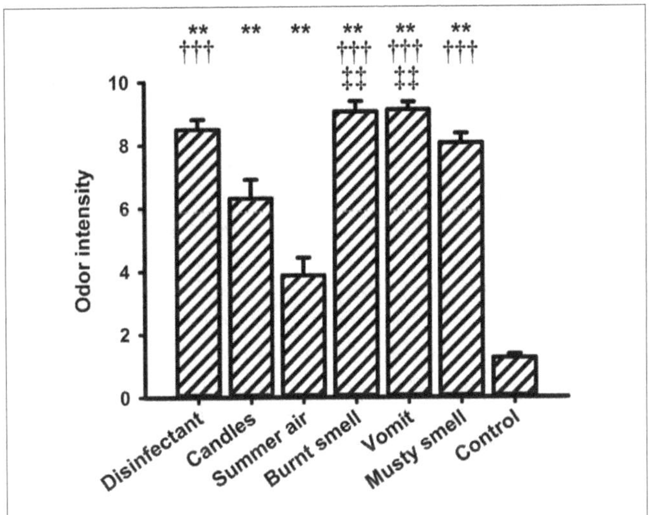

FIGURE 6 | Mean values (and s.e.m.) of the ratings of odor intensity. **Differs significantly ($P < 0.01$) from control, †††differs significantly ($P < 0.001$) from "summer air," ‡‡differs significantly ($P < 0.01$) from "candles."

observed for the control stimulus (i.e., odorless water). *Post-hoc* pairwise comparisons revealed significant differences between odorless water and all other fragrances ("disinfectant": $P = 0.000$, "candles": $P = 0.000$, "summer air": $P = 0.003$, "burnt smell": $P = 0.000$, "vomit": $P = 0.000$, and "musty smell": $P = 0.000$). "Summer air" also had a very low intensity rating and showed significant differences to "disinfectant" ($P = 0.000$), "burnt smell" ($P = 0.000$), "vomit" ($P = 0.000$), and "musty smell" ($P = 0.000$). "Summer air" further showed a marginally significant difference to "candles" ($P = 0.051$). The fragrance "candles" showed significant differences in intensity to "burnt smell" ($P = 0.003$) and "vomit" ($P = 0.009$).

With respect to the familiarity ratings the One-Way ANOVA also revealed a significant main effect for the within-subjects factor "odor" [$F_{(6, 90)} = 13.627$, $P = 0.000$]. The lowest familiarity rating was observed for the control stimulus (i.e., odorless water). *Post-hoc* pairwise comparisons showed significant differences between odorless water and all other fragrances ("disinfectant": $P = 0.000$, "candles": $P = 0.007$, "summer air": $P = 0.015$, "burnt smell": $P = 0.014$, "vomit": $P = 0.012$, and "musty smell": $P = 0.000$). "Disinfectant" received a very high familiarity rating and showed significant differences to "candles" ($P = 0.009$), "summer air" ($P = 0.005$), "burnt smell" ($P = 0.003$), and "vomit" ($P = 0.014$).

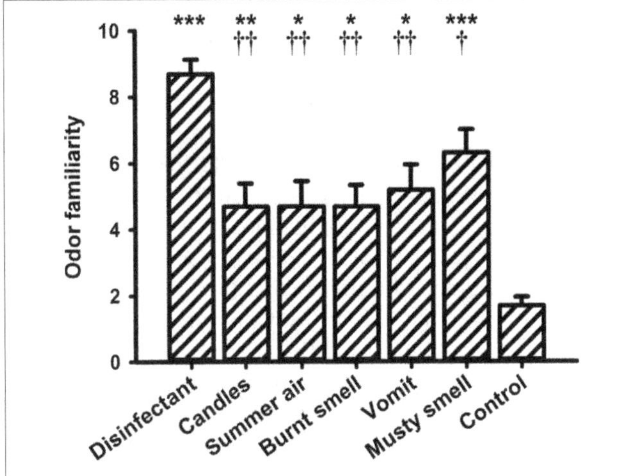

FIGURE 7 | Mean values (and s.e.m.) of the ratings of odor familiarity. *Differs significantly ($P < 0.05$) from control, **differs significantly ($P < 0.01$) from control, ***differs significantly ($P < 0.001$) from control, †differs significantly ($P < 0.05$) from "disinfectant," ††differs significantly ($P < 0.01$) from "disinfectant."

The correlation analysis showed a marginally significant negative correlation between the odor valence and intensity ratings ($N = 7$, $r = -0.723$, $P = 0.067$; **Figure 8A**). When this correlation was controlled for familiarity, it became highly significant ($N = 7$, $r = -0.951$, $P = 0.004$). Furthermore, a marginally significant, positive correlation between the intensity and familiarity ratings ($N = 7$, $r = 0.719$, $P = 0.068$; **Figure 8B**) was revealed. After controlling for the valence ratings, this correlation also became highly significant ($N = 7$, $r = 0.950$, $P = 0.004$). Finally, a partial positive correlation between the odor valence and familiarity ratings (controlled for intensity) was found ($N = 7$, $r = 0.895$, $P = 0.016$; uncontrolled $r = -0.090$, $P = 0.847$).

VERBAL LABELS

Table 2 shows the verbal descriptions of the olfactory stimuli given by the participants. In general, only about 25–50% of the subjects were able to put a name to the odors that were presented throughout the psychophysiological recordings even though the stimuli were presented again during the rating procedure. The only exception was "disinfectant" which was labeled by 24 out of 30 participants (80%). With respect to the labels, it is obvious that "disinfectant," "burnt smell," "musty smell," "vomit" and the control odor were described quite accurately, whereas "summer air" and "candles" were never labeled correctly. However, in the case of "summer air" which was represented by the so called leaf alcohol the verbal labels demonstrate that subjects identified the "green" note of the fragrance that reminds of leaves and freshly cut grass.

COGNITIVE ASSOCIATION BETWEEN OLFACTORY STIMULI AND BASIC EMOTIONS

The χ^2 test revealed that the odors "candles" ($\chi^2 = 31.6$, $P = 0.000$) and "summer air" ($\chi^2 = 17.2$, $P = 0.001$) were both associated specifically with the basic emotion "happiness," whereas "vomit" ($\chi^2 = 33.2$, $P = 0.000$) and "burnt smell" ($\chi^2 = 12.0$, $P = 0.017$) were both associated specifically with the basic emotion "disgust." The odors "disinfectant" und "musty smell" were not specifically related to a single basic emotion ($P > 0.1$). It is important to note that the control stimulus (i.e., odorless water) was specifically associated with no basic emotion ($\chi^2 = 62.8$, $P = 0.000$). Thus, four odors could be associated with a single basic emotion in this study, but only two of these odors ("vomit" and "summer air") could be associated with the hypothetical basic emotion (see **Table 3**).

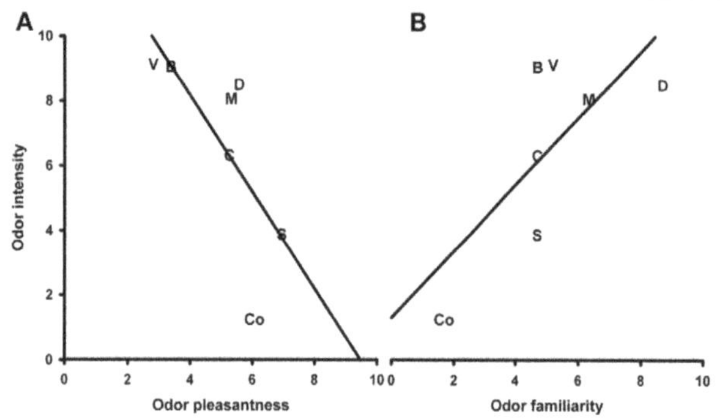

FIGURE 8 | Correlation between ratings of odor intensity and odor valence (A) and odor intensity and odor familiarity (B). S, Summer air; C, Candles; D, Disinfectant; B, Burnt smell; M, Musty smell; V, Vomit; Co, Control.

Table 2 | Number of participants ($N = 30$) who named the olfactory stimuli and verbal labels (with number of nominations) for all odors.

Odor	No.	Verbal labels
Summer air	14	Flowers/flower water/flowery meadow (8), conifer/fir tree (3), grass/grass clippings (3), lettuce (1), tomato (1)
Candles	8	Flowers/lilac/rose/cedar wood (6), banana (1), solvent (1)
Disinfectant	24	Disinfectant (13), alcohol/ethanol/isopropanol/solvent (11), doctor's office (2)
Burnt smell	13	Burnt smell/smoke/fire/lit match (6), wood/forest (4), leather (3), rubber (1), salami (1), dentist's office (1)
Musty smell	18	Soil/compost (8), musty/putrid/cellar (5), beet/carrot/asparagus/radish/red cabbage (6), flower (1), tires (1)
Vomit	12	Vomit/gastric acid/fermented/vinegar (5), peach/red currant/fruity (3), mold/organic waste (2), chewing gum (1), sweat (1), valerian (1)
Water (control)	7	Water (3), lotion with unobtrusive smell (1), no odor (1), paper (1), rose (1)

DISCUSSION

In the present study, we aimed to evaluate the emotional potency and distinctiveness of six odors that were connoted with the olfactory environment of the City of Vienna. Based on earlier reports on the induction of discrete emotions by odors (e.g., Alaoui-Ismaili et al., 1997a; Robin et al., 1999; Vernet-Maury et al., 1999) we hypothesized that urban odors elicit emotional responses that can be distinguished by physiological activity. Since the study of Robin et al. (1999) showed that the emotional response toward an odor is shaped by prior subjective experience, we sought to account for this finding when selecting the odors for the current investigation by taking into account autobiographical factors.

AUTONOMIC NERVOUS SYSTEM PARAMETERS AND SUBJECTIVE ODOR RATINGS

Our data did not show any emotion specific autonomic response patterns as a result of the olfactory stimulation. Although the parameters chosen in this study resemble those in the investigation of Ekman et al. (1983) and have also been used by others to detect emotion-specific autonomic activity in response to sensory stimuli (for details see Kreibig, 2010), our array of parameters differs from that of Alaoui-Ismaili et al. (1997a) in their olfactory studies. Thus, we may have failed to choose the appropriate set of physiological endpoints to detect olfactory induced emotions. This seems plausible as a recent investigation (Croy et al., 2013) demonstrated that systolic blood pressure responses differed depending on the sensory channel used to induce disgust. With regard to individual autonomic parameters, we found that the amplitude of the SCR varied as a function of odor presentation. In addition, hedonic odor valence was negatively correlated with the amplitude of the SCR. Thus, our results indicate that electrodermal activity differentiates between pleasant and unpleasant odors. These observations are in line with previous findings of Delplanque et al. (2009) but in contrast with the findings of Moller and Dijksterhuis (2003), who found no evidence for a relationship between odor pleasantness and the amplitude

Table 3 | Association (number of nominations) of the olfactory stimuli with the basic emotions.

Odor	Hap	Sur	Fea	Ang	Sad	Dis	Uns
Summer air	**16***	4	0	0	0	1	9
Candles	16*	**3**	1	0	1	5	4
Disinfectant	8	3	**3**	1	3	6	6
Burnt smell	3	7	3	**0**	0	13*	4
Musty smell	7	7	0	0	**0**	11	5
Vomit	1	4	0	0	0	**21***	4
Water (Control)	4	1	0	1	1	2	**21***

Numbers in bold indicate a match between the hypothetical and the observed association. Hap, happiness; Sur, surprise; Fea, fear; Ang, anger; Sad, sadness; Dis, disgust; Uns, no or unspecific association.

**Indicates that the verbal association was emotion-specific.*

of the SCR using four iso-intense non-trigeminal odors. Bensafi et al. (2002a) reported a marginal correlation between electrodermal activity and odor intensity which was also revealed in our study. The magnitude of the electrodermal response is believed to reflect the activation level of the sympathetic branch of the ANS (Critchley, 2002; Sequeira et al., 2009). Since hedonic odor valence and odor intensity ratings were strongly correlated in our study, we cannot fully rule out the possibility that the effect on electrodermal activity was driven by odor intensity or potential differences in the trigeminal activity of the odors.

In regard to cardiovascular activity, we found that HRV decreased as the fragrances were rated more intense and less pleasant. Similar relationships between heart rate variations and subjective ratings of odor pleasantness have been described by Bensafi et al. (2002a). Aue and Scherer (2008) reported smaller changes in heart rate in response to unpleasant as opposed to pleasant pictures. HRV has been linked with regulated emotional responding, and reduced overall, and parasympathetically mediated HRV has been observed in several forms of anxiety and depression (Appelhans and Luecken, 2006). Thus, our results could probably be interpreted in terms of diminished regulated emotional responding accompanying negative emotional states such as fear and sadness as the olfactory stimuli were perceived as more intense and less pleasant. An alternative explanation is that odors which were rated high in intensity and low in pleasantness induced sympathetic activation (Inoue et al., 2003) resulting in reduced HRV.

With respect to the ratings of perceived odor pleasantness, intensity, and familiarity, the results of the present study showed that the unpleasant odors "vomit" and "burnt smell" differed significantly from the pleasant fragrance "summer air" and from the control odor. Regarding intensity, all odors differed significantly from the weak odor "summer air" and from the control odor. Finally, "candles" rated intermediate in intensity differed from the very strong odors "vomit" and "burnt smell." The analyses of the familiarity ratings showed that both the most familiar odor, i.e., "disinfectant," as well as the least familiar control odor differed significantly from all other odors. The correlation between the change in ST and the odor familiarity ratings indicated that ST decreased with increasing odor familiarity. To the best of our knowledge such a relationship has never been observed before and more research is needed to interpret this finding.

VERBAL LABELS AND COGNITIVE ASSOCIATIONS

The analyses of the verbal responses showed that only 25–50% of the participants could produce a label for the presented odors. In addition, some odors were harder to name than others. In particular, verbal descriptions for "disinfectant," "burnt smell," "musty smell," "vomit," and the control odor were accurate in most cases, whereas none of the subjects used the labels "summer air" and "candles" for the respective fragrances. Difficulties in odor naming are a common finding (Cain, 1979) and are particularly relevant in verbal odor identification tasks. To account for this general deficit odor identification is often facilitated in such tasks by offering a number of alternatives from which the correct label must be chosen. As we were interested in free associations rather than correct identification in this study we decided against the use of verbal cues. The odor naming deficit is often observed even for very familiar odors (Olofsson et al., 2013). In the present study, however, the number of label use seemed to go hand in hand with the familiarity ratings. "Disinfectant" which received the highest familiarity rating was named by 80% of the participants and was followed in terms of labeling by several odors with similar familiarity ratings. The control odor which was rated least familiar also had the lowest count of labels used.

In regard to the verbal associations between the odors and the basic emotions it is obvious that fragrances with high pleasantness and low intensity ratings were associated with happiness, whereas those with low pleasantness and high intensity ratings were associated with disgust. Similar observations have also been made in the visual (Barrett and Niedenthal, 2004) and in the olfactory domain (Alaoui-Ismaili et al., 1997a; Robin et al., 1999; Weber and Heuberger, 2011). Levenson stated that when sensory stimuli are used for emotion induction subjects "report feeling emotions that [. . .] represent their judgments of the emotional qualities of the stimuli" rather than experiencing emotions (Levenson, 2003, p. 217). However, with the current experimental paradigm we can neither confirm nor reject this argument. We found that only four out of six odors, i.e., "summer air," "candles," "burnt smell," and "vomit" were uniquely assigned to a single basic emotion. Moreover, only two of the six emotions, i.e., happiness and disgust, were specifically associated with an odor. The latter finding is in line with previous observations on the relationship between basic emotions and verbal associations (Alaoui-Ismaili et al., 1997a; Bensafi et al., 2002b; Croy et al., 2011) and can be explained by the results of Chrea et al. (2009) and Delplanque et al. (2012). Nevertheless, the practical constraints in the odor selection process that have been outlined in the Introduction may also have contributed to these results.

In conclusion, our results suggest that urban odors may evoke specific cognitive concepts of basic emotions. Moreover, both autonomic activity and cognitive associations elicited by such odors seem to be related to odor hedonics and odor strength without being necessarily emotion specific. Our findings might be relevant in the field of urban design in that they underscore the emotional potency of odors connoted with an urban environment while at the same time they discourage ambitions to deliberately induce specific affective states utilizing ambient odors in public spaces.

AUTHOR CONTRIBUTIONS

Sandra T. Glass and Eva Heuberger conceived and designed the experiments, Sandra T. Glass and Elisabeth Lingg collected and analyzed the data, Sandra T. Glass and Eva Heuberger wrote the paper.

ACKNOWLEDGMENTS

This study was funded by a grant from Vienna Science and Technology Fund (grant no. CI06 009). We gratefully acknowledge the contributions of Theresa Förster-Streffleur and Christiane Weißinger in the selection and preparation of the olfactory stimuli. We also want to thank our panel of experts Stefanie Bail (Firmenich, Austria), Reinhild Eberhardt (Food Testing and Research Institute Vienna, Austria), Dorota

Majchrzak and Petra Rust (Department of Nutritional Sciences, University of Vienna, Austria), Heidrun Unterweger (AGES, Austria), Erich Leitner (Institute of Analytical Chemistry and Food Chemistry, Technical University Graz, Austria), and Erich Schmidt (Kurt Kitzing, Germany) for valuable advice on the chemical composition of the odor stimuli.

REFERENCES

Alaoui-Ismaili, O., Robin, O., Rada, H., Dittmar, A., and Vernet-Maury, E. (1997a). Basic emotions evoked by odorants: comparison between autonomic responses and self-evaluation. *Physiol. Behav.* 62, 713–720. doi: 10.1016/S0031-9384(97)90016-0

Alaoui-Ismaili, O., Vernet-Maury, E., Dittmar, A., Delhomme, G., and Chanel, J. (1997b). Odor hedonics: connection with emotional response estimated by autonomic parameters. *Chem. Senses* 22, 237–248. doi: 10.1093/chemse/22.3.237

Appelhans, B. M., and Luecken, L. J. (2006). Heart rate variability as an index of regulated emotional responding. *Rev. Gen. Psychol.* 10, 229–240. doi: 10.1037/1089-2680.10.3.229

Aue, T., and Scherer, K. R. (2008). Appraisal-driven somatovisceral response patterning: effects of intrinsic pleasantness and goal conduciveness. *Biol. Psychol.* 79, 158–164. doi: 10.1016/j.biopsycho.2008.04.004

Barrett, L. F., and Niedenthal, P. M. (2004). Valence focus and the perception of facial affect. *Emotion* 4, 266–274. doi: 10.1037/1528-3542.4.3.266

Bensafi, M., Rouby, C., Farget, V., Bertrand, B., Vigouroux, M., and Holley, A. (2002a). Autonomic nervous system responses to odours: the role of pleasantness and arousal. *Chem. Senses* 27, 703–709. doi: 10.1093/chemse/27.8.703

Bensafi, M., Rouby, C., Farget, V., Bertrand, B., Vigouroux, M., and Holley, A. (2002b). Psychophysiological correlates of affects in human olfaction. *Neurophysiol. Clin.* 32, 326–332. doi: 10.1016/S0987-7053(02)00339-8

Boucsein, W. (1988). *Elektrodermale Aktivität. Grundlagen, Methoden und Anwendungen*. Berlin: Springer Verlag. doi: 10.1007/978-3-662-06968-4

Brauchli, P., Ruegg, P. B., Etzweiler, F., and Zeier, H. (1995). Electrocortical and autonomic alteration by administration of a pleasant and an unpleasant odor. *Chem. Senses* 20, 505–515. doi: 10.1093/chemse/20.5.505

Cacioppo, J. T., Tassinary, L. G., and Fridlund, A. F. (1990). "The skeletomotor system," in *Principles of Psychophysiology: Physical, Social, and Inferential Elements*, eds J. T. Cacioppo and L. G. Tassinary (New York, NY: Cambridge University Press), 325–384.

Cain, W. S. (1979). To know with the nose: keys to odor identification. *Science* 203, 467–470. doi: 10.1126/science.760202

Chrea, C., Grandjean, D., Delplanque, S., Cayeux, I., Le Calve, B., Aymard, L., et al. (2009). Mapping the semantic space for the subjective experience of emotional responses to odors. *Chem. Senses* 34, 49–62. doi: 10.1093/chemse/bjn052

Christie, I. C., and Friedman, B. H. (2004). Autonomic specificity of discrete emotion and dimensions of affective space: a multivariate approach. *Int. J. Psychophysiol.* 51, 143–153. doi: 10.1016/j.ijpsycho.2003.08.002

Chu, S., and Downes, J. J. (2000). Odour-evoked autobiographical memories: psychological investigations of proustian phenomena. *Chem. Senses* 25, 111–116. doi: 10.1093/chemse/25.1.111

Chu, S., and Downes, J. J. (2002). Proust nose best: odors are better cues of autobiographical memory. *Mem. Cogn.* 30, 511–518. doi: 10.3758/BF03194952

Collet, C., Vernet-Maury, E., Delhomme, G., and Dittmar, A. (1997). Autonomic nervous system response patterns specificity to basic emotions. *J. Auton. Nerv. Syst.* 62, 45–57. doi: 10.1016/S0165-1838(96)00108-7

Critchley, H. D. (2002). Book review: electrodermal responses: what happens in the brain. *Neuroscientist* 8, 132–142. doi: 10.1177/107385840200800209

Croy, I., Laqua, K., Suess, F., Joraschky, P., Ziemssen, T., and Hummel, T. (2013). The sensory channel of presentation alters subjective ratings and autonomic responses towards disgusting stimuli—Blood pressure, heart rate and skin conductance in response to visual, auditory, haptic and olfactory presented disgusting stimuli. *Front. Hum. Neurosci.* 7:510. doi: 10.3389/fnhum.2013.00510

Croy, I., Olgun, S., and Joraschky, P. (2011). Basic emotions elicited by odors and pictures. *Emotion* 11, 1331–1335. doi: 10.1037/a0024437

Delplanque, S., Chrea, C., Grandjean, D., Ferdenzi, C., Cayeux, I., Porcherot, C., et al. (2012). How to map the affective semantic space of scents. *Cogn. Emot.* 26, 885–898. doi: 10.1080/02699931.2011.628301

Delplanque, S., Grandjean, D., Chrea, C., Aymard, L., Cayeux, I., Le Calve, B., et al. (2008). Emotional processing of odors: evidence for a nonlinear relation between pleasantness and familiarity evaluations. *Chem. Senses* 33, 469–479. doi: 10.1093/chemse/bjn014

Delplanque, S., Grandjean, D., Chrea, C., Coppin, G., Aymard, L., Cayeux, I., et al. (2009). Sequential unfolding of novelty and pleasantness appraisals of odors: evidence from facial electromyography and autonomic reactions. *Emotion* 9, 316–328. doi: 10.1037/a0015369

Ekman, P. (1992). Are there basic emotions? *Psychol. Rev.* 99, 550–553. doi: 10.1037/0033-295X.99.3.550

Ekman, P., Levenson, R. W., and Friesen, W. V. (1983). Autonomic nervous system activity distinguishes among emotions. *Science* 221, 1208–1210. doi: 10.1126/science.6612338

Etzel, J. A., Johnsen, E. L., Dickerson, J., Tranel, D., and Adolphs, R. (2006). Cardiovascular and respiratory responses during musical mood induction. *Int. J. Psychophysiol.* 61, 57–69. doi: 10.1016/j.ijpsycho.2005.10.025

Ferdenzi, C., Roberts, S. C., Schirmer, A., Delplanque, S., Cekic, S., Porcherot, C., et al. (2013). Variability of affective responses to odors: culture, gender, and olfactory knowledge. *Chem. Senses* 38, 175–186. doi: 10.1093/chemse/bjs083

Ferdenzi, C., Schirmer, A., Roberts, S. C., Delplanque, S., Porcherot, C., Cayeux, I., et al. (2011). Affective dimensions of odor perception: a comparison between Swiss, British, and Singaporean populations. *Emotion* 11, 1168–1181. doi: 10.1037/a0022853

Fowles, D. C., Christie, M. J., Edelberg, R., Grings, W. W., Lykken, D. T., and Venables, P. H. (1981). Committee report. Publication recommendations for electrodermal measurements. *Psychophysiology* 18, 232–239. doi: 10.1111/j.1469-8986.1981.tb03024.x

Friedman, B. H. (2010). Feelings and the body: the Jamesian perspective on autonomic specificity of emotion. *Biol. Psychol.* 84, 383–393. doi: 10.1016/j.biopsycho.2009.10.006

Goddard, L., Pring, L., and Felmingham, N. (2005). The effects of cue modality on the quality of personal memories retrieved. *Memory* 13, 79–86. doi: 10.1080/09658210344000594

Hosey, L. (2013 October 27). Scent and the city. *The New York Times*. (Accessed January 14, 2014).

Hummel, T., Sekinger, B., Wolf, S. R., Pauli, E., and Kobal, G. (1997). "Sniffin" sticks': olfactory performance assessed by the combined testing of odour identification, odor discrimination and olfactory threshold. *Chem. Senses* 22, 39–52. doi: 10.1093/chemse/22.1.39

Inoue, N., Kuroda, K., Sugimoto, A., Kakuda, T., and Fushiki, T. (2003). Autonomic nervous responses according to preference for the odor of jasmine tea. *Biosci. Biotechnol. Biochem.* 67, 1206–1214. doi: 10.1271/bbb.67.1206

Jellinek, J. S. (1997). Psychodynamic odor effects and their mechanisms. *Cosmet. Toiletries* 112, 61–71.

Koenig, S., and Mecklinger, A. (2008). Electrophysiological correlates of encoding and retrieving emotional events. *Emotion* 8, 162–173. doi: 10.1037/1528-3542.8.2.162

Kreibig, S. D. (2010). Autonomic nervous system activity in emotion: a review. *Biol. Psychol.* 84, 394–421. doi: 10.1016/j.biopsycho.2010.03.010

Levenson, R. W. (2003). "Autonomic specificity and emotion," in *Handbook of Affective Sciences*, eds R. J. Davidson, K. R. Scherer, and H. H. Goldsmith (New York, NY: Oxford University Press), 212–224.

Moller, P., and Dijksterhuis, G. (2003). Differential human electrodermal responses to odours. *Neurosci. Lett.* 346, 129–132. doi: 10.1016/S0304-3940(03)00498-1

Olofsson, J. K., Rogalski, E., Harrison, T., Mesulam, M.-M., and Gottfried, J. A. (2013). A cortical pathway to olfactory naming: evidence from primary progressive aphasia. *Brain* 136, 1245–1259. doi: 10.1093/brain/awt019

Robin, O., Alaoui-Ismaili, O., Dittmar, A., and Vernet-Maury, E. (1999). Basic emotions evoked by eugenol odor differ according to the dental experience. A neurovegetative analysis. *Chem. Senses* 24, 327–335. doi: 10.1093/chemse/24.3.327

Rousmans, S., Robin, O., Dittmar, A., and Vernet-Maury, E. (2000). Autonomic nervous system responses associated with primary tastes. *Chem. Senses* 25, 709–718. doi: 10.1093/chemse/25.6.709

Sarrami, N., Pemberton, M. N., Thornhill, M. H., and Theaker, E. D. (2002). Adverse reactions associated with the use of eugenol in dentistry. *Br. Dent. J.* 193, 253–255. doi: 10.1038/sj.bdj.4801539

Schandry, R. (1989). *Lehrbuch der Psychophysiologie.* Weinheim: Psychologie Verlags Union.

Sequeira, H., Hot, P., Silvert, L., and Delplanque, S. (2009). Electrical autonomic correlates of emotion. *Int. J. Psychophysiol.* 71, 50–56. doi: 10.1016/j.ijpsycho.2008.07.009

Stephens, C. L., Christie, I. C., and Friedman, B. H. (2010). Autonomic specificity of basic emotions: evidence from pattern classification and cluster analysis. *Biol. Psychol.* 84, 463–473. doi: 10.1016/j.biopsycho.2010.03.014

Stern, R. M., Ray, W. J., and Quigley, K. S. (2001). *Psychophysiological Recording.* Oxford: University Press.

Vernet-Maury, E., Alaoui-Ismaili, O., Dittmar, A., Delhomme, G., and Chanel, J. (1999). Basic emotions induced by odorants: a new approach based on autonomic pattern results. *J. Auton. Nerv. Syst.* 75, 176–183. doi: 10.1016/S0165-1838(98)00168-4

Weber, S. T., and Heuberger, E. (2008). The impact of natural odors on affective states in humans. *Chem. Senses* 33, 441–447. doi: 10.1093/chemse/bjn011

Weber, S. T., and Heuberger, E. (2011). "Smell and be well—influence of ambient odors on basic emotions and affect," in *Senses and the City: An Interdisciplinary Approach to Urban Sensescapes*, eds M. Diaconu, E. Heuberger, R. Mateus-Berr, and L. M. Vosicky (Vienna: Lit Verlag), 165–188.

Willander, J., and Larsson, M. (2007). Olfaction and emotion: the case of autobiographical memory. *Mem. Cognit.* 35, 1659–1663. doi: 10.3758/BF03193499

13

Olfactory LOVER: behavioral and neural correlates of autobiographical odor memory

Maria Larsson[1,2] *, Johan Willander[2], Kristina Karlsson[2] and Artin Arshamian[1,2]

[1] Gösta Ekman Laboratory, Department of Psychology, Stockholm University, Stockholm, Sweden
[2] Department of Psychology, Stockholm University, Stockholm, Sweden

***Correspondence:**
Maria Larsson, Gösta Ekman Laboratory, Department of Psychology, Stockholm University, Frescati Hagväg 9A, 106 91 Stockholm, Sweden
e-mail: marlar@psychology.su.se

Autobiographical memories (AMs) are personally experienced events that may be localized in time and space. In the present work we present an overview targeting memories evoked by the sense of smell. Overall, research indicates that autobiographical odor memory is different than memories evoked by our primary sensory systems; sight, and hearing. Here, observed differences from a behavioral and neuroanatomical perspective are presented. The key features of an olfactory evoked AM may be referred to the LOVER acronym—**L**imbic, **O**ld, **V**ivid, **E**motional, and **R**are.

Keywords: autobiographical memory, odor, smell, neuroanatomy, experience, applied psychology

Autobiographical memories (AMs) are personally experienced events that may be localized in time and space (Conway and Pleydell-Pearce, 2000). In general, knowledge regarding AM function is well documented, although most of the evidence is based on recollections following a verbal cuing. However, during the past decade a number of studies have targeted memories cued by the sense of smell (e.g., Chu and Downes, 2000; Larsson and Willander, 2009; Zucco et al., 2012). The bulk of this research indicates that olfactory evoked AM differ from memories evoked by our primary senses; sight, and hearing. In particular, odor-evoked AM are older, more emotional, vivid, and relatively rare. The main aim of the present paper is to provide an overview regarding the observed differences from a behavioral and neuroanatomical perspective and to discuss potential applications of this knowledge. Also, the key features of an olfactory evoked AM – **L**imbic, **O**ld, **V**ivid, **E**motional, and **R**are are referred to the acronym LOVER.

RETRIEVAL MODES IN AUTOBIOGRAPHICAL MEMORY

Autobiographical memories may be assessed differently depending on the research question. The most common method is the Galton–Crovitz method where individuals are given unimodal cues (e.g., words, pictures, or sounds) and asked to retrieve an AM for each cue (Crovitz and Schiffman, 1974). With successful retrieval, a short description of the event is provided along with ratings of experiential factors (e.g., vividness of the evoked memory, emotionality) of the recollected event. Typically, when all cues have been presented, the participant is asked to go back to each evoked event and date it (i.e., to indicate the age-at-event).

Evidence suggests that different retrieval strategies influence event selection and the age distribution of events (Conway and Pleydell-Pearce, 2000). Two modes of retrieval have been suggested: generative or direct (Moscovitch, 1995; Conway and Pleydell-Pearce, 2000; Conway, 2005). In generative retrieval, autobiographical information is validated in relation to an event description and the search process is intentional, iterative, and elaborative. In contrast, in direct retrieval, a cue activates a pattern of highly associated autobiographical information, resulting in an immediate and effortless recollection. Thus, selection is bypassed in the direct retrieval mode. It has been suggested that highly perceptual cues (e.g., odors) more often result in a direct recollection, whereas verbal information activate generative search strategies. Recent work has highlighted the functional neuroanatomy of direct and search oriented retrieval modes for autobiographical olfactory memories cued by odors and words (Arshamian et al., 2013). This study documented that both verbal and olfactory cues activated brain areas typically associated with retrieval of AM in general by recruiting prefrontal regions (e.g., dorsolateral prefrontal cortex), medial temporal lobe regions (e.g., parahippocampus), superior and middle temporal areas, fusiform gyrus, occipital areas, and the cerebellum (for reviews see, Svoboda et al., 2006; Cabeza and St Jacques, 2007). However, as compared to olfactory cues, the verbal cuing resulted in a substantially extended prefrontal activity where the right anterior prefrontal cortex, bilateral dorsolateral prefrontal cortex, middle frontal gyrus activation, and the left inferior frontal gyrus were recruited. These activations most likely reflect an increment of strategic retrieval demands induced by verbal labels as compared to odor cues that mapped directly on the olfactory memory representation (Conway and Pleydell-Pearce, 2000). In a related vein, Willander and Larsson (2007) reported that also the age distribution of memories might be affected by retrieval strategy. Here, the AMs triggered by olfactory information was localized in an earlier bump location (i.e., in childhood years) that may reflect an immediate recollection that bypass the retrieval selection process, whereas additional semantic information on the same odor cues resulted in a bump spanning both childhood and young adult age years, that may reflect a stimulation of a generative search process (cf. Conway and Pleydell-Pearce, 2000).

THE LOVER ACRONYM OF AUTOBIOGRAPHICAL ODOR MEMORY

As noted above, evidence shows that olfactory evoked personal information is different from information evoked by the primary senses. Below follows a description of the key features that differentiate odor-evoked AM from that triggered by other modalities. In the present work, these core features are referred to the acronym LOVER—**L**imbic, **O**ld, **V**ivid, **E**motional, and **R**are (see **Figure 1**).

LIMBIC ACTIVATIONS

The sense of smell is characterized by a unique intimacy with the limbic system, where amygdala is located only one synapse away from the olfactory receptors. Moreover its extended neural network involves a large portion of the limbic and paralimbic cortices, including piriform cortex, amygdala and entorhinal cortices (Gottfried, 2010). In the first neuroimaging study of AM targeting odors, Herz et al. (2004) asked five participants whether they could recall a positive memory in which both the sight and scent of a perfume occurred. Later the participants were presented with the odors and pictures of the recollected perfumes in the fMRI while intentionally retrieving the memories. The results showed that odor cued memories were related to stronger activations in the amygdala and hippocampal regions than picture cued recollections. Arshamian et al. (2013) demonstrated that alongside amygdala and hippocampus, odor-evoked AMs also activated the limbic and paralimbic cortices of piriform cortex and entorhinal cortex and an extended limbic network (Morgane et al., 2005) including parahippocampus, insular cortex, and the orbitofrontal cortex.

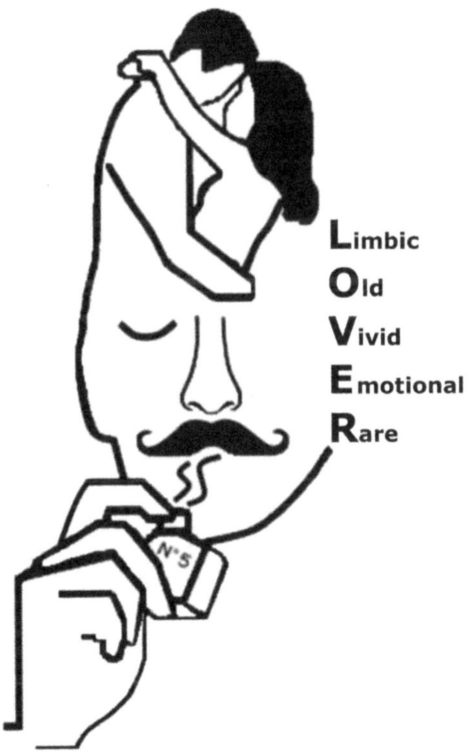

FIGURE 1 | Illustration of the acronym olfactory LOVER covering the core features of an autobiographical memory evoked by olfactory information. Memories triggered by the sense of smell rely on the integrity of the **L**imbicsystem and are typically **O**ld, more **V**ivid, often **E**motional, and relatively **R**are as compared to autobiographical information evoked by our primary sensory systems.

OLD MEMORIES

It is well documented that the age distribution of memories evoked by verbal information follows a distinct pattern involving three main components: the childhood amnesia, the bump, and recency. Childhood amnesia reflects the dramatic reduction of memories reported from early childhood. In contrast, a significantly larger number of memories are recalled from the ages of 10–30, a phenomenon that has been termed the bump. The third component, recency, reflects better retention of events occurring from the last years (Rubin, 1982). In the past decade, a number of studies have focused on the age distribution of odor-evoked memories. The overall results from these studies indicate that olfactory evoked autobiographical information is ontogenetically older than memories evoked by visual, auditory, and verbal information (Chu and Downes, 2002; Willander and Larsson, 2006, 2007; Willander et al., submitted). Specifically, the bump or the clustering of memories is localized to childhood that is the first decade of life (<10 years). Hence, distinct autobiographical episodes involving olfactory information are formed early in life than those comprising verbal and visual information. This observation supports research showing that associative odor learning begins very early in life, with events and experiences that may become accessible in old age through exposure to event-congruent olfactory information (Yeshurun et al., 2009). Targeting the neural correlates of olfactory evoked AM, Arshamian et al. (2013) investigated a group of adults with olfactory evoked AM. A comparison between evoked AMs from childhood (i.e., 3–10 years) and young adulthood (i.e., 11–20 years) revealed differences in brain activity. Specifically, odor memories derived from childhood were related to a stronger activity in the secondary olfactory cortex (i.e., orbitofrontal cortex), whereas olfactory evoked memories clustered in young adulthood were related to a more pronounced activity in the left inferior frontal gyrus, a brain region that supports semantic memory processing. Speculatively, it may be hypothesized that olfactory representations involved in the formation of AM initially may be more perceptually and imagery based, that with increasing age gradually shift to a more semantically driven consolidation.

VIVID RECOLLECTIONS

Odor-evoked AM also differ with regard to phenomenology. A typical finding is that odor-evoked events are accompanied by stronger feelings of being brought back in time to the occurrence of the events (Herz et al., 2004; Willander and Larsson, 2006). Also, Chu and Downes (2002) highlighted that olfactory cued memories evoked more vivid and detailed memories than representations evoked by other sensory modalities. Targeting aversive memories, Toffolo et al. (2012) reported that odor-evoked memories of aversive events were more detailed than memories evoked by auditory but not visual cues. Interestingly, mimicking experiential evidence, also the functional neuroanatomy of olfactory AM indicate that brain areas involved in visual vividness such as occipital gyrus and precuneus are recruited during recollection, activation patterns that were more pronounced than for a verbal cuing (Arshamian et al., 2013). It is also worth noting that experiences of vividness have been linked to emotion such that high vividness is associated with increased emotionality (Todd et al., 2013). Hence, the heightened vividness experience in olfactory AM may relate to the typical emotional potency associated with odor-evoked memory recollection.

EMOTIONAL EXPERIENCE

The olfactory sense is an emotional system (Lundström et al., 2010). Given that the olfactory nerves project directly to the amygdala complex, it has been proposed that odor-evoked AM are more emotional than memories cued by other modalities. Indeed, most studies suggest an emotional advantage of olfactory evoked AM over verbally and visually evoked memories (Herz and Cupchik, 1992; Herz, 1998; Larsson and Willander, 2009; but see Willander and Larsson, 2006; Toffolo et al., 2012; for different outcomes). In a recent study, Arshamian et al. (2013) explored the neural correlates of olfactory cued AM in an fMRI paradigm. The same odor-evoked memory was cued by either verbal or olfactory information. As compared to a verbal cue, an olfactory cued retrieval resulted in more activity in medial temporal lobe regions (e.g., parahippocampus, insula) and in the temporal poles. The latter activation is of particular interest as the temporal poles have been associated with positive memory processing (Piefke et al., 2003) that also was manifested among participants at the experiential level.

RARE OCCURENCE

In anecdotes, it is often stated that odors act as common reminders of past experiences than other types of stimuli. However, a review of the empirical evidence indicates the opposite, namely that odor cues produce fewer memories and are associated with longer response latencies (Rubin et al., 1984; Goddard et al., 2005; Willander and Larsson, 2007; Willander et al., submitted). These findings suggest that odors may be less efficient reminders of past experiences than verbal or visual information. It has been proposed that cue specificity may underlie this discrepancy. Odors are more specific cues than verbal or pictorial information. As a consequence, odors will match fewer representations than more generic cues such as words or pictures. Indeed, research shows that if semantic information is provided with the odor cue (i.e., the odor identity) or when the odor is identified, more memories will be retrieved (Willander and Larsson, 2007; Yamamoto, 2008).

Relatedly, it is of interest to highlight that memories evoked by the olfactory sense in general have been thought about less often than memories evoked by other sensory cues (Rubin et al., 1984; Willander and Larsson, 2006). The implicit nature of olfactory representations and the low frequency of AMs probably underlie the experienced "suddenness" of an odor-evoked memory that may bias the notion of its powerfulness.

UNIMODAL vs. MULTIMODAL CUING OF AUTOBIOGRAPHICAL ODOR MEMORIES

Almost all of the knowledge on odor-evoked AM is based on unimodal cuing, where an individual is presented to one odor and is subsequently asked to retrieve any personal associated information for that specific smell that may be defined in space and time. As noted, the results from this research indicate that odor-evoked AM are different from information triggered by verbal, visual, or auditory information. The observed differences are documented both at a behavioral and a neural level (e.g., Willander and Larsson, 2006; Arshamian et al., 2013; Karlsson et al., 2013; Willander et al., submitted).

A unimodal retrieval procedure (i.e., cues pertaining to one modality) entails that sensory information from different modalities is treated as separate entities rather than as a component of integrated multimodal representations. An important research question recently raised is therefore to determine the relative influence and hierarchy among modalities that are represented in a multimodal cue on the recollection of olfactory information (Karlsson et al., 2013; Willander et al., submitted).

Willander and Larsson (2007) indirectly addressed bimodal cues when individuals were asked to retrieve AM following single odors or odors presented in conjunction with their respective names. The results showed that semantic knowledge of an odor's name affected the age distribution such that the memory peak in childhood observed for only odors was attenuated. Specifically, the peak took an intermediate position between the age distributions obtained for verbal cuing and odor cuing only. Also, semantic knowledge of the odors resulted in that the experiential factors (emotionality, brought back in time) mimicked a verbal cuing of AM. Hence, this outcome indicated that the age and phenomenology of memories vary with the number and types of cues available at retrieval.

In this vein, it is of interest to highlight results from a recent study that targeted multimodal retrieval of AM (Willander et al., submitted). Here, participants were randomized across three unimodal (pictures, sounds, odors) and one multimodal condition (picture + sound + odor). To maximize ecological validity, cues from the three unimodal conditions were presented simultaneously, whereas in the unimodal conditions cues were presented separately. The unimodal cues were selected so that they could be combined into a multimodal naturalistic context. For example, the context harbor was represented by a photo of a harbor by the sea containing fishing boats; sounds from fishing boats, sea birds, sea waves; and the smell of fresh fish. The results indicated that the number of olfactory evoked memories were fewer than the number of memories evoked by visually and multimodally presented cues. The unimodal cuing of AM replicated previous findings by showing a significant clustering of odor memories in childhood, and peaks of memories following visual and auditory cuing in young adulthood (e.g., Larsson and Willander, 2009). As noted, the analysis of the evoked memories following a multimodal cuing indicated a significant clustering of memories in young adulthood, mimicking that observed for our primary sensory systems. Also, modeling of the semantic content of the retrieved memories indicated that the multimodal content differed from odor-evoked content but not from visual content (Karlsson et al.,

2013). Hence, these results suggest a hierarchy among modalities represented in multimodal cue information, and that the subordinate role that is played by the sense of smell may underlie the rare occurrence of odor-evoked AMs (Posner et al., 1976; Sinnett et al., 2007).

This outcome supports the notion of visual cue dominance in multimodal contexts. One important question in future research is to determine the role played by modality attention in multimodal settings.

APPLIED POSSIBILITIES OF ODOR-EVOKED AUTOBIOGRAPHICAL INFORMATION

The literature on potential applications of olfactory AMs is scarce and portrays a mixed pattern of findings. Greenberg et al. (2011) examined whether odors could be used as memory cues to promote memory recollection in patients with semantic dementia. The results showed that odor cues were less effective reminders of past experiences than were verbal and visual cues. This was most likely a reflection of the early degeneration of anterior temporal regions in the dementia process, as the same regions also are fundamental for the integrity of the olfactory system. Other research has highlighted that autonomic functions are affected by AM. For example, Masaoka et al. (2012) demonstrated that odors that evoked AMs lowered the respiratory frequency as compared to odors that were unrelated to memory evocation. Likewise, Matsunaga et al. (2011) reported a decrease in heart rate, and an increase in skin-conductance following odor-evoked AMs. For example, Matsunaga et al. (2011) showed that immune responses associated with systemic inflammation could be inhibited by odor-evoked AMs. Further, Matsunaga et al. (2013) demonstrated that these immune responses were negatively correlated with activations in orbitofrontal cortex, precuneus, and the posterior cingulate cortex as determined by PET. This could indicate that inhibition of inflammatory mechanisms decrease as a function of the vividness and emotionality of the evoked memories (c.f. Arshamian et al., 2013).

Interestingly, individual differences in mood and personality traits have been found to interact with odor-evoked AM. For example, Masaoka et al. (2012) reported that participants who where high in trait anxiety experienced stronger feelings of being brought back in time to the occurrence of the event, and showed increments in arousal level during retrieval of odor-evoked AMs. Also, Matsunaga et al. (2011) reported that odor-evoked AMs that were associated with positive emotions increased positive mood states, such as comfort and happiness, and decreased negative mood states, such as anxiety. Moreover, Reid et al. (2014) studied experiences of nostalgia in the context of odors. They demonstrated that participants reported most nostalgia when the odors were arousing, familiar, and evoked AMs. Furthermore, odors that only evoked nostalgia induced more positive emotions than both non-nostalgic odors that evoked AMs, and those that did not. Participants that were generally more prone to nostalgia reported more odor-evoked nostalgia, but not more autobiographical events. Taken together, the research cited above suggests that olfactory evocation of autobiographical information has the potential to affect our autonomic functions and emotional state.

AUTHOR CONTRIBUTIONS

Maria Larsson and Artin Arshamian jointly prepared the manuscript. Maria Larsson, Artin Arshamian, Johan Willander, and Kristina Karlsson wrote the manuscript. Artin Arshamian made the illustration.

ACKNOWLEDGMENT

This work was supported by a grant from the Swedish Research Council to Maria Larsson.

REFERENCES

Arshamian, A., Iannilli, E., Gerber, J. C., Willander, J., Persson, J., Seo, H. S., et al. (2013). The functional neuroanatomy of odor evoked autobiographical memories cued by odors and words. *Neuropsychologia* 51, 123–131. doi: 10.1016/j.neuropsychologia.2012.10.023

Cabeza, R., and St Jacques, P. (2007). Functional neuroimaging of autobiographical memory. *Trends Cogn. Sci.* 11, 219–227. doi: 10.1016/j.tics.2007.02.005

Chu, S., and Downes, J. J. (2000). Odour-evoked autobiographical memories: psychological investigations of proustian phenomena. *Chem. Senses* 25, 111–116. doi: 10.1093/chemse/25.1.111

Chu, S., and Downes, J. J. (2002). Proust nose best: odors are better cues of autobiographical memory. *Mem. Cognit.* 30, 511–518. doi: 10.3758/BF03194952

Conway, M. A. (2005). Memory and the self. *J. Mem. Lang.* 53, 594–628. doi: 10.1016/j.jml.2005.08.005

Conway, M. A., and Pleydell-Pearce, C. W. (2000). The construction of autobiographical memories in the self-memory system. *Psychol. Rev.* 107, 261–288. doi: 10.1037/0033-295 X.107.2.261

Crovitz, H. F., and Schiffman, H. (1974). Frequency of episodic memories as a function of their age. *Bull. Psychon. Soc.* 4, 517–518. doi: 10.3758/BF03334277

Goddard, L., Pring, L., and Felmingham, N. (2005). The effects of cue modality on the quality of personal memories retrieved. *Memory* 13, 79–86. doi: 10.1080/09658210344000594

Gottfried, J. A. (2010). Central mechanisms of odour object perception. *Nat. Rev. Neurosci.* 11, 628–641. doi: 10.1038/nrn2883

Greenberg, D. L., Ogar, J. M., Viskontas, I. V., Gorno Tempini, M. L., Miller, B., and Knowlton, B. J. (2011). Multimodal cuing of autobiographical memory in semantic dementia. *Neuropsychology* 25, 98–104. doi: 10.1037/a0021005

Herz, R. S. (1998). Are odors the best cues to memory? A cross-modal comparison of associative memory stimuli. *Ann. N. Y. Acad. Sci.* 855, 670–674. doi: 10.1111/j.1749-6632.1998.tb10643.x

Herz, R. S., and Cupchik, G. C. (1992). An experimental characterization of odor-evoked memories in humans. *Chem. Senses* 17, 519–528. doi: 10.1093/chemse/17.5.519

Herz, R. S., Eliassen, J., Beland, S. L., and Souza, T. (2004). Neuroimaging evidence for the emotional potency of odor-evoked memories. *Neuropsychologia* 42, 371–378. doi: 10.1016/j.neuropsychologia.2003.08.009

Karlsson, K., Sikström, S., and Willander, J. (2013). The semantic representation of event information depends on the cue modality: an instance of meaning-based retrieval. *PLoS ONE* 8:e73378. doi: 10.1371/journal.pone.0073378

Larsson, M., and Willander, J. (2009). Autobiographical odor memory. *Ann. N. Y. Acad. Sci.* 1170, 318–323. doi: 10.1111/j.1749-6632.2009.03934.x

Lundström, J. N., Boesveldt, S., and Albrecht, J. (2010). Central processing of the chemical senses: an overview. *ACS Chem. Neurosci.* 2, 5–16. doi: 10.1021/cn1000843

Masaoka, Y., Sugiyama, H., Katayama, A., Kashiwagi, M., and Homma, I. (2012). Slow breathing and emotions associated with odor-induced autobiographical memories. *Chem. Senses* 37, 379–88. doi: 10.1093/chemse/bjr120

Matsunaga, M., Bai, Y., Yamakawa, K., Toyama, A., Kashiwagi, M., Fukuda, K., et al. (2013). Brain–immune interaction accompanying odor-evoked autobiographic memory. *PLoS ONE* 8:e72523. doi: 10.1371/journal.pone.0072523

Matsunaga, M., Isowa, T., Yamakawa, K., Kawanishi, Y., Tsuboi, H., Kaneko, H., et al. (2011). Psychological and physiological responses to odor-evoked autobiographic memory. *Neuro. Endocrinol. Lett.* 32, 774–780.

Morgane, P. J., Galler, J. R., and Mokler, D. J. (2005). A review of systems and networks of the limbic forebrain/limbic midbrain. *Prog. Neurobiol.* 75, 143–160. doi: 10.1016/j.pneurobio.2005.01.001

Moscovitch, M. (1995). Recovered consciousness: a hypothesis concerning modularity and episodic memory. *J. Clin. Exp. Neuropsychol.* 17, 276–290. doi: 10.1080/01688639508405123

Piefke, M., Weiss, P. H., Zilles, K., Markowitsch, H. J., and Fink, G. R. (2003). Differential remoteness and emotional tone modulate the neural correlates of autobiographical memory. *Brain* 126, 650–668. doi: 10.1093/brain/awg064

Posner, M. I., Nissen, M. J., and Klein, R. M. (1976). Visual dominance: an information-processing account of its origins and significance. *Psychol. Rev.* 83, 157–171. doi: 10.1037/0033-295X.83.2.157

Reid, C. A., Green, J. D., Wildschut, T., and Sedikides, C. (2014). Scent-evoked nostalgia. *Memory* 1–10. doi: 10.1080/09658211.2013.876048 [Epub ahead of print].

Rubin, D. C. (1982). On the retention function for autobiographical memory. *J. Verbal Learning Verbal Behav.* 21, 21–38. doi: 10.1016/S0022-5371(82)90423-90426.

Rubin, D. C., Groth, E., and Goldsmith, D. J. (1984). Olfactory cuing of autobiographical memory. *Am. J. Psychol.* 97, 493–507. doi: 10.2307/1422158

Sinnett, S., Spence, C., and Soto-Faraco, S. (2007). Visual dominance and attention: the colavita effect revisited. *Percept. Psychophys.* 69, 673–686. doi: 10.3758/BF03193770

Svoboda, E., McKinnon, M. C., and Levine, B. (2006). The functional neuroanatomy of autobiographical memory: a meta-analysis. *Neuropsychologia* 44, 2189–2208. doi: 10.1016/j.neuropsychologia.2006.05.023

Todd, R. M., Schmitz, T. W., Susskind, J., and Anderson, A. K. (2013). Shared neural substrates of emotionally enhanced perceptual and mnemonic vividness. *Front. Behav. Neurosci.* 7:40. doi: 10.3389/fnbeh.2013.00040

Toffolo, M. B., Smeets, M. A., and van den Hout, M. A. (2012). Proust revisited: odours as triggers of aversive memories. *Cogn. Emot.* 26, 83–92. doi: 10.1080/02699931.2011.555475

Willander, J., and Larsson, M. (2006). Smell your way back to childhood: autobiographical odor memory. *Psychon. Bull. Rev.* 13, 240–244. doi: 10.3758/BF03193837

Willander, J., and Larsson, M. (2007). Olfaction and emotion: the case of autobiographical memory. *Mem. Cognit.* 35, 1659–1663. doi: 10.3758/BF03193499

Yamamoto, K. (2008). Influence of odor cueing on the retrieval processes for autobiographical memories. *Shinrigaku Kenkyu* 79, 159–165. doi: 10.4992/jjpsy.79.159

Yeshurun, Y., Lapid, H., Dudai, Y., and Sobel, N. (2009). The privileged brain representation of first olfactory associations. *Curr. Biol.* 19, 1869–1874. doi: 10.1016/j.cub.2009.09.066

Zucco, G. M., Aiello, L., Turuani, L., and Koster, E. (2012). Odor-evoked autobiographical memories: age and gender differences along the life span. *Chem. Senses* 37, 179–189. doi: 10.1093/chemse/bjr089

14

Pregnancy and olfaction

E. Leslie Cameron*

Department of Psychological Science, Carthage College, Kenosha, WI, USA

Correspondence:
E. Leslie Cameron, Department of Psychological Science, Carthage College, 2001 Alford Park Drive, Kenosha, WI 53140, USA
e-mail: lcameron@carthage.edu

Many women report a heightened sense of smell during pregnancy. Accounts of these anecdotes have existed for over 100 years, but scientific evidence has been sparse and inconclusive. In this review, I examine the literature on olfactory perception during pregnancy including measures of self-report, olfactory thresholds, odor identification, intensity and hedonic ratings, and disgust. Support for a general decrease in olfactory thresholds (increase in sensitivity) is generally lacking. There is limited evidence that some suprathreshold measures of olfactory perception, such as hedonic ratings of odors, are affected by pregnancy, but these effects are idiosyncratic. In this review, I explore the hypotheses that have been put forth to explain changes in olfactory perception during pregnancy and provide suggestions for further research.

Keywords: self report, odor identification, threshold, hedonics, pregnancy sickness, hormones, hyperosmia, hyperreactivity

INTRODUCTION

Anecdotal reports of heightened sense of smell during pregnancy are common, and the majority of pregnant women report increased olfactory sensitivity (Nordin et al., 2004; Cameron, 2007, 2014). However, the scientific literature on this topic is rather limited and inconclusive. Heightened sense of smell in pregnancy is an important topic because it has been hypothesized to be a trigger for nausea and vomiting (Erick, 1995; Heinrichs, 2002) and an evolutionary mechanism has been proposed – namely that increased olfactory sensitivity protects the developing embryo by reducing the likelihood that the mother will ingest toxins (Steiner, 1922; Profet, 1992). In this review, I summarize the literature on pregnancy and olfaction in humans and explore the possible mechanisms that could underlie the changes women often notice in their perception of odors during pregnancy.

SELF-REPORTED CHANGE IN SENSE OF SMELL DURING PREGNANCY

The most consistent source of evidence that the sense of smell of women changes during pregnancy comes from anecdotal reports and questionnaire studies. It is clear from perusing websites, reading popular books on pregnancy, and from discussions with pregnant women, that *something* in the perception of odors changes during pregnancy[1]. As early as 1895, Zwaardemaker documented that self-reported hyperosmia is common in pregnancy, although he also noted that empirical measurements of this phenomenon were lacking (Zwaardemaker, 1895). Steiner (1922) reported that almost all pregnant women report a stronger sense of smell, usually in the early months of pregnancy and particularly in the first pregnancy. Henssge (1930) described a case study in which a 27-year-old pregnant woman reported that her olfactory "sensitivity increased" and that odors that were "normally imperceptible were now unbearable." Henssge (1930) indicated, in that report, that he encountered frequent cases of such "hypersensitivity" in the early phases of pregnancy and although no psychophysical measurements were made, he stated that "Beyond doubt, the patients experienced these odors in response to genuine stimuli which were imperceptible to normal people"[2].

According to two more recent studies, approximately two-thirds of pregnant women rate their sense of smell as higher than normal (Cameron, 2007) or as abnormally sensitive (Nordin et al., 2004). A third study also found pregnant women to rate their sense of smell as more sensitive compared to controls, particularly later in pregnancy and even in the postpartum period (Ochsenbein-Kölble et al., 2007). Cameron (2007) found that 85% of pregnant women ($n = 60$) identified at least one odor to which they were more sensitive and Nordin et al. (2004) reported that, relative to non-pregnant women ($n = 76$), more of the pregnant women ($n = 144$) reported "stronger-than-normal smell sensation" of particular odors, including cooking odors, cigarette smoke, spoiled food, perfumes, spices, and coffee. This was particularly evident early in pregnancy. In a subsequent study using the Chemical Sensitivity Scale for Sensory Hypersensitivity (Nordin et al., 2003), Nordin et al. (2007) found self-reported hyperosmia (defined as "increased odor sensitivity during the past month compared to what is normal to that individual" p. 340) in pregnant women ($n = 95$) to be specific to a set of odors, such as cigarettes, prepared or spoiled food, coffee, gasoline, and perfumes.

While the preponderance of self-reports appear to reflect olfactory hypersensitivity, it should be noted that not all studies have found increased self-reported olfactory hypersensitivity in pregnancy. In fact, one early case study described a 25-year-old

[1]A sample blog post: ...*But there have been some changes [in pregnancy]. Namely, smell. I smell everything to an acute degree bordering on insanity. Let me clarify that. I smell everything bad and it's making me feel like a crazy woman! I smell garbage, gas, poo, chickens, old eggs, stinky breath, dirty sheets. But flowers and nice perfume? Nah, can't smell that.* (From http://www.rurallyscrewed.com).

[2]All quotes from English translation of the abstract.

pregnant woman with asthma who complained of experiencing nearly complete loss of sense of smell (and taste) in early pregnancy, which resolved later in pregnancy (Schmidt, 1925). Moreover, Gilbert and Wysocki (1991) noted in a sample of 13,610 pregnant and 277,228 non-pregnant women who were part of the National Geographic Smell Study, that pregnant women rated their own sense of smell significantly *lower* than non-pregnant women on a 5-point Likert scale. Kölble et al. (2001) reported no significant difference in self-rated sense of smell between 53 pregnant and 59 non-pregnant women. The reason for the disparate data on self-report is unclear, although it does perhaps reflect the idiosyncratic nature of olfaction in general and olfaction during pregnancy in specific.

HYPEROSMIA

Given that olfaction is important for detecting danger and enjoying food as well as for overall quality of life (Deems et al., 1991; Miwa et al., 2001; Hummel and Nordin, 2005), much research has focused on the causes and impact of loss of sense of smell, either hyposmia or anosmia. Relatively less research has explored heightened sense of smell or hyperosmia. But hyperosmia is important because, even if relatively rare, it is thought to be disruptive to normal functioning (e.g., Erick, 1995; Heinrichs, 2002; Nordin et al., 2005).

Hyperosmia refers to the condition in which there is an increase in olfactory sensitivity. Sensitivity is the inverse of threshold, which in the case of olfaction refers to the minimum concentration of an odor required for its detection. Therefore, an *increase* in olfactory sensitivity is equivalent to a *decrease* in the threshold for detection of an odor. Hyperosmia is relatively infrequently reported and true cases may be relatively rare. There are reports based on empirical testing that hyperosmia occurs in patients with temporal lobe epilepsy (Campanella et al., 1978; Grant, 2005), Addison's disease (Henkin and Bartter, 1966), and migraines (Hirsch, 1992). However, these findings are controversial. For example, West and Doty (1995) pointed out that there is considerable inconsistency in the epilepsy literature, Murphy et al. (2003) indicated that replications of the findings for Addison's disease have not been forthcoming and Demarquay et al. (2006) did not find hypersensitivity in patients with migraines. Moreover, patients with specific complaints of "chemical hypersensitivity" have normal olfactory thresholds for those stimuli that have been assessed, namely phenyl ethyl alcohol (PEA, a rose odor) and methyl ethyl ketone (a common solvent; Doty et al., 1988).

It is imperative to stress that most reports of "hyperosmia" or "olfactory hypersensitivity" are anecdotal and lack empirical verification. In light of evidence that self-reported chemosensory function can be unreliable (Nordin et al., 1995; Landis et al., 2003; Soter et al., 2008; Shu et al., 2009) it is important that olfactory sensitivity be measured in cases of suspected hyperosmia. Moreover, what is meant by "heightened sense of smell" or "heightened sensitivity" in the general public may not correspond to the same phenomenon as the hyperosmia defined by olfactory scientists. Steiner (1922) wondered whether the self-reported hypersensitivity might actually be a "subjective" experience.

HYPEROSMIA IN PREGNANCY?

Given that the self-report data suggest the presence of hyperosmia in pregnancy, it is important to distinguish between the measures used to assess olfaction in pregnant women, some of which, at least on the surface, do not appear to measure sensitivity *per se*. In general, it has been assumed that "heightened olfactory sensitivity" or "hyperosmia" refers to reduced olfactory detection thresholds, although this, in fact, need not be the case. This section reviews the literature on olfactory detection and recognition thresholds.

DETECTION THRESHOLDS

Several studies have examined the effect of pregnancy on olfactory detection thresholds. Kölble et al. (2001) found no significant difference in olfactory detection thresholds between non-pregnant women and women in the first trimester of pregnancy[3]. Thresholds were measured with the odor *n*-butanol, which has a window-cleaner like smell, using a staircase procedure in which the target odor had to be selected from triplets of stimuli (two "blanks" and one odorant). Savovic et al. (2002) measured olfactory detection thresholds for six odors, namely anethol (aniseed), vanillin, PEA, citral, menthol, and pyridine (a fishy odor), in 20 non-pregnant and 20 women in their first trimester of pregnancy using the Fortunato–Niccolini air-dilution olfactometer (Caruso et al., 2001). Thresholds were determined by the smallest volume of air, presented during normal inspiration, that resulted in the detection of an odor. There were no significant differences between the detection thresholds of pregnant and non-pregnant women. Laska et al. (1996) measured olfactory detection thresholds longitudinally across all three trimesters and found no significant systematic changes across trimesters, nor between the 20 pregnant and 20 non-pregnant women, although compared to controls, pregnant women's thresholds were significantly higher in the first trimester and significantly lower in the third trimester. Laska et al. (1996) also used the odorant *n*-butanol, but with a single ascending staircase technique. The finding from Laska et al. (1996) is consistent with Good et al. (1976) who, in a case study, found that the number of *false alarms* (responding that the musk-like compound Exaltolide was present when it was not) decreased as the woman came closer to parturition. Therefore, her d' (a measure of sensitivity derived from signal detection theory; see Green and Swets, 1966) was higher in the third than the second trimester. Ochsenbein-Kölble et al. (2007) also showed that olfactory detection thresholds for *n*-butanol decreased over the course of pregnancy in 39 women and were statistically lower in the last trimester and postpartum than that of 45 non-pregnant controls. While the decrease in detection threshold in late pregnancy is consistent with Laska et al. (1996) and Good et al. (1976), the postpartum results are surprising and are not consistent with other reports in the literature on olfactory thresholds in the postpartum period (see Recognition Thresholds). More recently, Cameron (2014) measured detection thresholds for PEA longitudinally across the three trimesters of pregnancy in 23 women and found

---

[3]Sample sizes are reported only once for studies that are discussed in multiple sections of this review. For example, sample sizes for this study were provided in Section "Self-reported Change in Sense of Smell During Pregnancy."

no significant differences in detection threshold between pregnant women and 25 non-pregnant controls. This study employed the standard 1-up, 2-down staircase method, as described by Doty (2000).

The only study in the literature that clearly demonstrated a significant decrease in olfactory detection thresholds in early pregnancy was conducted by Luvara and Murizi (1961). For each of four odors (anise, musk ketone, carnation, and citral), the authors established detection thresholds using the blast-injection technique (Elsberg and Levy, 1935). There were 47 women tested in this study, some of whom were tested twice (in two phases of pregnancy or during pregnancy and postpartum). I have plotted the data, provided only in tabular format in the original article, in **Figure 1**. Doty (1976) previously conducted statistical analyses of these data and reported that all comparisons were significant.

Of particular interest, with respect to the purported heightened sensitivity in early pregnancy, is that there is a significant difference in thresholds between the first trimester and the postpartum period. To my knowledge, this constitutes the only empirical support in the literature for lower olfactory detection thresholds in early pregnancy[4]. However, the blast-injection technique, unlike other measures of threshold, may reflect changes in nasal engorgement in the later stages of pregnancy (see Pregnancy and the Nose).

[4]It is worth noting that two unpublished works (Dastur, 2001; Broman et al., 2003) found decreased odor thresholds in pregnancy. Dastur (2001) reported, in a doctoral dissertation, that detection thresholds for PEA were significantly lower in 19 women tested longitudinally across all trimesters of pregnancy compared to 18 non-pregnant controls and the pregnant women tested in the postpartum period. Broman et al. (2003), in an abstract reported at the Association for Chemoreception Sciences, found decreased thresholds for pyridine (a fishy odor) in 30 women in the second trimester of pregnancy compared to 30 non-pregnant women.

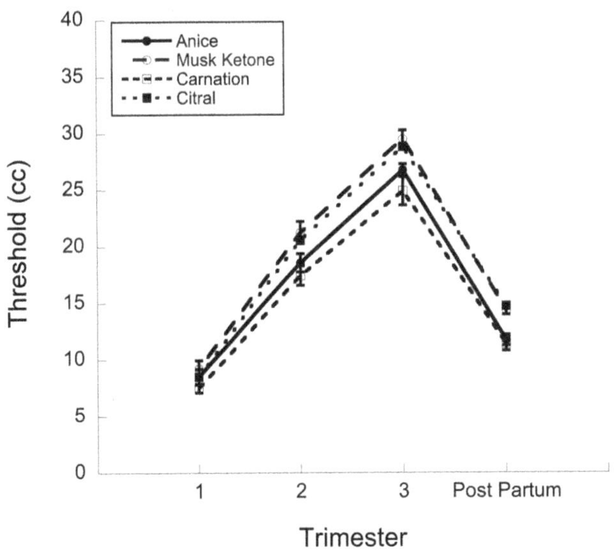

FIGURE 1 | Data from Luvara and Murizi (1961). Threshold (in cubic centimeter, as measured by the blast injection technique) across pregnancy trimester and postpartum. There were a total of 47 participants; 14–21 per session and some participated in more than one session.

It is worthy of note that all of the studies that have measured olfactory detection thresholds in pregnant women have employed validated methods for measuring thresholds; these methods are sensitive to differences in smell function between sexes and age groups (Doty et al., 1984a) and can identify some clinical populations, such as patients with Alzheimer's and Parkinson's (Doty, 2003). Thus, failure to observe changes in olfactory detection thresholds in pregnant women is unlikely due to the method employed. However, some cases of increased sensitivity to odors have been demonstrated using sensitive *signal detection* measures. For example, Doty et al. (1981) used such methods to demonstrate subtle changes in olfactory sensitivity across the menstrual cycle. Cameron (2014) adopted the same method as Doty et al. (1981) to measure olfactory sensitivity in pregnant women. After the assessment of their olfactory detection threshold, participants completed an additional 75 signal detection trials, using an odorant whose concentration was close to the participant's own threshold. On each trial two jars were presented – on half of the trials one of the jars contained the weak PEA odorant ("signal + noise") and the other the diluent alone ("noise") and on the other half of the trials both jars contained the diluent alone ("noise"). In this method, *hits* refer to trials in which the *signal* was present and the participant said it was and *false alarms* refer to trials in which the *signal* was not present but the participant said it was. Hits and false alarms were used to compute d' (sensitivity) and c (response bias)[5]. Cameron (2014) employed this signal detection paradigm, albeit with a smaller number of trials than used by Doty et al. (1981), and still found no significant increase in olfactory sensitivity (i.e., no increase in d') in pregnant women. The data suggest that pregnant women exhibit a more *liberal* criterion (i.e., made more *false alarms*) early in pregnancy, although the difference between pregnant and non-pregnant women was not statistically significant in this small sample. A more liberal criterion would be consistent with the greater number of *false alarms* reported in Good et al.'s (1976) case study.

In summary, there is only limited evidence for decreased in olfactory detection thresholds (hyperosmia) in pregnant women, even using sensitive measures and despite the self-reported increase in sensitivity.

RECOGNITION THRESHOLDS

Two studies have measured olfactory recognition thresholds in pregnant women. Hansen and Glass (1936), using a Zwaardemaker olfactometer and a method of ascending limits, tested 22 women and found that recognition sensitivity was lower at the end of pregnancy compared to two postpartum periods (2–3 days or 2–3 months after delivery) for all three odors tested (rubber, rose oil, and nitrobenzene (bitter almonds)). I have plotted these data in **Figure 2**. Doty (1976) reported that the differences between the thresholds in the two postpartum periods were not statistically significant, but that they were both significantly lower than thresholds at the end of pregnancy.

[5]Sensitivity (d') = Z (hit rate) − Z (false alarm rate); response bias (c) = −0.5 [Z (hit rate) − Z (false alarm rate)].

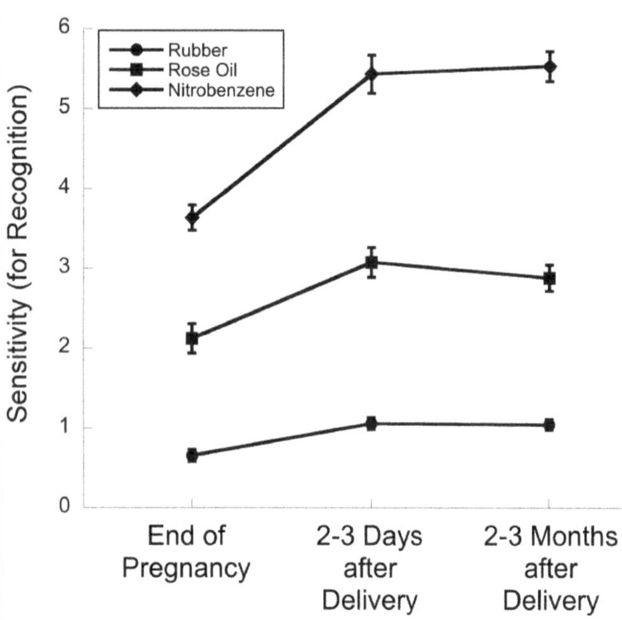

FIGURE 2 | Data from Hansen and Glass (1936). Sensitivity (inverse of threshold) for recognition for each of three odors, plotted for the end of pregnancy and two postpartum test sessions. Zwaardemaker olfactometer was used to measure thresholds of 22 participants who were followed longitudinally.

Noferi and Giudizi (1946) compared recognition thresholds for a lemon odor using the blast-injection technique in a cross-sectional study. **Figure 3** shows that thresholds were significantly higher in 15 women in late pregnancy compared to 15 non-pregnant controls and compared to 15 women who were within 2 weeks postpartum (Doty, 1976). Again, this may be due to the method of testing.

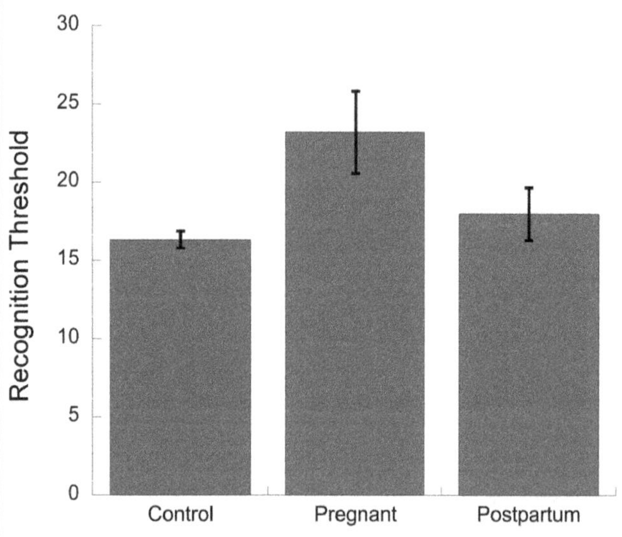

FIGURE 3 | Data from Noferi and Giudizi (1946). Recognition thresholds for non-pregnant, pregnant, and postpartum women. Blast olfactometer was used to determine recognition thresholds for lemon. There were 15 participants per group in a cross-sectional design.

In summary, the data on recognition thresholds suggests that late pregnancy is a period of low sensitivity (recognition thresholds are *high*) relative to the postpartum period. These results are inconsistent with the detection threshold results from Cameron (2014), Good et al. (1976), and Laska et al. (1996) but are consistent with a more recent report of decreased threshold sensitivity in the third trimester compared with controls (Ochsenbein-Kölble et al., 2007, using the same methods as Kölble et al., 2001).

OTHER MEASURES OF SMELL FUNCTION IN PREGNANCY

The inconsistency between the self-reported increased olfactory sensitivity in pregnant women and the lack of evidence of decreased olfactory (detection or recognition) thresholds begs the following questions: How is olfactory processing affected by pregnancy? Do pregnant women outperform non-pregnant women on other olfactory tasks, such as odor identification? And do pregnant women rate the intensity and hedonicity of odors differently than non-pregnant women? This section reviews the literature on the effect of pregnancy on several measures of olfaction other than thresholds.

ODOR IDENTIFICATION

Eight studies have assessed odor identification in pregnant women (Gilbert and Wysocki, 1991; Laska et al., 1996; Kölble et al., 2001; Savovic et al., 2002; Swallow et al., 2005a; Cameron, 2007; Ochsenbein-Kölble et al., 2007; Kim et al., 2011).

Gilbert and Wysocki (1991) compared odor identification in pregnant and non-pregnant women using six odors – isoamyl acetate (banana/pear), eugenol (the primary component of clove oil), rose, a mixture of mercaptans (smell added to natural gas), galaxolide (musky), and androstenone (musky/urine). Participants were instructed to scratch and sniff the odor and then to select one of the following words that best described the odor: no odor, floral, musky, urine, foul, ink, spicy, woody, fruity, burnt, sweet, and other. They found no significant general effect of pregnancy status on odor identification, except that pregnant women were able to identify clove significantly more readily. Laska et al. (1996) examined odor identification for 12 odors: all of the odors employed by Gilbert and Wysocki (1991) except for the mixture of mercaptans, as well as citronelle nitrile (lemon), peanut aroma, Chanel No. 5, anethole, linalool (lavender), n-butanol (described by the authors as oily, alcoholic) and a 12-component mixture. Participants sniffed the odors presented in squeeze bottles and were instructed to generate a name or attempt to describe the odor[6]. Despite different methods, the results were consistent with Gilbert and Wysocki (1991) in that pregnant women outperformed non-pregnant women in identifying eugenol. However, they were *less* able to provide appropriate descriptors or accurate names for peanut, banana, aniseed, and lemon.

Kölble et al. (2001) and Ochsenbein-Kölble et al. (2007) measured odor identification using the 16-item Sniffin' Sticks (odors include orange, peppermint, turpentine, cloves, leather, banana, garlic, rose, fish, lemon, coffee, anise, cinnamon, liquorice,

[6]No information is provided in that paper as to how those data were coded.

apple, and pineapple). Kölble et al. (2001) found that, relative to controls, women in the first trimester of pregnancy tended to perform more poorly and Ochsenbein-Kölble et al. (2007) found no significant change across pregnancy status compared to controls. No data were presented as to the relative ability to identify specific odors. Consistent with these studies, Kim et al. (2011) reported no significant difference between 35 pregnant and 40 non-pregnant women using the Korean Version of the Sniffin' Sticks (KVSS-II test) and Savovic et al. (2002) found no significant difference in odor identification performance of women in their first trimester compared to controls using the Fortunato–Niccolini olfactometer. Swallow et al. (2005a) tested odor identification for six odors (three "safe" – strawberry, vanilla, and melon and three "potentially harmful" – coffee, cabbage, and fish) and found no significant difference in odor identification among three groups – pregnant women ($n = 55$), non-pregnant women ($n = 42$), and men ($n = 48$) – except for the strawberry odor. Non-pregnant women outperformed pregnant women and men, but correct identification overall for strawberry was relatively poor and worse than for other odors (Swallow, personal communication). Finally, Cameron (2007) measured odor identification in pregnant women (20 in each trimester), 20 non-pregnant controls and 20 women in the postpartum period on the 40-item scratch and sniff University of Pennsylvania Smell Identification Test (UPSIT; Doty et al., 1984b) and found no overall effect of pregnancy status on odor identification. However, watermelon was identified significantly better by pregnant women[7].

In summary, odor identification has been explored in pregnant women using a wide range of odors, with several methods, and in a number of different cultural contexts. There is no evidence that pregnant women generally identify odors consistently better than non-pregnant controls. In fact, some studies have even reported a tendency for *worse* performance in pregnancy, at least for some odors (Laska et al., 1996; Kölble et al., 2001; Swallow et al., 2005a). Notwithstanding these negative findings, there is evidence that pregnant women identify some odors better than controls [clove by Gilbert and Wysocki (1991) and Laska et al. (1996); strawberry by Swallow et al. (2005a), and watermelon by Cameron (2007)], suggesting that perhaps there is an improved ability to identify some odors during pregnancy.

INTENSITY RATINGS

Olfactory perception in pregnant women has also been assessed by means of odor intensity ratings. Gilbert and Wysocki (1991) found that two odors (isoamyl acetate and a mixture of mercaptans) of six were rated as significantly more intense by pregnant women compared to controls, but they also found that two other odors (androstenone and galaxolide) were rated as significantly less intense by pregnant women compared to controls. Likewise, Cameron (2007) found that overall there was a trend for pregnant women, compared to controls, to rate odors as more intense in the first trimester (~75% of odors were rated as slightly more intense by pregnant women), but there was a statistically significant increase in intensity ratings for only three (leather, lemon, and natural gas) of 39 UPSIT odors.

Laska et al. (1996) reported that intensity judgments were relatively stable across test sessions and consistent between pregnant and non-pregnant women. Pregnant women rated only two (galaxolide and androstenone) of 12 odors to be statistically significantly more intense, but this was not consistent, nor stable across pregnancy. Kölble et al. (2001) and Ochsenbein-Kölble et al. (2007) had pregnant women rate the intensity of 10 common odors (deodorant, bacon, clove, cigarette butt, coffee, androstenone, acetic acid, rum, peanut butter, and chocolate). There were no statistically significant differences in the intensity ratings between pregnant women and controls in either study. Swallow et al. (2005a) found no overall difference between groups in ratings of odor "strength," although melon was rated to be statistically significantly stronger by pregnant women compared to non-pregnant women and men.

In a questionnaire study, Nordin et al. (2004) found the percentages of "stronger-than-normal sensations" to be high for women in the first two trimesters of pregnancy for most of the 14 odors investigated. It must be noted, however, that this was a self-report measure, and not one based on rating of odors that were being smelled at the time of testing.

In summary, although overall odor intensity ratings do not appear to be higher in pregnant than non-pregnant women, there is some evidence that odor intensity ratings for select odors are higher in pregnant women than in controls.

HEDONICS

Another metric of olfactory perception that has been employed to assess the impact of pregnancy on olfaction is hedonic or pleasantness ratings of odors. Six studies have examined the rating of odor hedonics in pregnancy (Gilbert and Wysocki, 1991; Laska et al., 1996; Kölble et al., 2001; Nordin et al., 2005; Swallow et al., 2005a; Cameron, 2007; Ochsenbein-Kölble et al., 2007). Gilbert and Wysocki (1991) reported that half of the odors they tested (galaxolide, eugenol, and mercaptans) were rated as significantly less pleasant by pregnant women and Kölble et al. (2001) reported that pregnant women found cigarettes, coffee, and rum to be significantly less pleasant than controls, although there were no differences between the groups for hedonic ratings of other odors. Ochsenbein-Kölble et al. (2007) reported that, compared to controls, pregnant women rated cloves and coffee to be less pleasant during pregnancy although the differences in ratings for coffee were only statistically significant in the first trimester. Cameron (2007) reported there was a tendency for pregnant women to rate most odors on the UPSIT as less pleasant than controls. Orange, grape, and natural gas were rated as significantly less pleasant by pregnant women compared to controls. Swallow et al. (2005a) reported that overall pregnant women rated odors to be significantly less pleasant than did men but that there were no specific odors that accounted for the result. Laska et al. (1996) reported considerable variability in hedonic ratings in pregnant women. Only peanut was statistically significantly rated to be less pleasant by pregnant women across all trimesters of pregnancy. There was no consistent pattern across the remainder of the odors.

[7] Dastur (2001) also found no difference between pregnant and non-pregnant women in UPSIT performance. Performance by odor was not reported in that study.

There are relatively few studies that report that pregnant women rate odors as more pleasant. Compared to the odors that are rated as less pleasant, there are relatively fewer odors that are rated as more pleasant, and the results are not consistent across pregnancy. Gilbert and Wysocki (1991) reported that androstenone was rated as significantly more pleasant in pregnant women (pregnancy phase not known). Cameron (2007) reported that only one of 39 odors (fruit punch) was rated to be marginally more pleasant in the first trimester of pregnancy, and Laska et al. (1996) indicated that clove, aniseed, and perfume were rated as significantly more pleasant in some trimesters (this varied with odor). Ochsenbein-Kölble et al. (2007) found that acetic acid was rated as significantly more pleasant during the second and third trimesters of pregnancy.

In addition to rating pleasantness, some studies have asked pregnant women to identify odors that they find particularly pleasant or unpleasant. Cameron (2007) reported that 90% of pregnant women identified odors that they found to be less pleasant. In addition to a range of food odors (e.g., meat, fish, and eggs), pregnant women indicated that noxious odors such as cigarettes, fumes, and garbage were particularly unpleasant. They also reported that some "social odors," such as body odor, baby odors, and perfume and colognes were unpleasant[8]. Cameron (2007) also reported that less than half as many odors were identified by pregnant women as being *more* pleasant, the vast majority of them being foods (e.g., pickles, fruits, and spices). It is worthy of note that Steiner (1922) quoted several women who cited many of these same items – e.g., burnt, spoiled or cooked food, cigarette smoke, and perfume – as being unpleasant, particularly during the early stages of pregnancy.

It is clear from the above that most studies have demonstrated changes in odor hedonics during pregnancy, typically resulting in a reduction in the ratings of pleasantness of odors, although this depends on odor. Anecdotally, pregnant women indicate that the hedonics of odors change, specifically that odors smell bad or that they are particularly aware of foul odors (see text footnote 1).

DISGUST

People's beliefs about the potential danger of exposure to certain chemicals and odors may be a factor that contributes to disgust. Rozin and Fallon (1987) defined disgust as "revulsion at the prospect of oral incorporation of offensive objects. These objects have contamination properties" (p. 23). To the extent that odors are related to these "offensive objects," they could be considered to be a source of contamination.

The finding that many of the odors that are identified as less pleasant during pregnancy are food related odors or "noxious" substances, such as cigarettes and smoke, is consistent with the idea that these odors could be thought by pregnant women to be contaminants. Moreover, given that there is a change in odor hedonics in pregnancy, it seems likely that pregnant women would score particularly high on a measure of disgust. Fessler et al. (2005) administered the Disgust Scale (Haight et al., 1994) to 496 pregnant women and reported that women in the first trimester scored significantly higher on this scale compared to the last two trimesters of pregnancy.

CLINICAL OR EVOLUTIONARY RELEVANCE

The consistent finding that pregnancy affects the hedonic valence of odors and the finding that disgust sensitivity is high, particularly early in pregnancy, leads to two important clinical and evolutionary questions: What is the relationship between olfaction and nausea and vomiting? And is there support for the embryo protective hypothesis?

HYPEROSMIA AND NAUSEA AND VOMITING IN PREGNANCY

Nausea and vomiting ("morning sickness") afflicts about three-quarters of pregnant women (e.g., Lacroix et al., 2000; Niebyl, 2010). The idea of a causal link between increased olfactory sensitivity and nausea and vomiting is compelling (e.g., Erick, 1995; Heinrichs, 2002; Niebyl, 2010). Such a link could be important for understanding and managing maternal nutritional status, which has a significant impact on fetal well-being and development. However, this link depends on a heightened sense of smell, which has yet to be documented. Nonetheless, Heinrichs (2002) reported a substantial decrease in reports of incidence of nausea and vomiting in pregnant women with congenital anosmia (only one of nine patients). Moreover, Cantoni et al. (1999) reported that 58% of 500 women responded that there were odors that caused nausea during pregnancy and Swallow et al. (2005b) found that, in a sample of 273 pregnant women, those who were adversely affected by odors scored higher on a measure of the severity of their nausea and vomiting. However, Hummel et al. (2002) found no significant correlation between the incidence of self-reported nausea and vomiting and performance on olfactory detection threshold, discrimination nor identification tasks in 53 women in the first trimester of pregnancy. The authors suggested that nausea and vomiting may not be strongly tied to basic olfactory function.

Classical conditioning could explain the relationship between the perception of odors and nausea and vomiting in pregnancy. Perhaps pregnant women rapidly condition to odors that are present during a moment of nausea and/or vomiting, as in the Garcia effect (conditioned taste aversion). Thus, a previously neutral, conditioned stimulus (an odor) becomes associated with an unconditioned stimulus (whatever instigated the nausea/vomiting) and the conditioned response of nausea/vomiting becomes elicited by the conditioned stimulus (the odor). Subsequent exposures to that neutral odor could invoke a rapidly conditioned response (nausea and vomiting). An important aspect of this hypothesis is that it does not require hyperosmia. The odor could be present and perceived at essentially any intensity level. Note that in a study published only in abstract form, Bartoshuk and Wolfe (1990) reported conditioned aversion that was induced by smell, but not by taste.

THE EMBRYO PROTECTIVE HYPOTHESIS

It has been argued that hypersensitivity to odors would provide a protective function for the embryo by limiting what the mother ingests, particularly early in pregnancy when the embryo/fetus is

[8] These data are in accord with a large retrospective self-report study by Cantoni et al. (1999) that was published only in abstract form. Approximately three-quarters of women reported that there were odors that smelled less pleasant during pregnancy (e.g., cigarettes, coffee, meat, food in general, diesel exhaust, and sweat). Less than a quarter of pregnant women reported that there were odors that smelled more pleasant (fruits, flowers, woodlands, and perfume).

most vulnerable. This notion was proposed as early as 1922 by Gabriel Steiner (Steiner, 1922) and elaborated more recently by Margie Profet (Profet, 1992). The hypothesis is that hyperosmia in pregnancy leads to nausea and vomiting and that this provides a protective function for the embryo, inhibiting the pregnant woman from ingesting teratogens during the phase of pregnancy when the embryo is most vulnerable (the first trimester).

This hypothesis has two significant limitations. First, the evidence for hyperosmia in pregnancy is weak, as demonstrated in this review. Thus, whatever changes occur in the olfactory system during pregnancy, it is does not appear to result in a generalized lowered detection threshold. Therefore, it seems unlikely that hyperosmia underlies the nausea and vomiting that would protect the embryo. Second, two studies have directly tested this hypothesis and neither one support it. Swallow et al. (2005a) explored odor ratings of liking, strength, and pleasantness for six odors, half of which were considered to be potentially dangerous. Pregnant women did rate odors as significantly less pleasant than non-pregnant women or men. However, there was no significant interaction between group and type of odor (safe or potentially harmful), which would have indicated that pregnant women were more averse to potentially harmful odors. Likewise, Brown et al. (1997) explored the relationship between the intake of bitter vegetables and other foods thought to be harmful (Profet, 1992) and the incidence of nausea and vomiting in a very large sample ($n = 549$). There were no significant differences in the intake of food thought to be harmful to the developing embryo between the group who had nausea and/or vomiting in early pregnancy and the group that did not.

MECHANISMS UNDERLYING CHANGES IN OLFACTION DURING PREGNANCY

Although the data do not support a general hyperosmia, there does appear to be a change in the perception of odors during pregnancy. Several mechanisms have been suggested to account for this result.

HORMONES AND SENSE OF SMELL

Levels of circulating gonadal hormones are often proposed as an explanation for heightened sense of smell. For example, hormone levels are widely believed to explain sex differences, changes in olfactory sensitivity across the menstrual cycle and for the purported changes in olfactory processing in pregnancy (for a review, see Doty and Cameron, 2009). Although olfactory detection thresholds are correlated with circulating levels of estrogen in normally cycling women, thresholds also vary similarly across the menstrual cycle in women taking oral contraceptives, calling into question whether this relationship is causal (Doty et al., 1981). Estrogen levels rise throughout pregnancy, reaching their peak shortly before parturition (Gard, 1998). Thus, one would predict that smell function should improve across pregnancy if estrogen, alone, were involved. This is neither what is observed in measures of olfactory perception, nor what is expected based on self-report. To the extent that one can rely on self-report, which indicates the largest changes in odor perception (particularly odor hedonicity) occur early in pregnancy, the changing levels of the hormone human chorionic gonadotropin (hCG) match the temporal profile of the self-reported changes (Gard, 1998; Niebyl, 2010; and see **Figure 4**). Thus, hCG might be considered to be a candidate underlying changes in olfactory perception, or at least changes in odor hedonicity. Interestingly, incidents of nausea and vomiting are also correlated with hCG levels in pregnancy (see **Figure 4**).

A potentially related condition to the experience of pregnant women's sense of smell and its relationship to hCG comes from people who are on the controversial hCG hormone diet. Developed by Simeons in the 1950s and sometimes recommended for treatment of obesity, this extremely low calorie diet (500 calories/day) is coupled with intramuscular injections of hCG. The hormone is thought to suppress hunger and allow people to remain on the diet for over a month. This diet gained popularity in the 1970s and had a resurgence several years ago. In the United States, the Food and Drug Administration has warned against the use of this diet because there are no scientific studies that have verified its effectiveness[9] and the Obesity Society recently published a position statement indicating that they do not condone its use[10].

People who are injected with hCG as part of this controversial diet and women who are injected with hCG for infertility treatment report, anecdotally, that their sense of smell is heightened. A perusal of blog postings indicates that the sort of self-report of this experience is very similar to the reports of some pregnant women, particularly in early pregnancy. For example, several people posted on HCG DIET INFO FORUMS (August 29, 2010):

> *... about the heightened sense of smell ... but I couldn't sleep on my left side last night because I could smell my husband's breath and I couldn't sleep on my right side because I could smell a sealed bottle of incense I had in my bedside table's drawer. It's ridiculous!!*
>
> *I thought it was just me with the extra sensitive nose lately. I've always had a good "sniffer" but lately I smell everything!*
>
> *I feel like a superhero or something with this new sense of smell and it is making me crazy!*

[9] USA Today, 12/6/2011

[10] http://www.obesity.org/images/TOSpositionPaperlHCGrxObesityRevised12-12_-_Final_Approved_1-23-13.pdf.

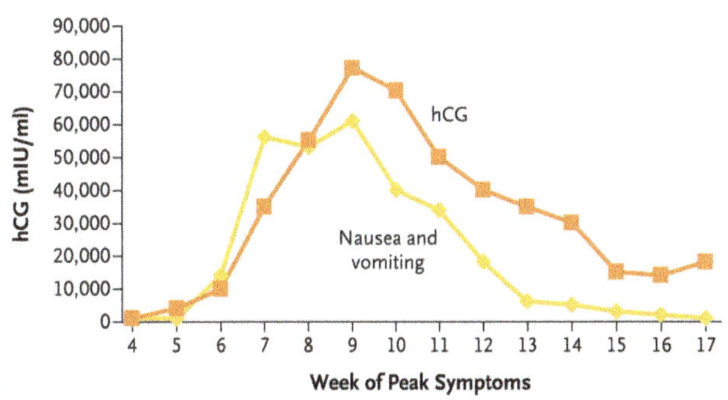

FIGURE 4 | Human chorionic gonadotropin (hCG) levels (and reports of nausea and vomiting) as a function of number of weeks of pregnancy. hCG level peaks during the first trimester. From Niebyl (2010), permission received.

These sorts of comments are reminiscent of comments by pregnant women, including the one reported at the start of this review[1]. Here are two responses to that posting:

> *I've always had a sensitive nose and it was magnified by my pregnancy as well. Horrible. I sometimes find being out in public overwhelming with all the perfumes and body odors and whatnot.*
>
> *My second pregnancy was a[n] olfactory nightmare. The dog stunk to high heaven, my firstborn was a diaper-wearing terror of wafting fumes, and I actually woke my husband up from a sound sleep to make him go brush his teeth in the middle of the night. Really.*

To my knowledge, no study has examined smell function in people on the hCG diet. Moreover, no study has measured hormone levels and smell function concomitantly during pregnancy, but the evidence so far does not suggest a strong correlation between estrogen and hyperosmia.

COGNITIVE/ATTENTIONAL MECHANISMS

Another possible explanation for the change in odor perception during pregnancy is that the effect is a more cognitive (high-level) than sensory (low-level) one. Such a high-level change in odor processing would not be expected to result in changes measured by most standard tests of smell function. Evidence for a high-level mechanism comes from event-related potential (ERP) data. Olofsson et al. (2005) measured chemosensory ERPs in 15 pregnant and 15 non-pregnant women and found no significant differences between groups in amplitude nor latency of N1 and P1 components (which reflect sensory processing), but rather a tendency for shorter latency and higher amplitude of the more perceptual/cognitive P3 component in the pregnant group. This suggests that changes may be observed for more central levels of olfactory processing. This is consistent with the results reported above that show that relative to later in pregnancy, pregnant women exhibited a more liberal criterion in an odor detection task using a signal detection paradigm in early pregnancy (Cameron, 2014).

It is worthy of note that pyridine, which has a trigeminal component, was used as the stimulus in Olofsson et al.'s (2005) study [and in the previously mentioned Broman et al.'s (2003) study that showed significantly reduced thresholds in pregnancy] and it has been suggested that perceived hyperosmia may be related to trigeminal function (Nordin et al., 2005). In addition, pyridine is an unpleasant odor, which may also have been a factor in the outcome of these studies.

HYPERREACTIVITY

The cognitive hypothesis is consistent with a hyperreactivity hypothesis: self-reported olfactory hypersensitivity in pregnant women could reflect a hyper-*awareness* of or irritation produced by many odors. This may be analogous to the literature on hyperosmia in migraines, as described by Demarquay et al. (2006) "In the field of migraine and MCS [multiple chemical sensitivity], this term [hypersensitivity or hyperacuity] is used in a broader sense, reflecting the discomfort perceived by the patient as an inappropriate and excessive odour-induced response." (Demarquay et al., 2006, p. 1128). Steiner (1922) suggested that perhaps the self-reported increased sensitivity in pregnancy was in fact an emotional reactivity. There is some evidence of this from questionnaire studies. Nordin et al. (2005, 2007) found that pregnant women, particularly in the first trimester of pregnancy, score higher on the Chemical Sensitivity Scale for Sensory Hyperreactivity (Nordin et al., 2003). This lead the authors to conclude that "pregnant women to a large degree are affected by odorous/pungent substances in their daily activities" (Nordin et al., 2007, p. 341). They also conclude that olfaction is the major contributor to this sensory hyperreactivity, and that this hyperreactivity does not extend to auditory stimuli.

The general decrease in pleasantness of odors during pregnancy may result in a change in the *awareness* of or *attention* to odors. Bad smells attract our attention. The awareness that is drawn to the odors may be incorrectly interpreted by pregnant women as hyperosmia. This is consistent with the correlation between self-rating of olfactory function and self-rating of odor annoyance in a sample of 1311 people (Knaapila et al., 2008).

Such a hyperreactivity or hyperawareness may be under relatively high-level, cognitive control. Dalton (1996) demonstrated that when participants were exposed to the odor isobornyl acetate (balsam) and told that the odor was a "natural, healthy extract," they adapted to it and rated its perceived intensity to be low and decreasing across exposure duration. On the other hand, when participants were exposed to the same odor and told that it was "potentially hazardous" they became sensitized to it and rated its perceived intensity to be relatively high, particularly toward the end of the exposure duration. Interestingly, detection thresholds remained constant, regardless of the nature of the information given. Risk perception appears to influence perceived odor intensity. Therefore, one possible explanation of self-reported olfactory hypersensitivity in pregnant women is that it reflects a hyperreactivity to odors that arises from beliefs about health risks associated with odors. Interestingly, beliefs about the health risks of exposure to certain odors may or may not occur at the level of conscious awareness (Dalton, 2012).

PREGNANCY AND THE NOSE

Although the first trimester appears to be the time during which the greatest changes in perception of odors occur, some of the detection and recognition threshold data reported above suggested impaired olfactory function at the end of pregnancy (Hansen and Glass, 1936; Noferi and Giudizi, 1946; Luvara and Murizi, 1961; Ochsenbein-Kölble et al., 2007). This may be accounted for by peripheral mechanisms. For example, nasal airflow varies as a function of pregnancy status. As with many tissues of the body the nose becomes more engorged and "stuffy" during pregnancy (Bende and Gredmark, 1999; Ellegard and Karlsson, 1999; Philpott et al., 2004). Nasal congestion occurs in the late stages of pregnancy and thus airflow is reduced, which reduces the ability to perceive odors.

SUMMARY AND SUGGESTED FURTHER RESEARCH

In this review, I have described all of the extant data on the effect of pregnancy on olfaction. There is no evidence for a general hyperosmia during pregnancy, although it must be noted that there remains a dearth of conclusive studies on this topic. This is surprising given the abundant anecdotal evidence. Therefore, it may be premature to draw strong conclusions.

Several aspects of olfaction and pregnancy require further study. Perhaps the central issue for further study is the effect of odorant-specificity on olfactory perception in pregnant women. Performance on a range of olfactory tasks depends upon the specific odors presented. Further research is necessary to explore this phenomenon in more detail, with carefully selected odors. First, detection and recognition thresholds and odor identification should be measured using a broader range of odors, taking into consideration the hedonic tone of the odors. Second, given the substantial individual differences in odor preference, further research is needed to explore whether there are odors that are commonly reported to be unpleasant by pregnant women (some evidence suggests that there are). Third, intensity ratings for a range of odors at a range of concentrations should be established. Finally, it is important to distinguish between odors that are purely olfactory and those that contain a trigeminal component. The differences in the processing of pyridine by pregnant women in the studies by Olofsson et al. (2005) and Broman et al. (2003) suggests that pregnancy may modify the processing of trigeminal stimuli. This idea deserves further investigation.

Pregnant women have been tested on both low-level threshold (detection) tasks and high-level suprathreshold (identification) olfactory tasks, but further research is needed using both types of task. It is important to distinguish between sensory and cognitive changes in the olfactory system that may be brought about by pregnancy. First, odor detection across a range of concentrations using the method of constant stimuli would enable an examination of differences between psychometric functions (e.g., differences in slopes) of pregnant and non-pregnant women. Second, suprathreshold measurements, such as cross-modal matching, could reveal differences that have not been demonstrated with more common methods of measuring olfactory perception. Future studies could examine performance on tasks that require olfactory cognition, such as tests of odor memory or attention.

Further research is needed to examine the complex relationship between hormones and smell function, particularly with respect to pregnancy. No study has measured hormone levels and smell function concomitantly in pregnant women, but the evidence so far does not suggest a clear and causal relationship between estrogen and hyperosmia given the discrepancy between the self-reported smell function during early pregnancy and the relatively lower levels of estrogen at that time in pregnancy. hCG is thought to stimulate the production of estrogen (Niebyl, 2010) and it is possible that there is a complex interaction among hormones that underlies olfactory perception, particularly in pregnant women.

It is compelling to suppose that there is a link between odors and the onset of nausea and vomiting in pregnancy. At present there is no scientific evidence for a direct link, and yet many women can identify odors that bring on nausea and vomiting. It is worthy of note that nausea is correlated with ratings of food disgust (Fessler et al., 2005) and nausea and vomiting is less common in people with anosmia or hyposmia than in normosmics. Clearly more study is needed in this area. A better understanding of the relationship between olfaction and nausea and vomiting in pregnancy could help the many women who suffer from these symptoms.

ACKNOWLEDGMENTS

The author wishes to thank Matthias Laska and Greg Baer for English translation of German articles.

REFERENCES

Bartoshuk, L. M., and Wolfe, J. M. (1990). Conditioned taste aversion in humans: are they olfactory aversions? *Chem. Senses* 15, 551.

Bende, M., and Gredmark, T. (1999). Nasal stuffiness during pregnancy. *Laryngoscope* 109, 1108–1110. doi: 10.1097/00005537-199907000-00018

Broman, D. A., Olofsson, J., Olsson, M. J., and Nordin, S. (2003). Olfactory differences between pregnant and non-pregnant women. *Chem. Senses* 28, 551.

Brown, J. E., Kahn, E. S., and Hartman, T. J. (1997). Profet, profits, and proof: do nausea and vomiting of early pregnancy protect women from "harmful" vegetables? *Am. J. Obstet. Gynecol.* 176, 179–181. doi: 10.1016/S0002-9378(97)80032-4

Cameron, E. L. (2007). Measures of human olfactory perception during pregnancy. *Chem. Senses* 32, 775–782. doi: 10.1093/chemse/bjm045

Cameron, E. L. (2014). Pregnancy does not affect human olfactory detection thresholds. *Chem. Senses* 39, 143–150. doi: 10.1093/chemse/bjt063

Campanella, G., Filla, A., and De Michele, G. (1978). Smell and taste acuity in epileptic syndromes. *Eur. Neurol.* 17, 136–141. doi: 10.1159/000114936

Cantoni, P., Hudson, R., Distel, H., and Laska, M. (1999). Changes in olfactory perception and dietary habits in the course of pregnancy: a questionnaire study. *Chem. Senses* 24, 58.

Caruso, S., Grillo, C., Agnello, C., Maiolino, L., Intelisano, G., and Serra, A. (2001). A prospective study evidencing rhinomanometric and olfactometric outcomes in women taking oral contraceptives. *Hum. Reprod.* 16, 2288–2294. doi: 10.1093/humrep/16.11.2288

Dalton, P. (1996). Odor perception and beliefs about risk. *Chem. Senses* 21, 447–458. doi: 10.1093/chemse/21.4.447

Dalton, P. (2012). "There's something in the air: effects of beliefs and expectations on response to environmental odors," in *Essays in Olfactory Cognition: Advances in Consciousness Research*, eds G. M. Zucco, R. S. Herz, and B. Schaal (Amsterdam: John Benjamins), 23–38.

Dastur, F. N. (2001). *A Controlled, Longitudinal Study of Olfactory Perception and Symptoms of Pregnancy Sickness.* Doctoral dissertation, Dartmouth University. Dissertations Abstracts International 62(6-B): 2986.

Deems, D. A., Doty, R. L., Settle, R. G., Moore-Gillon, V., Shaman, P., Mester, A. F., et al. (1991). Smell and taste disorders: a study of 750 patients from the University of Pennsylvania Smell and Taste Center. *Arch. Otolaryngol. Head Neck Surg.* 117, 519–528. doi: 10.1001/archotol.1991.01870170065015

Demarquay, G., Royet, J. P., Giraud, P., Chazot, G., Valade, D., and Ryvlin, P. (2006). Rating of olfactory judgements in migraine patients. *Cephalalgia* 26, 1123–1130. doi: 10.1111/j.1468-2982.2006.01174.x

Doty, R. L. (1976). "Reproductive endocrine influences upon human nasal chemoreception: a review," in *Mammalian Olfaction, Reproductive Processes and Behavior*, ed. R. L. Doty (New York: Academic Press), 295–321.

Doty, R. L. (2000). *The Smell Threshold Test Administration Manual.* Haddon Heights, NJ: Sensonics, Inc.

Doty, R. L. (2003). "Odor perception in neurodegenerative diseases," in *Handbook of Olfaction and Gustation*, 2nd Edn, ed. R. L. Doty (New York: Marcel Dekker Inc.), 479–502.

Doty, R. L., and Cameron, E. L. (2009). Sex differences and reproductive hormone influences on human odor perception. *Physiol. Behav.* 97, 213–228. doi: 10.1016/j.physbeh.2009.02.032

Doty, R. L., Deems, D. A., Frye, R. E., Pelberg, R., and Shapiro, A. (1988). Olfactory sensitivity, nasal resistance, and autonomic function in patients with multiple chemical sensitivities. *Arch. Otolaryngol. Head Neck Surg.* 114, 1422–1427. doi: 10.1001/archotol.1988.01860240072027

Doty, R. L., Shaman, P., Applebaum, S. L., Giberson, R., Siksorski, L., and Rosenberg, L. (1984a). Smell identification ability: changes with age. *Science* 226, 1441–1443. doi: 10.1126/science.6505700

Doty, R. L., Shaman, P., and Dann, M. (1984b). Development of the University of Pennsylvania Smell Identification Test: a standardized microencapsulated test of olfactory function. *Physiol. Behav.* 32, 389–502. doi: 10.1016/0031-9384(84)90269-5

Doty, R. L., Snyder, P., Huggins, G., and Lowry, L. D. (1981). Endocrine, cardiovascular, and psychological correlates of olfactory sensitivity changes during the human menstrual cycle. *J. Comp. Physiol. Psychol.* 95, 45–60. doi: 10.1037/h0077755

Ellegard, E., and Karlsson, G. (1999). Nasal congestion during pregnancy. *Clin. Otolaryngol. Allied Sci.* 24, 307–311. doi: 10.1046/j.1365-2273.1999.00264.x

Elsberg, C. A., and Levy, I. (1935). The sense of smell: I. A new and simple method of quantitative olfactometry. *Bull. Neurol. Inst. N. Y.* 4, 5–19.

Erick, M. (1995). Hyperolfaction and hyperemesis gravidarum: what is the relationship? *Nutr. Rev.* 53, 289–295. doi: 10.1111/j.1753-4887.1995.tb01479.x

Fessler, D. M. T., Eng, S. J., and Navarrete, C. D. (2005). Elevated disgust in the first trimester of pregnancy: evidence supporting the compensatory prophylaxis hypothesis. *Evol. Hum. Behav.* 26, 344–351. doi: 10.1016/j.evolhumbehav.2004.12.001

Gard, P. R. (1998). *Human Endocrinology*. London: Taylor & Francis.

Gilbert, A. N., and Wysocki, C. J. (1991). Quantitative assessment of olfactory experience during pregnancy. *Psychosom. Med.* 53, 693–700.

Good, P. R., Geary, N., and Engen, T. (1976). The effect of estrogen on odor detection. *Chem. Senses* 2, 45–50. doi: 10.1093/chemse/2.1.45

Grant, A. C. (2005). Interictal perceptual function in epilepsy. *Epilepsy Behav.* 6, 511–519. doi: 10.1016/j.yebeh.2005.03.016

Green, D. M., and Swets, J. A. (1966). *Signal Detection Theory and Psychophysics.* New York: Wiley.

Haight, J., McCauley, C. R., and Rozin, P. (1994). A scale to measure disgust sensitivity. *Pers. Individ. Differ.* 16, 701–713.

Hansen, R., and Glass, L. (1936). Über den Geruchssinn in der Schwangerschaft. *Klin. Wochenschr.* 15, 891–894. doi: 10.1007/BF01781122

Heinrichs, L. (2002). Linking olfaction with nausea and vomiting of pregnancy, recurrent abortion, hyperemesis gravidarum, and migraine headache. *Am. J. Obstet. Gynecol.* 186, S215–S219. doi: 10.1067/mob.2002.123053

Henkin, R. I., and Bartter, R. C. (1966). Studies on olfactory thresholds in normal man and in patients with adrenal cortical insufficiency: the role of adrenal cortical steroids and of serum sodium concentration. *J. Clin. Invest.* 45,1631–1639. doi: 10.1172/JCI105470

Henssge, E. (1930). Steigerung der Geruchsempfindlichkeit in der Schwangerschaft. *Psychol. Med.* 4, 206–207.

Hirsch, A. R. (1992). Olfaction in migraineurs. *Headache* 32, 233–236. doi: 10.1111/j.1526-4610.1992.hed3205233.x

Hummel, T., and Nordin S. (2005). Olfactory disorders and their consequences for quality of life. *Acta Otolaryngol.* 125, 116–121. doi: 10.1080/00016480410022787

Hummel, T., von Mering, R., Huch, R., and Kölble, N. (2002). Olfactory modulation of nausea during early pregnancy? *Int. J. Gynecol. Obstet.* 109, 1394–1397. doi: 10.1046/j.1471-0528.2002.02287.x

Kim, H. J., Park, H. J., Park, J. Y., Park, H. E., Lee, S. S., and Bae, J. H. (2011). The possibility of morning sickness from olfactory hyperacuity during pregnancy. *Kor. J. Otorhinolaryngol. Head Neck Surg.* 54, 473–476. doi: 10.3342/kjorl-hns.2011.54.7.473

Knaapila, A., Tuorila, H., Kyvik, K. O., Wright, M. J., Keskitalo, K., Hansen, J., et al. (2008). Self-ratings of olfactory function reflect odor annoyance rather than olfactory acuity. *Laryngoscope* 118, 2212–2217. doi: 10.1097/MLG.0b013e3181826e43

Kölble, N., Hummel, T., von Mering, R., Huch, A., and Huch, R. (2001). Gustatory and olfactory function in the first trimester of pregnancy. *Eur. J. Obstet. Gynecol. Reprod. Biol.* 99, 179–183. doi: 10.1016/S0301-2115(01)00408-0

Lacroix, R., Eason, E., and Melzack, R. (2000). Nausea and vomiting during pregnancy: a prospective study of its frequency, intensity, and patterns of change. *Am. J. Obstet. Gynecol.* 182, 931–937. doi: 10.1016/S0002-9378(00)70349-8

Landis, B., Hummel, T., Hugentobler, M., Giger, R., and Lacroix, J. S. (2003). Ratings of overall olfactory function. *Chem. Senses* 28, 691–694. doi: 10.1093/chemse/bjg061

Laska, M., Koch, B., Heid, B., and Hudson, R. (1996). Failure to demonstrate systematic changes in olfactory perception in the course of pregnancy: a longitudinal study. *Chem. Senses* 21, 567–571. doi: 10.1093/chemse/21.5.567

Luvara, A., and Murizi, M. (1961). Ricerche di olfattometria in gravidanze. *Boll. Mal. Orecch. Gola Naso* 79, 367–375.

Miwa, T., Furukawa, M., Tsukatani, T., Costanzo, R., DiNardo, L. J., and Reiter, E. R. (2001). Impact of olfactory impairment on quality of life and disability. *Arch. Otolaryngol. Head Neck Surg.* 127, 497–503. doi: 10.1001/archotol.127.5.497

Murphy, C., Doty, R. L., and Duncan, H. J. (2003). "Clinical disorders of olfaction," in *Handbook of Olfaction and Gustation*, 2nd Edn, ed. R. L. Doty (New York: Marcel Dekker Inc.), 461–478.

Niebyl, J. R. (2010). Nausea and Vomiting in Pregnancy. *N. Engl. J. Med.* 363, 1544–1550. doi: 10.1056/NEJMcp1003896

Noferi, G., and Giudizi, S. (1946). Le variazioni della sensibilita gustative in particolari situazioni fisiologiche ed in alcuni stati morbois. Nota IV. Le variazioni dellasoglia gustative per l'acido e della soglia olfattiva per l'odre limone durante la gravidanza. *Rev. Crit. Clin. Med.* 5, 89–100.

Nordin, S., Broman, D. A., Bringlöv, E., and Wulff, M. (2007). Intolerance to ambient odors at an early stage of pregnancy. *Scand. J. Psychol.* 48, 3990–3343. doi: 10.1111/j.1467-9450.2007.00572.x

Nordin, S., Broman, D. A., Olofsson, J. K., and Wulff, M. (2004). A longitudinal descriptive study of self-reported abnormal smell and taste perception in pregnant women. *Chem. Senses* 29, 391–402. doi: 10.1093/chemse/bjh040

Nordin, S., Broman, D. A., and Wulff, M. (2005). Environmental odor intolerance in pregnant women. *Physiol. Behav.* 84, 175–179. doi: 10.1016/j.physbeh.2004.10.003

Nordin, S., Millqvist, E., Löwhagen, O., and Bende, M. (2003). The Chemical Sensitivity Scale: psychometric properties and comparison with the noise sensitivity scale. *J. Environ. Psychol.* 23, 359–367. doi: 10.1016/S0272-4944(03)00002-1

Nordin, S., Monsch, A. U., and Murphy, C. (1995). Unawareness of smell loss in normal aging and Alzheimer's disease: discrepancy between self-reported and diagnosed smell sensitivity. *J. Gerontol. B Psychol. Sci. Soc. Sci.* 50, 187–192. doi: 10.1093/geronb/50B.4.P187

Ochsenbein-Kölble, N., von Mering, R., Zimmerman, R., and Hummel, T. (2007). Changes in olfactory function in pregnancy and postpartum. *Int. J. Gynecol. Obstet.* 97, 10–14. doi: 10.1016/j.ijgo.2006.12.009

Olofsson, J. K., Broman, D. A., Wulff, M., Martinkauppi, M., and Nordin, S. (2005). Olfactory and chemosomatosensory function in pregnant women assessed with event-related potentials. *Physiol. Behav.* 86, 252–257. doi: 10.1016/j.physbeh.2005.07.022

Philpott, C. M., Conboy, P., Al-Azzawi, F., and Murty, G. (2004). Nasal physiological changes during pregnancy. *Clin. Otolaryngol.* 29, 343–351. doi: 10.1111/j.1365-2273.2004.00815.x

Profet, M. (1992). "Pregnancy sickness as adaptation: a deterrent to maternal ingestion of teratogens," in *The Adapted Mind: Evolutionary Psychology and the Generation of Culture*, eds J. H. Barkow, L. Cosmides, and J. Tooby (New York: Oxford University Press), 327–365.

Rozin, P., and Fallon, A. E. (1987). A perspective on disgust. *Psychol. Rev.* 94, 23–41. doi: 10.1037/0033-295X.94.1.23

Savovic, S., Nincic, D., Lemajic, S., Pilija, V., Mandic, A., Rajovic, J., et al. (2002). Olfactory perception in women with physiologically altered hormonal status (during pregnancy and menopause). *Med. Pregl.* 55, 380–383. [Article in Croatian; abstract in English]. doi: 10.2298/MPNS0210380S

Schmidt, H. (1925). Transient loss of the sense of smell and taste during pregnancy. *Klin. Wochenschr.* 4, 1967–1968. doi: 10.1007/BF01734094

Shu, C.-H., Hummel, T., Lee, P.-L., Chiu, C.-H., Lin, S.-H., and Yuan, B.-C. (2009). The proportion of self-rated olfactory dysfunction does not change across the life span. *Am. J. Rhinol. Allergy* 23, 413–416. doi: 10.2500/ajra.2009.23.3343

Soter, A., Kim, J., Jackman, A., Tourbier, I., Kaul, A., and Doty, R. L. (2008). Accuracy of self-report in detecting taste dysfunction. *Laryngoscope* 118, 611–617. doi: 10.1097/MLG.0b013e318161e53a

Steiner, G. (1922). Psychische Untersuchungen an Schwangeren. *Arch. Psychiatr. Nervenkr.* 65, 171–190. doi: 10.1007/BF02029573

Swallow, B. L., Lindow, S. W., Aye, M., Masson, E. A., Alasalvar, C., Quantick, P., et al. (2005a). Smell perception during early pregnancy: no evidence of an adaptive mechanism. *BJOG* 112, 57–62. doi: 10.1111/j.1471-0528.2004.00327.x

Swallow, B. L., Lindow, S. W., Masson, E. A., and Hay, D. M. (2005b). Women with nausea and vomiting in pregnancy demonstrate worse health and are adversely affected by odours. *J. Obstet. Gynecol.* 25, 544–549. doi: 10.1080/01443610500230783

West, S. E., and Doty, R. L. (1995). Influence of epilepsy and temporal lobe resection on olfactory function. *Epilepsia* 36, 531–542. doi: 10.1111/j.1528-1157.1995.tb02565.x

Zwaardemaker, H. (1895). *Die physiologie des Geruchs.* Leipzig: Engelmann.

15

A "Misfit" Theory of Spontaneous Conscious Odor Perception (MITSCOP): reflections on the role and function of odor memory in everyday life

Egon P. Köster[1]*, Per Møller[2] and Jozina Mojet[3]

[1] Psychological Laboratory, Helmholtz Institute, Utrecht University, Utrecht, Netherlands
[2] Department of Food Science, University of Copenhagen, Frederiksberg, Denmark
[3] Wageningen – UR, Food and Biobased Research, Wageningen, Netherlands

Correspondence:
Egon P. Köster, Psychological Laboratory, Helmholtz Institute, Utrecht University, Wildforsterweg 4A, 3881 NJ Putten, Utrecht, Netherlands
e-mail: ep.koster@gmail.com

Our senses have developed as an answer to the world we live in (Gibson, 1966) and so have the forms of memory that accompany them. All senses serve different purposes and do so in different ways. In vision, where orientation and object recognition are important, memory is strongly linked to identification. In olfaction, the guardian of vital functions such as breathing and food ingestion, perhaps the most important (and least noticed and researched) role of odor memory is to help us not to notice the well-known odors or flavors in our everyday surroundings, but to react immediately to the unexpected ones. At the same time it provides us with a feeling of safety when our expectancies are met. All this happens without any smelling intention or conscious knowledge of our expectations. Identification by odor naming is not involved in this and people are notoriously bad at it. Odors are usually best identified via the episodic memory of the situation in which they once occurred. Spontaneous conscious odor perception normally only occurs in situations where attention is demanded, either because the inhaled air or the food smell is particularly good or particularly bad and people search for its source or because people want to actively enjoy the healthiness and pleasantness of their surroundings or food. Odor memory is concerned with novelty detection rather than with recollection of odors. In this paper, these points are illustrated with experimental results and their consequences for doing ecologically valid odor memory research are drawn. Furthermore, suggestions for ecologically valid research on everyday odor memory and some illustrative examples are given.

Keywords: incidental learning, implicit memory, olfactory perception, ecological validity

INTRODUCTION

According to Gibson (1966, 1979) our senses have developed as an answer to the world we live in and their diversity can be seen as the reaction to the different challenges our world poses. Thus, he describes the many senses involved in movement and kinesthesis (from skin pressure to joint angle sensitivity and vestibular orientation) as an answer to gravity. The intricate interplay of these sensory impressions remains implicit and escapes our conscious attention, making sure that we are never in doubt about our relative position with regard to the earth. The memory for our movements in relation to the weight of objects permits us to fulfill small wonders like making three pointers in basketball. Odor perception and odor memory are also most of the time implicit, but for a different reason. As Gibson indicated, smelling is an accompaniment of breathing, which is a vital function in all animals. As such it is sensitive to volatile "foreign substances" in the normally constant system of pure air that remains odorless. Here Gibson forgot to mention that the sense of smell is also watching over the foods we ingest by the retro-nasal stimulation occurring during eating. He only pays attention to the orthonasal stimulation and its function in food, mate finding, and in relation to prey/predator behavior. In doing so he adds to the conviction that identifying the odor source is the primary objective of olfaction. Before discussing odor perception and odor memory in more detail, it is perhaps useful to clarify the meaning of some of the terms used. Implicit perception and implicit memory refer too our unawareness of either perceiving something or having a memory of it. In everyday life our explicit and conscious perception and memory cover only a small part of what goes on. Memory is to a large part based on incidental learning that takes place without any intention to memorize and our memory is filled with knowledge that we use without special conscious attention. Olfactory memory is usually strongly, but implicitly linked to emotion and hedonic appreciation of our surroundings rather than to explicit odor source recognition. Thus, although it is true that odors may result in attraction or repellence and may have strong emotional and behavioral effects (Jacob and McClintock, 2000; Lundstrom et al., 2003; Chebat and Michon, 2003; Holland et al., 2005), it is doubtful that at least in human olfaction explicit or even implicit identification of the odor source necessarily plays a role. In fact, most well-known odors are not even consciously remarked and just provide a sense of safety. Only the odors that do not fit our memory based expectations, either because they deviate from the normal odor in that situation or by being particularly "good" or "bad," are spontaneously and consciously remarked in normal everyday life. All expected odors are usually not. Each room in our house and even each room corner smells differently but we do not notice the hundreds of odors in our daily surroundings (Keller, 2011). Of course it is possible to actively smell them by sniffing, but in contrast to most animals, humans do seldom use active smelling, since due to their erect posture, they are primarily oriented by vision and audition. If they do smell actively, it is usually to verify the safety of the surroundings or to enjoy sensual pleasures. Thus, olfactory memory seems to play a very special role in life: it helps people "not to notice" known odors, but to react to all unexpected ones. One does not smell the odors in one's own house, but notices the odors in the houses of friends. This might mean that, at least in humans, the implicit memory of odor perception could be more related to its passive function as a warning system for the breathing or ingestion of possibly dangerous odors or foods (see the section on incidentally learned food memory below), than to the active behavior of food and mate search that Gibson described. This passivity may perhaps also explain why odor evoked memories are more emotional than memories evoked by visual or verbal stimuli (Herz and Schooler, 2002; Herz, 2004). Only in special cases, when the odors are new or do not fit the situation (Herz, 1997) or when the situation is new or so exceptional that it puts all our senses on alert, will we note the odors, whereas under normal circumstances we do not. Nordin et al. (1995) showed that 77% of healthy elderly remain unaware of the fact that they have severe losses of olfactory sensitivity (even up to complete anosmia). White and Kurtz (2003) confirmed that elderly have little metacognitive awareness of their olfactory deficiencies and that this lack of awareness might be due to the slow disappearance of their sensitivity similarly to what occurs sometimes in loss of hearing. They also showed that metacognitive awareness of odor perception is also weak in young people who show a tendency to underestimate their olfactory capabilities. This seems to indicate that conscious odor perception is probably never such an important part of life as in hearing or vision where our communication with others and our environment depend on it. Complete loss of hearing or blindness would seldom go unremarked, but complete anosmia is often unnoticed. Along similar lines it can be explained why the bump in the autobiographical memory curve (i.e., the period of one's lifetime to which most memories go back) evoked by odors lies much earlier (before 10 years) than that for visually or verbally evoked memories [between 15 and 25 years; (Chu and Downes, 2000, 2002; Willander and Larsson, 2006, 2007, 2008)]. Once known, odors are simply not very easily remarked anymore in later phases of life. As a result the first impressions with them are not replaced by later events involving them. Furthermore, since most authors used only odors that were known by most of their subjects already as a child and were thereafter seldom consciously experienced, they reduced the chances of association of these odors with later events. Unfortunately, none of the authors did specify the results for the odors they used. Otherwise it might have been possible to date their first contacts with them. According to the theory developed below, the chances to be linked to an autobiographical memory at a later age are slimmer for odors that were already perceived regularly (or even occasionally) in childhood. In the Proust (Proust, 1922/1960) phenomenon it is the rather unique combination of the madeleine and linden tea that, when the same combination arrives many years later unexpectedly in a different situation, evokes the memory of the Sunday mornings before mass in his aunts bedroom. Ordinary daily odors that are encountered in many different situations could not do this. Therefore keeping track of the frequency of occurrence of the individual odors and of the moments of first encounter with them in the life of individual subjects seems important in autobiographical research.

Another indication that olfaction does not seem to be interested in known odors is the fact that olfaction is a sense with complete adaptation. It means that the sensitivity for sustained monotonous stimulation is completely lost after a few minutes and that recovery from adaptation after cessation of the stimulus is slow. Nevertheless the sensitivity to new other odors remains largely intact (Köster, 1971; Köster and De Wijk, 1991). Moreover, complete adaptation seems to indicate that permanent awareness of experienced odors is not important and that it may even be harmful in as far as it might make us less vigilant and less attentive to the arrival of new and potentially dangerous odors in the very complex olfactory environment we constantly live in. In senses that play an active role in spatial orientation and movement such as vision and audition complete adaptation does not occur.

On the basis of the foregoing, we would like to formulate what we could call "the misfit theory of spontaneous conscious odor perception" (MITSCOP), a form of "perception by exception" guided by olfactory memories via the expectations about the odors in the situation. It plays, next to more semantic forms of explicit memory, a large role in incidental learning and implicit odor memory and is based on the following principles.

- In everyday life almost all odors are incidentally and unconsciously associated to the situation in which they occur and are stored as implicit expectations about their occurrence and not as precise recollections of the odor itself.
- An incidentally learned odor will not be spontaneously perceived consciously if it fits our implicit expectations in the situation, but if there is a misfit it will.
- Misfits may occur in different forms:
    a. A novel or changed odor will be presented in the same situation
    b. The original odor will be presented in a new situation.
    c. The originally encountered odor or situation may acquire a new emotional value due to state dependent factors in the perceiver (hunger, emotional shock, extreme odor intensity perception, etc.)
- Explicit odor perception and memory are important only in a few instances of normal life (gas detection, cooking, etc.), but are of great significance in the work of odor and flavor experts. With respect to the normal role and function of odors in human everyday life, the ecological validity of explicit intentional odor perception and memory experiments involving the identification of odors as such, might be questioned.

In this paper, we will provide further evidence for such a view and we will discuss the existing literature on odor perception and memory research critically. Finally, we will formulate criteria for ecologically valid odor perception and memory research and we will try to indicate ways in which these criteria can be met. MITSCOP is proposed as a more parsimonious explanation of the fact that conscious olfaction is rare than the idea of a "constant state of olfactory change blindness" proposed by Sela and Sobel (2010) which can't explain many of the phenomena discussed here. Their theory is based on the idea that sniffing is the only way in which odors become effective. Thus, it seems to exclude retronasal food perception and the many instances where subliminal odors influence behavior unconsciously.

CONSCIOUS ATTENTION TO ODORS

Once an odor has been perceived for the first time in a certain situation we tend to pay no more attention to it in that situation, probably because it does not provide a threat and its implicit perception results in feelings of well-being and safety without conscious perception of the odor itself. This idea is one of the corner stones of MITSCOP. Although it may seem that this is just an instance of a very general attentional theory and not specific for olfaction, it should be pointed out that the role of familiarity and novelty detection seems to be different in olfaction and in vision. People are extremely sensitive to off-odors and off flavors (Nijssen, 1991) in very complex odor mixtures, but easily overlook changes in the visual surroundings and spend a long time finding the 10 differences in two-picture-puzzles or to locate Wally in "Where is Wally?" pictures. Conscious attention in odor perception and its necessity for effectiveness in present or later behavior has also been a subject of discussion. Herz (1997) insisted on drawing people's attention to the odor during the encoding of her context-dependent memory tasks, whereas others (Kirk-Smith et al., 1983; Degel et al., 2001; Holland et al., 2005; Li et al., 2007; Zucco et al., 2009; Gaillet et al., 2013) carefully avoided drawing attention to the presence of odor in their incidental learning sessions. These latter authors clearly showed that conscious odor awareness is not a prerequisite for its effectiveness in behavioral modulation. Along another line, even the possibility to selectively direct one's attention to olfaction has been doubted on the basis of the fact that olfactory information bypasses the thalamus, but Spence et al. (2000, 2001) have clearly established the possibility of modulating behavioral responses by selective attention to odors. The relationship between attention and olfactory consciousness was also extensively discussed in a review article by Keller (2011). In line with MITSCOP, he points out that "with almost every breath we inhale air containing odors at relatively high concentrations; yet olfactory experiences are very rare." Furthermore, he points out that the involuntary increase in attention to odors which women may experience during pregnancy without change of olfactory acuity (Doty and Cameron, 2009) is probably an adaptive response to the fetuses' special sensitivity to poison. There are also large differences in attention to olfaction among non-pregnant individuals. Nevertheless, it is true that in everyday life almost all people pay little conscious attention to odors and it remains surprising how little research has been done on the effects of unattended and unconscious odor perception.

INCIDENTALLY LEARNED MEMORY FOR FOODS

Perhaps the most extensive evidence for the misfit theory comes from food memory. The results of a number of different experiments (Morin-Audebrand et al., 2012) showed that memory for incidentally learned food properties (texture, flavor, taste) was based on detection of change rather than on recollection of the previous experience with the food. All experiments were based on a paradigm developed by Mojet and Köster (2002, 2005), in which people were exposed incidentally to foods and/or drinks during another experiment or a quasi-accidental meal without any reference to a memory task and were later unexpectedly asked to recognize these foods amidst distractors consisting in slight variations of that food which still had the same basic flavor, but in which one of the components (e.g., the sweetness, the fattiness, or the flavor, etc.) had been changed by a small, just detectable, amount. In these experiments the participants could not indicate the original food better than by chance, but they could detect very clearly that the distractors were not the ones they had had before. In other words they noted the misfits readily, but could not identify the earlier perceived food itself (see **Figure 1**).

To counter the idea that these results were based on a response bias on the part of the participants that favors the correct rejection of the variants and diminishes the hit rate, the certainty of the respondents in uttering their responses was also measured in most experiments. It showed that the participants were significantly more certain of their correct rejections of the variants than of any of the other three possible responses (Hits and Misses: saying yes or no to the earlier experienced one; False alarms: saying yes to a variant). Support for the fact that novelty detection prevails over recollection comes also from the work of Jehl et al. (1995), who showed that familiarization with odors did not affect the hit rate for these odors in a memory experiment, but significantly improved correct rejection of the distractors as shown in reduced false alarm rates. A similar support for novelty detection dominance was obtained in the interference experiments of Zucco (2003), who found that odor memory (in contrast to visual and auditory memory) was not affected by interference. In the discussion Zucco remarks "The assumption that people lack a conscious representation for odors could successfully explain any of these effects." On the basis of recent incidental learning and recognition experiments (see below), the present authors take the more radical viewpoint that correct rejection of the distractors on the basis of their novelty in the experimental situation suffices to explain the results and that characteristics of the olfactory engram do not come into play in recognition at all. In other words, what is not there (the engram or recollection) cannot be interfered with or forgotten, but novelty (of distractors) is always functional. This might also explain the longevity of odor memory in recognition experiments (e.g., Engen and Ross, 1973) and why many authors fail to find serial position effects in odor memory (see overview Miles and Hodder, 2005). In most memory tests (visual as well as olfactory) the authors have used a two alternative forced choice test to measure the memory performance. Unfortunately this made it impossible to know whether the memory was based on recollection of the earlier experienced stimulus or on rejection of the distractor as being novel (see also the criticisms on the

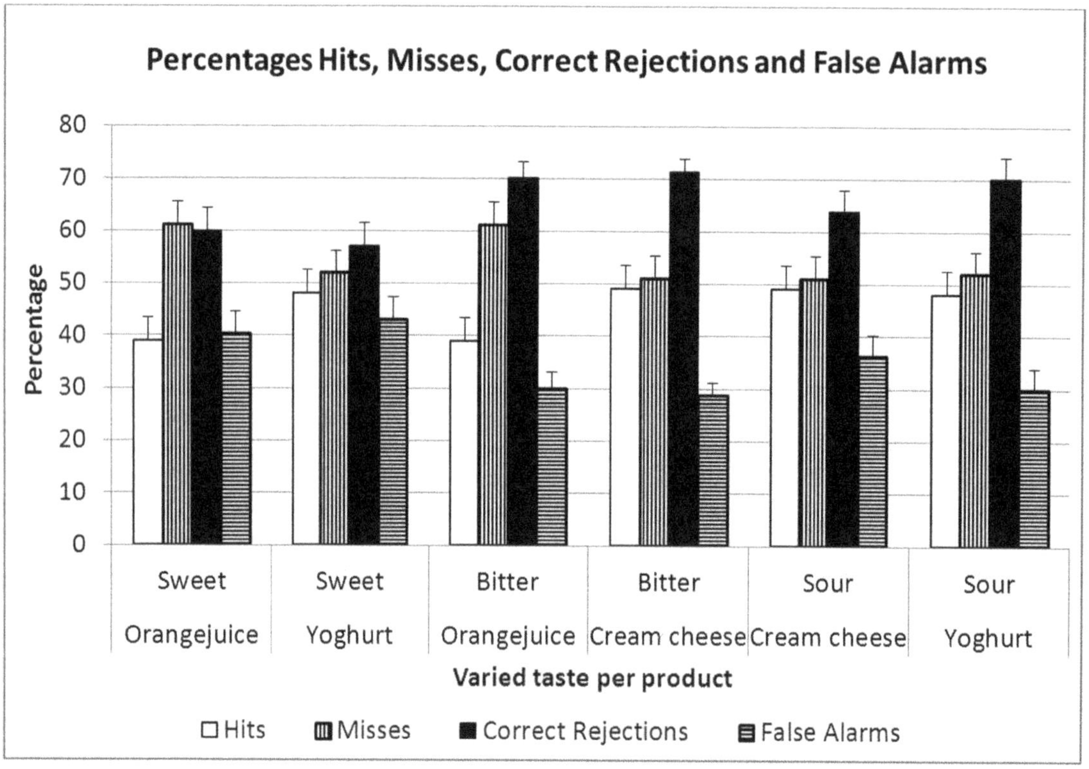

FIGURE 1 | Percentages of the four response types in each of six taste memory tests by Köster et al. (2004).

use of Signal Detection Theory in memory research discussed below). Thus, odors in the laboratory may not be remembered as such, but merely become linked to the experimental situation. When the situation is repeated only the distractors will be detected by their novelty in that situation and there is no need for recollection or re-activation of the engram characteristics of the earlier experienced stimuli. Indeed, it has been shown that incidentally presented odors are not even better remembered than by chance guessing, unless they are associated with a name or with an emotional event, but the new distractors are correctly rejected with great certainty and account for the memory performance (see below Degel et al., 2001; Møller et al., 2004, 2007; Morin-Audebrand et al., 2012).

Not having a specific memory of the odor characteristics is indeed perhaps also the best way to prevent extinction or loss under counter-conditioning as in the experiments of Stevenson (2001a,b,c). Again, what is not functional or is not even present can't be lost or affected by new information. In vision and audition, where conscious representation is possible and recollection seems to prevail, interference occurs probably because the representations of the remembered and the new stimuli compete at the same level (Zucco, 2003). In vision there is also evidence of a dissociation between familiarity based and content related memories (Brown and Aggleton, 2001; Daselaar et al., 2006a,b,c), but since there are only few data on truly incidentally learned visual memory, it is not clear whether "feelings of not-knowing" play the same role as in olfaction. Novel events and the neural mechanisms for detecting and remembering them have also been discussed by Ranganath and Rainer (2003) distinguishing stimulus novelty and contextual novelty.

The findings in olfaction and eating behavior were interpreted (Köster, 2005) as indications that whereas identification of a possible danger source is important in vision where it may help to choose adequate action (hiding, aggression, submission, etc.), it is not important in olfaction, where only one possible reaction (holding one's breath and fleeing, or spitting out in the case of food) is possible and time allowed for adequate reaction is short, because the stimulus is already at or in the body. Novelty and change detection might therefore have priority over identification. We are not only bad at odor identification, knowing the name of an odor may also make it lose its intimate connections to the situations in which it was first perceived, as the results of Willander and Larsson (2007), studying autobiographical memories, suggest. They compared memories evoked by respectively odors alone, odor names alone, and odors with their names and found that the high percentage of early autobiographical memories that came in the odor alone condition was very significantly reduced if the name was given with the odor. This suggests that "objectifying" the odor by naming it, makes it lose the emotional bond with specific life situations, which is so typical for the effects of odors in everyday life.

A further argument for MITSCOP was found in an extensive same-different judgment experiment with odors (Møller et al., 2012) showing that, contrary to same–different experiments carried out under comparable circumstances in vision where same detection is a bit faster than difference detection (Farell, 1985; Luce, 1986; Posner, 1986), in olfaction detecting a difference between two odors (a misfit) is much faster than detecting sameness. This strongly suggests that identification is important in vision but not in olfaction, where fast change detection is more important.

IMPLICIT MEMORY FOR INCIDENTALLY LEARNED ODOR-PLACE ASSOCIATIONS

The most convincing demonstration that odor identification, being the most outspoken form of explicit awareness, is not a necessary prerequisite in odor memory comes from experiments demonstrating the memory relationship between odors and the places where they were present without being consciously noticed (Degel and Köster, 1998, 1999; Degel et al., 2001; Köster et al., 2002). It was shown that people who had been unknowingly exposed to very slight and consciously unnoticed odors in rooms in which they performed a psychological test, would later, in a seemingly unrelated experiment on room odor selection indicate the exposure odor as fitting the room much better than people who had not been exposed to odor in that room, but only when they could not identify the odor by name. If they did know the name of the odor the situational spell was broken and they reacted in the same way as the people who had not been exposed to odor in the room or had never been in it (see **Table 1**).

These results clearly show that objectifying odors by identifying and naming them makes them lose their probably most important function of secretly connecting us via memory to places and situations in our life that have emotional meaning. Others (Li et al., 2007) have also illustrated loss of function by conscious awareness of the odors. They showed that odors only had emotional effects on the judgment of faces when they were not consciously perceived. Furthermore it is well-known in the perfume industry that many ingredients (e.g., musk, civet) lose their effectiveness in a mixture at concentrations where they begin to be perceived (Köster and Degel, 2000). Such results also show us that we may be mistaken if we see odor identification as the penultimate goal of odor memory and they may help us understand the importance of the silent implicitness of odor memory in making us at home in our world. Odors are not meant to be objectified and identified and therefore we are so bad at it.

Table 1 | Ratings of fit of the odors to the rooms by non-identifiers, identifiers, and non-exposed subjects (Degel et al., 2001).

Room	Room A	Room A	Room B	Room B	Total
Odor	Lavender	Orange	Lavender	Orange	
Non-identifiers	1.49[a]	0.83[a]	1.68[a]	1.31[a]	1.33[a]
Identifiers	0.61[b]	0.44[b]	0.89[b]	0.80[b]	0.69[b]
Non-exposed	0.62[b]	0.48[b]	0.76[b]	0.99[b]	0.73[b]

Ratings with different letters in the columns are significantly different ($P < 0.05$).

TRADITIONAL ODOR MEMORY RESEARCH: FLAWS AND VIRTUES

If our misfit theory is right, most odor memory remains implicit using its "conscious perception effacing" function to make us feel well and safe by not noticing the expected. Therefore, one may ask why most odor memory research has been directed at explicit recognition and identification of odors that usually were learned in objectified form during explicit learning sessions. For even if no explicit memorizing demand is made, a laboratory session in which odors are presented as separate items in bottles (or by an olfactometer), is far removed from the incidental learning situations in normal life, where odor often is an ephemeral epiphenomenon of an otherwise attention demanding situation. In most laboratory experiments odors are treated as things independent of any situation at learning and, in analogy to memory for visual objects, memory for them is tested by asking for their recognition via recollection and identification amidst completely unrelated other odor items. Such an approach is not only ecologically invalid, but it differs also fundamentally from the methods for studying food memory described above. Nevertheless, it may provide insights in the working of odor perception and memory under such abnormal conditions, compared to those in other sensory modalities tested under the same conditions and help to elucidate differences between people in their odor sensitivity, discrimination and memory due to gender and age. It has been shown for instance that the time-curves of memory and forgetting for thus presented single odors resembles that of non-identifiable and unstructured visual shapes (Lawless, 1978) and differs from those found for identifiable visual pictures or words (Engen and Ross, 1973). In an experiment associating odors with two different pictures, Lawless and Engen (1977) also found that the first association was better remembered than the second one. They interpreted this finding as an indication of strong proactive inhibition. At the same time all these findings fit well in the misfit theory and the unimportance of odor identification.

Research with itemized single odors has also clarified important differences between implicitly and explicitly learned odor memory. In an experiment with very uncommon odors, chosen to avoid the possible influence of verbal memory, groups of elderly and young people were either incidentally exposed to the odors and judged them on pleasantness or were exposed under the instruction to remember them in view of a later test (Møller et al., 2004). It could be shown that the incidentally learned odor memory of the elderly was at least as good as and even slightly better than that of the young subjects, but that the young outdid the elderly significantly in the intentional learning condition. This result was later confirmed in an ecologically more appropriate experiment with soups and more natural incidental learning conditions (Møller et al., 2007). Thus, it can be seen that the unnatural conditions in the laboratory may be very informative, but that it is nevertheless good to verify their external validity by more ecologically based means. Perhaps the worst mistakes are based on the idea that explicit odor perception and odor memory are the normal ways of dealing with odors. Especially in the learning phase it is necessary to arrange things in a normal way without attracting extra attention to the odor and without any reference to memory. Thus, it might not be a good idea to ask people how often in their life they have encountered certain odors as the learning phase in an implicit odor memory experiment using repetition priming as Olsson (1999) and Olsson and Cain (2003) did. It invokes the thought of memory even if it does not contain a direct hint that the odors should be remembered. On the other hand, Olsson (1999) used a very good method trying to avoid the possible influence of semantic memory on the results in the later testing of the memory for the odor. Instead of asking people to recognize the previously presented and non-presented controls while measuring their reaction times, he familiarized the subjects with a special comparison stimulus and asked in the final test whether the presented stimulus was the comparison stimulus or not. He then compared the reaction times to the "no" responses given to the earlier primed stimuli and non-primed control stimuli. Under these conditions no overall priming effect was found, but further analysis of the data after the participants had also performed an identification test, showed that primed identifiable odor stimuli did significantly worse than identifiable control odors, whereas with unidentifiable odors the reverse was true, the primed ones showing shorter reaction times. This is in line with the data of Degel et al. (2001) on the effects of odor identification in incidentally learned memory for room odors (see **Table 1** above).

As indicated, it is often difficult to separate veridical odor memory (i.e., memory for the smell itself) from the semantic memory for the *odor's* name. Unfortunately, the overwhelming majority of odor memory studies falls prey to this confound (see Larsson, 1997). Investigations of veridical odor memory should not provide subjects with the possibility of remembering an odor by some verbal label. This can be avoided by using targets and distractors which belong to the same odor-category and which subjects would label in the same way, while still being able to perceptually discriminate between them. The methods used in the studies of food memory mentioned above (Morin-Audebrand et al., 2012) can easily be applied to other odor memory research. Another way to minimize the use of verbal labels is to apply stimuli which subjects do not have names for. An example of this is provided by Møller et al. (2004). Those who are fascinated by the question why it is so difficult to identify odors by name (Cain, 1982; Cain et al., 1998) or those who think that naming odors is the ultimate goal in odor memory studies (Lehrner et al., 1999), have long dominated the field of odor memory and contributed much to the distinction between the two forms of memory, but have often neglected to study veridical odor memory itself. One of the most recent and extreme examples is a study by Cessna and Frank (2013) in which they tried to answer the question whether odor knowledge or an odor naming strategy mediates the relationship between odor naming and recognition memory. Although this question may be of academic interest and the methods used to provide an answer to it were ingenious, one may wonder about their relevance for everyday life where we almost never name odors and the odors that are most important to us (odors of our surroundings and of people we know) are usually non-nameable. The fascination for identification as the way to do "object memory" research in the same way as in visual and verbal memory studies has in a way estranged the researchers of their subject. The few nameable odors in our life are almost certainly the ones that have lost their intimate relationship with places and situations and although to many authors nameable odors seem to be also ecologically most relevant, according to the MITSCOP they are much less interesting than the non-nameable odors that surround us but are not consciously remarked because they fit our expectations in the situation. Such odors are seldom used in odor memory experiments. The exceptions are collected air samples from odor polluted areas or from sick buildings, but these are usually only used to determine their detection thresholds and to characterize their intensity. To study veridical odor memory, it might be interesting to present subjects with the odors collected from rooms in their house and to check how well they could localize them. The nearest attempt to do something like this was that of Balez (2001) in France, who collected stories about the odors emanating from the different places in a shopping mall and about how regular visitors of the mall felt they could orient themselves and knew their position in the mall on the basis of them. Unfortunately, she did not verify their actual memory based orientation by presenting the odors to them and asking questions about their imagined position in the mall. It would have been a better proof of the way people use odor in their orientation than the highly artificial, but otherwise interesting and amusing experiment on scent-tracking by human subjects (Porter et al., 2005, 2007). They showed that people could follow a chocolate oil odor trail and that they probably used the lateral differences in odor intensity between the two nostrils. This reopened the old debate about the localization of odorant sources by birhinal differences in olfactory (Von Skramlik, 1924; Von Békésy, 1964) or in trigeminal (Kobal et al., 1989) stimulation. It was argued that active sniffing versus passive stimulation might play an important role in the question. Kobal et al., using passive sniffing, claimed that only odorants that also stimulated the trigeminal nerve showed localization and that purely olfactory stimulation did not. Stimulus concentration (Cometto-Muniz and Cain, 1990; Hummel et al., 2003; Frasnelli and Hummel, 2005; Frasnelli et al., 2009) or overall stimulus mass concentration (Cometto-Muniz and Cain, 1984) and/or the influence of stimulus volume (Frasnelli et al., 2011) were also indicated as possible factors. According to these authors, the role of active versus passive smelling in localization depended on the odorants used. Thus, mixed olfacto-trigeminal stimulants were better localized under passive conditions, but a pure odorant was better localized under active sniffing, probably due to increased olfactory attention as suggested by Zelano et al. (2005). In this connection it should be remarked that all experiments (both passive and active) were carried out under explicit perceptual conditions, but that there is of course a definite intentional difference between active sniffing and waiting for a stimulus to come. If one thinks about the difference between touching and being touched, one can easily imagine that in the case of olfaction the difference might also be important even in explicit experimental conditions. Of course there is also a large difference between the attention given to the stimulus in explicit laboratory experiments and the implicit and often unnoticed encounters with odors in everyday life. After all sniffing is usually limited to the few situations in which unexpected odors or new surroundings have to be inspected. In this respect almost all laboratory experiments are atypical for normal olfactory behavior and it will demand quite drastic steps on a number of aspects to bring the two closer together in order to provide ecologically valid insight in the role odor perception and memory play in our life.

DO'S AND DON'TS IN ECOLOGICALLY VALID ODOR MEMORY RESEARCH

Generally speaking ecologically valid memory research should be based on incidental learning in an everyday situation and on implicit memory measurement. Apart from the earlier mentioned experiments by Degel and Köster (1999), Degel et al. (2001), only a few recent experiments meet these demands. Holland et al. (2005) showed the influence of incidental smelling of cleaning spirit on cleaning behavior and research in waiting rooms of Dutch hospitals showed that unnoticed odors can reduce aggressiveness and promote the perception of friendliness (LEV Report, 2012). The experiments on incidentally learned food memory did not respect the demand of implicit memory measurement. They asked people explicitly to recognize the food they had eaten under everyday circumstances and without any special attention and had people compare their memory of the food with new samples of the same food and slight variations of it. Although this type of measurement is not implicit, it provides much information about the implicit memory for incidentally learned food impressions. Thus, it has been shown, that the memory for sweetness and fattiness, may be distorted in some products whereas for other sensory aspects it remains intact (Mojet and Köster, 2002, 2005; Köster et al., 2004). Especially the method of relative memory measurement, in which people are asked to tell whether the presented samples are more, less or equally strong compared to the earlier incidentally eaten food, provides much information about changes in appreciation and perception of the food occurring in memory. It is difficult to obtain such information with purely implicit memory methods and responses to questions like "Is this product now worse or better liked than it was?" may nevertheless tell much about the way in which the memory was implicitly retained (e.g., whether the memory of the sweetness has faded, while the memory of the bitterness did not).

The more implicit ways of testing memory such as measuring preference and/or decision time in free choice among a set of alternatives after previous incidental exposure to one of them, or registering behavioral and facial changes to incidental stimuli (Fedoroff et al., 1997, 2003; Holland et al., 2005; Papies and Hamstra, 2010; Soussignan et al., 2012; Gaillet et al., 2013) often fail to provide such more detailed information. Thus, in order to do ecologically relevant memory research, it is perhaps more important to make sure that learning is truly incidental or takes place in the same way as in everyday life than to comply with the rule of implicit memory that no explicit link may be made with the learning event. In the case of Gaillet et al. (2013), who exposed people, who were waiting to take part in a meal, to afaint and unnoticed fruit odor, variation of that odor was used to show the specificity of the reaction. Melon odor led to the choice of more vegetable rich appetizers, whereas pear odor changed the dessert choices toward fruits and away from rich and fatty items. Such category specific reactions provide interesting and truly ecological information, but do not provide insight in memory distortions of the food itself as explicit relative memory measurements would. Of course, it is preferable to have an implicit memory measure first before asking explicit questions. Since subjects who have been exposed to explicit questions have lost their naivety and cannot be used again in incidental learning and implicit memory experiments, one should limit the use of such questions to the moment one is sure not to need the subject again. This limits the experimental possibilities. Thus, it is only possible to do within-subject research if the subject was incidentally exposed to different stimuli in the same session or in comparable sessions before the memory was tested, even with implicit methods (e.g., reaction time measurements). It is also important to avoid methods that imply identification of the stimuli either by name or otherwise and that objectify the odor in some form. As shown above in the experiments by Degel and Köster (1999), Degel et al. (2001), odors that can be identified by name, become "things" and tend to lose their intimate connections with the situations in which they occurred in a person's life and therewith their main function. Odors are probably not meant to be identified. They are the silent emotional reminders of the surroundings and situations with which they are linked by unconscious association and they are powerful evokers of the feelings that belonged to these events. In fact, we have stored many thousands odors in that associative and unconscious way and we have perhaps only names for at most 50 of them (Schab, 1991; Sulmont et al., 2002). Usually, we even determine the name of the odor and its source by remembering first the situation in which we earlier encountered the odor (why does this odor make me think of the attic in the house of my grand-parents when I was looking for fishing gear? Ah, there were apples drying. It is the odor of drying apples!). Objectifying odors into objects is denying them an essential part of their function in life and although it may be useful in the study of olfactory perception mechanisms and in the industrial application of chemicals in the perfume industry, it destroys the possibility of studying their normal function in human life. The proponents of odor-object theories overlook this in their search for odor identification and discrimination as the end goal of all odor research. If odors are indeed not meant to be identified, but should, as stated in the misfit theory, be recognized as the ephemeral and unnoticed providers of feelings of safety and comfort, unless they are unknown and unexpected or out of place, we may need to devote more time to emotional effects of odor associations and to the investigation of incidentally learned situational odor memories instead of investigating how "odor objects" are constructed and changed by odor-odor and odor-taste learning under laboratory conditions with odors from bottles or olfactometers.

If indeed MITSCOP is right, situational experience with an odor will reduce the conscious perception of that odor upon repetition in the same surroundings or foods, but may remain unchanged or might even be enhanced in other environments or eating situations. The consequence for research is fundamental. It means that single measurements of the emotional effects of odors are not predictive of the longer term odor effects and that these effects are not odor-object dependent, as is often assumed, but are strongly linked to associations and depend on situational congruence. Perhaps only in artificial laboratory situations where the odors are presented explicitly as particular items alone or in combination with other odor or taste items as in the experiments on odor-odor learning or odor-taste learning (Stevenson, 2001a,b,c;

Stevenson and Boakes, 2003) can the influence of situational effects be excluded or at least controlled. The external validity of that type of research could be questioned however. Within the limitations of the laboratory situation, the odors or flavors of the other items are the only situational context elements available and odors are therefore almost inevitably associated with them. Nevertheless, the same mechanisms seem to function in the real world as is illustrated by cross-cultural studies, which show that different cultural settings not only lead to differences in preference for flavors, but also to genuine differences in perception and discrimination (Ayabe-Kanamura et al., 1998).

In this respect the research by Baeyens et al. (1996) is perhaps most revealing. They incidentally exposed people to scented toilets in one experiment and to scented massage oil in another and showed that the liking for the odor was strongly dependent on the situational appreciation of the subjects, irrespective of whether they had consciously noted the odors during the exposure or not. Rozin et al. (1998) on the other hand tried to repeat this type of evaluative conditioning in a laboratory setting and had very little success. They ascribed their lack of success mainly to the laboratory surroundings and to the fact that the neutral odors they used might be particularly resistant to picking up emotional associations. The use of squeeze bottles for the explicit presentation of the odors and the use of very well-known odors (related to many different previous situations) may also have contributed to their failure.

Table 2 presents a summary of the do's and don'ts in performing ecologically relevant odor memory research.

The first four of these recommendations have been amply discussed above, but some of the comments in the table might need more clarification. Thus, avoiding memory references means that people should not be aware of participating in a memory experiment and that all allusions to memory should be avoided [see discussion on Olsson and Cain (2003) above]. Furthermore it is important to ask the people, who, after finishing the experiment, know that it was about memory, not to divulge this knowledge to others and to corroborate this demand by explaining that there is a prize for the person who has the best memory results and that telling others would reduce their chances of winning it. Providing a representative situational link by making people think of a situation in their life (either by providing images or telling them a story) may help to verify the influence of the appropriateness of the stimulus in this situation on the odor memory. Of course letting them participate in a real situation is preferable but imagination can work well especially via stories in which the subjects can imagine the situation in their own familiar surroundings.

Incidental learning in natural situations as in the Baeyens et al. experiments or by presenting the odors in a perceptible, but not spontaneously noted, way as in the experiments of Degel and Köster (1999), Degel et al. (2001), Fedoroff et al. (1997, 2003), Holland et al. (2005) and of Gaillet et al. (2013) is perhaps the best way to assess ecological validity of the results. Other forms of stimulus exposure (even in the laboratory from bottles or an olfactometer) may also be used as long as they are so well disguised as part of another research subject, that even the thought of them being

Table 2 | Overview of recommendations in ecologically valid odor memory research.

Feature	Do	Don't	Comment (see also text below)
Learning exposure	Present stimuli incidentally in a natural situation	Draw attention to the target stimulus in any way	Avoid memory references
Subject choice	Select people that are naïve to memory experiments	Use the same people again after a memory test	Ask secrecy of your subjects
Stimulus selection	Choose situationally relevant stimuli	Choose very well-known and /or nameable stimuli	Provide imagined situational link
Stimulus presentation	Present naturally or at unnoticed strength	Present from odor bottles or olfactometers	Pre-tests necessary
Memory verification (implicit)	Give priority to implicit measurements	Present test stimuli in a way different from learning	Prepare natural alternatives of same category
Memory verification (explicit)	Absolute and relative memory measurements	Fatigue subjects with long questionnaires and why's?	Select attributes for relative memory tests
Data treatment	Look for segments in your subject population	Average without looking for behavior differences	Prior analysis of behavioral differences
Data analysis	Analyze your hits, misses, false alarms, correct rejections	Calculate composites (d') without verifying hits, correct rejections	Hit rate as smaller, larger, or equal to chance? Verify!
Characterization of memory effects	Verify distortions in relative memory	Forget to check differences in rel. attribute memory	Check memory mode: recollection or change detection
Repeated exposure effects	Use different subject groups. Vary amount of learning exposure	Expect that more exposure will have no effect on both liking and perception	Check influence of perceived complexity

used as memory targets does not arise in the experimental subjects. Thus, asking people in a laboratory setting to judge odors or flavors on their pleasantness or intensity and later presenting some of these odors in a relative memory test among slightly modified variations of them as distractors, might still provide ecologically valid information about the stability or distortion of the memory for them, even if the proper situational circumstances are not respected. The information obtained in this way is more limited however. If it relies on explicit memory verification as proposed here, this might perhaps be preceded or accompanied by implicit measurements such as face reading or psychophysiological measurements (heart rate, electro-dermal responses). If the emotions raised by the memory should be measured, it should be done before the explicit memory measurement and preferable in an implicit way (e.g., in a seemingly non-related projection test taken under the influence of the stimuli under the same unnoticed conditions). Once memory testing is made explicit, the emotional value of the stimulus will probably change and loose its ecological relevance.

DATA TREATMENT

In treating the data, one should look for possible segments in the population that may differ in their behavior with regard to the stimuli involved or in the importance they attribute to them. Thus, it is known that with respect to eating chocolate the population is divided into two groups, those who bite and chew their chocolate and those who suck it, and the difference in the perception and memory of chocolate in these groups makes it difficult to make chocolate that is satisfying both groups. Averaging over such groups should therefore be avoided and prior segmentation on the basis of stimulus-related behavior is a prerequisite of good ecologically valid research. Experience with odors and flavors in a certain domain will also be an important criterion for segmenting. People who collect wines and keep them for aging and special occasions will appreciate and remember them differently than do wine novices.

In analyzing perceptual detection and memory data, Signal Detection Theory has played a predominant role over the last few decades and in many cases, the results are only presented in the form of the composite statistic d' or similar measures. In the case of perceptual detection, where there is no doubt about what is the signal and what is noise, this use is obvious, but in incidentally learned odor memory where all signs point in the direction of novelty and change detection rather than recollection of the earlier encountered stimulus (Morin-Audebrand et al., 2012), the situation is less clear and in this case it is advisable to look at the components (hits, misses, false alarms, and correct rejections) as well as at the composite. Furthermore, it is worthwhile to compare the certainty of the subjects about their different statements. If indeed novelty prevails over recollection in this form of memory, correct rejection should be seen as the signal and it is not surprising that it is also the response the subjects are more certain of than of their hits, which they seem not to detect any better than by chance. Since this may truly reflect a mode of remembering (and one that fits well in the misfit theory), it seems important not to hide it under composites like d'. Verification whether the hit rate is better than chance and how sure the people are of their different responses is to be recommended as a first step in the verification of the form of the memory involved. As already described above, more detailed information about the memory effects can be obtained from relative memory measurements that involve comparison of the actual and remembered target.

That memory measurement necessarily involves a repeated encounter with the earlier learned stimulus may also have an influence on the memory content because repeated exposure to an odor may change the perceived quality of it, especially when the odor is new and complex (Köster and Mojet, 2007; Mojet and Köster, 2013). It may therefore be of interest to compare the memory for odors in a group that has been incidentally exposed only once to the odor with that of a group that has been exposed to it more (5–10) times. Especially when new odors are involved, it may well be that the memory of such a repetition group provides a more realistic image of the memorability of the odor when used more frequently in normal everyday life.

RELEVANT ODOR MEMORY RESEARCH PARADIGMS

Three examples of ecologically relevant research paradigms are described, one devoted to pre-launch research for the introduction of a new flavor, one dedicated to possible uses as an environmental odor, and one directed at reduction of aggression or stimulation of pleasant behavior in public places. These examples stem from applied work that we have carried out and that have led to successful solutions. Here they are presented as suggestions for more relevant research. In our case they worked well, but much may depend on the circumstances and the people involved. In some of the cases described there was simply no funding and no time to do elaborate research comparing experimental and control groups. We hope that suggestions like these might stimulate readers to come out of their laboratories and to try some more ecologically relevant methods to answer real problems.

ODOR OR FLAVOR MEMORY AS A PREDICTIVE ELEMENT IN PRE-LAUNCH RESEARCH

Suppose one had to choose between two alternative new formulas (A and B) for a product to be launched in an already existing market in which a competitor product (CP) is the market leader, how could flavor memory help in reaching the best decision? In answering this question we suppose that all traditional measures have been taken and that the three products A, B and CP (which serves as a benchmark) have been extensively described by a well-trained descriptive panel and have already been judged positively on a hedonic scale by a representative consumer panel or by different segments of the consumer population such as product users and non-users, or groups that differ in their use of the product (due to habit, age, etc.). In some cases, depending on the implicitness of the way the hedonic information was obtained, these groups could be used again for the memory testing. They might again be invited under a false pretense (e.g., an unrelated experiment) and then inadvertently be exposed to the three stimuli and a number of small variants of each of them in an absolute memory test in which they simply indicated whether they had recognized the one they had judged in the earlier session. After this they were confronted with a newly coded set of the same stimuli for a relative memory test in which they indicated whether the now presented stimuli were nicer, less nice or equally nice (and intense on a number of relevant attributes) as the similar shaped ones they had judged some time (a day, a week) ago. On the basis of the hit and correct rejection rates of the answers in the absolute memory, one could draw conclusions about the prevailing mode of the memory (recollection or change and novelty detection) and the relative memory would make it possible to see whether the product was more positively or negatively remembered and which of the significant attributes might have contributed to eventually found memory distortions. This provides important information for possible product improvements. In combination with some repeated presentation measurements (extended boredom test as described in (Köster and Mojet, 2007; Mojet and Köster, 2013), the comparison of the memory results for the new products with that of the benchmark in both user and non-user groups will provide better predictive information about the future market success of the new products than the simple first impression measurements on which most present pre-launch consumer research is based and may help reducing the risk of market flops considerably (see Köster and Mojet, 2012a,b).

USE OF ODOR MEMORY IN THE IMPROVEMENT OF LIVING PLEASURE FOR MENTALLY HANDICAPPED OR VISUALLY HANDICAPPED PERSONS

In institutions for mentally or visually handicapped people, odors can be used quite effectively in several ways.

Finding one's way

In an institution for mentally handicapped persons in The Netherlands, a problem arose from the fact that several different corridors to the dormitory units had their access via a large hall and many of the inhabitants got lost trying to find their way home. Odorizing the different corridors with hardly detectable and spontaneously not noticed odors solved the problem. People "smelled home" at the corridor entrance and were hardly ever mistaken. In the same way odors have been used at corridor crossings in institutes for the visually handicapped. They learned very quickly what turn they should make.

Preparing for routines

Personnel working with mentally handicapped people often have difficulty obtaining their clients cooperation in the preparation for daily (meals) or regularly recurring events (going to the swimming pool). Hardly noticeable food odors or swimming pool odors have been used with success in making clients more cooperative by giving them an anticipatory pleasure that could not be matched by any other source of stimulation.

REDUCING AGGRESSION AND STIMULATION OF PLEASANT BEHAVIOR IN PUBLIC PLACES

In emergency waiting rooms in hospitals where aggression and unfriendliness may arise easily from the fact that some later arrivals are treated more rapidly than others on account of their more acute need as judged by the staff, weak and not spontaneously noticed odors have been used with success to reduce aggressive behavior and stimulate friendliness between visitors and toward the personnel (LEV Report, 2012). The odors were chosen on the basis of a photographic projection test developed for judging the influence of unnoticed odors and of the presence of flowers on the appreciation of rooms and meals (Mojet, Holthuysen, Van Veggel, de Wijk and Köster, in preparation). The odors are also employed to try to reduce unpleasant behavior in public transport.

FINAL CONCLUSIONS ON THE ROLE OF ODOR MEMORY IN EVERYDAY LIFE: MISFIT AND FIT

Odors guard our lives while not being noticed consciously most of the time. Thus they provide feelings of safety and comfort with the surroundings without demanding attention for themselves. They are not there to be named or identified, but to silently link us to the world and to our history of lived situations. When identified, odors lose this function. Most odors that fit our expectations remain unnoticed. Misfits are noted. Although it is also important, intentional smelling and the pleasures and displeasures it may provide is disproportionately overrepresented in olfactory research compared to its role in daily life. Applied research should be further developed, taking the special characteristics and functions of incidental odor memory into account.

AUTHOR CONTRIBUTIONS

Egon P. Köster drafted, Per Møller and Jozina Mojet co-drafted the manuscript. All authors were involved in developing the first draft of the manuscript into the final version suitable for publication and they all approved the final manuscript.

REFERENCES

Ayabe-Kanamura, S., Schicker, L., Laska, M., Hudson, R., Distel, H., Kobayakawa, T., et al. (1998). Differences in perception of everyday odors: a Japanese-German cross cultural study. *Chem. Senses* 23, 31–38. doi: 10.1093/chemse/23.1.31

Baeyens, F., Wrzesniewskl, A., De Houwer, J., and Eelen, P. (1996). Toilet rooms, body massages, and smells: two field studies on human evaluative odor conditioning. *Curr. Psychol. Dev. Learn. Pers. Soc.* 15, 77–96. doi: 10.1007/BF02686936

Balez, S. (2001). *Ambiances Olfactives Dans l'espace Construit (Odoursurroundings in the Builtenvironment)*. Doctoral thesis, Ecole Polytechnique de l'Université de Nantes, France.

Brown, M. W., and Aggleton, J. P. (2001). Recognition memory: what are the roles of the perirhinal cortex and hippocampus? *Nat. Rev. Neurosci.* 2, 51–61. doi: 10.1038/35049064

Cain, W. S. (1982). Odor identification by males and females: predictions vs. performance. *Chem. Senses* 7, 129–142. doi: 10.1093/chemse/7.2.129

Cain, W. S., De Wijk, R., Lulejian, C., Schiet, F., and See, L. C. (1998). Odor identification: perceptual and semantic dimensions. *Chem. Senses* 23, 309–326. doi: 10.1093/chemse/23.3.309

Cessna, T. C., and Frank, R. (2013). Does odor knowledge or an odor naming strategy mediate the relationship between odor naming and recognition memory? *Chem. Percept.* doi: 10.1007/s12078-013-9139-y

Chebat, J.-C., and Michon, R. (2003). Impact of ambient odors on mall shoppers' emotions, cognition, and spending. A test of competitive causal theories. *J. Business Res.* 56, 529539. doi: 10.1016/S0148-2963(01)00247-8

Chu, S., and Downes, J. J. (2000). Long live Proust: the odour-cued autobiographical memory bump. *Cognition,* 75, B41–B50. doi: 10.1016/S0010-0277(00)00065-2

Chu, S., and Downes, J. J. (2002). Proust nose best: odors are better cues of autobiographical memory. *Mem. Cognit.* 30, 511–518. doi: 10.3758/BF03194952

Cometto-Muniz, E., and Cain, W. S. (1984). Temporal integration of pungency. *Chem. Senses* 8, 315–327. doi: 10.1093/chemse/8.4.315

Cometto-Muniz, J. E., and Cain, W. S. (1990). Thresholds for odor and nasal pungency. *Physiol. Behav.* 48, 719–725. doi: 10.1016/0031-9384(90)90217-R

Daselaar, S. M., Fleck, M. S., Prince, S. E., and Cabeza, R. (2006a). The medial temporal lobe distinguishes old from new. *J. Neurosci.* 26, 5835–5839. doi: 10.1523/JNEUROSCI.0258-06.2006

Daselaar, S. M., Fleck, M. S., Prince, S. E., and Cabeza, R. (2006b). Triple dissociation in the medial temporal lobes: recollection, familiarity and novelty. *J. Neurophysiol.* 96, 1902–1911. doi: 10.1152/jn.01029.2005

Daselaar, S. M., Fleck, M. S., Dobbins, I. G., Madden, D. J., and Cabeza, R. (2006c). Effects of healthy aging on hippocampal and rhinal memory functions: an event related FMRI study. *Cereb. Cortex* 16, 1771–1782. doi: 10.1093/cercor/bhj112

Degel, J., and Köster, E. P. (1998). Implicit memory for odors: a possible method for observation. *Percept. Mot. Skills* 86, 943–952. doi: 10.2466/pms.1998.86.3.943

Degel, J., and Köster, E. P. (1999). Odors: implicit memory and performance effects. *Chem. Senses* 24, 317–325. doi: 10.1093/chemse/24.3.317

Degel, J., Piper, D., and Köster, E. P. (2001). Implicit learning and implicit memory for odors: the influence of odor identification and retention time. *Chem. Senses* 26, 267–280. doi: 10.1093/chemse/26.3.267

Doty, R. L., and Cameron, E. L. (2009). Sex differences and reproductive hormone influences on human odor perception. *Physiol. Behav.* 97, 213–228. doi: 10.1016/j.physbeh.2009.02.032

Engen, T., and Ross, B. M. (1973). Long-term memory of odors with and without verbal descriptions. *J. Exper. Psychol.* 100, 221–226. doi: 10.1037/h0035492

Farell, B. (1985). "Same–Different" judgments: a review of current controversies in perceptual comparisons. *Psychol. Bull.* 98, 419–456. doi: 10.1037/0033-2909.98.3.419

Fedoroff, I. C., Polivy, J., and Herman, C. P. (1997). The effect of pre-exposure to food cues on the eating behavior of restrained, and unrestrained eaters. *Appetite* 28, 33–47. doi: 10.1006/appe.1996.0057

Fedoroff, I. C., Polivy, J., and Herman, C. P. (2003). The specificity of restrained versus unrestrained eaters' responses to food cues: general desire to eat, or craving for the cued food? *Appetite* 41, 7–13. doi: 10.1016/S0195-6663(03)00026-6

Frasnelli, J., Charbonneau, G., Collignon, O., and Lepore, F. (2009). Odor localization and sniffing. *Chem. Senses* 34, 139–144. doi: 10.1093/chemse/bjn068

Frasnelli J. and Hummel T. (2005). Olfactory dysfunction and daily life. *Eur. Arch. Otorhinolaryngol.* 262, 231–235. doi: 10.1007/s00405-004-0796-y

Frasnelli, J., Hummel, T., Berg, J., Huang, G., and Doty, R. L. (2011). Intranasal localizability of odorants: influence of stimulus volume. *Chem. Senses* 36, 405–411. doi: 10.1093/chemse/bjr001

Gaillet, M., Sulmont-Rossé, C., Issanchou, S., Chabanet, C., and Chambaron, S. (2013). Priming effects of an olfactory food cue on subsequent food-related behavior. *Food Qual. Pref.* 30, 274–281. doi: 10.1016/j.foodqual.2013.06.008

Gibson, J. J. (1966). *The Senses Considered as Perceptual Systems.* Boston: Houghton-Mifflin.

Gibson, J. J. (1979). *The Ecological Approach to Visual Perception.* Boston: Houghton-Mifflin.

Herz, R. S. (1997). The effects of cue distinctiveness on odor-based context-dependent memory. *Mem. Cognit.* 25, 375–380. doi: 10.3758/BF03211293

Herz, R. S. (2004). A naturalistic analysis of autobigraphical memories triggered by olfactory, visual and auditory stimuli. *Chem. Senses* 29, 217–224. doi: 10.1093/chemse/bjh025

Herz, R. S., and Schooler, J. W. (2002). A naturalistic study of autobiographical memories evoked by olfactory and visual cues: testing the Proustian hypothesis. *Am. J. Psychol.* 115, 21–32. doi: 10.2307/1423672

Holland, R. W., Hendriks, M., and Aarts, H. (2005). Smells like clean spirit. Nonconscious effects of scent on cognition and behavior. *Psychol. Sci.* 16, 689–693. doi: 10.1111/j.1467-9280.2005.01597.x

Hummel, T., Futschik, T., Frasnelli, J., and Hüttenbrink, K. B. (2003). Effects of olfactory function, age, and gender on trigeminally mediated sensations: a study based on the lateralization of chemosensory stimuli. *Toxicol. Lett.* 140–141, 273–280. doi: 10.1016/S0378-4274(03)00078-X

Jacob, S., and McClintock, M. K. (2000). Psychological state and mood effects of steroidal chemosignals in women and men. *Horm. Behav.* 37, 57–78. doi: 10.1006/hbeh.1999.1559

Jehl, C., Royet, J. P., and Holley, A. (1995). Odor memory and recognition memory as a function of familiarization. *Percept. Psychophys.* 56, 658–668. doi: 10.3758/BF03208359

Keller, A. (2011). Attention and olfactory consciousness. *Front. Psychol.* 2:380. doi: 10.3389/fsyg.2011.00380

Kirk-Smith, M. D., Van Toller, C., and Dodd, G. H. (1983). Unconscious odour conditioning in human subjects. *Biol. Psychol.* 17, 221–231. doi: 10.1016/0301-0511(83)90020-0

Kobal, G., Van Toller, T., and Hummel, T. (1989). Is there directional smelling? *Experientia* 45, 130–132. doi: 10.1007/BF01954845

Köster, E. P. (1971). *Adaptation and Cross-Adaptation in Olfaction.* Published Doctoral Thesis, Bronder Offset, Utrecht.

Köster, E. P. (2005). Does olfactory memory depend on remembering odors? *Chem. Senses* 30(Suppl. 1), i236–i237. doi: 10.1093/chemse/bjh201

Köster, E. P., Degel, J., and Piper, D. (2002). Proactive and retroactive interference in implicit odor memory. *Chem. Senses* 27, 191–207. doi: 10.1093/chemse/27.3.191

Köster, E. P., and De Wijk, R. A. (1991). "Olfactory adaptation," in *The Human Sense of Smell*, eds D. G. Laing, R. L. Doty, and W. Breipohl (Berlin: Springer-Verlag), 199–215. doi: 10.1007/978-3-642-76223-9_10

Köster, E. P., and Degel, J. (2000). Are weak odors stronger than strong odors? The influence of odor on human performance. *Aromachology* 9, 9–11.

Köster, E. P., and Mojet, J. (2007). "Boredom and the reasons why some new products fail," in *Consumer-led Food Product Development*, ed. H. J. H. MacFie (Abbington: Woodhead Publishing), 262–280. doi: 10.1533/9781845693381.2.262

Köster, E. P., and Mojet, J. (2012a). Analysis of Flops: a useful tool for future innovations. Part 1: the diagnostic phase. *Agro Food Indus. Hi-Tech*, 23, 6–9.

Köster, E. P., and Mojet, J. (2012b). Analysis of Flops: a useful tool for future innovations. Part 2: the reduction of future flop risks. *Agro Food industry Hi-Tech* 23, 6–10.

Köster, M. A., Prescott, J., and Köster, E. P. (2004). Incidental learning and memory for three basic tastes in food. *Chem. Senses* 29, 441–453. doi: 10.1093/chemse/bjh047

Larsson, M. (1997). Semantic factors in episodic recognition of common odors in early and late adulthood: a review. *Chem. Senses* 22, 623–633. doi: 10.1093/chemse/22.6.623

Lawless, H. T. (1978). Recognition of common odors, pictures and simple shapes. *Percept. Psychophys.* 24, 493–495. doi: 10.3758/BF03198772

Lawless, H., and Engen, T. (1977). Associations to odors: interference from, mnemonics, and verbal labeling. *J. Exper. Psychol. Hum. Learn. Mem.* 3, 52–59. doi: 10.1037/0278-7393.3.1.52

Lehrner, J., Gluck, J., and Laska, M. (1999). Odor identification, consistency of label use, olfactory threshold and their relationships to odor memory over the human lifespan. *Chem. Senses* 24, 337–346. doi: 10.1093/chemse/24.3.337

LEV Report. (2012). *Vriendelijkegeuren op de spoedeisendehulp (in Dutch: Friendly odors in the emergency ward), LandelijkeExpertisegroepVeiligheidspercepties (National Expert group Safety perception)*, Amsterdam.

Li, W., Moallem, I., Paller, K. A., and Gottfried, J. A. (2007). Subliminal smells can guide social preferences. *Psychol. Sci.* 18, 1044–1049. doi: 10.1111/j.1467-9280.2007.02023.x

Luce, R. D. (1986). *Response Times.* New York, Oxford University Press.

Lundstrom, J. N., Goncalves, M., Esteves, F., and Olsson, M. J. (2003). Psychological effects of subthreshold exposure to the ptative human pheromone 4,16 androstadien-3-one. *Horm. Behav.* 44, 395–401; 1303–1314. doi: 10.1016/j.yhbeh.2003.06.004

Miles, C., and Hodder, K. (2005). Serial position effects in recognition memory for odors: a reexamination. *Mem. Cognit.* 33, 1303–1314. doi: 10.3758/BF03193230

Mojet, J., and Köster, E. P. (2002). Texture and flavour memory in foods: an incidental learning experiment. *Appetite* 38, 110–117. doi: 10.1006/appe.2001.0460

Mojet, J., and Köster, E. P. (2005). Sensory memory and food texture. *Food Qual. Pref.* 16, 251–266. doi: 10.1016/j.foodqual.2004.04.017

Mojet, J., and Köster, E. P. (2013). "Dynamics of liking," in *Time Dependent Measures of Perception in Sensory Evaluation*, eds J. Hort, S. Kemp, and T. Hollowood (Chichester: John Wiley & Sons).

Møller, P., Köster, E. P., Dijkman, N., De Wijk, R. A., and Mojet, J. (2012). Same-different reaction times to odors: some unexpected findings. *Chemosens. Percept.* 5, 158–171. doi: 10.1007/s12078-012-9124-x

Møller, P., Mojet, J., and Köster, E. P. (2007). Incidental and intentional flavour memory in young and older subjects. *Chem. Senses* 32, 557–567. doi: 10.1093/chemse/bjm026

Møller, P., Wulff, C., and Köster, E. P. (2004). Do age differences in odour memory depend on differences in verbal memory? *Neuroreport* 15, 915–917. doi: 10.1097/00001756-200404090-00036

Morin-Audebrand, L., Mojet, J., Chabanet, C., Issanchou, S., Møller, P., Köster, E. P., et al. (2012). The role of novelty detection in food memory. *Acta Psychol.* 139, 233–238. doi: 10.1016/j.actpsy.2011.10.003

Nijssen, B. (1991). "Off-flavors," in *Volatile Compounds in Foods and Beverages*, eds B. Nijssen and H. Maarse (New York: Marcel Dekker), 689–735.

Nordin, S., Monsch, A. U., and Murphy, C. (1995). Unawareness of smell loss in normal aging and Alzheimer's disease: discrepancy between self-reported and diagnosed smell sensitivity. *J. Gerontol. B Psychol. Sci. Soc. Sci.* 50, P187–P192. doi: 10.1093/geronb/50B.4.P187

Olsson, M. J. (1999). Implicit testing of odor memory: instances of positive and negative priming. *Chem. Senses* 24, 347–350. doi: 10.1093/chemse/24.3.347

Olsson, M. J., and Cain, W. S. (2003). Implicit vs. explicit memory for odors: hemispheric differences. *Mem. Cognit.* 31, 44–50. doi: 10.3758/BF03 196081

Papies, K., and Hamstra, P. (2010). Goal priming and eating behavior: enhancing self-regulation by environmental cues. *Health Psychol.* 29, 384–388. doi: 10.1037/a0019877

Porter, J., Anand, T., Johnson, B., Khan, R. M., and Sobel, N. (2005). Brain mechanisms for extracting spatial information from smell. *Neuron* 47, 581–592. doi: 10.1016/j.neuron.2005.06.028

Porter, J., Craven, B., Khan, R. M., Chang, S.-J., Kang, I., Judkewicz, B., et al. (2007). Mechanisms of scent-tracking in humans. *Nat. Neurosci.* 10, 27–29. doi: 10.1038/nn1819

Posner, M. I. (1986). *Chronometric Explorations of Mind.* (2nd Revised Edn). Oxford: Oxford University Press.

Proust, M. (1922/1960). *Swann's Way (Part 1)* (Trans. C. K. Scott Moncrieff). London: Chatto & Windus.

Ranganath, C., and Rainer, G. (2003). Neural mechanisms for detecting and remembering novel events. *Nat. Rev. Neurosci.* 4, 193–202. doi: 10.1038/nrn1052

Rozin, P., Wrzesniewski, A., and Byrnes, D. (1998). The elusiveness of evaluative conditioning. *Learn. Motiv.* 29, 397–415. doi: 10.1006/lmot.1998.1012

Schab, F. R. (1991). Odor memory: taking stock. *Psychol. Bull.* 109, 242–251. doi: 10.1037/0033-2909.109.2.242

Sela, L., and Sobel, N. (2010). Human olfaction: a constant state of change-blindness. *Exp. Brain Res.* 205, 13–29. doi: 10.1007/s00221-010-2348-6

Soussignan, R., Schaal, B., Boulanger, V., Gaillet, M., and Jiang, T. (2012). Orofacial reactivity to the sight and smell of food stimuli – evidence for anticipatory liking related to food reward cues in overweight children. *Appetite* 58, 508–516. doi: 10.1016/j.appet.2011.12.018

Spence, C., Kettenmann, B., Kobal, G., and McGlone, F. P. (2000). Selective attention to nthe chemosensory modality. *Percept. Psychophys.* 62, 1265–1271. doi: 10.3758/BF03212128

Spence, C., McGlone, F. P., Kettenmann, B., and Kobal, G. (2001). Attention to olfaction: a psychophysical investigation. *Exp. Brain Res.* 138, 432–437. doi: 10.1007/s002210100713

Stevenson, R. J. (2001a). The acquisition of odor quality. *Quart. J. Exp. Psychol. Hum. Exp. Psychol.* 54, 561–578.

Stevenson, R. J. (2001b). Associative learning and odor quality perception: how sniffing an odor mixture can alter the smell of its parts. *Learn. Motiv.* 32, 154–177. doi: 10.1006/lmot.2000.1070

Stevenson, R. J. (2001c). Perceptual learning with odors: implications for psychological accounts of odor quality perception. *Psychon. Bull. Rev.* 8, 708–712. doi: 10.3758/BF03196207

Stevenson, R. J., and Boakes, R. A. (2003). A mnemonic theory of odor perception. *Psychol. Rev.* 10, 340–364. doi: 10.1037/0033-295X.110.2.340

Sulmont, C., Issanchou, S., and Köster, E. P. (2002). Selection of odorants for memory tests on the basis of familiarity, perceived complexity, pleasantness, similarity and identification. *Chem. Senses* 27, 307–317. doi: 10.1093/chemse/27.4.307

Von Békésy, G. (1964). Olfactory analogue to directional hearing. *J. Appl. Physiol.* 19, 369–373.

Von Skramlik E. (1924). Über die Lokalisation der Empfindungen bei den niederen Sinnen. *Zeitschr. Sinnesphysiol.* 56, 69.

White, T. L., and Kurtz, D. B. (2003). The relationship between metacognotive awareness of olfactory ability and age in people reporting chemosensory disturbances. *Am. J. Psychol.* 116, 99–110. doi: 10.2307/1423337

Willander, J., and Larsson, M. (2006). Smell your way back to childhood: autobiographical odor memory. *Psychon. Bull. Rev.* 13, 240–244. doi: 10.3758/BF03193837

Willander, J., and Larsson, M. (2007). Olfaction and emotion: the case of autobiographical memory. *Mem. Cognit.* 35, 1659–1663. doi: 10.3758/BF03193499

Willander, J., and Larsson, M. (2008). The mind's nose and autobiographical odor memory. *Chemosens. Percept.* 1, 210–215. doi: 10.1007/s12078-008-9026-0

Zelano, C., Bensafi, M., Porter, J., Mainland, J., Johnson, B., Bremner, E., et al. (2005). Attentional modulation in human primary olfactory cortex. *Nat. Neurosci.* 8, 114–120. doi: 10.1038/nn1368

Zucco, G. (2003). Anomalies in cognition: olfactory memory. *Eur. Psychol.* 8, 77–86. doi: 10.1027//1016-9040.8.2.77

Zucco, G. M., Paolini, M., and Schaal, B. (2009). Unconscious odour conditioning 25 years later: revisiting and extending 'Kirk-Smith, Van Toller and Dodd'. *Learn. Motiv.* 40, 364–375. doi: 10.1016/j.lmot.2009.05.001

16

How incorporation of scents could enhance immersive virtual experiences

Matthieu Ischer[1,2], Naëm Baron[1,2], Christophe Mermoud[3], Isabelle Cayeux[4], Christelle Porcherot[4], David Sander[1,2] and Sylvain Delplanque[1,2]*

[1] Swiss Center for Affective Sciences, University of Geneva, Geneva, Switzerland
[2] Department of Psychology, University of Geneva, Geneva, Switzerland
[3] Department of Medicine, University of Geneva, Geneva, Switzerland
[4] Firmenich, S.A., Geneva, Switzerland

***Correspondence:**
Sylvain Delplanque, Swiss Center for Affective Sciences, University of Geneva, Campus Biotech, Chemin des Mines 9, Case Postale 60, 1211 Genève 20, Switzerland
e-mail: sylvain.delplanque@unige.ch

Under normal everyday conditions, senses all work together to create experiences that fill a typical person's life. Unfortunately for behavioral and cognitive researchers who investigate such experiences, standard laboratory tests are usually conducted in a nondescript room in front of a computer screen. They are very far from replicating the complexity of real world experiences. Recently, immersive virtual reality (IVR) environments became promising methods to immerse people into an almost real environment that involves more senses. IVR environments provide many similarities to the complexity of the real world and at the same time allow experimenters to constrain experimental parameters to obtain empirical data. This can eventually lead to better treatment options and/or new mechanistic hypotheses. The idea that increasing sensory modalities improve the realism of IVR environments has been empirically supported, but the senses used did not usually include olfaction. In this technology report, we will present an odor delivery system applied to a state-of-the-art IVR technology. The platform provides a three-dimensional, immersive, and fully interactive visualization environment called "Brain and Behavioral Laboratory—Immersive System" (BBL-IS). The solution we propose can reliably deliver various complex scents during different virtual scenarios, at a precise time and space and without contamination of the environment. The main features of this platform are: (i) the limited cross-contamination between odorant streams with a fast odor delivery (< 500 ms), (ii) the ease of use and control, and (iii) the possibility to synchronize the delivery of the odorant with pictures, videos or sounds. How this unique technology could be used to investigate typical research questions in olfaction (e.g., emotional elicitation, memory encoding or attentional capture by scents) will also be addressed.

Keywords: virtual reality, olfactory display, olfactometer, emotion, scent

INTRODUCTION

The replication of everyday life environments in laboratory experiments is crucial in behavioral sciences because it directly improves the ecological validity of the results, especially when subtle and complex interactions are concerned (Spooner and Pachana, 2006). For instance, in affective sciences, many theories postulate that the elicitation and the differentiation of emotions are determined by continuous and recursive evaluations of events (see Ellsworth and Scherer, 2003 for an overview on appraisal models of emotions). Evaluation of the environment through smell, taste, sight, hearing, touch, temperature, and balance perception contributes to the extraordinary changeability and the high degree of qualitative differentiation of emotional experiences, as well as individual differences in emotional reactions. Consequently, being able to simulate a rich environment is a key point to investigate a large variety of affective behaviors. However, standard laboratory tests in humans are typically conducted in nondescript rooms in front of two-dimensional environments displayed on flat computer screens and are very far from replicating the complexity of real world experiences.

Advances in Immersive Virtual Reality (IVR) technologies have recently opened a new range of possibilities in empirical research. IVR technologies provide virtual environments that mimic the complexity of the real world and at the same time grant scientists with many control and monitoring capabilities. It has become a promising framework to immerse people into a close-to-reality environment that involves more human senses. The capacity to completely control the environment fulfills the experimental criteria required in many behavioral sciences. Owing to the latest advancement in computer technologies, the subject's immersion in a three-dimensional (3D) experimental scenario is constantly improved. Consequently, the "sense of presence"[1] that leads to a direct engagement from the subject in interactivity with the 3D world is increasing. These close-to-reality experiences could possess a considerable potential in research, either to obtain better treatment options for people showing behavioral and cognitive deficits or to investigate fundamental hypotheses.

To date, real everyday life auditory and visual perceptions can be almost perfectly replicated in IVR environments. Since senses work together to create the overall sensory experience, increasing the quality of the represented environment as well as implementing more senses remain worth pursuing (Nakamoto et al., 2008). This idea has already been empirically supported (Dinh et al., 1999), but it almost never includes chemoperception (Craig et al., 2009). Because olfaction is more complex to implement and control, its uses in IVR environments remain more the exception than the rule.

Several attempts have been made to implement controlled scent delivery systems (olfactory display[2], OD) in virtual reality environments (e.g., Richard et al., 2006). For instance, Tortell et al. (2007) used a system able to deliver four different odorants by evaporation of different chemical compounds presented on scented collars. With this methodology, the authors brought experimental elements showing that presentation of scents is a promising method by which a user's attention is devoted to the IVR environment exploration, heightening their sense of presence. However, to obtain a reliable and controlled olfactory stimulation, the OD should satisfy very important constraints, such as being able to produce reproducible releases of various kinds of compounds over multiple trials, without contamination from one trial to the other, at known time, localization and strength, and without additional noise or tactile stimulations in the nose.

So far, standard olfactory delivery systems do not propose a rich repertoire of compounds, which limits the variety and the subtlety of situations the participant can be exposed to. In order to avoid this issue, available systems (Yamanaka et al., 2002; Weiling et al., 2010) create blends of odors by mixing basic predefined sets of odors. Albeit ingenious, these solutions cannot propose a rich variety of realistic odors that are often composed of thousands of different molecules. Exception to this olfactory poverty exists. For example, Sezille et al. (2013) developed a portable OD dedicated to fMRI experiments, which satisfies most of the constraints described above and can deliver up to 15 odorants. Nakamoto and Minh (2007) designed an OD which can deliver up to 30 odorants at constant flow rate. In this configuration, the main tubes manifold (along with the bank of odorants) and the solenoid valves are attached together. As the noise of the solenoid valves could give clues to the participant about the delivery of odorants, this solution requires using long distance common odorant-bearing tubes or wearing additional headphones. These constraints increase the risks of contamination of one odorant by remaining traces of the preceding one (i.e., cross-contamination) or the weight and the number of apparatuses users should wear. Since unencumbering systems are important in IVR, Yanagida et al. (2004) proposed an OD that does not require the user to attach anything on the head. The main device involves an "air cannon" which projects scented air puffs near the user's nose. In order not to deflect the trajectory of the scented air puff, ventilation and air extraction are not integrated in the display. Unfortunately, this technical solution increases the likelihood of odor contamination in the ambient air. Users had to limit the use of this display with four low-concentrated scents delivered with short emissions, which could thus sometimes be undetectable to users. Furthermore, a contamination between odorant sources in the "air cannon" at continuous use compromised the reproducible releases of various kinds of compounds over multiple trials. Sato et al. (2009) showed that synchronizing the delivery of odors with the user's breathing pattern could prevent ambient contamination. However, the disadvantage of the setup is that users have to stay still and close to the fixed OD, which largely complicates its implementation in IVR environments where head movements, at least, should not be restricted. Yamada et al. (2006) developed another miniaturized system to be worn by the participant in an outdoor environment. This OD can deliver 3 different odors at different strengths according to a virtual "*odor field*," but the variation of the odorant's strength is mainly controlled by an increase of the airflow. The main disadvantage associated with such a design is the possible changes in tactile sensations in the nose (due to airflow fluctuations) that are irrelevant to the odorant perception. Lastly, latencies between the order to deliver an odorant and its effective delivery to the nose (see also Narumi et al., 2011 for another head mounted OD) are often not strictly controlled or reported (Brkic et al., 2009; Ramic-Brkic and Chalmers, 2010) and it appears very difficult to rapidly and dynamically adjust the amount/intensity of odor according to the recipients' needs.

In this technology report, we will present an odor delivery solution applied to a state-of-the-art IVR technology that provides a 3D, immersive, and fully interactive visualization environment called BBL-IS (Brain and Behavior Laboratory—Immersive System). After exposing the basic principles of the system, we will present several studies that demonstrate its efficiency to deliver a large number of different odorants in the virtual environment: (i) in total safety for the subjects, (ii) reliably and in a reproducible manner, at a low and constant flow rate among subjects and without other perceptible changes (i.e., noise or tactile), (iii) with a limited cross-contamination between odorant streams, and (iv) with an easily and controllable interface. How this unique technology could be used to investigate typical research questions in olfaction (e.g., emotional elicitation, memory encoding or attentional capture by scents) will also be addressed.

MATERIALS AND METHODS

THE OLFACTORY DISPLAY

Design

The OD is based on a series of 32 computer-controlled solenoid valves. A schematic diagram of the OD is presented in **Figure 1**.

[1]The sense of presence is defined by the fact that participants forget that their perception is mediated by technology. Main criteria for a good sense of presence are; a) the sensation of being in a real place (place illusion) and b) the illusion that the scenario being depicted is actually occurring (plausibility illusion; Slater, 2009).

[2]In describing our apparatus, we will use the term "OD", defined as "*...a collection of hardware, software, and chemicals that can be used to present olfactory information to the virtual environment participant*" (Barfield and Danas, 1995).

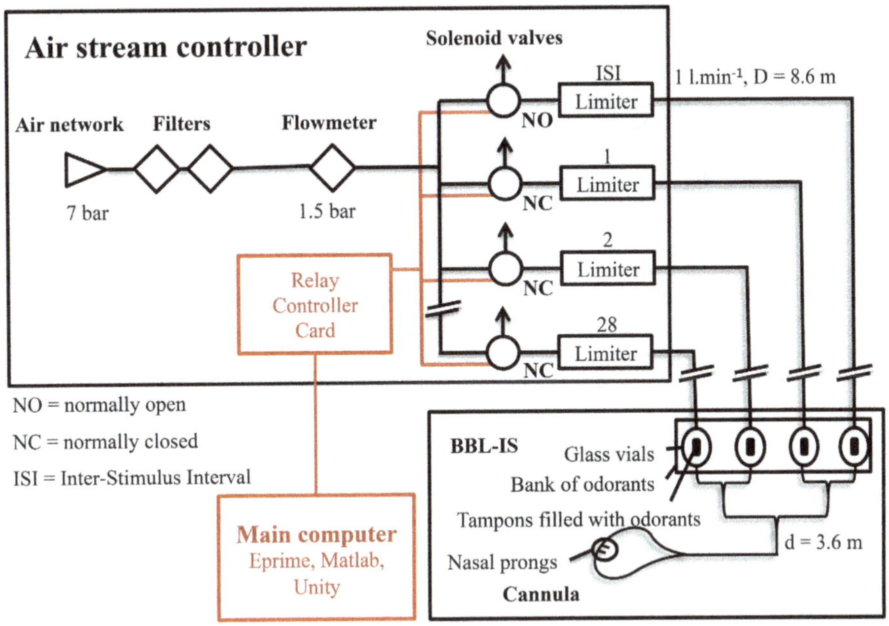

FIGURE 1 | Schematic diagram of the OD. For clarity reasons, channels 3 to 27 are not represented.

Individual solenoid valves are numerated from 1 to 28, the four remaining valves being attributed to air delivery during inter-stimulus intervals (ISI), and CO_2 at different concentrations (not described in this report).

The OD is connected to the medical air supply of the building (an internal compressor is also available) and is filtered using charcoal filters. Thus, no extraneous odorant or particle can contaminate the airstream that enters in the main flow meter, which can be manually adjusted according to the experimental design. Then, the air is distributed to different solenoid valves. Opening and closure of the valves are rapidly controlled via a relay controller card (National Control Device®, ProXR RS-232 E3C). The control of the card is performed via a custom-developed library that can be run by various software (e.g., Eprime®, Matlab® and Unity®). In the non-active state, the inter-stimuli interval (ISI) air valves are open so that clean air is delivered to the nose. During odor delivering, ISI valves are automatically switched off and the corresponding odor valves are switched on. Consequently, manipulation and control are simple, even with up to 28 different odors. Each channel's flow rate can be manually regulated by limiters and is usually fixed around $1\,l.min^{-1}$. This low-intensity airflow simplifies the system because it is no longer necessary to humidify or to heat the air for participants' comfort (e.g., Lorig et al., 1999). Since both ISI and odorant flows are setup to the same level, the flow rate perceived in the nose remains constant (see below for an empirical demonstration); only the noise coming from the valves might give external clues about the olfactory stimulation. In order to avoid this issue, the airstream controller is situated outside the experiment room (see **Figure 2**).

Airflows leaving the airstream controller are conveyed through small diameter polyurethane plastic tubes (inside diameter: 2.5 mm) of equal length to ensure accurate timing of odorant delivery. They reach the bank of odorants made up of custom-made glass vials positioned on the top of the IVR system via custom-made support (see **Figure 2**). Odorant vials in this design are made of small glass cylinders (22 mm of diameter × 120 mm high). Odorants are placed inside each vial using pen's tampon (Burghart® GmbH) filled with different quantities of pure odorants or odorants dissolved in solvents (e.g., propylene glycol or mineral oil). Odorant molecules evaporate in the vial, creating a headspace of constant volume. The availability of many glass vials allows the use of the same molecule at many different concentrations or many different molecules at a known concentration. This design also intends to mimic a natural environment in which different odors are present separately or as a combination.

Glass vials are positioned as close as possible to the participants' nose (**Figure 2**) in order to reduce the cross-contamination between odorants. The proximity between the nose and the odorants, associated with the small diameter of the tubes connected to the air stream controller allow the rapid delivery of odorant molecules into the participants' nose within a short delay (as empirically demonstrated below). All tubes (PTFE) are gathered using Y push-in fittings (Festo®) and the final delivery piece is a light and easy replaceable nasal cannula directly positioned at the entrance of the nostrils. This light device tends to be unnoticed by users after a few minutes and delivers small quantities of odorant directly into the nose, minimizing the pollution of the ambient air. Cannulas' prongs are sized so as not to obstruct the nose, allowing the subject to breathe normally.

In order to avoid olfactory contamination of the room by the odorant releases, a first air-extractor ($125\,m^3.h^{-1}$, not

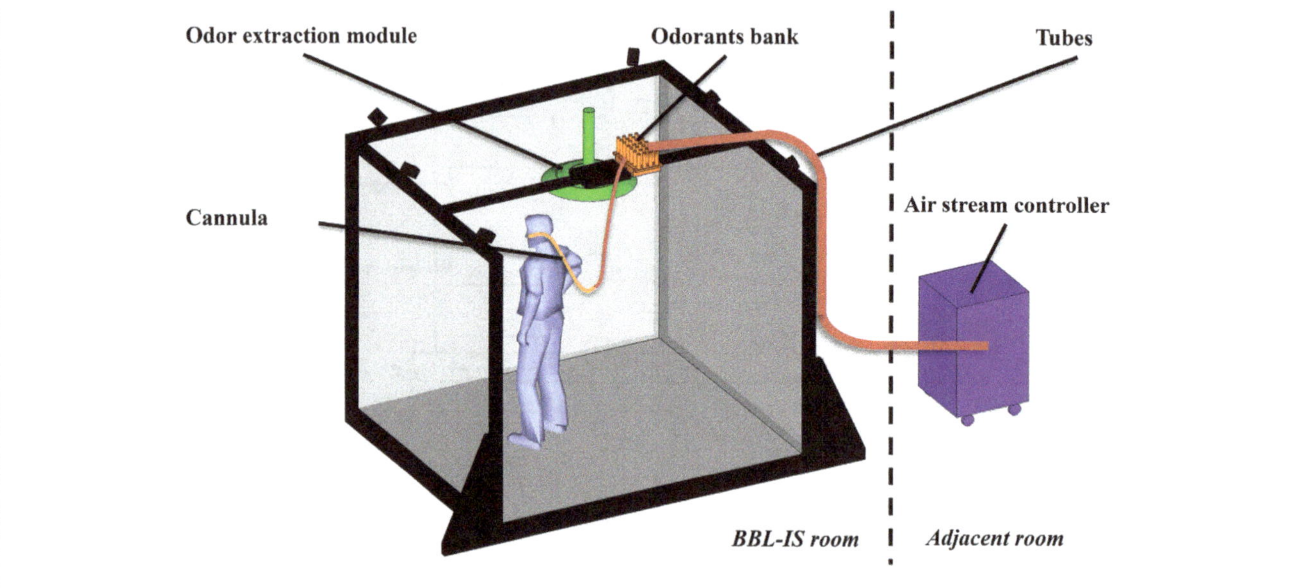

FIGURE 2 | Schematized illustration of the OD integrated in the BBL-IS.

represented in **Figure 2**) is located on the ceiling of the room and guarantees a global air renewal. A second air-extraction system is positioned close to the participants' head without hindering their movements. This module is composed of a collector shaped as a flattened cone (diameter 50 cm) linked to the global air extraction system of the building (125 $m^3.h^{-1}$). Room temperature is regulated around 22°C.

To summarize and as illustrated in **Figure 2**, the OD setup comprises four parts: the bank of odorant located in the BBL-IS as close as possible to the user; the air stream controller placed in an adjacent room to the BBL-IS; the tubes connecting the air stream controller to the bank of odorants and then to the nose of the participants; and the odor extraction module located above the BBL-IS.

We set up the olfactory device to be safe and comfortable for the subjects, to deliver air with or without odorants at a constant rate in a reliable and reproducible manner. The switch between odors and inter-stimulus air should be almost instantaneous without other perceptible stimuli. We tried to reduce cross-contamination between odorant streams and odorant contamination of the experimental room. Our OD is also set up to deliver various and easily changeable odorants in a controllable and easy way. To demonstrate that we reached those objectives, we present a couple of validation studies (see section Performance Tests) after introducing the immersive environment.

THE "BBL-IS" SYSTEM

The IVR system, which provides a 3D, immersive and fully interactive visualization environment, is installed in the Brain and Behavior Laboratory (BBL) of Geneva. This system, called BBL-IS (BBL-Immersive System http://bbl.unige.ch/ResearchModules/BBL-IS.html) is shaped as a room-sized cube, using four walls as screens on which images are projected by several synchronized video projectors (see **Figure 3**).

Technical specification

The BBL-IS has 4 sides presenting seamless and perspective coherent 3D images for user wearing IVR glasses (**Figure 3**). Seven video projectors (Digital Projections®, TITAN QUAD 3D WUXGA) project high-resolution images (1920*1200 pixels) at 120 frames per second. Projection is performed on the four acrylic coated screens (DaLite®, 2.8 m wide and 2.4 m high) with a high contrast ratio and brightness (1600 $cd.m^{-2}$ per screen). An optical motion tracking system composed of eight infrared cameras (Vicon®, Bonita 3) is used to capture the participant movements. These movements' parameters are integrated in the virtual scenario to create a fully interactive environment. In our configuration, an infrared reflective sensor is positioned on the virtual reality glasses to mimic the position of the nose. This position will be recorded on line and used to trigger the odorant delivery. The environment rendering is provided by a cluster of workstations. Further technical information is available at http://bbl.unige.ch/ResearchModules/BBL-IS.html.

This platform allows researchers to benefit from the state-of-the-art in virtual reality for creating and using immersive scenarios. More particularly, fully controlled manipulations of visual, auditory and olfactory stimulations coupled with the possibilities to track eyes, head and body movements of one participant allow scientists to investigate complex behaviors and emotional responses in realistic scenes.

INTEGRATION OF THE OLFACTORY DEVICE

Control of odorant delivery

The control of the OD can be performed manually via a simple software or computer-controlled via a custom made software toolkit (Geneva Virtual Reality Elements, GeVRE). The latter brings IVR related features to existing interactive 3D software,

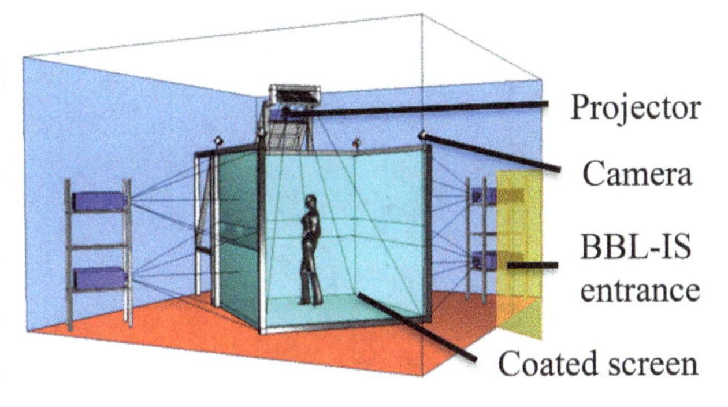

FIGURE 3 | Schematic representation of the "BBL-IS" system.

mainly in Unity3D®[3]. GeVRE extends the capabilities of classical 3D software by adding the features needed to build and run IVR environments (e.g., displaying synchronized images with perceivable depth, allowing cluster computing, adjusting the images perspective to the user's point of view, integrating various devices such as position tracker, haptic devices, joystick, etc.). GeVRE also provides modules for scientific studies, like event coding to synchronize external recording devices, accurate binocular gaze data recording and OD control functions. More importantly for our purpose, GeVRE allows researchers to use Unity3D® to build a complex virtual environment comprising smells. The basic principle is as follows: the researcher defines olfactory sources that possess different parameters such as the odorant type, the shape and size of olfactory volumes, and their position. All those features are defined directly using the interface of Unity3D® (**Figure 4**). This option makes the control of the OD easy and flexible.

More precisely, the experimenter specifies the attributes of the world that permit the definition of the complex olfactory environment: (1) the object that represents the nose for the system and that is tracked on line via the motion tracking system, (2) the type of odorant (up to 28 possibilities), (3) the position and the shape of the olfactory volume (i.e., from spheres to complex geometric figures), and (4) the behavior of the olfactory source (e.g., transient or permanent delivery, moving source).

After the communication between the OD and GeVRE has been established, an odorant is triggered according to the user's nose position estimated from the BBL-IS tracking system. When the nose enters one of the olfactory volumes defined by the user, the command is sent to the OD to deliver the corresponding odor. Multiple olfactory volumes can be used on the same object to create an odor gradient and recreate a natural scene (see **Figure 5**).

A custom-made dynamic link library, which provides predefined functions to send activation or deactivation commands for a specific odorant to the relay controller card, achieves the communication. One of the advantages of this GeVRE toolkit is its modular design allowing to implement another OD with ease (more information are available upon request).

[3]www.Unity3D.com.

PERFORMANCE TESTS

The objective of this report is to present an OD solution that is efficient to reliably deliver a large number of different odorants in the IVR environment in a reproducible manner, at a low and constant flow rate among all subjects, without other perceptible changes (i.e., noise or tactile) and without cumbersome apparatus attached to the participant. The following sections present results of different tests performed on the OD to demonstrate its efficiency to reliably deliver odors in the BBL-IS.

GAS DETECTOR ANALYSES

The extremity of the OD was connected to a photo-ionization detector (miniPID 200B, Aurora scientific inc.) which monitors concentration changes of an input gas or vapor across time, at a millisecond resolution. The output (in Volts) is proportional to the concentration of sampled compounds and was recorded for offline analyses using Biopac® system with a sampling rate of 1000 Hz. Five blocks of fifty odor pulses (classical shampoo fragrance diluted in dipropylene glycol at 10%, flow rate 1 $l.min^{-1}$) were triggered with a constant inter stimulus interval (ISI) of 5 s. Within each block, the duration of pulses was constant and increases by 250 ms steps, beginning at 1000 ms up to 2000 ms. Those durations were chosen as they could be used inside a unique inspiration phase. Within each block and for each pulse, the latency of the response onset as well as the maximum of concentration changes and its latency were extracted with the Acknowledge® software (Biopac® System). The averaged (across the 50 trials) output responses are presented in **Figure 6**.

Latency calculation

Latency between the command to deliver the odorant and the actual delivery at the nostrils level is a key aspect of every OD. If the participants realize that the olfactory scenario being depicted is not actually occurring, they will lose the sense of presence. As participants' movements in the direction of an olfactory source can be unpredictable, the latency must be as short as possible. The concentration of the compound starts increasing at latencies varying from 433 to 455 ms after the valve was opened, reaching its maximum between 1500 and 1748 ms, depending on pulse duration. The biggest onset latency fluctuation between different pulse durations represents a time variation of around 5% of the mean. Ninety-five percent of onset latencies values are situated within an averaged time margin of $\pm$ 6.36% of the mean onset value. These analyses demonstrated that, despite the 13 m length of the tubing part and the passage of the air through the glass vials, the system is able to deliver the compounds as early as 440 ms after the triggering command. Even for long aperture durations with a short ISI (5 s) the maximum of concentration is reached during the first 2 s for this particular compound. In sum, the OD is fast enough to provide a puff within a unique inspiration phase.

Concentrations reliability

We also measured the maximum amplitude of the gas detector output signal (i.e., the maximal concentration) of the compound for each of the 50 pulses. Gas sensor output values as a function of the pulse duration are represented in **Figure 7**.

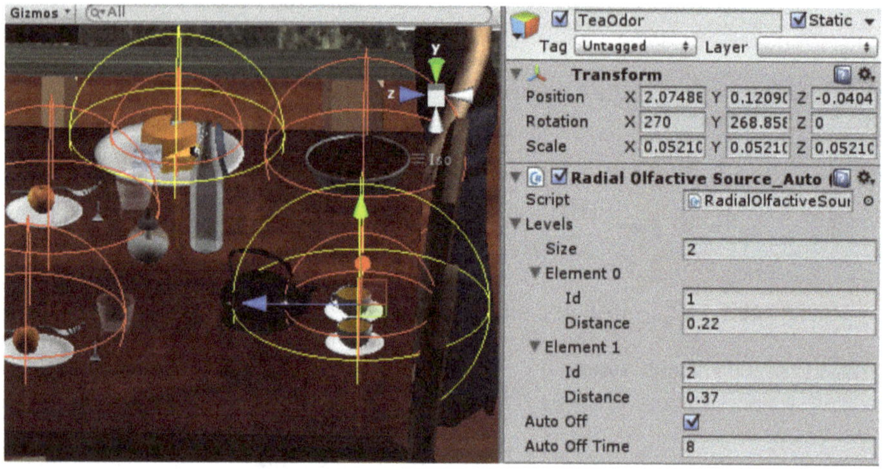

FIGURE 4 | Screenshot of the Unity3D editor while building a virtual kitchen with odorant objects (e.g., tea, cheese etc.) and 3D olfactory volumes (in red and yellow).

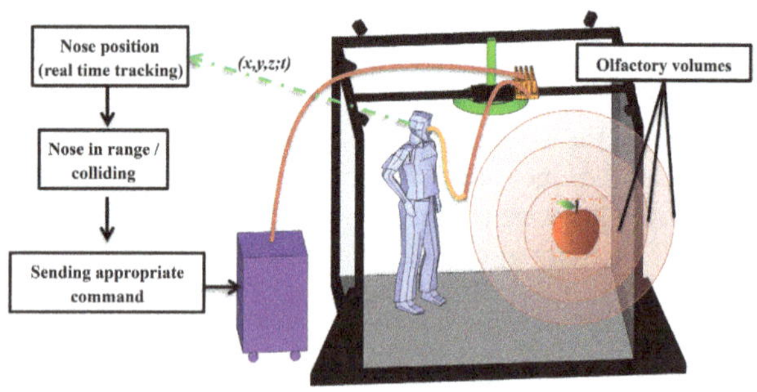

FIGURE 5 | Schema of the control protocol.

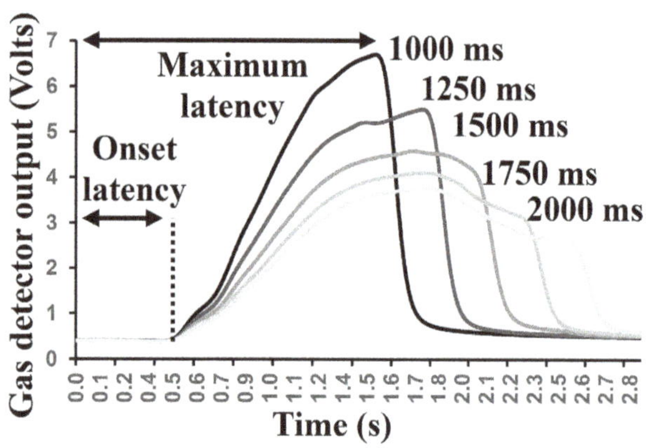

FIGURE 6 | Averaged gas detector response changes across all 50 pulses (ISI = 5 s) for each pulse duration condition.

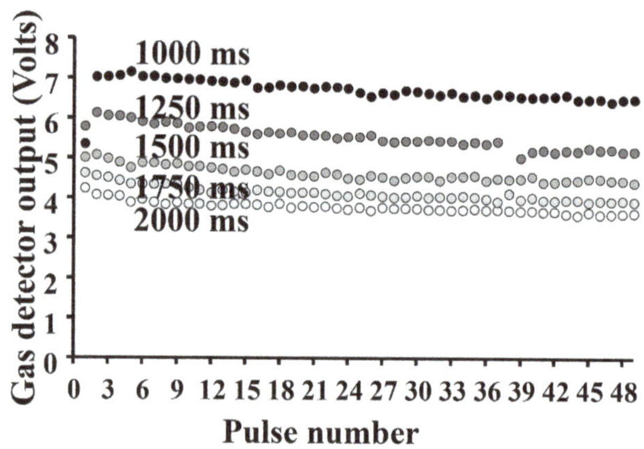

FIGURE 7 | Gas sensor output values for each of the 50 pulses as a function of the pulse duration.

For a given pulse duration, the reproducibility of odor delivery across the successive pulses was very satisfying. Ninety-five percent of maximum amplitude values are situated within an average margin of ± 4.82% of the mean maximum value. The measures also revealed a decrease in maximum concentration available as a function of the increase in duration of valve aperture. This relation is represented in **Figure 8**. The high quadratic regression coefficient indicates that maximum concentration tends to stabilize as the aperture time increases. These changes in concentration as a function of aperture duration are linked to the fixed ISI we employed. Indeed, the longer the aperture duration, the longer the time needed to recover the initial headspace.

To address this issue, we performed a supplementary test during which we measured gas detector output values during sequences of 10 pulses of another odorant (apple aroma B diluted in dipropylene glycol at 20%, 1000 ms duration). Eight sequences with fixed ISI of 2, 4, 6, 8, 10, 12, 14, and 16 s were launched. Each new sequence was separated from the preceding one by 2 min to allow the recovery of the headspace. We then measured the maximum amplitude of the gas detector output signal during the odorant delivery. Then, for each pulse, we calculated the percentage of change according to the maximum amplitude of

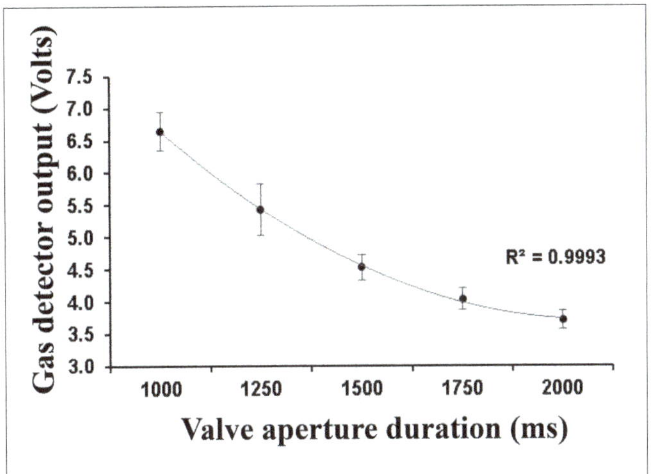

FIGURE 8 | Mean gas sensor maximum amplitude values as a function of the duration of valve aperture. Error bars indicates the 95% confidence interval. The quadratic correlation coefficient is also indicated.

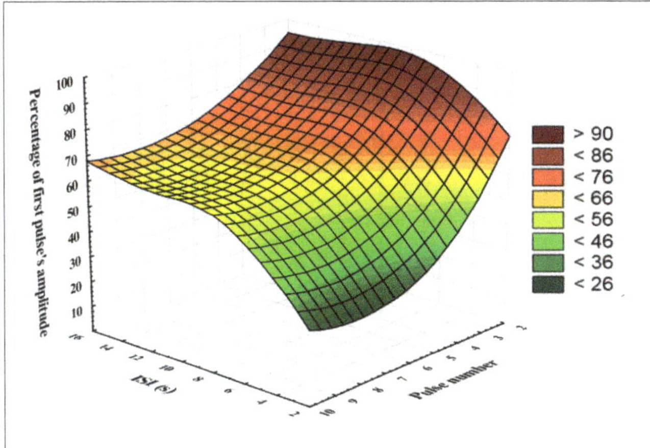

FIGURE 9 | Percentage of gas detector output changes as a function of the pulse number and the ISI.

the first pulse of the sequence. In **Figure 9**, we then reported those percentages of change as a function of the pulse number and the ISI. This graph reveals that the shorter the ISI, the stronger the initial reduction in maximal signal output. For instance, 2 s ISI leads to a reduction of more than 60% in quantity of compounds after four pulses. Fortunately, those conditions are unlikely to occur in a virtual environment since it requires the participants to cross the same olfactory area every 2 s four consecutive times. Concentration reliability if far better for ISI superior to 8 s and stabilizes around 70% of the maximum quantity of compound after 5 pulses. For ISI equal or superior to 8 s and for less than 5 consecutive pulses, the quantity of compound delivered is around 90% of the quantity of the first pulse. This latter condition will constitute the majority of the situations participants will be exposed to inside the virtual environment. So as suspected, the number and the interval between consecutive pulses of odorant can have an impact on the quantity of product released. Consequently, the time the individual will spend sampling the odorant, the number of samples and the interval between consecutive samples will clearly affect the quantity of compound he will be exposed to. All those variables should be recorded to perform appropriate statistical corrections if needed.

Cross-contamination test

Another key issue in olfactory displays fabrication is to minimize cross-contamination. Cross-contamination corresponds to the contamination of one odorant by remaining traces of the preceding one. This cross-contamination depends on the compound properties (i.e., volatility, interaction with tubing material) and the ability of the system to evacuate remaining odorant molecule during the ISI. Observed gas detector values at the closure of the valves seem to reach their pre-aperture values after a delay of around 500 ms (see **Figure 6**). This descriptive result suggests that any other odorant delivered after this recovery period is unlikely to be contaminated by the preceding odorant. To investigate this point more thoroughly, we measured the gas detector output values for 15 different odors (see **Figure 10** for the name of the odorants). Each odorant was delivered 10 times at 1 l.min^{-1} flow rate for 2 s with an ISI duration of 4 s. Gas sensor output values obtained for one sequence of 15 odorants delivery are represented in **Figure 10**. The gas detector output values averaged 500 ms before each valve aperture were used as baselines for each trial. For each odorants, we averaged the gas detector values within successive 500 ms periods across the 10 trials during the 3 s following valve aperture. The resulting gas detector mean values averaged across odorants are represented in **Figure 11**. Non-parametric tests (Sign Test) were used on those averaged values to statistically compare each of the 6 periods to the baseline. To address the problem of multiple comparisons, we applied the Bonferroni correction to all analyses (for $n = 6$ comparisons, the new significance level is set to $0.05/n = 0.0083$). Results indicated that the mean gas detector values were significantly different from the baseline for 0.5 to 1 s, 1 to 1.5 s, and 1.5 to 2 s periods (all $Z_s = 3.61$; $p_s < 0.001$). Gas detector values obtained just before and just after the delivery of the odorant are not significantly different from baseline values (see **Figure 11**). This result indicates that the level of ionization obtained just after the delivery of the molecules is similar to the level before, rendering the cross-contamination highly unlikely. However, since cross contamination could depend on many other factors like the valves' aperture time, this test should be systematically performed before any new experiment.

PSYCHOPHYSICS OF FLOW DETECTION

The objective of this test was to investigate whether participants were able to detect flow changes potentially occurring during odor delivery at 1 l.min^{-1}. Indeed, when an odor is delivered, the OD switches from the inter-stimulus airflow to the odor flow. This change could produce differences in the net flow that may create a perceptible tactile stimulation in the nose. In order to control this potential problem, we performed a supplementary flow detection task.

Procedure

Twelve volunteers (29.8 ± 6.8 years old; 5 females, 7 males) performed the detection task. When requested, they had to

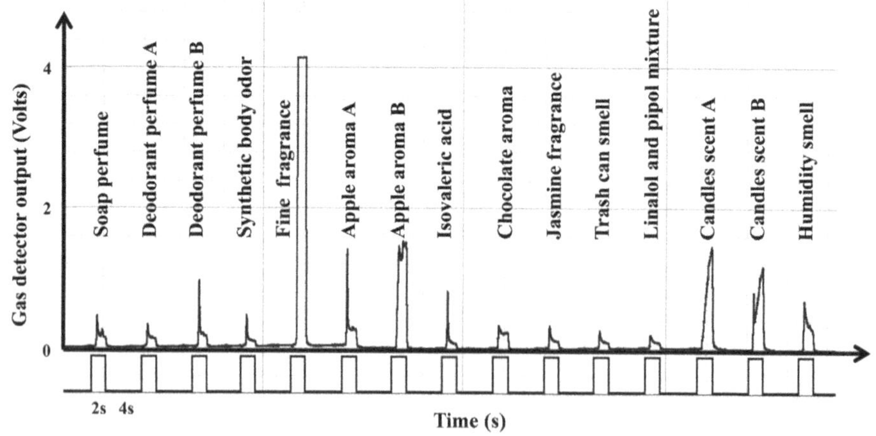

FIGURE 10 | Gas sensor output values obtained for one sequence of 15 different odorants delivery.

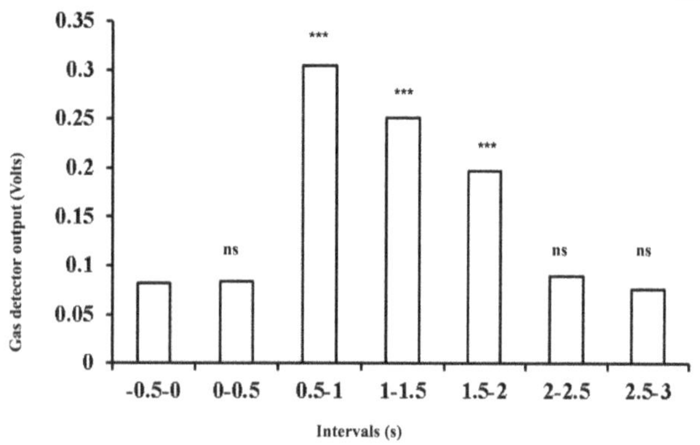

FIGURE 11 | Mean gas detector output values for the six 500 ms periods and the baseline. ns, non-significant, *** = $p < 0.001$

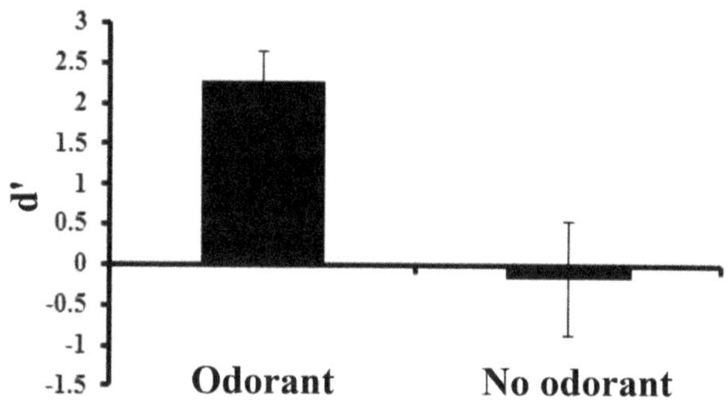

FIGURE 12 | Mean d′ (± *SD*) in the two conditions.

concentrate on any sensation that they could perceive in their nose while they were connected to the OD receiving the different stimulations (airflow fixed at 1 $l.min^{-1}$). After each trial, participants had to report to the experimenter whether they perceive any change in their nose sensations. They were presented with three kinds of trials: (1) no change at all, (2) opening of a valve with the same airflow as the ISI airflow for 1 s or (3) opening of one valve with the pure odorant (orange aroma) for 1 s. The task comprised a total of 10 trials per condition presented at random.

Analysis

For each individual, we calculated a sensitivity measure (d′) based on hit rate and false alarm rate. A hit was recorded when the opening of a valve occurred and was detected by the participant, a false alarm was recorded when no change occurred but was falsely detected by the participant as such. The greater the participants discrimination abilities, the higher the d′ values (zero meaning no discrimination).

Results

The mean d′ calculated for each condition (odorant and no-odorant vial) is presented in **Figure 12**. In the no-odorant condition, d′ did not differ from zero (Test of means against reference constant, t-value $= -1.45$; $df = 11$; $p = 0.18$). This result indicates that participants were not able to perceive a change during valve switching. By contrast, when the odorant is added in the flow, participants clearly detect a difference (test of means against zero, t-value $= 10.81$; $df = 11$; $p < 0.001$). This psychophysical experiment shows that under the normal condition of use (ISI airflow similar to odor airflow), participants should only detect changes in the nose due to odorants.

SPATIALIZED DETECTION TEST

At the perceptive level, cross-contamination results in the perception of a mixed odor while different odorants are actually delivered at separate moments in time. To investigate whether the present OD suffers from cross-contamination at a perceptive level, we developed an olfactory two-alternative forced-choice task (2AFC). Since the originality of our platform is to be able to spot odor sources in 3D environments, we focused on consequences of cross-contamination on the ability to discriminate odor sources in space. We aim at testing whether different virtual olfactory objects can be rapidly and accurately distinguished from one another, even if they are close in the virtual space as could be real olfactory sources. This distinction can be really impaired if there is cross-contamination in the OD.

Procedure

Nine healthy volunteers (31.6 ± 4.3 years old; 5 females, 4 males) participated in the test. After being connected to the OD via the cannula, they were immersed into a simple dark immersive virtual environment made of a floor composed of a white grid pattern (a video presenting the test in the BBL-IS is presented at http://www.affective-sciences.org/virolfac). Two virtual white spheres with a radius of 50 mm, and respective center points located at 150 mm distance from each other were presented in the virtual environment. Those olfactory virtual spheres were thus separated in space by only 50 mm. Participants move into the virtual world to reach the spheres and were requested to smell each sphere rapidly and to determine which one contained a randomly assigned target odorant. The two odors (orange and soap-like) were randomly assigned across the trials. Each odorant was delivered for 500 ms. Participants had to select the correct sphere with a remote control. After each trial ($n = 8$), participants had to wait 20 s before another couple of spheres appears in the virtual world.

Results

The binomial distribution is used to set our criteria for the correct odor detection; specifically, the minimum numbers of correct judgments to establish significance for the 2AFC test (one-tailed, $\alpha < 0.05$, probability of guessing $p = 1.2$) is calculated. For $n = 8$ tests, the minimum numbers of correct judgments is seven. Six participants obtained eight correct answers and three participants seven correct answers. All participants could discriminate the target odor above chance. In total, the percentage of correct response was 95.83% (± 6.25). For indicative purposes, we also calculated the time elapsing between the samplings of the two spheres. Participants spent on average 6.48 s (± 2.28) to smell the two spheres. All the participants reported noticeable and clear perception of the two odorants.

Conclusion

This psychophysical test reveals that participants accurately distinguish two different olfactory objects separated in space by only 50 mm. Participants performance and subjective reports indicate that cross-contamination is very unlikely to occur with this olfactory design. However, as the cross-contamination is also dependent on the molecules used, this should be formally measured before each experiment.

DISCUSSION

The objective of this report was to present an olfactory display connected to an IVR system that is efficient to deliver a large number of different odorants in the virtual environment: (i) at a low and constant flow rate among subjects and without other perceptible changes (i.e., noise or tactile sensations), (ii) with limited cross-contamination between odorant streams, and (iii) with an easily and controllable interface. The platform, combining a new state-of-the-art BBL-IS system and a high-performance OD, offers excellent characteristics for researchers in behavioral sciences. As demonstrated by the different tests we performed, the OD rapidly (~ 440 ms) releases various kinds of compounds (up to 28) over multiple trials, with almost no contamination from one trial to the other, at known timings, localization and strength, and without noticeable supplementary noise or tactile stimulations in the nose. By being shorter than the inspiration and the expiration phases, those latencies would allow to synchronize the odorant delivery and the participant breathing pattern.

Several caveats and limitations of this olfactory platform need to be mentioned. The first important limitation of the system is its cost. The availability of such IVR environment is far from being worldwide. Only few research centers are equipped, increasing the difficulty to reproduce the results and potentially decreasing the scope of the conclusions. One can only hope that the current and future technological advances in this domain will allow easier and less expensive immersive virtual environment implementation in many different laboratories. A second important point is that it remains unclear whereas such complex experimental settings will really help researchers to answer fundamental and/or applied questions, when compared to classical experimental setups. Although a benefit is clearly expected, further quantitative and qualitative studies will be needed to directly compare those two situations. A third limit worth mentioning is that the reliability of the OD we present in this report is highly dependent on factors that are modified as a function of the research question and the experimental procedure. For instance, increasing odorants' concentration and the number of olfactory sources in the virtual environment will increase the likelihood of cross-contamination. This should be controlled with gas detector analyses as well as psychophysical tests before each new experiment. Moreover, we demonstrated that concentration release is dependent on the duration of the stimulation, the number of successive presentations of the same odorant and the interval between those presentations. Since in most virtual reality applications, participants' sampling behavior will condition those parameters, it will thus be necessary to measure them during the experiment.

Being able to provide visual, auditory and olfactory stimulations in a fully controllable and close to reality environment should allow researchers to study complex and multisensory interactions. For instance, a key research question in olfactory literature remains how and to what extent chemosensory preferences can be modulated. It is now well accepted that needs, goals, values, learning and exposure deeply influence odorant perception and preferences (see Coppin and Sander, 2011 for a recent review). Future studies could be conducted in the immersive virtual environment to investigate more thoroughly the role of the perceptual changes as well as social interactions on odors evaluation or emotional reaction. The richness and the closeness to reality quality of the environment should help researchers to better understand how the different senses work together to elicit subtle, personal and variable emotional reactions or to shape implicit or explicit olfactory memories. All those research questions can be addressed simultaneously at the cognitive, behavioral and physiological level. For instance, the platform can easily integrate and be synchronized with wireless psychophysiological recording systems. In addition to the recording of the breathing pattern that is so important in olfaction research, several peripheral psychophysiological measures (e.g., electromyography, electrocardiography, electrodermal activity, skin temperature) can be recorded and analyzed off line or even used in real-time to modify virtual world. Associated with covert behavioral responses like action tendencies, investigation times, eye position and also participant's overt subjective responses, this platform constitutes a unique opportunity to study complex, multi-level phenomena like emotions.

In addition to the fundamental research questions that could potentially be addressed with such platforms, immersive reality olfactory environments offer a potentially very power tool for clinical applications. For instance, promising virtual reality therapy exists to reduce pain and anxiety of burn victims (Morris et al., 2009), to help restoring memory deficits in people with acquired brain injury (Yip and Man, 2013) or to enhance behavioral treatments of compulsive eating related disorders (Cesa et al., 2013). Using the powerful effect of odors on moods and emotions (Schiffman et al., 1995; Rétiveau et al., 2004) during those virtual therapies could increase their efficiency. Other authors have already stressed how useful could be the inclusion of olfaction in immersive virtual environment for virtual therapy in post-traumatic stress disorder resulting from military assault or combat (Pair et al., 2006).

Virtual reality environments coupled with olfactory displays could foster new researches in development departments of many companies worldwide and revolutionize many steps of a product design. For instance, sensory research departments of fragrances and flavors aim at providing products that people prefer, and at understanding how emotions are elicited and measured. Given that direct product experience is generally the optimal method for consumers to learn about products, looking for verisimilitude in sensory research is a key objective. Mimicking normal everyday conditions in a controlled virtual environment could increase understanding how the senses work together to create the overall product experience including emotional experience that fills a typical person's life.

The replication of everyday life environments in laboratory experiments is crucial in behavioral sciences because it directly improves the ecological validity of the results, especially when complex interactions are concerned. Virtual reality environments provide both the complexity of the real world that could elicit vivid human experiences and the control of the experimental variables that is a prerequisite to produce reliable conclusions in behavioral research. In that sense, every attempt to include the olfactory modality in virtual environments should be actively fostered.

ACKNOWLEDGMENT

We wish to thank Dr. C. Steinberger and Ms. S. Trznadel for giving helpful advice.

REFERENCES

Barfield, W., and Danas, E. (1995). Comments on the use of olfactory displays for virtual environments. *Presence* 5, 109–121.

Brkic, B. R., Chalmers, A., Boulanger, K., Pattanaik, S., and Covington, J. (2009). "Cross-modal affects of smell on the real-time rendering of grass," in *Proceedings of the 25th Spring Conference on Computer Graphics* (Budmerice, Slovakia: ACM).

Cesa, L. G., Manzoni, M. G., Bacchetta, M., Castelnuovo, G., Conti, S., Gaggioli, A., et al. (2013). Virtual reality for enhancing the cognitive behavioral treatment of obesity with binge eating disorder: randomized controlled study with one-year follow-up. *J. Med. Internet Res.* 15, e113. doi: 10.2196/jmir.2441

Coppin, G., and Sander, D. (2011). "The flexibility of chemosensory preferences," in *The Neuroscience of Preference and Choice,* eds R. J. Dolan and T. Sharot (Elsevier Publishing), 257–275. doi: 10.1016/B978-0-12-381431-9.00021-8

Craig, A. B., Sherman, W. R., and Will, J. D. (2009). *Developing Virtual Reality Applications: Foundations of Effective Design.* Burlington, MA; Oxford: Morgan Kaufmann; Elsevier Science distributor.

Dinh, H. Q., Walker, N., Hodges, L. F., Chang, S., and Kobayashi, A. (1999). "Evaluating the importance of multi-sensory input on memory and the sense of presence in virtual environments," in *Proc. of the IEEE Virtual Reality Conf.* 222–228. doi: 10.1109/VR.1999.756955

Ellsworth, P. C., and Scherer, K. R. (2003). "Appraisal processes in emotion," in *Handbook of Affective Sciences,* eds R. Davidson, K. R. Scherer, and H. H. Goldsmith (New York, NY: Oxford University Press), 572–595.

Lorig, T., Elmes, D., Zald, D., and Pardo, J. (1999). A computer-controlled olfactometer for fMRI and electrophysiological studies of olfaction. *Behav. Res. Methods Instrum. Comp.* 31, 370–375. doi: 10.3758/bf03207734

Morris, L. D., Louw, Q. A., and Grimmer-Somers, K. (2009). The effectiveness of virtual reality on reducing pain and anxiety in burn injury patients: a systematic review. *Clin. J. Pain* 25, 815–826. 10.1097/AJP.1090b1013e3181aaa1909

Nakamoto, T., and Minh, H. P. D. (2007). "Improvement of olfactory display using solenoid valves," in *Proc. of the IEEE Virtual Reality Conf.* 179–186. doi: 10.1109/VR.2007.352479

Nakamoto, T., Otaguro, S., Kinoshita, M., Nagahama, M., Ohinishi, K., and Ishida, T. (2008). Cooking up an interactive olfactory game display. *IEEE Comput. Graph. Appl.* 28, 75–78. doi: 10.1109/MCG.2008.3

Narumi, T., Kajinami, T., Nishizaka, S., Tanikawa, T., and Hirose, M. (2011). "Pseudo-gustatory display system based on cross-modal integration of vision, olfaction and gustation," in *Proc. of the IEEE Virtual Reality Conf.* 127–130. doi: 10.1109/VR.2011.5759450

Pair, J., Allen, B., Dautricourt, M., Treskunov, A., Liewer, M., Graap, K., et al. (2006). "A virtual reality exposure therapy application for Iraq war post traumatic stress disorder," in *Proc. of the IEEE Virtual Reality Conf.* 67–72. doi: 10.1109/VR.2006.23

Ramic-Brkic, B., and Chalmers, A. (2010). "Virtual smell: authentic smell diffusion in virtual environments," in *Proceedings of the 7th International Conference on Computer Graphics, Virtual Reality, Visualisation and Interaction in Africa.* (Franschhoek: ACM).

Rétiveau, A. N., Iv, E. C., and Milliken, G. A. (2004). Common and specific effects of fine fragrances on the mood of women. *J. Sens. Stud.* 19, 373–394. doi: 10.1111/j.1745-459x.2004.102803.x

Richard, E., Tijou, A., Richard, P., and Ferrier, J. L. (2006). Multi-modal virtual environments for education with haptic and olfactory feedback. *Virtual Real.* 10, 207–225. doi: 10.1007/s10055-006-0040-8

Sato, J., Ohtsu, K., Bannai, Y., and Okada, K. (2009). "Effective presentation technique of scent using small ejection quantities of odor," in *Proc. of the IEEE Virtual Reality Conf.* 151–158. doi: 10.1109/VR.2009.4811015

Schiffman, S. S., Sattely Miller, E. A., Suggs, M. S., and Graham, B. G. (1995). The effect of environmental odors emanating from commercial swine operations on the mood of nearby residents. *Brain Res. Bull.* 37, 369–375. doi: 10.1016/0361-9230(95)00015-1

Sezille, C., Messaoudi, B., Bertrand, A., Joussain, P., Thevenet, M., and Bensafi, M. (2013). A portable experimental apparatus for human olfactory fMRI experiments. *J. Neurosci. Methods* 218, 29–38. doi: 10.1016/j.jneumeth.2013.04.021

Slater, M. (2009). Place illusion and plausibility can lead to realistic behaviour in immersive virtual environments. *Philos. Trans. R. Soc. Lond. B Biol. Sci.* 364, 3549–3557. doi: 10.1098/rstb.2009.0138

Spooner, D. M., and Pachana, N. A. (2006). Ecological validity in neuropsychological assessment: a case for greater consideration in research with neurologically intact populations. *Arch. Clin. Neuropsychol.* 21, 327–337. doi: 10.1016/j.acn.2006.04.004

Tortell, R., Luigi, D. P., Dozois, A., Bouchard, S., Morie, J. F., and Ilan, D. (2007). The effects of scent and game play experience on memory of a virtual environment. *Virtual Real.* 11, 61–68. doi: 10.1007/s10055-006-0056-0

Weiling, L., Jingling, B., Kehua, Z., Changjian, L., Liyuan, W., and Yan, X. (2010). Computer-controlled olfactometer for quantitative study of odor concentration measurement. *Biomed. Eng. Inform.* 4, 1440–1443. doi: 10.1109/BMEI.2010.5639404

Yamada, T., Yokoyama, S., Tanikawa, T., Hirota, K., and Hirose, M. (2006). "Wearable olfactory display: using odor in outdoor environment," in *Proc. of the IEEE Virtual Reality Conf.* 199–206. doi: 10.1109/VR.2006.147

Yamanaka, T., Matsumoto, R., and Nakamoto, T. (2002). Study of odor blender using solenoid valves controlled by delta–sigma modulation method for odor recorder. *Sens. Actuators B Chem.* 87, 457–463. doi: 10.1016/S0925-4005(02)00300-3

Yanagida, Y., Kawato, S., Noma, H., Tomono, A., and Tesutani, N. (2004). "Projection based olfactory display with nose tracking," in *Proc. of the IEEE Virtual Reality Conf.* 43–50. doi: 10.1109/VR.2004.1310054

Yip, B. C. B., and Man, D. W. K. (2013). Virtual reality-based prospective memory training program for people with acquired brain injury. *Neurorehabilitation* 32, 103–115. doi: 10.3233/nre-130827

17

Visual attention for a desktop virtual environment with ambient scent

Alexander Toet [1,2] * _and Martin G. van Schaik_ [1]

[1] *TNO, Soesterberg, Netherlands*

[2] *Department of Information and Computing Sciences, University Utrecht, Utrecht, Netherlands*

Correspondence:
Alexander Toet, TNO, Kampweg 5, 3769 DE Soesterberg, Netherlands
e-mail: lex.toet@tno.nl; lextoet@gmail.com

In the current study participants explored a desktop virtual environment (VE) representing a suburban neighborhood with signs of public disorder (neglect, vandalism, and crime), while being exposed to either room air (control group), or subliminal levels of tar (unpleasant; typically associated with burned or waste material) or freshly cut grass (pleasant; typically associated with natural or fresh material) ambient odor. They reported all signs of disorder they noticed during their walk together with their associated emotional response. Based on recent evidence that odors reflexively direct visual attention to (either semantically or affectively) congruent visual objects, we hypothesized that participants would notice more signs of disorder in the presence of ambient tar odor (since this odor may bias attention to unpleasant and negative features), and less signs of disorder in the presence of ambient grass odor (since this odor may bias visual attention toward the vegetation in the environment and away from the signs of disorder). Contrary to our expectations the results provide no indication that the presence of an ambient odor affected the participants' visual attention for signs of disorder or their emotional response. However, the paradigm used in present study does not allow us to draw any conclusions in this respect. We conclude that a closer affective, semantic, or spatiotemporal link between the contents of a desktop VE and ambient scents may be required to effectively establish diagnostic associations that guide a user's attention. In the absence of these direct links, ambient scent may be more diagnostic for the physical environment of the observer as a whole than for the particular items in that environment (or, in this case, items represented in the VE).

Keywords: attention, ambient odor, semantic congruency, affective congruency, virtual environment

INTRODUCTION

BACKGROUND

Desktop virtual environments (VEs) are increasingly deployed to study future design plans and the possible effects of environmental qualities and interventions on human behavior and feelings of safety in built environments with signs of public disorder (Cozens et al., 2003; Park et al., 2008, 2010; Toet and van Schaik, 2012). Desktop VEs offer cost-effective, safe, controlled, and flexible environments that allow to investigate human response to a wide range of environmental factors without the constraints, distractions, and dangers of the real world (e.g., Nasar and Cubukcu, 2011). They are relatively cheap, widely available, and easy to use, while most users are familiar with these displays and their interaction devices. Desktop VEs are also preferred for communication of design and intervention plans because they can be made accessible to a large numbers of users in internet applications (Dang et al., 2012). For these applications it is essential that users perceive the desktop VE in a similar way as they would perceive its real world counterpart. Previous studies have shown that environmental characteristics like lighting, sound, and dynamic elements similarly affect the perception of desktop VEs and real environments (Bishop and Rohrmann, 2003; Houtkamp et al., 2008). Ambient scent is another important environmental characteristic that is currently lacking in most VEs. Ambient scent is known to significantly affect our perception of real environments (Wrzesniewski et al., 1999), and people have strong expectations about the way an environment should smell (Henshaw and Bruce, 2012). It has also been shown that ambient odor can increase the sense of presence in immersive VEs (Dinh et al., 1999; Washburn et al., 2003; Tortell et al., 2007). Thus, ambient odors may be an effective tool to tune the user perception of less immersive desktop VEs (e.g., by evoking implicit associations).

Despite the importance of scent in our everyday life olfaction is rarely applied in the scope of VEs (Baus and Bouchard, 2010). Recent technological developments enable the effective and localized dispersion and control of scents (Yanigada et al., 2003, 2004, 2005; Yu et al., 2003; Oshima et al., 2007; for reviews see Richard et al., 2006; Riener and Harders, 2012), thereby providing VE researchers and developers with the ability to utilize scent to create compelling VEs (Tomono et al., 2011). Enhancing VEs with olfactory stimuli may enhance user experience by heightening the sense of reality (Chalmers et al., 2009; Ghinea and Ademoye, 2011). It has indeed been shown that the addition of olfactory cues to an immersive VE can increase the user's sense of presence, memory and perceived realism of the simulated environment (Dinh et al., 1999; Washburn et al., 2003; Tortell et al., 2007). However, it is still unknown if ambient scents can influence the attention for details in a desktop VE (Ghinea and Ademoye, 2011).

In a previous study we found that signs of disorder influence the affective appraisal of a desktop VE to a large degree in a similar way as the appraisal of its real world counterpart (Toet and van Schaik, 2012). However, it appeared that participants focused more on signs of disorder in a desktop VE than in a similar real world environment. This finding, which may seriously degrade the ecological validity of VEs for the aforementioned applications, was partly reduced by the addition of a realistic soundscape to the VE simulation. We argued that in the real world the saliency of signs of public disorder is typically modulated by various environmental factors which are typically lacking in a desktop VE, such as ambient sounds, tactile or olfactory cues. For instance, their saliency may be ameliorated by the sound of birds, a soft warm breeze, sun, and pleasant ambient smells of fresh air and vegetation, or enhanced by loud noise, strong cold wind, or unpleasant (e.g., garbage and urine) smells. In this study we investigated if ambient odors can influence the visual attention for these details in a desktop VE.

VISUAL-OLFACTORY INTERACTIONS

Interactions between olfaction and vision appear to be widespread. Neuroimaging studies have shown that interaction between olfaction and vision occurs at multiple levels of information processing (Gottfried and Dolan, 2003; Österbauer et al., 2005; Walla, 2008; Seubert et al., 2013). Also, it was found that stimulation of the human visual cortex enhances odor discrimination (Jadauji et al., 2012). Linking the perceptions of odors and colors appears to occur mainly in the amygdala and the orbitofrontal cortex (OFC; Gottfried and Dolan, 2003; Österbauer et al., 2005).

The amygdala is a central perceptual node where information from olfactory, visual, auditory, and tactile modalities converges (Zald, 2003). It is an integral component of a distributed affective circuit in the mammalian brain that mediates both positive and negative affect and the processing of reward-predicting cues (Murray, 2007). Recent evidence suggests that the amygdala also plays a central causal role in the modulation of visual attention (Vuilleumier, 2005; Williams et al., 2005; Duncan and Feldman Barrett, 2007; for a recent overview see Pourtois et al., 2013). The amygdala enhances the visual saliency of affective targets (Duncan and Feldman Barrett, 2007). This implies that the activation state of the amygdala determines whether affective features or objects are prioritized. Since the amygdala responds to both positive and negative valenced odors (but not to neutral odors: Winston et al., 2005), olfactory induced amygdala activity may boost visual attention for affectively congruent (potentially threatening or rewarding) targets (Vuilleumier, 2005; Mohanty et al., 2009; Jacobs et al., 2012).

There is ample evidence for the visual modulation of olfactory perception. A neutral suprathrehold odor is rated significantly more pleasant after viewing positive pictures and significantly less pleasant and more intense after seeing unpleasant pictures (Pollatos et al., 2007). A visual feature that has a particular strong influence on odor perception is color (Zellner, 2013). Color enhances the perceived intensity of odors (independent of color appropriateness: Zellner and Kautz, 1990). Color also modulates the hedonic value of odors: both neural response in brain area encoding the hedonic value of smells (Österbauer et al., 2005) and the subjectively judged pleasantness of color-odor combinations (Zellner et al., 1991) increase with perceived color-odor appropriateness. Odors are detected faster and more accurately in the presence of semantically congruent colors (Zellner et al., 1991) or pictures (Gottfried and Dolan, 2003; Demattè et al., 2009), while incongruent colors and shape cues reduce odor discrimination accuracy (Demattè et al., 2009). Color-smell associations can be so compelling that color can even completely change the quality of the perceived odor (a white wine is perceived as having the odor of a red wine when artificially colored red: Morrot et al., 2001). Visual-olfactory interactions appear to be automatic: color and shape cues affect the accuracy of odor discrimination, even when the information is task irrelevant and when participants are explicitly instructed to ignore these cues (Demattè et al., 2009). Specific odor components of complex odor mixtures that are congruent with a presented color are perceived as more prominent, suggesting that color directs olfactory attention to color-associated components (Arao et al., 2012). Functional magnetic resonance imaging studies have shown neurophysiological correlates of olfactory response modulation by color cues: activity in caudal regions of the OFC and in the insular cortex increase progressively with perceived odor-color congruency (Österbauer et al., 2005).

In contrast to the large amount of evidence for the visual modulation of olfactory perception, there are less reports on the reverse. However, recently evidence was presented that olfactory input can indeed modulate visual perception. Fear-related chemical signals modulate visual emotion perception in an emotion-specific way (Zhou and Chen, 2009), while unpleasant odors reduce perceived attractiveness of faces (Demattè et al., 2007). Olfactory cues also bias the dynamic process of binocular rivalry: an odorant that is congruent with one of the competing images prolongs the time that image is visible and shortens its suppression time (Zhou et al., 2010, 2012). Finally, subliminal olfactory cues modulate visual sex discriminations made on the basis of biological motion cues: ambiguous point-light walkers are more often judged as males in the presence of unconsciously perceived male sweat (Hacker et al., 2013). Hence, there is now sufficient evidence for the modulation of visual perception by olfactory input.

OLFACTION AND VISUAL ATTENTION

An organism continuously and simultaneously receives an overload of multisensory input from its environment. Because of limitations in processing capacity, simultaneous stimuli cannot be fully analyzed in parallel and thus compete for processing resources in order to gain access to higher cognitive stages and awareness. Attention serves as a gating mechanism to prioritize and enhance sensory information that is relevant for survival such as threats (Fox et al., 2002; Koster et al., 2004; Williams et al., 2006; Lin et al., 2009) or rewards (Anderson, 2013), while suppressing irrelevant information. Attentional selection is typically driven by stimulus saliency, novelty, and reward-related associations (Anderson, 2013). Attention acts upon and modulates information in each sensory modality (visual, auditory, olfactory, etc.; Woldorff et al., 1993; Zelano et al., 2005). Information from different sensory modalities is pre-attentively integrated into a unified coherent percept, resulting in multimodal internal representations in which attention can be directed (Driver and Spence, 1998). As a result, tactile (Van der Burg et al., 2009), auditory (Van der Burg et al., 2008), and olfactory (Seo et al., 2010; Tomono et al., 2011; Seigneuric et al., 2012; Chen et al., 2013; Durand et al., 2013) cues can boost the saliency of visual features, even when the cues provide no information about the location or nature of the visual feature. Thus, ambient odors (even at sub-threshold levels) can modulate visual attention (Morrin and Ratneshwar, 2000; Michael et al., 2003, 2005; Chen et al., 2013), even in 4-month-old infants (Durand et al., 2013). Recent studies have shown that odors can reflexively direct visual attention to *semantically congruent* visual objects (Seo et al., 2010; Tomono et al., 2011; Seigneuric et al., 2012; Chen et al., 2013). Objects that are semantically congruent with a presented odor are looked at faster and more frequently than other objects in a scene (Seo et al., 2010; Chen et al., 2013), even if participants are not aware that an odor has been presented (Seigneuric et al., 2010). It appears that crossmodal odor-object associations are automatically activated, without the need for explicit odor identification (Seigneuric et al., 2012), thus boosting the saliency of the corresponding visual object (Chen et al., 2013). Ambient odors also bias visual attention to favor stimuli that are *affectively congruent* to their hedonic quality (a case of affect-biased attention: Todd et al., 2012). Pleasant odors facilitate the processing of positive visual cues (Leppänen and Hietanen, 2003), while unpleasant odors facilitate the processing of negative cues (Ehrlichman and Halpern, 1988) and inhibit the processing of positive cues (Leppänen and Hietanen, 2003). The pre-attentive affective bias induced by ambient unpleasant odors probably serves the ecological purpose of facilitating threat detection (Krusemark and Li, 2012).

CURRENT STUDY

The current study was performed to test if exposure to ambient odor can modulate the visual attention to signs of disorder in a desktop VE representing an urban area. Participants performed a walking tour through the VE while being exposed to either room air (control group), tar (typically perceived as unpleasant and frequently associated with burned or waste material), or the odor of freshly cut grass (typically perceived as pleasant and frequently associated with natural or fresh material). Whenever they noticed signs of disorder during their walk they reported their detection and their emotional response. The scent of cut grass had semantically congruent visual and auditory representations in the simulation, since the VE showed abundant greenery and contained the occasional sound of grass mowers in the associated soundtrack. The scent of tar could be associated with the occasional sounds of construction activities (e.g., hammering, sawing) in the soundtrack of the VE, and was affectively congruent with derelict areas in general. Since people tend to respond to an environment as a whole (a "molar" environment) rather than to its individual features (Bitner, 1992; Bell et al., 2010; Brosch et al., 2010; Houtkamp, 2012), and since affective qualities are prioritized in this categorization process (Brosch et al., 2010), the presence of an ambient scent with an affective (pleasant or unpleasant) loading was expected to bias the visual attention (away from or toward) for signs of disorder in the VE. More specifically, it was hypothesized that (H1) participants in the ambient tar (unpleasant) odor condition would report more signs of public disorder than participants in the control condition, because the unpleasant odor would bias visual attention to visual cues with a negative affective connotation. In contrast, it was expected that (H2) participants in the cut grass (pleasant) odor condition would report less signs of public disorder than participants in the control condition, because the smell of cut grass would bias their attention to the – semantically congruent – greenery and thereby distract them from the negative cues.

MATERIALS AND METHODS

VIRTUAL ENVIRONMENT

A small area in the town of Soesterberg, The Netherlands (with a rectangular shape and a total extent of about 200 m × 200 m; coordinates 52°; 7′ N, 5°; 17′34″ E:) was simulated in 3D using the Unreal Tournament 2004 game-engine v2.5 (Epic Games Inc.; for further details on the VE model and its contents see Toet and van Schaik, 2012). The area is enclosed by roads on four sides and contains blocks of houses, two squares with parking places, benches, and statues, two playgrounds with benches, and a network of pathways connecting the squares and playgrounds (see **Figure 1**). All houses have a garden in the back, typically enclosed with a wooden fence, with an exit door to a pathway. The pathways are typically covered with tarmac, and bordered on both sides with trees and shrubs. The houses are generally well maintained and quite uniform. The pathways and parks are reasonably well kept. The walking route (designated by arrows drawn on the ground) had no intersections and covered most of the area. To simulate a state of public disorder 42 test items were distributed over 34 different locations in the VE. The items signaled three different classes of social incivilities: Neglect (24 items), Vandalism (one item), and Crime (17 items: see **Table 1**; Perkins et al., 1992; Caughy et al., 2001), and had social connotations ranging from indifference (e.g., litter, trash, dog droppings) and loitering (e.g. empty beer cans, cigarette butts, fast food wrappers) to vandalism (broken bus shelter windows) and predatory crime (smashed car windows, crime watch signs, CCTV cameras, and camera surveillance signs).

The simulation was performed on Dell Precision 490 PC computers, equipped with Dell 19″ monitors. Logitech Rumblepad 2 Gamepads were used for navigation. User movement in the VE was from a first-person viewing perspective with walking motion supporting forward and backward movements and left and right rotation movements. User movement speed was fixed and collision detection enabled to prevent users from walking through objects. A non-repeating soundscape that was characteristic for the environment was composed from sounds (birds twittering, cars passing by, children shouting, hammering and drilling, and dogs barking) recorded at several locations and at different times in the corresponding real environment. The soundscape was presented through Sennheiser eH 150 headphones. A previous study showed that this soundscape effectively increased the ecological validity of the VE (Toet and van Schaik, 2012).

ODOR SELECTION

The scent of freshly cut grass was selected as a semantically congruent pleasant odor in this study. This scent is generally considered

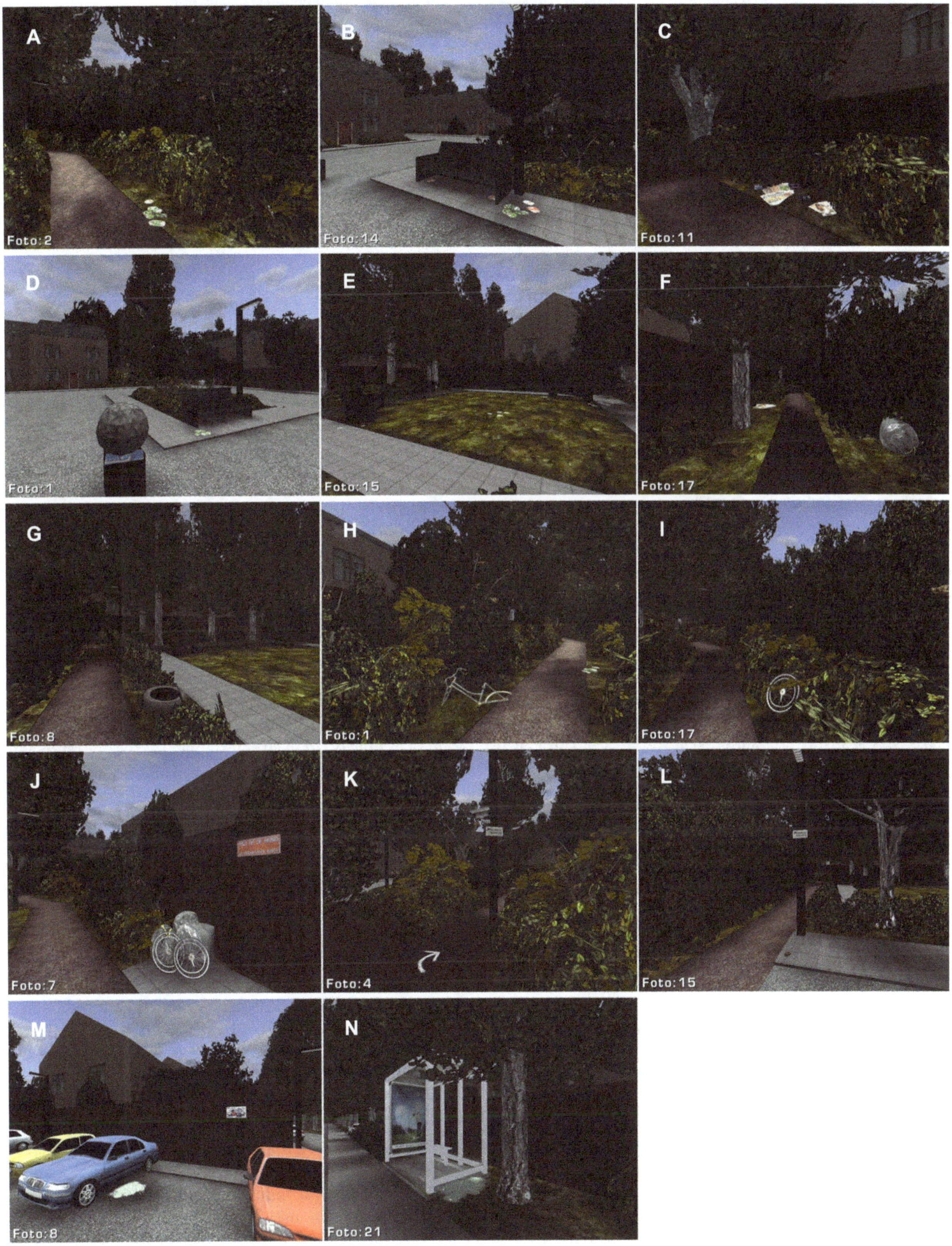

FIGURE 1 | Screen shots of the virtual environment, showing locations with litter (A–E), garbage (F,J), bicycle- and car parts (G–J), warning signs (J–M), cameras (K), and evidence of car burglary (M) and vandalism (N).

Table 1 | Experimental items, their connotations of physical and social disorder, and the experimental classification.

Experimental items (no.)	Social connotations	Experimental class (no. of items)
Garbage bags (2)	Neglect, indifference (Litter)	Neglect (24)
Cardboard boxes (1)		
Newspapers, flyers (2)		
Plastic shopping bags (2)		
Dog droppings (3)		
Bicycle frame (1)		
Bicycle wheels (2)		
Cigarette butts (1)		
Empty beer cans (7)		
Fast-food wrappers, boxes, paper cups (1)		
Old car tires (2)		
Bus shelter with broken windows (1)	Vandalism	Vandalism (1)
Smashed car windows and signs warning for car burglary (6)	Car burglary	Crime (17)
Neighborhood crime watch signs (3)	Home burglary	
Signs that homes are protected by private security services (2)		
Signs that homes are protected by dogs (2)		
CCTV security cameras and signs (4)	Predatory crime	

Numbers in brackets indicate the number of test items present in the VE.

to be stimulating and refreshing (the smell of freshly cut grass ranks among the top five preferred smell in several recent independent large scale polls in Britain: Reynolds, 2012; Henning, 2013). Since the VE used in this study shows a lot of grass and vegetation, the scent of grass may direct attention toward the greenery (Seo et al., 2010; Tomono et al., 2011; Seigneuric et al., 2012). The smell of cut-grass was created by mixing ethanol with cis-3-hexenol (leaf alcohol) in a 9:1 ratio. The associations that could be elicited by this scent in combination with the VE were investigated by presenting it to a panel of 10 participants while they were viewing the VE. The scent was presented in small glass tubes containing a cotton swab with three to four drops of the solution and sniffed by the participants approximately 5″ from their nose. About 9 out of 10 participants reported associations with greenery (four mentioned grass, three named freshly cut leaves and one mentioned broken twigs). All participants judged the scent to be pleasant.

An affectively congruent unpleasant scent was selected in a pilot test from a set of eight candidate aversive smells. The candidate smells were respectively Burned Wood (RS/420), Reptile (RS/424), Diesel Fumes (RS/423), Metal (RS/426), Dusty (RS/425), Tar (RS/401), Cow Manure, and Natural Gas (all obtained from RetroScent, Rotterdam, The Netherlands: www.geurmachine.nl). The scents were identified by randomly assigned numbers, presented in small glass tubes containing a cotton swab with 3–4 drops of aroma oil, and sniffed by the 10 participants of the pilot test in random order, approximately 5″ from their nose, while viewing the VE. The degree to which each scent fitted the VE (how environmentally appropriate the scent was for the VE) was evaluated on a 11 point Likert scale (ranging from 0 = *absolutely not* to 10 = *definitely*). Tar received the highest mean score (7.4), followed by Dusty (5.7). In addition, although the exact the nature of the tar smell was not identified by any of the testers, 8 out of 10 spontaneously reported associations with fire and burned material, while it was unanimously judged to be a very unpleasant scent that could occur in an environment as the one represented by the VE.

A second pilot test served to investigate the spontaneous associations that may be elicited by the two selected scents (grass and tar) independent of visual feedback. Three small glass tubes containing a cotton swab with three to four drops of either the grass odor solution, the tar aroma oil or clear tap water were presented in random order to 10 participants (who did not take part in the first pilot test). The tap water condition served as a control condition. The participants sniffed the samples approximately five inches from their nose, and rated respectively their pleasantness and familiarity on five point Likert scales (ranging from 0 = *absolutely not* to 4 = *very much*). The grass smell received the highest mean pleasantness rating (3.6), followed by tap water (2.6), while the tar smell received the lowest mean pleasantness rating (0.2). The tar smell received the highest mean familiarity score (2.9), followed by tap water (2.0), and grass (1.9). For the tar smell, 6 out of 10 participants reported associations with smoke, fire, and burned material, while two participants associated this smell with industrial activities, and two others had respectively associations with garages and garbage dumps. For the grass smell, 5 out of 10 participants reported associations with nature, flowers, pine trees, or leafs, one was reminded of fruit, while four participants associated it with air refreshers or cleaning material. Hence, the tar smell was frequently perceived as an unpleasant smell and associated with negative (burned or waste) material, while the grass smell was predominantly considered a pleasant smell associated with positive (natural) material.

ODOR DIFFUSION

Scents were diffused in the room (about 25 m^2) through a commercial electronic dispenser (1-3 RS-Classic Scentvertiser, RetroScent, Rotterdam, The Netherlands: www.geurmachine.nl). No odor was applied in the control condition. The dispenser was placed out of the participant's sight behind a screen. The participants could not hear the sound of the dispenser when they wore their headphones and listened to the soundscape of the VE. The experimenter turned on the dispenser after the participants had started their tour through the VE and he turned it off before they were instructed to take off their headphones. Odor was intermittently diffused (with a cycle period of 1 min) during the experiment so that the participants received fluctuating concentrations over time, thus preventing full adaptation.

It is likely that both aversive and pleasant odors turn on the sensory-driven attentional systems even at subthreshold levels to facilitate the detection and analysis of behavioral relevant stimuli (Krusemark and Li, 2012). In this study olfactory stimulation was therefore intentionally performed at a near-threshold level to preclude the possibility of top-down influence on visual perception (e.g., the use of explicit search strategies), thereby narrowing the effects down to bottom-up sensory driven attentional systems facilitating threat or reward detection. Ideally, the odor intensity should be sufficiently strong to be just noticeable when attended to. The odor intensity used in this study was between low and intermediate, corresponding to a mean level between 3 and 5 on a 10-point scale. A pilot experiment was performed to determine a setting of the dispenser and a duty cycle that resulted in a mean rating of 5.

The room in which the test was performed was well ventilated prior to each session. Only one scent per day was diffused to avoid mixing odors, and the lab was fully ventilated overnight to remove any lingering trace of the scent. Before beginning the study each morning, the room was "sniff-tested" by the two experimenters; no odors were detected to have remained in the room.

INSTRUMENTS

General questionnaire

As the results may be influenced by the characteristics of the participants, they were asked to complete a *General Questionnaire* including socio-demographic measures (sex, age, and education). Education was clustered into four groups: middle and higher level education, academic education, and other types of education.

Mental state questionnaire

A 7-item *Mental State Questionnaire* (adapted from Spielberger, 1983), consisting of four negative (*agitated, angry, anxious, distressed*), two neutral (*calm, relaxed*), and one positive (*cheerful*) emotional terms served to assess the emotions elicited by the individual incivilities. On each encounter with a sign of disorder during their walk participants reported their emotional reaction by selecting one of the seven items ("*I feel...*").

Post-experiment questionnaire

A 4-item *Post-Experiment Questionnaire* contained three questions investigating the extent to which the ambient temperature, illumination, and atmosphere in the room were characteristic for the VE (these three items were scored on a 5-point Likert scale, ranging from 1 = *completely disagree* to 5 = *completely agree*) and an open question ("*Was there anything else you noticed during the experiment?*") to test if the participants had noticed the ambient scent in the room.

EXPERIMENTAL PROCEDURE

After their arrival at the laboratory, the participants first read and signed an informed consent form. Next, they filled out the *General Questionnaire*. Then they read the following instructions:

"*The experiment concerns an area of Soesterberg near the TNO lab, and will take about 45 minutes. Citizens living in this area are concerned about the increasing social disorder in their neighborhood. They intend to draft a plan of action to confront this problem. After making an inventory of the different types of incivilities occurring in their neighborhood, the citizens will prioritize the order in which these should be addressed. To enable a large number of people to give their opinion on the social disorder in this area, the concerned citizens have commissioned a realistic and highly detailed computer model of their neighborhood.*

It is your task to make a tour through this virtual model and assess the social disorder in this neighborhood. Your route is marked by arrows drawn on the ground. Each time you notice signs of incivilities (e.g., litter, dog droppings, broken car windows, etc.) during your inspection tour, you are requested to:

1. *Make a snapshot of each sign of incivilities you notice (by pressing key F12).*
2. *Enter a brief description of the incivility on your questionnaire.*
3. *Report your current mental state by choosing one of the 7 emotional terms on the 'Mental State Questionnaire' (agitated, angry, anxious, distressed, calm, relaxed, cheerful).*"

Next, the experimenter verified if the participants had understood their instructions, and started the simulation. The experimenter then explained the function of the gamepad, and gave the participant the opportunity to practice maneuvering through the VE for about 5 min. At the end of this practice period the experimenter checked if the participant was able to perform the required maneuvers, and whether the participant paid attention to the arrows on the ground and the signs of disorder. Then, the experimenter gave the participants the printed questionnaires which they could use to fill out their reports, and positioned the point-of-view in the VE at the starting location, facing the direction of the route. The participants then put on their headphones and started their walkthrough, which they performed at their own pace. Each time the participants noticed signs of disorder during their walk they reported the item they had noticed and their current mental state. During the test, the experimenter was seated behind a screen in the room and intermittently turned on the odor dispenser at one minute intervals, maintaining a slightly fluctuating near threshold ambient odor level. Finally, after finishing their walkthrough, the participants filled out the *Post-Experiment Questionnaire*.

The experimental protocol was reviewed and approved by the TNO internal review board on experiments with human participants (TNO Toetsings Commissie Proefpersoon Experimenten, Soesterberg, The Netherlands), and was in accordance with the Helsinki Declaration of 1975, as revised in 2000 (World Medical Association, 2000). The participants provided their written informed consent prior to testing. The participants received a modest financial compensation for their participation.

PARTICIPANTS

The experiment was performed by 69 participants (3 groups of 23 each) that were selected from the TNO database of volunteers: 39 males and 30 females, aged 43 ± 18 years. The selection criteria guaranteed that they were not familiar with the urban area represented by the VE, that they had no problems with their sense of smell, and that they all had normal (or corrected to normal) vision with no color deficiencies. Also, they were unaware of the aim of the experiment. The participants' mean age, level of education, and computer proficiency and game experience were approximately the same for all three (no-ambient smell, ambient tar odor, and ambient grass odor) experimental conditions.

DATA ANALYSIS

The emotional responses reported for the detected signs of disorder (from the *Mental State Questionnaires*) were clustered for each of the three classes of experimental items: neglect, vandalism, and crime. Analysis of variance (ANOVA) was used to test the relationships between the main variables. Chi-squared tests were performed to determine whether observed frequencies were significantly different from expected frequencies. The statistical analyses were performed with IBM SPSS 20.0 for Windows. For all analyses a probability level of $p < 0.05$ was considered to be statistically significant.

RESULTS

Chi-squared tests showed a significant difference ($\chi^2 = 18.94$; df $= 4$; $p \leq 0.05$) between the observed and expected frequencies of the emotional responses (negative, neutral, or positive) associated with the reported items (signs of incivilities) in the classes Neglect, Vandalism, and Crime. Items in the classes Vandalism and Crime were more frequently associated with negative emotional responses than items in the class Neglect.

Figure 2 lists the detection performance for items signaling *Neglect* and *Crime* in each of the three experimental conditions. To enable a comparison of the performance between the different experimental classes (that were each represented by a different number of test items) the results are expressed in percentages (for the sake of completeness this figure also provides the mean number of detected items for each condition). **Figure 2** clearly shows that the relative detection performance is lower for signals of crime than for signals of neglect in all conditions.

A one-way ANOVA showed that the mean numbers of detected items signaling respectively *Neglect* and *Crime* did not differ significantly between the three ambient odor conditions. More specifically, there were no significant differences between the *Control* and *Grass* (respectively $F_{1,42} = 0.57$, $p = 0.45$ and $F_{1,37} = 1.76$, $p = 0.19$), *Control* and *Tar* (respectively $F_{1,45} = 3.10$, $p = 0.09$ and $F_{1,36} = 0.96$, $p = 0.33$) and between the *Tar* and *Grass* (respectively $F_{1,42} = 0.79$, $p = 0.38$ and $F_{1,38} = 0.01$, $p = 0.93$) conditions. Hence, the hypotheses (H1 and H2) that participants in the (un)pleasant odor condition would notice (more) less signs of disorder than participants in the (odorless) control condition is not supported by the present data. Compared to the control (odorless) condition, participants reported the same mean number (percentage) of signs of disorder in both (tar and grass) ambient odor conditions. In addition, there appears to be no effect of the hedonic tone of the ambient odor on visual attention toward neglect or crime objects. Also, ambient scent did not affect participants' subjectively reported emotional state. Since there were no main or interaction effects of age and level of education, these factors were omitted from later analyses.

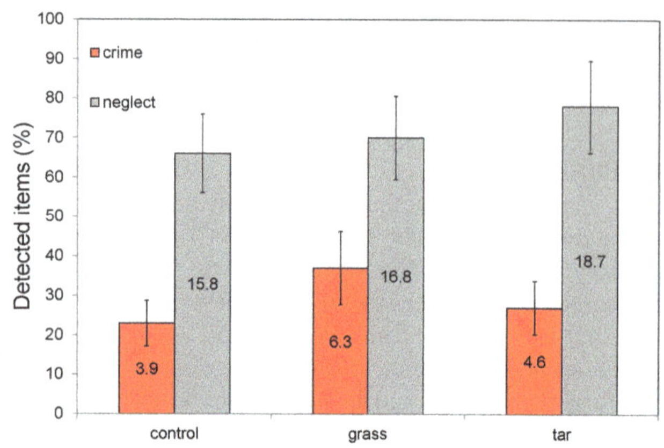

FIGURE 2 | Percentage of detected items signaling *Neglect* (a total of 24 items) and *Crime* (a total of 17 items) in each of the three experimental ambient scent conditions (no odor, grass odor, tar odor). The labels inside the bars represent the mean number of detected items. The error bars represent the standard error in the mean.

The VE contained multiple objects representing *Neglect* and *Crime*, but only a single object signaling *Vandalism* (a broken bus shelter). Since this item was rather conspicuous it was never missed by any of the participants. Hence, the results for this item have no discriminative value and are therefore not further discussed in this study.

In response to the open question in the *Post-Experiment Questionnaire* one participant (out of 23) claimed to have noticed a Lysol smell in the room in the control condition. In the tar odor condition one participant (out of 23) reported to have noticed a smell, but he was unable to identify its nature, and did not link the odor to the exploration task. No participant noticed a smell in the grass odor condition.

DISCUSSION

Based on the present we cannot conclude whether a subliminal ambient scent can affect the perception of the VE. The finding that ambient scent did not seem to affect participants' subjectively reported emotional state agrees with similar findings from related earlier studies who observed that pleasant ambient scents did not affect self-reported mood and arousal (Morrin and Ratneshwar, 2000, 2003; Teller and Dennis, 2011).

Contrary to our expectations the presence of the ambient odors also did not bias the participants' attention for the experimental items. Thus, we found no indication that ambient smell of a given nature selectively biases visual attention to details in a desktop VE. The design of the current study does not allow to determine whether the fact that we did not observe an effect is due to (1) the absence of an effect or (2) the limited power of the study design itself. In any case, it appears that ambient smell may only have limited effectiveness as a tool to direct a user's attention to specific details in a desktop VE. This result is somewhat surprising given the substantial amount of evidence that odors draw visual attention to congruent visual objects (e.g., Seo et al., 2010; Tomono et al., 2011; Seigneuric et al., 2012; Chen et al., 2013). However, the present result agrees with earlier reports that ambient scent has no effect on shopping behavior (Schifferstein and Blok, 2002; Teller and Dennis, 2011). It has in fact been argued that previous reports of significant effects of ambient scents on perception, emotions, and behavior in shopping environments need to be taken with care since most previous studies typically did not control for different sources of bias (Teller and Dennis, 2011). Our results also agree with those of Schifferstein and Blok (2002), who found that the scent of freshly cut grass did not affect sales of thematically (in-) congruent products. They argue that ambient scent is probably more diagnostic for the physical environment of the observer than for the particular items in that environment. This suggests that ambient scent may only effectively guide visual attention when there is a close link between the affective or semantic qualities of the scent and visual features in the VE. Although there may be a semantic link between the scent of cut grass and the greenery shown in the VE, the link between the scent of tar and signs of disorder is probably less evident. Also, more immersive VEs may be required to automatically establish associations between ambient scents and the VE itself. In case of desktop VEs, a close spatiotemporal link between the contents of the desktop VE and the scents with which they are supposed to be associated may be required to effectively establish diagnostic associations (i.e., smells and visual features may need to appear and disappear together to effectively induce the illusion that the smells actually emanate from the objects shown on the screen) that guide a user's attention.

Experimental items signaling vandalism (e.g., a damaged bus shelter) and crime (e.g., home protection signs and cameras) more frequently evoked negative affective appraisals than items representing neglect (e.g., litter, dog droppings, old bicycle parts). This finding agrees with the discriminant validity of different types of perceptual incivilities that is also found in the real world (e.g., between crime and social incivilities: Worrall, 2006; Armstrong and Katz, 2010). In reality, signs of crime are also more likely to evoke negative appraisals since they are typically associated with the risk of personal victimization (Phillips and Smith, 2004). This finding suggests that the affective appraisal of the VE had at least some ecological validity.

In all experimental conditions, the relative detection performance for signals of crime was lower than for signals of neglect. This is probably due to the fact that most signals of crime (i.e., the warning signs and CCTV cameras) were positioned at eye height or higher in the VE (e.g., attached to trees, lamp posts, or walls), while the signals of neglect were on the ground or on low supports (statues). Although participants were informed about the nature of the signals of disorder, and shown examples during their introduction to the experiment, they may have focused primarily on the signs of neglect on the ground and may have paid less attention to signals higher up in the scene. The fact that the walking route was indicated by arrows drawn on the ground may also have induced a bias for downward perception.

Summarizing, the present study does not allow us to conclude whether ambient odors may be an effective tool to direct a user's attention to specific (congruent) objects in a desktop VE (e.g., by evoking implicit associations).

LIMITATIONS OF THE PRESENT STUDY

In previous studies on the effects of odor on visual attention participants freely inspected visual scenes without any explicit instructions, and odor induced attentional bias became manifest in spontaneous fixation behavior (Seigneuric et al., 2010; Seo et al., 2010). In the current study the participants were explicitly instructed to look for signs of disorder in the VE. The cognitive effort associated with this strict assignment may have overruled any odor induced attentional bias effects. However, the fact that only a fraction of the targets was actually noticed suggests that there was still room for odor modulated performance enhancement.

The walking route through the VE was indicated by arrows drawn on the ground, which may have induced a bias for visual search near the ground. Unfortunately, fixation behavior was not measured in this study, so this hypothesis cannot be verified.

The scent of grass had an explicit visual representation in the VE, while the scent of tar could only implicitly be linked to visual (litter) and auditory (construction sounds) elements in the VE. Future studies should preferably employ scents that have explicit and unequivocal visual counterparts in the VE. Also, a range of both (1) neutral odors or odors with the same valence but different semantic connotations, and (2) odors of different valence but without any semantic counterparts in the VE should be deployed to enable a distinction between effects induced by hedonic or semantic congruency.

There was only one sign of vandalism in this study (the broken bus shelter) which was also highly salient. As a result this item had no discriminant value. Future studies should include a larger number of test items for each experimental class, with different (including low) visual saliencies. The attention enhancing effects of olfactory cues may be more prominent for targets with low visual saliencies.

The participants in this study reported that they had no problems with their sense of smell at the time of this experiment. Also, there were no entries in the TNO database of volunteers that any olfactory deficiencies had been noted during their participation in previous smell experiments. However, since we did not explicitly test their sense of smell in the current experiment there is no guarantee that they all had normal olfactory function.

SUGGESTIONS FOR FUTURE RESEARCH

It would be interesting to test whether the finding that specific odors can reflexively direct visual attention to *semantically congruent* visual objects (Seo et al., 2010; Tomono et al., 2011; Seigneuric et al., 2012; Chen et al., 2013) can also be replicated with dynamic desktop VEs. To effectively guide a user's attention dynamic olfactory displays are probably required so that a close spatiotemporal link may be established between the contents of the VE and the scents with which they are supposed to be associated.

Future studies should also register eye movements, since human fixation behavior may provide valuable additional information to subjectively reported results. Also, future studies should track the exact path of the participants through the VE. It is in principle possible that participants use scent cues to adjust their distance to certain items in the VE (e.g., that they show an approach or avoidance behavior, maintaining a larger distance to unpleasant smelling items, and coming closer to pleasant smelling items). Since distance affects the visual saliency and detectability of targets this may affect the results. Path deviations are not likely to be a significant confounding factor in the present study, since most parts of the route were rather narrow and did not leave much room for deviations.

It has previously been shown that the addition of olfactory cues to an immersive VE increases the user's sense of presence and perceived realism of the simulated environment, and ultimately his memory for details therein (Dinh et al., 1999; Washburn et al., 2003; Tortell et al., 2007). It would therefore be interesting to investigate whether an odor induced visual attention bias may also become manifest for desktop VEs when memory for details is tested instead of the number of detections. From the abovementioned previous studies we expect that participants in an (un)pleasant odor condition will remember (more) less signs of disorder than participants in an odorless control condition after completing their inspection tour of the VE.

REFERENCES

Anderson, B. A. (2013). A value-driven mechanism of attentional selection. *J. Vis.* 13, 7. doi: 10.1167/13.3.7

Arao, M., Suzuki, M., Katayama, J., and Akihiro, Y. (2012). An odorant congruent with a colour cue is selectively perceived in an odour mixture. *Perception* 41, 474–482. doi: 10.1068/p7152

Armstrong, T., and Katz, C. (2010). Further evidence on the discriminant validity of perceptual incivilities measures. *Justice Q.* 27, 280–304. doi: 10.1080/07418820802506198

Baus, O., and Bouchard, S. (2010). The sense of olfaction: its characteristics and its possible applications in virtual environments. *J. Cyber Ther. Rehab.* 3, 31–50.

Bell, P. A., Greene, T. C., Fisher, J. D., and Baum, A. (2010). *Environmental Psychology.* 5th Edn. London: Lawrence Erlbaum Associates.

Bishop, I. D., and Rohrmann, B. (2003). Subjective responses to simulated and real environments: a comparison. *Landsc. Urban Plan.* 65, 261–277. doi: 10.1016/S0169-2046(03)00070-7

Bitner, M. J. (1992). Servicescapes: the impact of physical surroundings on customers and employees. *J. Mark.* 56, 57–71. doi: 10.2307/1252042

Brosch, T., Pourtois, G., and Sander, D. (2010). The perception and categorisation of emotional stimuli: a review. *Cogn. Emot.* 24, 377–400. doi: 10.1080/02699930902975754

Caughy, M. O., O'Campo, P. J., and Patterson, J. (2001). A brief observational measure for urban neighborhoods. *Health Place* 7, 225–236. doi: 10.1016/S1353-8292(01)00012-0

Chalmers, A., Debattista, K., and Ramic-Brkic, B. (2009). Towards high-fidelity multi-sensory virtual environments. *Vis. Comput.* 25, 1101–1108. doi: 10.1007/s00371-009-0389-2

Chen, K., Zhou, B., Chen, S., He, S., and Zhou, W. (2013). Olfaction spontaneously highlights visual saliency map. *Proc. Biol. Sci.* 280, 1–7. doi: 10.1098/rspb.2013.1729

Cozens, P., Neal, R., Whitaker, J., and Hillier, D. (2003). Investigating personal safety at railway stations using "virtual reality" technology. *Facilties* 21, 188–194. doi: 10.1108/02632770310489936

Dang, A., Liang, W, and Chi, W. (2012). "Review of VR application in digital urban planning and managing," in *Geospatial Techniques in Urban Planning*, ed. Z. Shen (Berlin: Springer), 131–154.

Demattè, M. L., Osterbauer, R., and Spence, C. (2007). Olfactory cues modulate facial attractiveness. *Chem. Sens.* 32, 603–610. doi: 10.1093/chemse/bjm030

Demattè, M. L., Sanabria, D., and Spence, C. (2009). Olfactory discrimination: when vision matters? *Chem. Sens.* 34, 103–109. doi: 10.1093/chemse/bjn055

Dinh, H. Q., Walker, N., Hodges, L. F., Song, C, and Kobayashi, A. (1999). "Evaluating the importance of multi-sensory input on memory and the sense of presence in virtual environments," in *Proceedings of the Virtual Reality Annual International Symposium* (Piscataway, NJ: IEEE Press), 222–228.

Driver, J., and Spence, C. (1998). Cross-modal links in spatial attention. *Phil. Trans. R. Soc. B Biol. Sci.* 353, 1319–1331. doi: 10.1098/rstb.1998.0286

Duncan, S., and Feldman Barrett, L. (2007). The role of the amygdala in visual awareness. *Trends Cogn. Sci.* 11, 190–192. doi: 10.1016/j.tics.2007.01.007

Durand, K., Baudouin, J. Y., Lewkowicz, D. J., Goubet, N., and Schaal, B. (2013). Eye-catching odors: olfaction elicits sustained gazing to faces and eyes in 4-month-old infants. *PLoS ONE* 8:e70677. doi: 10.1371/journal.pone.0070677

Ehrlichman, H., and Halpern, J. N. (1988). Affect and memory: effects of pleasant and unpleasant odors on retrieval of happy and unhappy memories. *J. Pers. Soc. Psychol.* 55, 769–779. doi: 10.1037/0022-3514.55.5.769

Fox, E., Russo, R., and Dutton, K. (2002). Attentional bias for threat: evidence for delayed disengagement from emotional faces. *Cogn. Emot.* 16, 355–379. doi: 10.1080/02699930143000527

Ghinea, G., and Ademoye, O. A. (2011). Olfaction-enhanced multimedia: perspectives and challenges. *Multimed. Tools Appl.* 55, 601–626. doi: 10.1007/s11042-010-0581-4

Gottfried, J. A., and Dolan, R. J. (2003). The nose smells what the eye sees: cross-modal visual facilitation of human olfactory perception. *Neuron* 39, 375–386. doi: 10.1016/S0896-6273(03)00392-1

Hacker, G., Brooks, A., and van der Zwan, R. (2013). Sex discriminations made on the basis of ambiguous visual cues can be affected by the presence of an olfactory cue. *BMC Psychol.* 1:10. doi: 10.1186/2050-7283-1-10

Henning, E. (2013). *Britain's Favourite Smells.* Available at: http://blog.ambius.com/britains-favourite-smells

Henshaw, V., and Bruce, N. (2012). "Smell and sound expectation and the ambiances of English cities," in *Proceedings of the 2nd International Congress on Ambiances* (Montreal), 449–454.

Houtkamp, J. M. (2012). *Affective Appraisal of Virtual Environments.* Ph.D. Thesis. University Utrecht, Utrecht. Available at: http://igitur-archive.library.uu.nl/dissertations/2012-0620-200449/UUindex.html

Houtkamp, J. M., Schuurink, E. L., and Toet, A. (2008). "Thunderstorms in my computer: the effect of visual dynamics and sound in a 3D environment," in *Proceedings of the International Conference on Visualisation in Built and Rural Environments BuiltViz'08*, eds M. Bannatyne and J. Counsell (Los Alamitos: IEEE Computer Society), 11–17.

Jacobs, R. H., Renken, R., Aleman, A., and Cornelissen, F. W. (2012). The amygdala, top-down effects, and selective attention to features. *Neurosci. Biobehav. Rev.* 36, 2069–2084. doi: 10.1016/j.neubiorev.2012.05.011

Jadauji, J. B., Djordjevic, J., Lundström, J. N., and Pack, C. C. (2012). Modulation of olfactory perception by visual cortex stimulation. *J. Neurosci.* 32, 3095–3100. doi: 10.1523/JNEUROSCI.6022-11.2012

Koster, E. H., Crombez, G., Van Damme, S., Verschuere, B., and De Houwer, J. (2004). Does imminent threat capture and hold attention? *Emotion* 4, 312–317. doi: 10.1037/1528-3542.4.3.312

Krusemark, E., and Li, W. (2012). Enhanced olfactory sensory perception of threat in anxiety: an event-related fMRI study. *Chemosens. Percept.* 5, 37–45. doi: 10.1007/s12078-011-9111-7

Leppänen, J. M., and Hietanen, J. K. (2003). Affect and face perception: odors modulate the recognition advantage of happy faces. *Emotion* 3, 315–326. doi: 10.1037/1528-3542.3.4.315

Lin, J. Y., Murray, S. O., and Boynton, G. M. (2009). Capture of attention to threatening stimuli without perceptual awareness. *Curr. Biol.* 19, 1118–1122. doi: 10.1016/j.cub.2009.05.021

Michael, G. A., Jacquot, L., Millot, J.-L., and Brand, G. (2003). Ambient odors modulate visual attentional capture. *Neurosci. Lett.* 352, 221–225. doi: 10.1016/j.neulet.2003.08.068

Michael, G. A., Jacquot, L., Millot, J.-L., and Brand, G. (2005). Ambient odors influence the amplitude and time course of visual distraction. *Behav. Neurosci.* 119, 708–715. doi: 10.1037/0735-7044.119.3.708

Mohanty, A., Egner, T., Monti, J. M., and Mesulam, M. M. (2009). Search for a threatening target triggers limbic guidance of spatial attention. *J. Neurosci.* 29, 10563–10572. doi: 10.1523/JNEUROSCI.1170-09.2009

Morrin, M., and Ratneshwar, S. (2003). Does it make sense to use scents to enhance brand memory? *J. Market. Res.* 40, 10–25. doi: 10.1509/jmkr.40.1.10.19128

Morrin, M., and Ratneshwar, S. (2000). The impact of ambient scent on evaluation, attention, and memory for familiar and unfamiliar brands. *J. Bus. Res.* 49, 157–165. doi: 10.1016/S0148-2963(99)00006-5

Morrot, G., Brochet, F., and Dubourdieu, D. (2001). The color of odors. *Brain Lang.* 79, 309–320. doi: 10.1006/brln.2001.2493

Murray, E. A. (2007). The amygdala, reward and emotion. *Trends Cogn. Sci.* 11, 489–497. doi: 10.1016/j.tics.2007.08.013

Nasar, J. L., and Cubukcu, E. (2011). Evaluative appraisals of environmental mystery and surprise. *Environ. Behav.* 43, 387–414. doi: 10.1177/0013916510364500

Oshima, C., Wada, A., Ando, H., Matsuo, N., Abe, S., and Yanigada, Y. (2007). "Improved delivery of olfactory stimukus to keep drivers awake," in *Workshop on DSP for in-Vehicle and Mobile Systems*, Istanbul.

Österbauer, R. A., Matthews, P. M., Jenkinson, M., Beckmann, C. F., Hansen, P. C., and Calvert, G. A. (2005). The color of scents: chromatic stimuli modulate odor responses in the human brain. *J. Neurophysiol.* 93, 3434–3441. doi: 10.1152/jn.00555.2004

Park, A. J., Calvert, T., Brantingham, P. L., and Brantingham, P. J. (2008). The use of virtual and mixed reality environments for urban behavioural studies. *Psychnol. J.* 6, 119–130.

Park, A. J., Spicer, V., Guterres, M., Brantingham, P. L., and Jenion, G. (2010). "Testing perception of crime in a virtual environment," in *Proceedings of the 2010 IEEE International Conference on Intelligence and Security Informatics (ISI)* (Piscataway, NJ: IEEE Press), 7–12.

Perkins, D. D., Meeks, J. W., and Taylor, R. B. (1992). The physical environment of street blocks and resident perceptions of crime and disorder: implications for theory and measurement. *J. Environ. Psychol.* 12, 21–34. doi: 10.1016/S0272-4944(05)80294-4

Phillips, T., and Smith, P. (2004). Emotional and behavioral responses to everyday incivility: challenging the fear/avoidance paradigm. *J. Sociol.* 40, 378–399. doi: 10.1177/1440783304048382

Pollatos, O., Kopietz, R., Linn, J., Albrecht, J., Sakar, V., Anzinger, A., et al. (2007). Emotional stimulation alters olfactory sensitivity and odor judgment. *Chem. Sens.* 32, 583–589. doi: 10.1093/chemse/bjm027

Pourtois, G., Schettino, A., and Vuilleumier, P. (2013). Brain mechanisms for emotional influences on perception and attention: what is magic and what is not. *Biol. Psychol.* 92, 492–512. doi: 10.1016/j.biopsycho.2012.02.007

Reynolds, E. (2012). Our favourite smells: cut grass, aftershave, a freshly cleaned house, baking and a Sunday roast. *Daily Mail.* Available at: http://www.dailymail.co.uk/femail/article-2157519/ (accesses June 11, 2012).

Richard, E., Tijou, A., Richard, P., and Ferrier, J.-L. (2006). Multi-modal virtual environments for education with haptic and olfactory feedback. *Virtual Reality* 10, 207–225. doi: 10.1007/s10055-006-0040-8

Riener, R., and Harders, M. (2012). "Olfactory and gustatory aspects," in *Virtual Reality in Medicine*, eds R. Riener and M. Harders (London: Springer), 149–159.

Schifferstein, H. N. J., and Blok, S. T. (2002). The signal function of thematically (in)congruent ambient scents in a retail environment. *Chem. Sens.* 27, 539–549. doi: 10.1093/chemse/27.6.539

Seigneuric, A., Durand, K., Jiang, T., Baudouin, J. Y., and Schaal, B. (2010). The nose tells it to the eyes: crossmodal associations between olfaction and vision. *Perception* 39, 1541–1554. doi: 10.1068/p6740

Seigneuric, A., Durand, K., Jiang, T., Baudouin, J. Y., and Schaal, B. (2012). The nose tells it to the eyes: crossmodal associations between olfaction and vision. *Perception* 39, 1541–1554. doi: 10.1068/p6740

Seo, H. S., Roidl, E., Müller, F., and Negoias, S. (2010). Odors enhance visual attention to congruent objects. *Appetite* 54, 544–549. doi: 10.1016/j.appet.2010.02.011

Seubert, J., Freiherr, J., Djordjevic, J., and Lundström, J. N. (2013). Statistical localization of human olfactory cortex. *Neuroimage* 66, 333–342. doi: 10.1016/j.neuroimage.2012.10.030

Spielberger, C. D. (1983). *State-Trait Anxiety Inventory for adults.* Mountain View, CA: Consulting Psychologists Press, Inc.

Teller, C., and Dennis, C. (2011). The effect of ambient scent on consumers' perception, emotions and behaviour: a critical review. *J. Mark. Manage.* 28, 14–36. doi: 10.1080/0267257X.2011.560719

Todd, R. M., Cunningham, W. A., Anderson, A. K., and Thompson, E. (2012). Affect-biased attention as emotion regulation. *Trends Cogn. Sci.* 16, 365–372. doi: 10.1016/j.tics.2012.06.003

Toet, A., and van Schaik, M. G. (2012). Effects of signals of disorder on fear of crime in real and virtual environments. *J. Environ. Psychol.* 32, 260–276. doi: 10.1016/j.jenvp.2012.04.001

Tomono, A., Kanda, K., and Otake, S. (2011). Effect of smell presentation on individuals with regard to eye catching and memory. *Electron. Comm. Jpn.* 94, 9–19. doi: 10.1002/ecj.10319

Tortell, R., Luigi, D. P., Dozois, A., Bouchard, S., Morie, J. F., and Ilan, D. (2007). The effects of scent and game play experience on memory of a virtual environment. *Virtual Real.* 11, 61–68. doi: 10.1007/s10055-006-0056-0

Van der Burg, E., Olivers, C. N., Bronkhorst, A. W., and Theeuwes, J. (2008). Pip and pop: nonspatial auditory signals improve spatial visual search. *J. Exp. Psychol. Hum. Percept. Perform.* 34, 1053–1065. doi: 10.1037/0096-1523.34.5.1053

Van der Burg, E., Olivers, C. N., Bronkhorst, A. W., and Theeuwes, J. (2009). Poke and pop: tactile-visual synchrony increases visual saliency. *Neurosci. Lett.* 450, 60–64. doi: 10.1016/j.neulet.2008.11.002

Vuilleumier, P. (2005). How brains beware: neural mechanisms of emotional attention. *Trends Cogn. Sci.* 9, 585–594. doi: 10.1016/j.tics.2005.10.011

Walla, P. (2008). Olfaction and its dynamic influence on word and face processing: cross-modal integration. *Prog. Neurobiol.* 84, 192–209. doi: 10.1016/j.pneurobio.2007.10.005

Washburn, D. A., Jones, L. M., Satya, R. V., Bowers, C. A., and Cortes, A. (2003). Olfactory use in virtual environment training. *Model. Simulat. Mag.* 2, 19–25.

Williams, L. M., Palmer, D., Liddell, B. J., Song, L., and Gordon, E. (2006). The 'when' and 'where' of perceiving signals of threat versus non-threat. *Neuroimage* 31, 458–467. doi: 10.1016/j.neuroimage.2005.12.009

Williams, M. A., McGlone, F., Abbott, D. F., and Mattingley, J. B. (2005). Differential amygdala responses to happy and fearful facial expressions depend on selective attention. *Neuroimage* 24, 417–425. doi: 10.1016/j.neuroimage.2004.08.017

Winston, J. S., Gottfried, J. A., Kilner, J. M., and Dolan, R. J. (2005). Integrated neural representations of odor intensity and affective valence in human amygdala. *J. Neurosci.* 25, 8903–8907. doi: 10.1523/JNEUROSCI.1569-05.2005

Woldorff, M. G., Gallen, C. C., Hampson, S. A., Hillyard, S. A., Pantev, C., Sobel, D., et al. (1993). Modulation of early sensory processing in human auditory cortex during auditory selective attention. *Proc. Natl. Acad. Sci. U.S.A.* 90, 8722–8726. doi: 10.1073/pnas.90.18.8722

World Medical Association. (2000). World Medical Association Declaration of Helsinki: ethical principles for medical research involving human subjects. *J. Am. Med. Assoc.* 284, 3043–3045. doi: 10.1001/jama.284.23.3043

Worrall, J. L. (2006). The discriminant validity of perceptual incivility measures. *Justice Q.* 23, 360–383. doi: 10.1080/07418820600869137

Wrzesniewski, A., McCauley, C., and Rozin, P. (1999). Odor and affect: individual differences in the impact of odor on liking for places, things and people. *Chem. Sens.* 24, 713–721. doi: 10.1093/chemse/24.6.713

Yanigada, Y., Adachi, T., Miyasato, T., Tomono, A., Kawato, S., Noma, H., et al. (2005). "Integrating a projection-based olfactory display with interactive audio-visual contents," in *HCI International 2005*, Las Vegas.

Yanigada, Y., Kawato, S., Noma, H., Tetsutani, N., and Tomono, A. (2003). "A nose-tracked, personal olfactory display," in *International Conference on Computer Graphics and Interactive Techniques. ACM SIGGRAPH 2003 Sketches & Applications* (New York: ACM), 1.

Yanigada, Y., Kawato, S., Noma, H., Tomono, A., and Tetsutani, N. (2004). "Projection-based olfactory display with nose tracking," in *Proceedings of IEEE Virtual Reality 2004* (Piscataway, NJ: IEEE), 43–50.

Yu, J., Yanigada, Y., Kawato, S., and Tetsutani, N. (2003). "Air cannon design for projection-based olfactory display," in *Proceedings of the 13th International Conference on Artificial Reality and Telexistence*, Tokyo, 136–142.

Zald, D. H. (2003). The human amygdala and the emotional evaluation of sensory stimuli. *Brain Res. Rev.* 41, 88–123. doi: 10.1016/S0165-0173(02)00248-5

Zelano, C., Bensafi, M., Porter, J., Mainland, J., Johnson, B., Bremner, E., et al. (2005). Attentional modulation in human primary olfactory cortex. *Nat. Neurosci.* 8, 114–120. doi: 10.1038/nn1368

Zellner, D. A. (2013). Color odor interactions: a review and model. *Chemsens. Percept.* 1–15. doi: 10.1007/s12078-013-9154-z

Zellner, D. A., Bartoli, A. M., and Eckard, R. (1991). Influence of color on odor identification and liking ratings. *Am. J. Psychol.* 104, 547–561. doi: 10.2307/1422940

Zellner, D. A., and Kautz, M. A. (1990). Color affects perceived odor intensity. *J. Exp. Psychol. Hum. Percept. Perform.* 16, 391–397. doi: 10.1037/0096-1523.16.2.391

Zhou, W., and Chen, D. (2009). Fear-related chemosignals modulate recognition of fear in ambiguous facial expressions. *Psychol. Sci.* 20, 177–183. doi: 10.1111/j.1467-9280.2009.02263.x

Zhou, W., Jiang, Y., He, S., and Chen, D. (2010). Olfaction modulates visual perception in binocular rivalry. *Curr. Biol.* 20, 1356–1358. doi: 10.1016/j.cub.2010.05.059

Zhou, W., Zhang, X., Chen, J., Wang, L., and Chen, D. (2012). Nostril-specific olfactory modulation of visual perception in binocular rivalry. *J. Neurosci.* 32, 17225–17229. doi: 10.1523/JNEUROSCI.2649-12.2012

18

Dynamics of autonomic nervous system responses and facial expressions to odors

Wei He[1,2], Sanne Boesveldt[2], Cees de Graaf[2] and René A. de Wijk[1]*

[1] Consumer Science and Intelligent Systems, Food and Biobased Research, Wageningen University and Research Centre, Wageningen, Netherlands
[2] Division of Human Nutrition, Sensory Science and Eating Behaviour, Wageningen University, Wageningen, Netherlands

***Correspondence:**
René A. de Wijk, Consumer Science and Intelligent Systems, Food and Biobased Research, Wageningen University and Research Centre, PO Box 17, Bornse Weilanden 9, 6700 AA Wageningen, Netherlands
e-mail: rene.dewijk@wur.nl

Why we like or dislike certain products may be better captured by physiological and behavioral measures of the autonomic nervous system (ANS) than by conscious or classical sensory tests. Responses to pleasant and unpleasant food odors presented in varying concentrations were assessed continuously using facial expressions and responses of the ANS. Results of 26 young and healthy female participants showed that the unpleasant fish odor triggered higher heart rates and skin conductance responses, lower skin temperature, fewer neutral facial expressions and more disgusted and angry expressions ($p < 0.05$). Neutral facial expressions differentiated between odors within 100 ms, after the start of the odor presentation followed by expressions of disgust (180 ms), anger (500 ms), surprised (580 ms), sadness (820 ms), scared (1020 ms), and happy (1780 ms) (all *p*-values < 0.05). Heart rate differentiated between odors after 400 ms, whereas skin conductance responses differentiated between odors after 3920 ms. At shorter intervals (between 520 and 1000 ms and between 2690 and 3880 ms) skin temperature for fish was higher than that for orange, but became considerable lower after 5440 ms. This temporal unfolding of emotions in reactions to odors, as seen in facial expressions and physiological measurements supports sequential appraisal theories.

Keywords: skin conductance, skin temperature, heart rate, ANS responses, odor, valence, concentration, facial expressions

INTRODUCTION

Up to 80% of all new food products fail in the marketplace, despite the fact that they are typically subjected to a large number of sensory and consumer tests before their market introduction (Crawford, 1977). This suggests that the "standard" sensory and consumer tests, which typically include sensory analytical profiling and liking tests, have a low predictive validity with respect to general product performance. Possibly, consumer food choice outside the laboratory may be less based on cognitive information processing and rational reasoning, and more on unarticulated/unconscious motives and associations (Wansink, 2004). Reasons for likes or dislikes of specific foods are typically difficult to articulate but may determine much of our food choice. Unarticulated/unconscious motives and associations are not very well captured by traditional tests based on conscious cognitive processes, and may be better captured by physiological and behavioral measures (e.g., facial expressions) of the autonomic nervous system (ANS) which do not require conscious processes (Greenwald, 2009).

Physiological measures have been used extensively to capture responses of the ANS to various types of stimuli such as film clips, personalized recall of specific situations, and odors. In a previous study, Alaoui-Ismaïli et al. (1997) related various autonomic parameters to the pleasantness of five odorants, and found that unpleasant odors were associated with increased heart rate (HR) and longer skin conductance responses (SCR) compared to pleasant odors. Bensafi et al. (2002) related ANS measures to rated pleasantness, arousal, intensity, and familiarity for a set of six odorants and found that their results could be explained by two main factors: pleasantness, inversely related to HR (similar to Alaoui-Ismaïli et al., 1997) and arousal, positively related to skin conductance and rated intensity. Delplanque et al. (2009) found stronger SCR and higher HR for unpleasant compared to pleasant odors. They also established that HR differences between pleasant and unpleasant odors occurred relatively late in the deceleration phase, approximately 5–8 s after odor presentation. Considerable faster odor-specific responses were found for facial expressions; facial muscle activity associated with positive and negative facial expressions showed different activities for pleasant and unpleasant odors as soon as 400–500 ms after odor presentation (Delplanque et al., 2009).

Facial expressions have also been used extensively by others to measure emotional responses to food-related stimuli. Well-known are the positive facial expressions of new-borns toward liked (sweet) and the negative expressions toward disliked (bitter) basic tastes, extensively documented by Steiner (1973). More recently, an automated tool, FaceReader, has been developed and used to analyze more diverse, universal facial expressions. Using different food stimuli, it was found that happy expressions were not systematically related to liking scores, in contrast to neutral, angry, and disgusted expressions (Danner et al., 2014), and that stronger facial expressions to disliked foods compared to liked foods were already detected at the first visual encounter with the food (De Wijk et al., 2012).

The dynamic features over time of physiological responses and facial expressions have typical been outside the scope of most studies, even though they play a key role in several modern theories on emotion, the so-called componential appraisal models (see Ellsworth and Scherer, 2003 for an overview). The models assume that the elicitation and the differentiation of emotions are determined by appraisals, the continuous, recursive evaluations of events, Delplanque et al. (2009) investigated the appraisal of odor novelty and pleasantness and consequent emotional responses by measuring facial muscle activity and HR. They demonstrated that odors were detected as novel or familiar before being evaluated as pleasant or unpleasant (Distel et al., 1991; Royet et al., 1999). In addition, their results also argued in favor of a dynamic construction of facial expressions providing support for sequential appraisal theories (Ellsworth and Scherer, 2003). For example, early reactions, such as raising the eyebrows and opening the eyes, were related to the detection of a novel or unexpected stimulus, which is associated with increased alertness and attention. After this novelty detection, assessment of pleasantness may lead to avoidance when the stimulus is aversive or threatening, or approach when a pleasant response is activated.

The present study will expand on previous studies by using (food) odors delivered by an olfactometer, offering a high degree of control over timing and concentrations, and by incorporating additional ANS measures [skin temperature (ST)] and other types of facial expressions. Similar to Delplanque et al. (2009) the present study will also focus on the temporal development of each measure instead of the more commonly used time-averaged means (e.g., De Wijk et al., 2012; Danner et al., 2014). Physiological responses and facial expressions will be measured continuously and analyses will be based on time-averaged means (similar to most of the previous studies) as well as on their temporal development. It is hypothesized that the results based on time-averaged means will replicate the findings of similar studies by others, i.e., higher HR and skin conductance, lower ST and more negative facial expressions after exposure to the unpleasant odor compared to exposure to the pleasant odor. It is further hypothesized that ANS responses are slower than facial expressions, but that both follow sequential appraisal processes of evaluating the stimuli.

MATERIALS AND METHODS

PARTICIPANTS

Twenty-six young healthy female participants (mean age: 22.6 ± 1.5 years, range: 20–25 years, $18.5 < \text{BMI} < 25\,\text{kg/m}^2$) were recruited from the subject pool of Food and Biobased Research, part of Wageningen University and Research Center. Participants self-reported their BMI and if they had actual/previous history of smell or taste disorders known to affect chemosensory function. Detailed information regarding the experiment was given and an informed consent form was signed by all participants prior to testing. The study was approved by the Medical Ethical Committee of the Wageningen University.

ODOR STIMULI AND PRESENTATION

As described elsewhere (He et al., under review), two food odors were selected on the basis of their relatively negative (fish odor) or positive (orange odor) valence (Boesveldt et al., 2010). The orange (cold-pressed Californian orange oil, Sigma Aldrich, St. Louis, MO, USA) and fish (Fish flavor oil, Givaudan Inc., Geneva, Switzerland) odors were diluted with mineral oil (to 70%, v/v) and 1,2-propanediol (to 27%, v/v), respectively. With a dynamic olfactometer based on air-dilution (OM2s, Burghart instruments, Wedel, Germany), each odor was delivered in three different concentrations (low, medium, or high), correspondingly perceived at different intensities in a pilot study. The olfactometer allows the presentation of odorous stimuli within a continuous humidified (80%) and warmed (37°C) airstream of 8 L/min, which does not alter the mechanical or thermal conditions at the nasal mucosa (Kobal and Hummel, 1988). These stimuli were delivered through a nosepiece for 1 s with an inter stimulus interval of 60 s. Each block of six stimuli (i.e., orange odor in three concentrations and fish odor in three concentrations) was randomized and presented five times, for a total of 30 stimuli.

PROCEDURE

The experimental sessions took place in the physiological laboratory of the Restaurant of the Future located in Wageningen, the Netherlands. The experiment leader explained the experiment to the participant, allowed ample time for questions and asked the participant to sign the inform consent form (which they had received by e-mail prior to the experimental session) after which the electrodes were placed. Participants were seated in a comfortable chair, fitted with the olfactometer nosepiece, and oriented toward an adjustable computer monitor set with a webcam at eye-level (1 m viewing distance). They were asked to look directly toward the camera while receiving the odor stimulus to ensure recognition by the FaceReader software. Each trial started with an auditory attention signal to remind the participant to pay attention to the upcoming odor. The pleasantness and intensity of each odor was rated subsequently on a paper questionnaire 10 s after stimulation. The procedure is also shown schematically in **Figure 1**. The whole experiment lasted 45 min in total. **Photograph 1** shows the set-up as used in this study.

MEASUREMENTS

Physiological ANS measures

Physiological measures included:

1. Skin conductance response (SCR) measured in μSiemens with electrodes placed on the palm of the non-dominant hand of the participant.
2. Heart rate (HR) measured in beats per minute with electrodes placed on the chest.
3. Skin temperature (ST) measured in degrees Celsius with an electrode placed on the palm of the non-dominant hand of the participant.

The physiological data were collected at 200 Hz via a MindWare Acquisition data acquisition system (MindWare Technologies, Inc.) with separate filter settings for the electrocardiogram, finger temperature and electrodermal (SCR) activity. Filter settings were low-pass 0.5 Hz, high-pass 45 Hz for HR frequency, low-pass 1 Hz, high-pass 45 Hz for SCR, and low-pass 10 Hz, high-pass

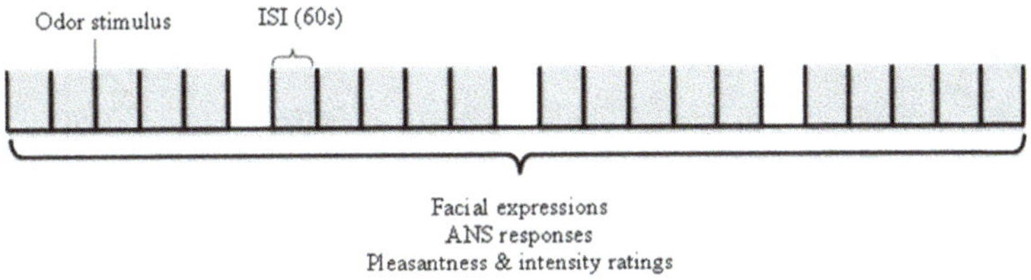

FIGURE 1 | Schematical representation of the experimental procedure followed during one experimental session.

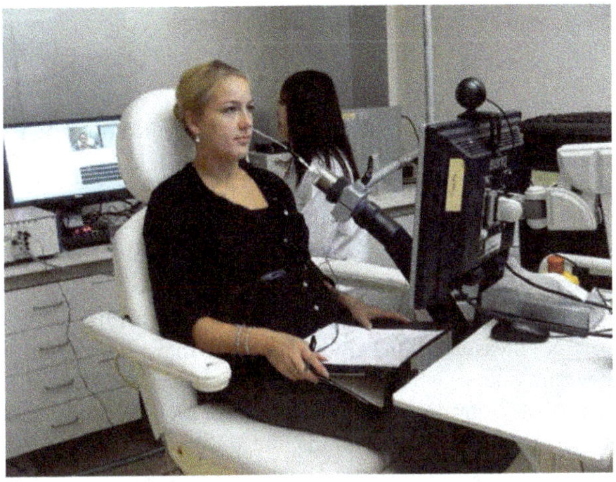

Photograph 1 | Set-up used in this study showing the participant and the experimenter, the arm of the olfactometer for odor presentation, and the monitor used for instructions with a camera used for facial expressions.

45 Hz for ST. Electrodes were used with a surface of 4.1 cm^2 and filled with 1% Chloride wet gel. Signals were transferred to the Acquisition Unit (16-bit A/D conversion) and stored on computer hard disk (sampling rate 500 Hz/s). Electrocardiographic R waves were detected offline, and intervals between heartbeats were converted to HR, expressed in beats per minute (BPM). SCR activity was recorded (high-pass filter: 0.025 Hz.) by the constant voltage method (0.5 V). The signal was amplified by 1000 and low-pass filtered (30 Hz).

Facial expressions

Facial expressions were automatically analyzed using FaceReader software version 4.0 (Noldus Information Technology B.V.). FaceReader works in three steps: (1) face finding, (2) face modeling, and (3) face classification. During face finding an accurate position of the face is found using the Active Template Method. During modeling, the Active Appearance Model is used to synthesize an artificial face model, which describes the location of 491 key points as well as the texture of the face. The actual classification of the facial expressions is done by training an artificial neural network as training material nearly 2000 manually annotated images were used. The network was trained to classify the six basic or universal emotions described by Ekman (1992): happy, sad, angry, surprised, scared, and disgusted and a neutral state. FaceReader analyzed the facial expressions on a frame-by-frame basis, i.e., at 25 Hz. Previous studies showed that FaceReader results corresponded between 71% (angry) to 99% (neutral) of all cases, with an average of 87%, with results from human observers (Terzis et al., 2012). FaceReader happiness scores correlated significantly ($r = 0.79$) with objectively measured activity in the *zygomaticus supercilli* or cheek muscle, a muscle that is activated during expressions of happiness (D'Arcey et al., 2012). A more detailed description of the science behind FaceReader can be found at: http://info.noldus.com/free-white-paper-on-facereader-methodology/.

Ratings of pleasantness and intensity

A visual analog scale of 10 cm was used to rate pleasantness and intensity after each odor presentation, ranging from "not perceivable" (left-hand end = 0 cm) to "extremely strong" (right-hand end = 10 cm), or from "very unpleasant" (left) to "neutral" (middle of the scale = 5 cm) to "very pleasant" (right). In this study, orange odors were rated more pleasant [$F_{(1, 25)} = 99.86$, $p < 0.001$] and less intense [$F_{(1, 25)} = 17.27$, $p < 0.001$] than fish odors by the participants (see **Table 1**). Furthermore, odor intensity increased with concentration [$F_{(2, 50)} = 47.15$, $p < 0.001$].

DATA ANALYSIS

The processed images with the facial expressions were combined with raw physiological data in Observer XT 10.5 software (Noldus Information Technology) for further analyses. The moments that odors were presented to the participants were marked automatically using the "trigger-out" signal from the olfactometer that signals the start of each odor presentation. The physiological measures SCR, HR, and ST were analyzed per odor presentation. The video images of the facial expressions were processed per odor presentation with FaceReader 4.0 software (Noldus Information Technology). Due to a technical malfunction, absolute ST values were not recorded, but the results can still be used to assess changes over time in ST per odor presentation. Results from some participants had to be removed from the analysis due to a large number of artifacts. The number of participants that is included in the analysis is 21 (HR), 22 (skin conductance and ST), and 24 (facial expressions).

Two types of statistical analyses were used: one based on post-odor time-averaged responses to verify systematic effects of odor and concentration, and one based on pre- and post-odor time-series of responses to verify the post-odor time at which responses become odor-specific. Details of each type of analysis

Table 1 | Average ratings (0–10, with standard deviation) of fish and orange odors diluted to different concentrations.

Odor	Concentration	Air-diluted to (%)	Intensity		Pleasantness	
			Mean	*SD*	Mean	*SD*
Fish (27% v/v)	Low	10	6.2	1.9	1.5	1.3
	Medium	25	6.7	1.6	1.5	1.3
	High	50	7.1	1.7	1.3	1.1
Orange (70% v/v)	Low	50	4.8	1.7	6.4	1.1
	Medium	80	6.0	1.7	5.6	1.6
	High	100	6.6	1.7	5.4	1.3

Ratings were made on a visual analog scale of 10 cm length. For intensity, 0 indicates "not perceivable" and 10 indicates "extremely strong"; For pleasantness, 0 indicates "very unpleasant," 5 indicates "neutral," and 10 indicates "very pleasant."

are given below. In addition, correlational analysis was used to verify systematic associations between measures.

1. Repeated measures ANOVAs (IBM SPSS Statistics 19.0, IBM Corporation, Armonk, USA) were conducted on post-odor time-averaged facial expressions, ANS responses with odor and concentration as within-subject variables. A p-value of 0.05 was considered significant.
2. To verify the time at which time-series ANS responses and facial expressions become odor-specific (i.e., differ significantly between odors), absolute deltas between orange and fish odors were calculated together with the standard deviations for the 2.5 s interval preceding odor presentation to establish a pre-odor baseline. Subsequently, post-odor times were identified at which the absolute delta between the odors exceeded the pre-odor average plus three times the pre-odor standard deviation.

RESULTS

EFFECTS OF ODOR AND CONCENTRATION

Physiological measures

Time-averaged means for HR [$F_{(1, 20)} = 18.7$, $p < 0.001$] and skin conductance [$F_{(1, 21)} = 6.3$, $p < 0.05$] were significantly higher for the unpleasant fish odor compared to the pleasant orange odor (**Figures 2A,B**). Skin temperature did not vary systematically with odor [$F_{(1, 21)} = 2.0$, n.s.; **Figure 2C**]. Heart rate also increased systematically with concentration [$F_{(2, 40)} = 5.3$, $p < 0.01$]. Concentration did not affect skin conductance [$F_{(1, 21)} = 0.6$, n.s.] or ST $F_{(1, 21)} = 0.9$, n.s.).

Facial expressions

Time-averaged means of facial expressions to the fish compared to the orange odor were significantly less neutral [$F_{(1, 23)} = 21.25$, $p < 0.001$; **Figure 2D**] and more disgusted [$F_{(1, 23)} = 9.63$, $p < 0.01$], and angry [$F_{(1,23)} = 4.00$, $p < 0.05$]. Moreover, facial expressions intensified at higher concentrations resulting, depending on the odor, in weaker neutral expressions [odor by concentration effect: $F_{(2, 46)} = 3.25$, $p < 0.05$] and stronger scared expressions [odor by concentration effect: $F_{(2, 46)} = 3.51$, $p < 0.05$].

Associations between physiological measures, facial expressions, and ratings are summarized by correlational analysis based on 24 stimuli (two odors × three concentrations × four replicates) averaged across participants (**Table 2**).

TIME-SERIES RESPONSES: WHEN DO RESPONSES BECOME ODOR SPECIFIC?

Physiological measures

Prior to the odor presentation, but after the warning signal is given, ANS measures show gradual changes that are independent of the odor valence whereby skin conductance and HR gradually increase and ST gradually decreases (**Figure 3**). Skin conductance continues to increase for seconds after odor presentation independent of the specific odor. After approximately 3 s, SCR for orange decreases whereas that for fish continues to increase. The difference in SCR becomes significant after 3920 ms (**Figure 3B** and **Table 3**). Heart rate for the unpleasant fish odor increases almost instantaneously after the odor is presented whereas HR for the pleasant orange odor shows much smaller effects (**Figure 3A** and **Table 3**). The difference in HR response between the odors becomes significant after 400 ms. Skin temperature follows a different, irregular pattern with higher temperatures for fish odor at shorter intervals (between 520 and 1000 ms and between 2690 and 3880 ms) and lower temperature at longer intervals (after 5440 ms) (**Figure 3C** and **Table 3**) compared to orange odor.

Facial expressions

Neutral expressions become odor-specific after less than 100 ms. Disgusted expressions take approximately another 100 ms to become odor-specific. Angry, surprised, sad, and scared become after 500–1000 ms odor-specific, whereas happy expression become odor-specific after more than 1700 ms (**Figure 4** and **Table 3**). **Table 3** summarizes the times at which ANS responses and facial expressions significantly differentiate between the unpleasant fish and pleasant orange odor.

DISCUSSION

Human responses to pleasant and unpleasant food odors presented in varying concentrations were assessed with facial expressions and responses of the ANS. Analysis were carried out on results with and without averaging over time, and showed partly overlapping and partly different results.

ANOVAs on time-averaged results showed that the unpleasant fish odor triggered higher HR and SCR, lower ST, fewer neutral facial expressions and more disgusted and angry expressions

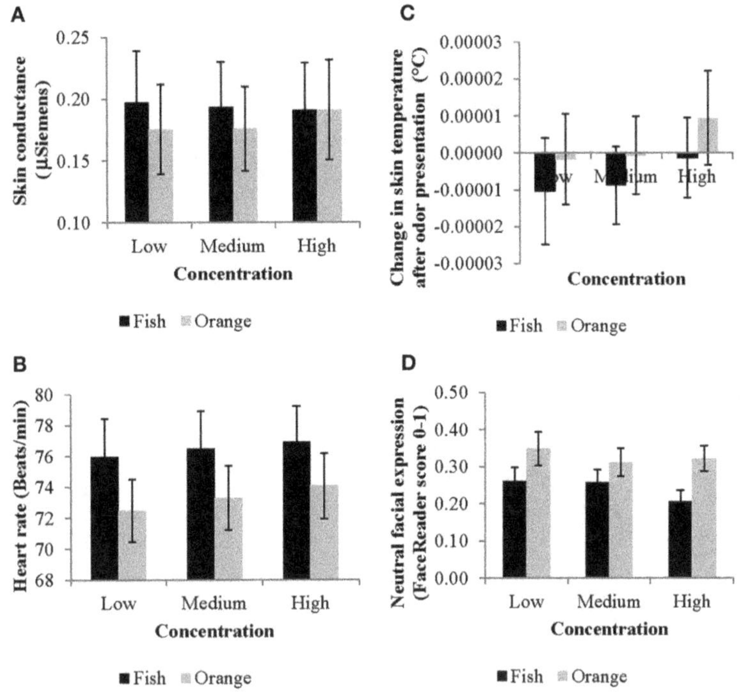

FIGURE 2 | Effects of odor and concentration on (A) skin conductance responses, (B) heart rate, (C) skin temperature, and (D) neutral facial expressions (averaged across time and bars indicate standard errors).

Table 2 | Pearson correlation coefficients between facial expressions, ratings and physiological measures for 24 stimuli averaged across participants.

		Facial expressions							Ratings		Physiological measures		
		Angry	Disgusted	Happy	Neutral	Sad	Scared	Surprised	Pleasantness	Intensity	HR	SCR	ST
Facial expressions	Angry	1	,49	,61*	−,65*	0.07	,50	−0.36	−,71*	,49	,61*	−0.09	0.02
	Disgusted		1	,40	−,78*	,48	,57*	−,59*	−,71*	,56*	,61*	0.04	−0.02
	Happy			1	−,52*	−0.04	0.31	−0.18	−,55*	,57*	,50	−0.21	0.12
	Neutral				1	−,43	−,58*	,48	,83*	−,55*	−,73*	0.15	0.19
	Sad					1	,43	−0.33	−,41	,41	,45	,56*	−0.23
	Scared						1	−0.23	−,61*	,52*	,50	0.06	−0.10
	Surprised							1	,65*	−0.35	−,62*	−0.22	−0.03
Ratings	Pleasantness								1	−,61*	−,93*	−0.08	0.21
	Intensity									1	,67*	0.07	0.17
Physiological measures	HR										1	0.23	−0.16
	SCR											1	0.11
	ST												1

**Correlation is significant at the 0.005 level (2-tailed).*

compared to the pleasant orange odor. Overall, our results were similar to the ones found in studies by others for HR (Alaoui-Ismaïli et al., 1997; Bensafi et al., 2002; Delplanque et al., 2009), skin conductance (Alaoui-Ismaïli et al., 1997; Delplanque et al., 2009), and ST (see Köster, 2009), indicating that these averaged physiological measurements are mainly responsive to the valence of a stimulus, and less to intensity, whereas facial expressions appear to demonstrate more concentration-specific effects.

Correlational analyses based on time-averaged results shows positive associations between odor liking and neutral/surprised

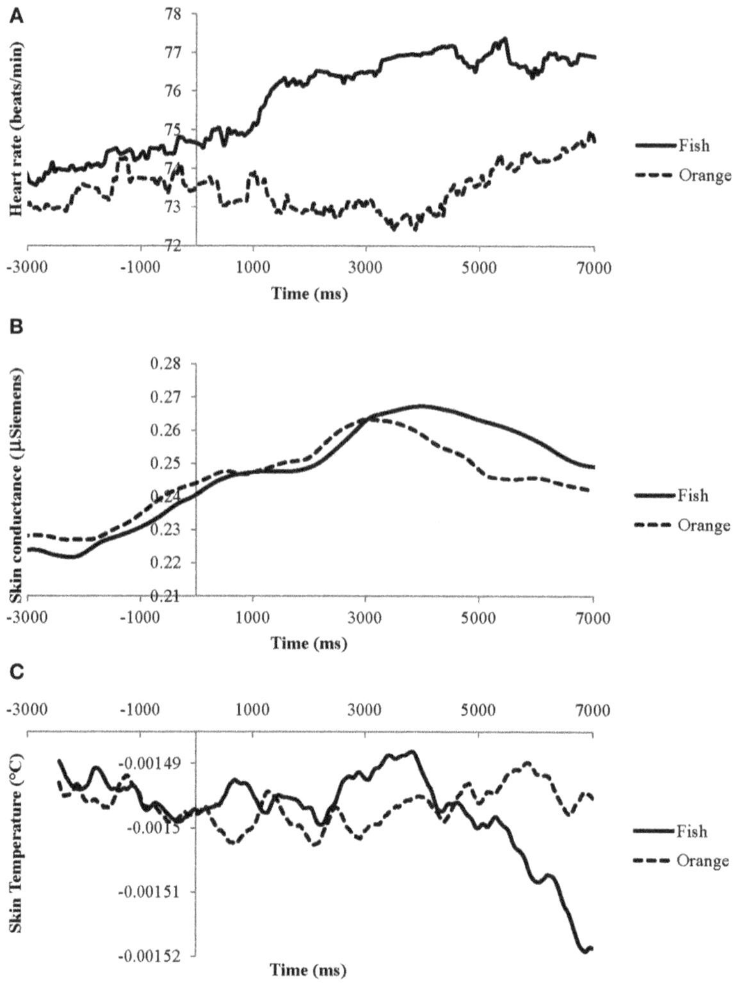

FIGURE 3 | Effects of odor (averaged across concentrations) on (A) heart rate, (B) skin conductance, and (C) skin temperature. Absolute skin temperatures are incorrect due to a technical malfunction.

Table 3 | Intervals in ms following odor presentation at which responses become odor-specific.

Measures		Odor-specific time (ms)
Facial expressions	Neutral	<100-end
	Happy	1780-end
	Sad	820-end
	Angry	500-end
	Surprised	580-end
	Scared	1020-end
	Disgusted	180-end
ANS responses	HR	400-end
	SCR	3920-end
	ST	520–1000
		2640–3880
		5440-end

facial expressions, and negative associations between odor liking and all other facial expressions, including happiness. Negative associations between odor liking and happy facial expressions have also been reported previously by others (Zeinstra et al., 2009; Danner et al., 2014; He et al., under review) suggesting that happy expressions cannot discriminate liked or disliked foods implicitly. Facial expressions of happiness are rarely displayed when one is alone and social interactions are absent suggesting that these expressions serve a social function (see also Gilbert et al., 1987 and Parkinson, 2005). The fact that they did occur in this study in the presence of experimental staff suggests that the happy facial expressions may serve some kind of social signaling function, e.g., to signal the staff that one is OK despite the previous display of negative expressions associated with disliked odors.

When results are not averaged across time, analyses demonstrate that facial expressions and physiological responses become

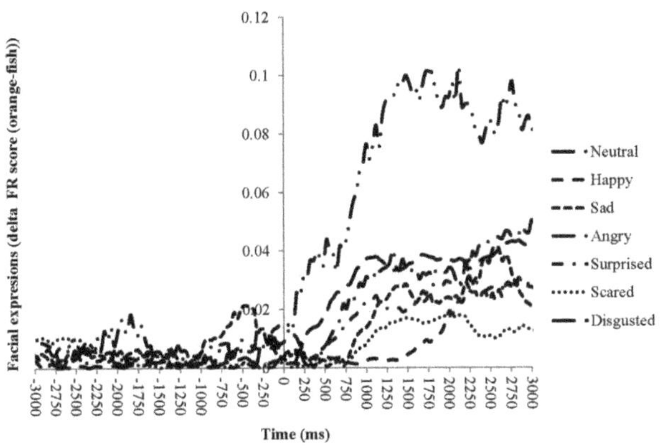

FIGURE 4 | Sequential unfolding of differences in facial expressions between the unpleasant fish odor and the pleasant orange odors for seven emotional facial expressions over time following the odor presentation.

rapidly odor-specific and are dynamic in nature. Responses such as skin conductance already start before the actual odor presentation These responses are obviously odor non-specific and probably reflect anticipatory processes, Almost immediately after the onset of the odor presentation, neutral facial expressions decrease followed after 100 ms by an increase in facial expressions of disgust. Within 400 ms HR for the unpleasant odor increase (similar to rapid acceleration in HR observed for negative emotions by Levenson, 1988), ST briefly increases, followed between 500 and 1000 ms by facial expressions of angry, surprised, sad, and scared, and after 1700 ms by happy expressions. During all this time, skin conductance gradually increases for both odors until approximately 3 s when skin conductance for the pleasant odor starts to decrease whereas that for the unpleasant odor continues to increase. Finally, after more than 4 s, skin conductance for the unpleasant odor decreases together with ST for the unpleasant odor. Combined these time-related results show that most facial expressions and physiological responses are fast reacting and odor-specific.

Our results correspond well with those found in previous studies; Delplanque et al. (2009) found odor-specific activities in two types of facial muscle activities 400–500 ms after odor presentation, which coincides approximately with sad, angry, and surprised expressions in the present study. These values also concur with the values found for other stimulus modalities such as vision; Dimberg et al. (2002) found facial responses to positive or negative visual stimuli after approximately 400–500 ms. In addition, we found other expressions that were triggered even faster, such as disgust, or slower, such as happy.

Response times for HR and for most of the facial expressions are well within 1 s after the odor is presented, and are often shorter than for example response time for odor detection (approximately 800 ms, De Wijk, 1989) or response time to decide whether or not an odor is more pleasant than a previous one (approximately 850 ms, Olofsson et al., 2012), where conscious action is needed. These differences in timing are possibly related to automated vs. conscious processes in the central nervous system. Facial expressions and ANS responses probably reflect automated processing of the central nervous system (see Dimberg et al., 2002 for automated processes and facial expressions), whereas decisions regarding detection and pleasantness/unpleasantness require also time-consuming conscious processing. The fact that automated emotional odor-response times may be as fast as response times in the visual domain despite the relatively slow peripheral and peri-peripheral processing of odors may reflect the anatomical overlap between CNS structures involved in olfaction and emotions; the peripheral and central olfactory system are only separated by one relay (glomerulus of the olfactory bulb) after the odor interacts with the primary olfactory neurons. Next, olfactory information is conducted to other olfactory structures, some of which are also involved in emotions (hippocampus, anterior cingulate cortex, orbitofrontal cortex and parts of the amygdala and insula Lundström et al., 2011; Soudry et al., 2011). Given the close correspondence of CNS structures involved in olfaction and emotions and the fact that these structures are activated simultaneously to when information becomes available for conscious, higher order cognitive processing in the cortex, it is no longer surprising that automated emotional odor response times are often faster than odor response times that involve conscious processing.

Combined the time-series responses found in this study show that most facial expressions and physiological responses are fast reacting and odor-specific. Moreover, different facial expressions and physiological measures develop at their own specific rate over time. Consequently, responses to the same stimulus may produce very different patterns of results depending on the time at which they are assessed. For example, fast responses around 500 ms, may be dominated by negative facial expressions such as disgust, increased HR and increased ST, whereas slower responses may be dominated by positive facial expressions, lower HR and decreased ST. The fast responses may be automated reflexes to novel and potentially dangerous stimuli, as observed by Delplanque et al. (2009), whereas the later responses may reflect a conscious processing of a sequence of different emotions, each resulting from a different appraisal of the stimulus by the observer (e.g., Ellsworth and Scherer, 2003). Results from the same laboratory indicate that conscious evaluative ratings of participants are associated with ANS responses and facial expressions between one and three seconds after stimulation (He et al., under review). This supports the notion that the fast responses, with response times of less than one second, are automated and relatively independent of evaluative ratings, whereas slower responses reflect conscious processing that form the basis for evaluative ratings and facial expressions of happiness for communicative purposes.

The present study has its obvious limitations; only a small number of odors were investigated, and their effects were investigated under controlled laboratory conditions with female participants. Nevertheless, the results may have some implications for consumer behavior in the real world. For example, visitors to supermarkets may have approximately 45 min to select their weekly groceries from up to 30,000 products. This task becomes even more daunting considering the fact that many of these selections are not planned but made in the supermarket. Given this abundance of choices consumers need a fast and partly automated selection mechanism that combines affect, appraisal, action readiness and autonomic arousal. This fast selection mechanism may be based on fast and probably automated ANS responses and facial expressions similar to the ones found in the present study. These fast responses may not only be triggered by odors, but also product packages and brand names. To explore real-life applications, future studies will measure ANS responses and facial expressions in relation to consumer choice behavior. Initially, consumer behavior will be assessed in the semi-real-life test environment of a virtual supermarket, followed by real-life assessment in an actual supermarket. Such studies will allow a proper evaluation of ANS measures and facial expressions as tools for marketing (research) because their associations with consumer product interactions and purchasing behaviors will be tested directly.

In summary, physiological and facial responses to odors prove to be fast and dynamic and the balance between these responses is continuously changing depending on their timing. This changing balance may reflect different sequential appraisals of emotions. This study along with other recent studies (e.g., Delplanque et al., 2009) shows the necessity of taking the time dimension into account and future studies should further explore the relation between dynamic responses and appraisals.

ACKNOWLEDGMENTS

We acknowledge the important contributions of Leanne Loijens and Patrick Zimmerman from Noldus Information Technology for their critical help in setting up the hardware and software necessary to conduct the study successfully.

REFERENCES

Alaoui-Ismaïli, O., Vernet-Maury, E., Dittmar, A., Delhomme, G., and Chanel, J. (1997). Odor hedonics: connection with emotional response estimated by autonomic parameters. *Chem. Senses* 22, 237–248. doi: 10.1093/chemse/22.3.237

Bensafi, M., Rouby, C., Farget, V., Bertrand, B., Vigouroux, M., and Holley, A. (2002). Autonomic nervous system responses to odours: the role of pleasantness and arousal. *Chem. Senses* 27, 703–709. doi: 10.1093/chemse/27.8.703

Boesveldt, S., Frasnelli, J., Gordon, A. R., and Lundström, J. N. (2010). The fish is bad: negative food odors elicit faster and more accurate reactions than other odors. *Biol. Psychol.* 84, 313–317. doi: 10.1016/j.biopsycho.2010.03.006

Crawford, C. (1977). Marketing research and the new product failure rate. *J. Marketing* 41, 55–61. doi: 10.2307/1250634

Danner, L., Sidorkina, L., Joechl, M., and Duerrschmid, K. (2014). Make a face! Implicit and explicit measurement of facial expressions elicited by orange juices using face reading technology. *Food Qual. Prefer.* 32, 167–172. doi: 10.1016/j.foodqual.2013.01.004

D'Arcey, T., Johnson, M., and Ennis, M. (2012). "Assessing the validity of FaceReader using facial electromyography," in *Proceedings of APS 24th annual meeting* (Chicago, IL).

Delplanque, S., Grandjean, D., Chrea, C., Coppin, G., Aymard, L., Cayeux, I., et al. (2009). Sequential unfolding of novelty and pleasantness appraisals of odors: evidence from facial electromyography and autonomic reactions. *Emotion* 9, 316–328. doi: 10.1037/a0015369

De Wijk, R. A. (1989). *Temporal Factors in Human Olfactory Perception.* Doctoral dissertation, State University of Utrecht, The Netherlands.

De Wijk, R. A., Kooijman, V., Verhoeven, R. H. G., Holthuysen, N. T. E., and de Graaf, C. (2012). Autonomic nervous system responses on and facial expressions to the sight, smell, and taste of liked and disliked foods. *Food Qual. Prefer.* 26, 196–203. doi: 10.1016/j.foodqual.2012.04.015

Dimberg, U., Thunberg, M., and Grunedal, S. (2002). Facial reactions to emotional stimuli: automatically controlled emotional responses. *Cogn. Emot.* 16, 449–471. doi: 10.1080/02699930143000356

Distel, H., Ayabe-Kanamura, S., Martínez-Gómez, M., Schicker, I., Kobayakawa, T., Saito, S., et al. (1991). Perception of everyday odors—correlation between intensity, familiarity and strength of hedonic judgement. *Chem. Senses* 24, 191–199. doi: 10.1093/chemse/24.2.191

Ekman, P. (1992). Facial expressions of emotion: an old controversy and new findings. *Philos. Trans. R. Soc. Lond. B Biol. Sci.* 335, 63–69. doi: 10.1098/rstb.1992.0008

Ellsworth, P. C., and Scherer, K. R. (2003). "Appraisal processes in emotion," in *Handbook of Affective Sciences*, eds R. J. Davidson, K. R. Scherer, and H. H. Goldsmith (New York, NY: Oxford University Press), 572–595.

Gilbert, A. N., Fridlund, A. J., and Sabini, J. (1987). Hedonic and social determinants of facial displays to odors. *Chem. Senses* 12, 355–363. doi: 10.1093/chemse/12.2.355

Greenwald, A. (2009). Supplemental material for understanding and using the implicit association test: III. Meta-analysis of predictive validity. *J. Pers. Soc. Psychol.* 97, 17–41. doi: 10.1037/a0015575

Kobal, G., and Hummel, C. (1988). Cerebral chemosensory evoked potentials elicited by chemical stimulation of the human olfactory and respiratory nasal mucosa. *Electroencephalogr. Clin. Neurophysiol.* 71, 241–250. doi: 10.1016/0168-5597(88)90023-8

Köster, E. (2009). Diversity in the determinants of food choice: a psychological perspective. *Food Qual. Prefer.* 20, 70–82. doi: 10.1016/j.foodqual.2007.11.002

Levenson, R. (1988). "Emotion and the autonomic nervous system: a prospectus for research on autonomic specificity," in *Social Psychophysiology and Emotion: Theory and Clinical Applications*, ed H. L. Wagner (London: John Wiley and Sons), 17–42.

Lundström, J. N., Boesveldt, S., and Albrecht, J. (2011). Central processing of the chemical senses: an overview. *ACS Chem. Neurosci.* 2, 5–16. doi: 10.1021/cn1000843

Olofsson, J. K., Bowman, N. E., Khatibi, K., and Gottfried, J. A. (2012). A time-based account of the perception of odor objects and valences. *Psychol. Sci.* 23, 1224–1232. doi: 10.1177/0956797612441951

Parkinson, B. (2005). Do facial movements express emotions or communicate motives? *Pers. Soc. Psychol. Rev.* 9, 278–311 doi: 10.1207/s15327957pspr0904_1

Royet, J. P., Koenig, O., Gregoire, M. C., Cinotti, L., Lavenne, F., Le Bars, D., et al. (1999). Functional anatomy of perceptual and semantic processing for odors. *J. Cogn. Neurosci.* 11, 94–109. doi: 10.1162/089892999563166

Soudry, Y., Lemogne, C., Malinvaud, D., Consoli, S.-M., and Bonfils, P. (2011). Olfactory system and emotion: common substrates. *Eur. Ann. Otorhinolaryngol. Head Neck Dis.* 128, 18–23. doi: 10.1016/j.anorl.2010.09.007

Steiner, J. (1973). The gustofacial response: observation on normal and anencephalic newborn infants. *Symp. Oral Sens. Percept.* 4, 254–278.

Terzis, V., Moridis, C. N., and Economides, A. A. (2012). The effect of emotional feedback on behavioral intention to use computer based assessment. *Comput. Educ.* 59, 710–721. doi: 10.1016/j.compedu.2012.03.003

Wansink, B. (2004). Environmental factors that increase the food intake and consumption volume of unknowing consumers. *Annu. Rev. Nutr.* 24, 455–479. doi: 10.1146/annurev.nutr.24.012003.132140

Zeinstra, G. G., Koelen, M., Colindres, D., Kok, F. J., and de Graaf, C. (2009). Facial expressions in school-aged children are a good indicator of "dislikes", but not of "likes." *Food Qual. Prefer.* 20, 620–624. doi: 10.1016/j.foodqual.2009.07.002

19

Smelly primes – when olfactory primes do or do not work

M. A. M. Smeets[1,2]* and G. B. Dijksterhuis[1,3]

[1] Unilever R&D, Vlaardingen, Netherlands
[2] Faculty of Social and Behavioural Sciences, Utrecht University, Utrecht, Netherlands
[3] Section for Sensory and Consumer Science, Faculty of Science (FOOD), University of Copenhagen, Copenhagen, Denmark

***Correspondence:**
M. A. M. Smeets, Faculty of Social and Behavioural Sciences, Utrecht University, Heidelberglaan 1, 3584 Cs Utrecht, Netherlands
e-mail: m.a.m.smeets@uu.nl

In applied olfactory cognition the effects that olfactory stimulation can have on (human) behavior are investigated. To enable an efficient application of olfactory stimuli a model of how they may lead to a change in behavior is proposed. To this end we use the concept of olfactory priming. Olfactory priming may prompt a special view on priming as the olfactory sense has some unique properties which make odors special types of primes. Examples of such properties are the ability of odors to influence our behavior outside of awareness, to lead to strong affective evaluations, to evoke specific memories, and to associate easily and quickly to other environmental stimuli. Opportunities and limitations for using odors as primes are related to these properties, and alternative explanations for reported findings are offered. Implications for olfactory semantic, construal, behavior and goal priming are given based on a brief overview of the priming literature from social psychology and from olfactory perception science. We end by formulating recommendations and ideas for a future research agenda and applications for olfactory priming.

Keywords: olfaction, priming, cognition and emotion, behavior, valence

INTRODUCTION

There is a substantial literature from social cognition on priming, demonstrating the sometimes substantial and unexpected effects that environmental stimuli can have on information processing and behavior. Due to the traditional emphasis in psychological science on visual and auditory perception and language, only few priming studies employ olfactory primes. In contrast, there is a bountiful literature from the chemical senses community on the effects of olfactory stimuli on perceptual and cognitive processing that could be conceived of as priming research, but is not always discussed within a priming framework. These literatures seem somehow disconnected. In this review we intend to forge a connection between the two in order to explore how conceiving of odors as primes can help us make better sense of their potential for influencing human information processing and behavior. Secondly, we propose guidelines for how odors are best used as primes based on the intrinsic and sometimes unique properties of the olfactory system that can be seen as opportunities but also as limitations. More systematic research on odor priming could be envisioned to realize its full potential for applications if both properties and limitations are taken into account. We will formulate a possible research agenda for such research.

We will start by addressing what we actually mean by priming and primes.

PRIMING IN THE SOCIAL SCIENCES

Priming refers to the phenomenon that incidental stimuli have been shown to influence higher-order cognitive and behavioral outcomes without the individual's awareness or appreciation of this influence (Bargh et al., 2010). Interestingly, such "incidental" priming stimuli can be manipulated in the context of experimental studies to achieve effects in participants in a mere passive, inactive manner. This is opposite to earlier (social) cognitive approaches in which experimental manipulations used to be brought to the conscious attention of participants to study how they affected decision-making (Bargh, 2006). To illustrate the former, Bargh (2006) gives the example of how polite behavior can be studied in an experiment in which the concept of politeness is passively manipulated by embedding adjectives related to politeness in a scrambled word test disguised as a language test, which is then followed by an opportunity to behave politely. Thus, priming research allows us to investigate how higher mental processes such as judgment and social behavior can be triggered and then operate in the absence of conscious awareness (Bargh and Morsella, 2008).

The notion that environmental stimuli can prime behavior is interesting, as it implies that there is a bridge between perception of the stimulus (e.g., a *word* related to politeness) and motor behavior (the polite *behavior* of waiting for someone to finish speaking instead of interrupting) possibly in the form of an activated mental *concept* of politeness. Specifically, by presenting words or images, the underlying related *concept* becomes accessible – an associative process – for further information processing (cf. Loersch and Payne, 2011). The mental content that has thus become available is now likely to be used as a source of information in subsequent information processing and behavior. Loersch and Payne (2011) distinguish between four types of priming: semantic priming (category identification), construal priming (judgment), behavior priming (action), and goal priming (motivation). Whichever type of priming occurs depends on whether the current situation invites, e.g., judgment rather than behavior or vice versa, and on other attributes such as a person's attitudes toward a primed category, personal goals and interests or constraints of the situation. A good example of the latter is an experiment by Cesario et al. (2010) in which participants who were in a enclosed booth when primed with a social stereotype of aggression, chose for a fight-like behavioral response, whereas those who were seated in an open field chose for a flight-like behavioral response.

An important consequence of Loersch and Payne's situated inference model of priming is that single primes can have multiple effects (i.e., as either one or more types of priming), but also that these effects are not the same for everybody or in all situations. This has special relevance for applications of priming in the real world, where individuals and situations will differ greatly.

In addition to the four types of priming that are central to the Loersch and Payne framework, we can distinguish between *perceptual* priming, *repetition* priming, and *affective* priming which bear relevance to odor priming. We speak of perceptual priming when prime and target share perceptual attributes. This is not the same as semantic priming. For example, Koenig et al. (2000) found that while odors presented during a learning phase acted as perceptual primes when participants were presented with these odors again during a test phase, there was no such priming effect when odor names – rather than odors themselves – had been used during the learning phase. The explanation for the difference may lie in the fact that perceptual priming involves modality-specific subsystems in memory, whereas semantic priming involves associative (amodal) subsystems in memory (Koenig et al., 2000). Repetition priming refers to the phenomenon that a stimulus can act as its own prime. When presented again, an odor is processed faster because its representation in memory was activated just before, and there is still a memory trace available. For odors, this was discussed by Olsson et al. (2002). They conclude that in some of the older repetition priming literature it is hard to disentangle purely olfactory priming from semantic priming – which is related to the previously mentioned distinction between perceptual priming and semantic priming. In Olsson (1999) even negative priming occurred when odors that were correctly identified were proven to be processed more slowly than odors that had not been identified. Identification of odors allowed for verbal labeling and may have led to semantic overshadowing (cf. Melcher and Schooler, 1996). Finally, in affective priming there is an unintentional influence of a first evaluative (affective) response, acting as a prime, on the subsequent processing of a target stimulus. For example, the positive affective tone of primes (often words) may activate affectively congruent material in memory (Klauer, 1997). Explanations have been sought in affective congruency between prime and target (both "positive" or "negative"), but also in congruency in response tendency. Consequently, positive affective primes would facilitate (congruent) approach responses, and negative affective primes would facilitate (congruent) avoidance responses to affectively congruent targets (Förster and Liberman, 2007). Odors may be potent affective primes as will be highlighted later in Section "Priming via valence".

Central to many explanations of *how* activated concepts can prime behaviors is William James' *ideo-motor action* principle which holds that activation of a cognitive representation of an action increases the likelihood of that action being carried out, via the triggering of active behavior representations, which cause movement of relevant muscles (Schröder and Thagard, 2013). Deliberate choice or motivation is not considered to be necessary. Priming effects, then, occur as a result of the *spreading of activation*, by which activation of one node in memory automatically spreads to another. Thus, priming effects are effortless and uncontrollable. For a more detailed account of how this might work involving computational modeling and neural networks, the reader is referred to Schröder and Thagard (2013).

Priming effects are supposed to take place outside of awareness. Social and cognitive psychologists have somewhat different perspectives on this. In cognitive psychology, awareness in this context would be equated with ability to perceive. For example, individuals could only be presumed to be unaware of a stimulus if stimulus intensity or duration would be below perceptual threshold (hence, at subliminal levels). According to Bargh (1992), it does not matter much from a social psychologist perspective whether someone is aware of the stimulus event, as long as the individual remains unaware of the ways in which the stimulus is interpreted and of the influence of this awareness on subsequent processing. Both subliminal as well as supraliminal primes have been proven to be effective primes (Bargh and Morsella, 2008). Goal or need state play an important role: for example Karremans et al. (2006) demonstrated that subliminal priming with a brand drink name such as Lipton Ice Tea positively affected participants' choice for and intention to drink the primed drink, but only for those who were thirsty.

To conclude, subliminality of stimulation could be important but only because if the individual is unaware of the stimulus event we can be sure they are unaware of the potential influence it has on their behavior. And, even when people are able of perceiving a priming stimulus, we might still conclude its subsequent effects on behavior take place outside of awareness.

So far we have seen that priming refers to the ability of "incidental" environmental stimuli to influence higher order cognitive processing and behavioral outcomes, and that these influences occur outside of awareness, effortlessly, and automatically. Mental representation of concepts play an important role, as activation of such a concept by a prime can lead to the simultaneous triggering of other cognitive, motivational, and behavioral processes by spreading of activation in memory. Both supraliminal as well as subliminal stimuli have been shown to be effective primes. Before we continue to look at the suitability and effectivity of odors as primes, we will first explore the unique properties of the sense of smell.

UNIQUE PROPERTIES OF OLFACTION

We are about to make claims about the suitability of contextual odors as primes. We start by introducing an important distinction: that between *odor* and *odorant*. The term *odorant* refers to the volatile chemical substance that is capable of eliciting the experience of an *odor* – it can be a single compound as well as a mixture consisting of a large number of compounds. The *odor* exclusively refers to an individual's experience, it is a percept. The olfactory experience (an "odor") is in all likelihood elicited by an *odorant*, but there have been occasions in which odor experiences have been reported even in the absence of an odorant. In a study by Knasko et al. (1990) the presence of an odor was strongly suggested by the context. Participants who were given the suggestion of a pleasant odor being in the room reported a more positive mood. A more extreme example is reported by O'Mahony (1978) who told a compelling story on TV which resulted in people calling the TV station stating that they had indeed smelled an odor emanating from their TV set. Furthermore, it is possible that a certain odor, experienced as resulting from a specific odorant, is not experienced by 100% of the subjects. Some subjects may perceive another odor, based on, for example, prior (lack of) experience with the odor.

Odors in memory are also referred to as *odor objects*, that, even when consisting of ten or hundreds of volatile components (the *odorant*) are perceived as unitary perceptual events (the *odors*) against a continually shifting olfactory background (Stevenson and Wilson, 2007). This goes to illustrate that there is not a necessary relation between the chemical properties, or even the presence, of an odorant, and the odor perceived as resulting from it (cf. Wilson and Stevenson, 2006). A focus on the so called "stimulus problem" (Stevenson and Boakes, 2003) will likely lead to incomplete theories and remain insufficient to understand olfactory perception in its entirety.

SENSE OF SMELL IS AN IMPLICIT SENSE

The sense of smell has also been alluded to as a hidden or *implicit* sense (Köster, 2002). Because vision is usually in the center of our attention, it is presumed to be the dominant sense, followed by the senses of hearing and touch. As a result, people tend to be less aware of odorants in their environment. Odorants, after all, cannot be seen or heard, and they can only be felt if they are at high enough concentrations to stimulate the trigeminal nerve innervating the nose, throat, mouth, and eyes, which induces sensations of tingling, prickling, burning, or even pain (Doty et al., 2004). There are large individual differences in the tendency to be aware of odors such that some people never seem to notice any, and would go to sleep without problem on a mattress on which the cat had just peed, whereas others are quick to notice any unpleasant or pleasant odors and would avoid them or seek them out purposefully (Smeets et al., 2008). Regardless, odorants –and their odors – are in general unlikely to draw attention unless they are especially pleasant, overly strong or an assault to the senses, or if they signal danger (fire, gas leak) or contamination (rotten foods, cadavers). According to Stevenson (2010) these are events which we have been "programmed" to attend to and as a result related approach or avoid-behaviors are hard-wired in the brain. Odors can also draw attention if they are especially meaningful to a person, i.e., they are learned to carry significance, be they approach or avoidance triggering (e.g., the perfume of your ex who left you).

There are several factors possibly contributing to odors taking a backseat among our sensory systems. One is that odorants spread, become diluted and are hard to pinpoint to a particular source. Thus adapted odorants cannot be easily localized and form a background for novel odor objects to figure against (Stevenson and Wilson, 2007).

With relevance to olfactory priming, odors appear to be perceived under different awareness circumstances:

1. Attentively: identifiable using verbal label: "I smell banana," or not identifiable: "I smell something, but I don't know what it is."
2. Semi-attentively: noticing there is something special, but not being able to pinpoint it (e.g., when one notices there's something different about a colleague –"Do you have new glasses?" and finding out he grew a mustache). With ambient odors this could be: "There's something special with this room today, but I can't really tell what it is."
3. Inattentively: subjects show no evidence of being aware of something in particular ("...").

ODORS QUICKLY ADAPT

Odor receptors are *quick to adapt*, Adaptation here refers to the "waning of response with stimulus repetition" (Dalton, 2000, p. 488) often referring to peripheral and physiological sensory processes, though "central adaptation," occurring in higher nervous centers can occur too (habituation). In olfaction peripheral adaptation is the much more common and stronger process. The adaptation process typically leads to a reduction in perceived intensity which can occur with even a few breaths of air containing an odorant (Dalton, 2000). The advantage of adaptation lies in a flexibility of the system to quickly tune into change. So, by current odor experiences merging with the background, chances of detecting novel odorants (e.g., by their odor) are much enhanced. The fact that olfactory adaptation is quick to set in, does not mean the olfactory stimulus ceases to have an effect on information processing after its onset. We recently observed effects of being exposed to sweat odor on facial emotional expressions (in this case fear and disgust) measured using facial EMG-electrodes lasting for at least 6 min, which is well beyond the time in which adaptation to the smell would have occurred (De Groot et al., 2012). The perception of the odor may have set in motion other processes that persist even after olfactory adaptation has set in.

So, to summarize, with one of the requirements for successful priming being that the individual is unaware of priming effects, the fact that humans are hardly aware of odors at all, and are quick to adapt to the sensation, makes odors good candidates for effective priming.

ODORS ARE STRONG TRIGGERS OF EMOTIONAL MEMORY

Another interesting characteristic of odors is that they are *strong triggers of emotions*. This is also known as the Proust effect, referring to the experience described by Marcel Proust in *A la Recherche du Temps Perdu* (Proust, 1913 in Jellinek, 2004) of his protagonist Swann feeling overcome with melancholy and emotion when experiencing the smell (and taste) from biting into a Madeleine after dipping it into tea. Inspired by this phenomenon many scientists devoted themselves to answering the question of whether odors are in fact stronger triggers of emotional memories than perception in other modalities. Note that Proust needed several pages to describe the mental search before finding the reason for the emotion. This illustrates the fact that the link between the prime and its effect normally escapes awareness. While the final judgment is still out on this (Jellinek, 2004; Gilbert, 2008; Toffolo et al., 2012), the ability of odors to trigger emotions make them suitable *affective* primes.

HUMAN ODOR CATEGORIZATION AND IDENTIFICATION: AMATEUR AT BEST

The connection between odors and language is a problematic one. Most individuals experience *odor-naming problems*. Even when an odor is common or seems very familiar, verbalizing it can be difficult (Cain, 1979); the tip-of-the-nose phenomenon (Lawless, 1977). People can classify odors into categories such as fruity, floral, and putrid, but there is little consensus on what the basic categories are (Wise et al., 2000; Auffarth, 2013), or even if they meaningfully exist. Categorization would be based on coarse perceptual features with boundaries between categories being rather fluid.

This problem with verbalizing odors may be related to the poor relation between the piriform cortex in which odor objects and categories are encoded, and the language network, e.g., cortical areas mediating odor naming and identification (Olofsson et al., 2013). It could be that from an evolutionary point of view, naming odors was never very important – performing immediate motor-induced actions either to approach or avoid was. Based on research in patients with semantic primary progressive aphasia, who suffer from extensive temporal lobe atrophy, Oloffson et al. posited that odor object information – even in healthy humans- is still relatively coarse and unprocessed compared to visual object information by the time it arrives at the lexical-semantic network in the brain. This would be due to fewer unimodal areas available for object processing in the olfactory than in the visual system prior to its arrival at the lexical-semantic network via the temporal lobe which constitutes a bridge into this network. The results may be mapping imprecision and object mismatch of odor objects. The authors conclude that because of this, odor object identification is more vulnerable to perceptual ambiguity. This phenomenon might have serious consequences for odor priming, as it casts into question the very ability of odors to link into specific, and unified, concepts which is central to conceptual (semantic) priming.

MOST IMPORTANT DIMENSIONS OF ODOR INFORMATION PROCESSING

Valence – varying from unpleasant to pleasant – is considered to be the most important odor dimension (Engen, 1982; Kaeppler and Mueller, 2013). Other dimensions considered as primary and employed in many studies (Kermen et al., 2011; Kaeppler and Mueller, 2013) are intensity, edibility and familiarity. Classifications of odors, relying on approaches asking subjects to engage in sorting, similarity judgments or sensory profiling have not led to universally agreed odor classes (Wise et al., 2000). One of the problems is that untrained subjects have great difficulty disregarding the valence dimension when asked to rate or classify odors (Kaeppler and Mueller, 2013) which in fact confirms its primacy in odor judgment. The dimensions of valence, intensity, edibility and familiarity seem to support the three major functions of olfaction as distinguished by Stevenson (2010), with digestion (i.e., appetite regulation) as first function being followed by avoiding environmental hazards (such as fires or rotten food) and social communication. All three functions, from an evolutionary perspective, subserve approach and avoidance behavior aimed at enhancing an individual's chance of survival.

ODOR PRIMING: WHAT'S DIFFERENT?

As previously noted, priming relies in large part on improving accessibility of conceptual representations for further information processing as a result of "incidental" perceptual stimulation. The question lying before us is whether priming with odors is in any way different from priming with visual stimulation in the form of images or words? We will reflect on the four types of priming distinguished by Loersch and Payne (2011): semantic priming (category identification), construal priming (judgment), behavior priming (action), and goal priming (motivation), and because of its special relevance here, to affective priming.

OBSERVATIONS ON BEHAVIORAL AND GOAL PRIMING WITH ODORS

When it comes to action priming or motivation priming, it seems obvious that odors are just as potent as (and sometimes even more potent than) visual stimuli. For example, immediately removing oneself from dangerous situations (a fire or a gas leak) or rotten food is a behavioral response that is in the interest of avoiding environmental hazards [Stevenson's (2010) second function of olfaction] and which relates to the primary dimensions of odor such as valence, edibility and familiarity. Although such reactions may not qualify as primes when individuals are aware of the link between the odor and the emotional (fear or disgust) and behavioral (moving away from the source) response, they are very much automatic. In a classical conditioning study, the low-level and briefly presented unpleasant odors of "rotten egg" and "sweaty socks" were successfully employed as aversive unconditioned stimuli to change expectations to a conditioned stimulus in the form of a human face (Gottfried and Dolan, 2004). This demonstrates how salience and automaticity of odor stimuli can affect information processing even when awareness of the odor must have been low. Semantic processing of the stimulus need not necessarily be invoked to yield action effects.

Odors are also effective as *goal* primes. Delicious food odors, in line with Stevenson's first function of olfaction – digestion and appetite regulation – may subconsciously divert a person from pursuing an ongoing goal and tempt people to start eating. Food courts in airports tend to have these effects and food odors – typically freshly baked bread – deliberately spread in supermarkets could lead to purchasing behavior. The first author, who on her daily train travel to work passes by a coffee factory spreading coffee roasting odors, has often observed other passengers formulating a desire for coffee or concrete plans to purchase some at the next station. In Gaillet et al. (2013) the odor of melon or of pear was unobtrusively presented. In a later choice test the group exposed to the melon odor chose more starter items consisting of fruit and vegetables, and the other (pear) group chose more desserts with fruit. Only the melon group had shown a decreased reaction time in a Lexical Decision Task for the word "melon." The effect on menu choice can be seen as goal priming, where melon – a typical starter item in France, the country of the study – led to an increase in choices for fruit/vegetable starters, and pear – a typical dessert item – led to an increase of choices of fruit desserts. Obviously we see here an odor priming effect, but rather than to conclude that it involved a semantically mediated concept of "pear" (which did occur for "melon"), both odors resulted in effective goal priming.

In a different domain, Miller and Maner (2011) showed that scent cues associated with female fertility (T-shirts worn by women in the late follicular versus luteal phase) enhanced reported perceptions of womens' sexual arousal in odor-sensitive males which the authors interpreted in the context of goal pursuit. The major dimensions of odor perception, valence, and edibility, can facilitate goal priming responses, again without semantic processing being required. It is thus safe to conclude that odors make for very effective behavioral and goal primes.

OBSERVATIONS ON SEMANTIC AND CONSTRUAL PRIMING WITH ODORS

Semantic and construal priming via odors, in view of the specific characteristics of odor just listed, is more complicated. Can the odor of camembert cheese, for example, prime words related to other typically French food products or a typically French sports event such as the Tour de France? Since we have seen that categorization and identification of odors is problematic, and since the semantic route partially relies on, or most certainly benefits from, such processes, semantic odor priming cannot simply be assumed to take place. For example, we might expect that *seeing* a picture of a camembert cheese likely activates mental representations of other foods (French) cheeses, other typical French food products such as baguettes, or even other French words, via conceptual links with the product, once recognized or identified. However, we cannot simply assume the odor of camembert to accomplish the same. We might expect the odor to be categorized as belonging to the food category, and even as cheese. Thus, via the semantic route, the odor of camembert might be a good prime for other food or cheese concepts (like beer can prime – a desire for – pretzels; Hyde and Witherly, 1993). However, many people would not be able to categorize the smell as (French) cheese or identify it as camembert. Due to the ambiguity inherent to the sense of smell, some might misconstrue it as body odor which would lead to another priming outcome altogether than would be the case if a visual prime of cheese had been used. Depending on the interpretation of the odor prime, the subsequent effects on judgment of an object or situation will be vastly different. Note that De Araujo et al. (2005) showed a difference in perceived valence depending on whether the odor was labeled as a body odor or as cheddar cheese.

This brings us to the fact that the characteristic odor of French cheeses can elicit *affective* reactions. The cheese odor represents an edible food product that is liked or disliked. As valence may be the primary dimension along which priming occurs in this camembert example, individuals may now have easier mental access to other well-liked or disliked products, or may show behavioral responses of approach of avoidance, respectively. But: would we expect the *odor* of camembert to cause shorter reaction times to French words – as, e.g., measured with a Lexical Decision Task – than to other language words in a priming task, which we would if *pictures* of camembert were used as primes? Probably not. Instead, priming with camembert *odor* might enhance the mental processing of words of other *liked* food products (or liked products in general) in a cheese-lover, create an approach response toward anything that follows such priming, or enhance the possibility for positive construal of an object, person, or situation.

Aside from a valence-route for priming with camembert odor, an individual who once enjoyed camembert with friends during a wonderful vacation in France might re-experience that memory and find themselves taken back there. Now priming may occur based on the content of the *autobiographical memory*. Thinking back of how lovely the French countryside was, would cause a spreading of activation to the concepts "France," "countryside," and "French countryside." A subject might now show a fast response to words related to the Tour de France on this basis, as it is now the memory providing the link to language and visual mental representations. Likewise, they may show speeded recognition of contextual features such as red-white checkered tablecloths because such a tablecloth happened to be part of their memory. Someone who did not have such a memory, would not show such a response, which makes this response differ strongly across individuals and almost impossible to systematically investigate.

Finally, there is a possible priming route that involves *mood*. This is in line with literature demonstrating that mood at the time of judgment can be used as information by an individual to reach a judgment, for example on how happy or satisfied one is (Schwarz and Clore, 1983, 2003). On a similar note, effects of odors on feelings of wellbeing and health in aromatherapy have been contributed to changes in mood caused by a strong liking for the odor (Stevenson and Boakes, 2003; Herz, 2009). This implies that the pleasant aromas do not directly reduce stress and increase relaxation via physiological changes induced by odorant inhalation. Rather, feelings of stress and relaxation are influenced in the same way as being in a good mood would, with the odor being the mood-enhancer. Liking camembert may put someone in a good mood when smelling it. Priming via mood might help explaining effects such as seen in the famous "the smell of helping" study by Baron (1997) in which it was demonstrated that passersby in a shopping mall were more inclined to help a same-sex accomplice (e.g., by picking up a dropped pen) when a pleasant ambient odor (e.g., of baked cookies) was present then in the absence of such an odor. Here, the odor of baked cookie primed the act of picking up a pen. It is unlikely that this involved a semantic route. After all, there is no clear conceptual relation between baked cookies and helping behavior. Would seeing pictures of cinnamon buns act as primes to helping others in the same way? It could if you really love cinnamon buns, and the mere sight of it improves your mood, but the odor may be a more direct route into mood and emotion, as previously argued. Thus, while semantic priming via odors can be problematic, effects that suggest semantic odor priming may be explained by alternative routes into the concept, such as via priming of memories that facilitate spreading of activation to any concepts related to that memory. As a consequence, substantial individual differences are expected, as autobiographical memories are unique. Likewise, odor primes intended to be semantic primes may inadvertently lead to affect (valence or mood) priming, thus yielding behavioral effects that never involved the underlying (semantic) concept. We would conclude that odors do not make for good semantic primes, but can nevertheless have effects that may be interpreted as such, by spreading of activation traveling via indirect "autobiographical" routes or via valence transfer, that eventually can be linked to semantic concepts indirectly. Of course, behavioral and goal priming could result via similar mechanisms.

RECOMMENDATIONS AND APPLICATIONS FOR ODOR PRIMING

PRIMING VIA VALENCE

One of the conclusions reached so far held that odors can make for good behavioral and goal primes along the primary dimension of valence. This is strongly related to the notion of *affective* priming, previously discussed in Section "Priming in the Social Sciences." Affective priming phenomena may have an adaptive function, in that they serve to quickly serve opportunities and threats in the environment (Klauer, 1997). Odors, generally evaluated primarily in terms of affect (good or bad) may therefore constitute important affective primes. For reasons of ease of comprehension, we propose to include all influences of odor valence priming under the header of affective priming for our current purpose. This is irrespective of whether the affect association originated from the various types of learning involving odors (Stevenson and Boakes, 2003), or from congruent mood, and irrespective of the underlying mechanisms (e.g., congruency of stimulus and response). This type of affective priming is prevalent in applied settings such as stores, parking garages, public transportation, health care settings, the workplace, etc., where positively valenced odors have been dispersed to trigger approach behavior (consumption, purchase), positive feelings (safety), a sense of wellbeing, work engagement, and so on. A few comments are in order: in many cases strong odors are used. When odors are strong and easy to notice, their influences on human cognition and behavior cannot be classified as primes under the definition that requires effects to take place outside of awareness. Strong odors tend to be disliked by people who are sensitive to strong stimulations (Doty et al., 2004) or score high on the avoidance scale of the Odor Awareness Scale (Smeets et al., 2008). Furthermore, odor quality tends to differ with concentration (Gross-Isseroff and Lancet, 1988) such that an odorant that has shown effective priming at lower concentrations may be associated with a different odor perception at higher concentrations. Thus, we recommend that in order to achieve the presumed effects to use odors at low intensities (cf. Köster and Degel, 2000).

SEMANTIC PRIMING

Priming via words can yield specific effects, as words would be used to pinpoint specific members and sub members of a taxonomy. Thus, the word "butterfly" could in theory be an effective prime for processing other words not just denoting insects, but specifically insects with wings. It will be clear from the above that such specific priming is unlikely to work using odors as primes. It would require not only that the odor is appropriately categorized but probably also identified by name. Knowing that individuals categorize odors in terms of, e.g., "fruity" should caution the experimenter not to use multiple fruity odors as primes. While pictures of a lemon, grapefruit and lime would possibly be easily identified by most people, this cannot be expected for the odors these fruits produce. They may be categorized as "fruity," or "citrus." This does not necessarily imply individuals could not discriminate between the odors at the perceptual level, but being unable to assign these odors to different categories may result in ineffective odor priming at the subcategory level.

Thus, if some form of semantic priming is intended, it is recommended to use an odor that fits a often-used category such as floral or fruity, and is a good prototype for the category (e.g., orange for citrus). Also, to ensure the priming effect was semantic/categorical there would have to be an appropriate control, for example for affective priming via odor valence. It would be good to include an odor that is equally liked or disliked but clearly does not belong to the same semantic odor category. To illustrate this we refer to a series of studies reported in Holland et al. (2005). Evidence of semantic olfactory priming was shown in a study where exposure to a citrus (cleaning agent) smell prompted subjects to express more cleaning behaviors than in the no-odor condition. Holland et al. (2005) used a Lexical Decision Task to show that a cleaning related concept had been activated through the exposure to the citrus scent. In a more applied study De Lange et al. (2012) used a similar citrus odor to show that train wagons scented with it were less littered by than unscented wagons. The activation of a cleaning related concept is held responsible for the behavioral effect of the odor prime in this study. The task in the testing phase is a behavioral one in both studies, and in addition a Lexical Decision Task in Holland et al. (2005). The authors claim that the odor activates a cleaning concept based on a past learned association of the odor with cleaning, resulting in an increased likelihood of cleaning related behavior (and faster recognition of cleaning related words in the Lexical Decision Task). However, as their studies only used one type of odor, alternative explanations related to, e.g., the valence of the odor cannot be ruled out.

In a recent study (Dijksterhuis et al., 2013), modeled after the Holland et al. (2005) study, we primed subjects with three odors of different nature. An orange odor (a citrus odor, pleasant, but with no *a priori* expected association to cleaning), a grass odor (also pleasant, but with no *a priori* association to cleaning), and a sulfur odor (unpleasant, and also not related to cleaning). The odors were presented at very low intensities in a neutral testing room, so that they were not attentively noticed. In the test phase of this study the "rusk eating task" as introduced by Holland et al. (2005) was used. The subjects were to cut and eat a rusk in a sham sensory study, and their behavior was observed to asses if and how much spontaneous cleaning actions (like wiping the table, picking up crumbs, etc.) subjects displayed under the different odor conditions. It turned out that under the sulfur condition our subjects displayed less table wiping actions than under the grass and orange odor. What this study shows is that other types of priming, than semantic priming, may be at play. The sulfur odor is unlikely to carry a semantic connotation to cleaning (more to dirt, in fact), nor do the grass and orange odors, yet they differ in the amount of cleaning behaviors they afford. We pose that the affective value of the odor can provide an alternative mechanism to explain the priming power of odors. We point out that the Dijksterhuis et al. (2013) study would have to be replicated including a no odor condition.

While on the topic of semantic odor priming it is of interest to note that Degel et al. (2001) posit that in fact, being able to verbally label an odor, seriously *interferes* with implicit priming effects. This may be due to the fact that cognitive processing of language may be disruptive to the implicit processing of odor, as the use of labels would cause a spreading of activation causing different cognitive and behavioral effects than spreading of activation solely by odor stimulation would.

Semantic priming via autobiographical memory

We have seen that odor priming via specific autobiographical memories can be potent and provide a gateway into semantic priming via concepts elicited by such memories. Clearly, odor priming via memory could be a very powerful application to entice consumers into buying products. The problem is that autobiographical memories are by definition personal. An odor experience that emotes one person may not do much for someone else. There are two approaches to this. One is to focus on odor experiences that are strongly linked to universally pleasant events and occasions and use these as primes to create an attraction to a product. For example, the smell of suntan lotion – often a fragrance heavy on coconut – has been reported as being associated with being on vacation in sunny locations. Thus, anecdotally, we have heard that some travel companies subtly fragrance their promotional material with coconut fragrance or provide pouches with suntan lotion along with it. This way, smelling the lotion might intensify the desire to take a vacation thus lowering the threshold for actually booking one. Likewise, parents have reported to experience feelings of melancholy and warmth when smelling the fragranced baby products (lotion, shampoo) they tended to use on their offspring, as it reminds them of nurturing their children when they were still babies. That such smells can in fact be good behavioral primes was demonstrated in an explorative study in which we first combined a novel fruity or floral odor with watching a movie in which parents interact with their babies in a loving way. In an unrelated session we later found that the smell that had been previously associated with watching the movie yielded a higher nurturing behavior score on a baby-doll than an unrelated equally pleasant smell (Smeets et al., 2010).

The second way in which learnings from the Proust effect can be used for application is by creating a memory by cleverly pairing an odorant with a certain experience so as to impart the nature of the experience onto the odorant. A subsequent encounter with that odorant would then be expected to act as prime for the experience. In their paper Degel and Köster (1999) describe an odor priming study including a learning phase. They had subjects perform a task in some rooms where an ambient odor was present. It was explicitly assessed afterward, that the subjects had not attentively perceived the odor while they were in the room. In the test phase subjects were to score the fit of the odors, now presented in jars, to environments – including the rooms they had been in – presented on photographs. A higher fit of the odor to the room the subjects had encountered the odor in was found for two out of three odors, illustrating a clear case of olfactory (repetition) priming. This cannot be attributed to some sort of a recognition effect as this would imply an explicit evaluation (recognition is an explicit function), which the authors preclude by making sure the subjects did not consciously perceive the odor in the room, with a judgment task in the test phase of the study that may be linked to the *familiarity* primary dimension of odor perception.

This result is related to the Olsson (1999) research that showed that negative priming occurred when odors that were correctly identified were proven to be processed more slowly than odors that had not been identified.

MULTI-MODAL PRIMING

During the multiple experiments we have conducted over the past years we have found that presenting odorants in typical lab experiments did not yield the expected effects. Odorants from very different sources – rotten eggs, pizza, brownie, etc., – when asked, often gave rise to labels as "sweaty," "computer-smell," "rubber," "stale-lab smell," which was sometimes bewildering. Clearly, laboratory environments are not meaningful contexts when trying to establish an appropriate understanding of odorants and their sources. Although theoretically it is possible that odors connect up with the appropriate concepts in the brain even when subjects cannot describe them, in everyday situations we rarely ever encounter odors completely in isolation and without proper context. Thus, odors probably need help channeling to the concept of interest (Wilson and Stevenson, 2006). An obvious solution would seem to pair ambiguous odors with positive or negative labels such as "parmesan cheese" or "vomit" as Herz and von Clef (2001) did, but that would make the odor and its quality explicit thereby potentially ruining the odor priming effect. Thus, an alternative solution could be to establish cross-modality correspondences using inconspicuous combinations of olfactive and other-modality stimuli (Stevenson et al., 2012), in order to help bring out a property of the jointly presented odor such as, e.g., "softness". Likewise, Gottfried and Dolan (2003) empirically demonstrated that semantically congruent visual information facilitated low level odor detection in congruent odor – picture pairs. Another solution is to provide context in other ways. For example if the intention is to convey the meaning of green grass and not just positive valence when presenting a green grass odor, one could put up a poster of a soccer field or have copies of soccer magazines in the waiting room to the experiment. By already making the concept accessible this way, the odor would be more likely to act as semantic prime, rather than as an affect prime, during subsequent testing. This approach is in line with the recommendations by Degel and Köster (1998) for effective odor priming:

1. the test does not supply explicit information about the stimuli,
2. the test acknowledges the nonverbal character of odor perception and memory,
3. the test allows perception of odors in a situation which is for the most part a biotic, normal everyday situation.

The latter point would explain why priming with odors in laboratories out of context is often bound to fail.

TO CONCLUDE: A FUTURE RESEARCH AGENDA FOR EFFECTIVE ODOR PRIMING

The goal of this review was to evaluate the suitability of odors as primes. The unique properties of the sense of smell make odors both more, as well as less, suitable as primes than, e.g., visual primes (depending on the type of priming). Since most people show a natural inclination to pay more attention to visual than olfactory attributes of the environment, olfactory stimuli tend to stay outside of awareness when considering complex environments. This is especially true when they are present at low levels, where they are expected to be more evocative than at high levels. On top of this, there is the fact that the sense of smell adapts rapidly to stimulation. All these properties would lead us to conclude that environmental odors may be considered to be even more suitable to act as primes that subconsciously affect information processing and behavior than visual stimuli. Especially in relation to food, odor primes would be expected to be very powerful, as we have seen that edibility is one of the primary dimensions of odor perception. For example, when smelling an odor, people might say they like the odor, to quickly follow up by saying it is the smell of food.

Olfaction may be conceived of as a sense whose purpose, if you will, is to act as a conduit quickly channeling the olfactory input to guide approach and avoidance behavior to or away from foods, mates, predators and toxic materials. After stimulation, emotions and memory traces are rapidly evoked to facilitate such channeling in a powerful manner in the interest of survival. Where the function of olfaction, then, seems to be to discriminate at a relatively coarse level between what environmental elements either sustain or threaten survival, the visual sense acts to add detail, and subject what is in the environment to more fine-grained analysis. As a result, olfactory primes are prone to do well when priming emotionally loaded cognitive processes and behaviors, but not so well when the processing requires analyses with high levels of detail. From these features, it may be inferred that odors make for great behavioral and goal primes, but presumably not for great semantic primes. Construal priming much depends on how the odor prime is interpreted, which cannot always be reliably predicted. Adding subtle contextual features to help channel the prime to the intended concept, or create an emotional experience around the odor prime, that will result in an emotional memory that, once associated with the prime, will assist channeling the prime to concepts encoded in memory.

To find effective odor primes for applied purposes, we advocate the following research agenda. Firstly, to investigate whether effective odor primes are successful because the underlying effect is one of affective priming versus semantic priming, a supposedly semantic odor prime should always be compared to another odor prime, matched for valence but unrelated to the intended semantic category. If it is found that other similarly valenced odors are equally effective, priming can be extended to include many other odor primes than only the one believed to have specific meaning.

Furthermore, the role of odorant concentration (and its perceptual pendant odor intensity) is very important. With increasing concentrations, odorants become detectable ("There is something."), then recognizable in terms of general quality or category ("It is fruity."), then potentially identifiable ("It is orange."). Now on the one hand identifiability might act as an aid to semantically channeling the odorant input to a concept, thus making it a semantic prime. On the other hand, as soon as the odor is strong people become aware, then, priming is unlikely to take place. This is in line with Loersch and Payne (2011) observations that extreme primes are less likely to have the expected priming effects, but instead, may even lead to contradictory outcomes. In addition, as soon as an odor is verbally labeled, cognitive processing is no longer implicit or automatic. Likewise, sensory profiles of odors tend to change with increasing concentrations of odorants. While the odorant composition is still the same, the mental representation associated with it, is not. Thus, research systematically investigating effects of changes in concentration of the odorant leading to the odor prime on the efficiency of the prime would help us find the most effective concentrations for priming. Because of a misunderstanding that odors must be strong and clearly perceivable, many intended odor primes are probably not as effective as they could be.

Finally, we expect that odors can become semantic primes with a little help from other-modality friends. After all, in accordance with the situated inference model, the nature of the prime depends on the situation (Loersch and Payne, 2011). Again, subtlety is king. Including some not-too-obvious cues can help give meaning to an odor prime while adding to the effect of the other-modality cue thus making it more effective (cf. Degel and Köster, 1998). Moreover, by linking the odor to an emotional experience around relevant concepts, it may be expected that the experience is encoded as a memory, encoding the odor along with it thus increasing the likelihood that the odor will act as semantic prime to these concepts on a subsequent encounter.

Olfactory priming exists. That is: the literature provides much support for the notion that odor priming in terms of an "effect" (i.e., odors activating related representations, all linked together in a conceptual network of mental representations) is a reality. However, the specific psychological and physiological processes responsible for the effects still need to be elucidated. The mechanism underlying priming may not be the same for visual and odor priming. In discussing matters of olfactory perception we have to beware not to mix the concepts odorant and odor, as there is not a one-to-one relationship between the two. There are several specific properties of the sense of smell that need closer scrutiny. Some properties make the olfactory sense a good or a not-so-good sense for priming depending on the type of priming. The nature of the odor, its intensity, and the context in which an odorant is presented has a great influence on the specific priming effect that will be experienced. Finally, the extent to which olfactory priming can be conceived of as semantic priming as opposed to affective priming providing the more parsimonious explanation, needs to be further explored.

We have taken first steps in setting an applied research agenda for olfactory priming, listing some topics of both theoretical and practical relevance. If we do it right, olfactory priming holds great promise.

AUTHOR CONTRIBUTIONS

The first author was invited to submit this article and contributed to the idea and main structure of the paper. The second author contributed specific texts and both authors subsequently shaped the paper.

REFERENCES

Auffarth, B. (2013). Understanding smell – the olfactory stimulus problem. *Neurosci. Biobehav. Rev.* 37, 1667–1679. doi: 10.1016/j.neubiorev.2013.06.009

Bargh, J. A. (1992). "Why subliminality does not matter to social psychology: awareness of the stimulus versus awareness of its effects," in *Perception Without Awareness: Cognitive, Clinical, and Social Perspectives,* eds R. Bornstein and T. Pittman (New York, NY: Guilford), 236–255.

Bargh, J. A. (2006). What have we been priming all these years? On the development, mechanisms, and ecology of nonconscious social behaviour. *Eur. J. Soc. Psychol.* 36, 147–168. doi: 10.1002/ejsp.336

Bargh, J. A., and Morsella, E. (2008). The unconscious mind. *Perspect. Psychol. Sci.* 3, 73–79. doi: 10.1111/j.1745-6916.2008.00064.x

Bargh, J. A., Williams, L. E., Huang, J. Y., Song, H. J., and Ackerman, J. M. (2010). From the physical to the psychological: Mundane experiences influence social judgment and interpersonal behaviour. *Behav. Brain Sci.* 33, 267. doi: 10.1017/S0140525X10000993

Baron, R. A. (1997). The sweet smell of...helping: effects of pleasant ambient fragrances on prosocial behaviour in shopping malls. *Personal. Soc. Psychol. Bull.* 23, 498–503. doi: 10.1177/0146167297235005

Cain, W. S. (1979). To know with the nose: keys to odour identification. *Science* 203, 467–470. doi: 10.1126/science.760202

Cesario, J., Plaks, J. E., Hagiwara, N., Navarrete, C. D., and Tory Higgins, E. (2010). The ecology of automaticity: how situational contingencies shape action semantics and social behavior. *Psychol. Sci.* 21, 1311–1317. doi: 10.1177/0956797610378685

Dalton, P. (2000). Psychophysical and behavioural characteristics of olfactory adaptation. *Chem. Senses* 25, 487–292. doi: 10.1093/chemse/25.4.487

De Araujo, I. E., Rolls, E. T., Velazco, M. I., Margot, C., and Cayeux, I. (2005). Cognitive modulation of olfactory processing. *Neuron* 46, 671–679. doi: 10.1016/j.neuron.2005.04.021

De Groot, J. H. B., Smeets, M. A. M., Kaldewaij, A., Duijndam, M. J. A., and Semin, G. R. (2012). Chemosignals communicate human emotions. *Psychol. Sci.* 23, 1417–1424. doi: 10.1177/0956797612445317

De Lange, M. A., Debets, L. W., Ruitenburg, K., and Holland, R. W. (2012). Making less of a mess: scent exposure as a tool for behavioural change. *Soc. Influence* 7, 90–97. doi: 10.1080/15534510.2012.659509

Degel, J., and Köster, E. (1998). Implicit memory for odors: a possible method for observation. *Percept. Mot. Skills* 86, 943–953. doi: 10.2466/pms.1998.86.3.943

Degel, J., and Köster, E. (1999). Odors: implicit memory and performance effects. *Chem. Senses* 24, 317–325. doi: 10.1093/chemse/24.3.317

Degel, J., Piper, D., and Köster, E. P. (2001). Implicit learning and implicit memory for odors: the influence of odor identification and retention time. *Chem. Senses* 26, 3, 267–280. doi: 10.1093/chemse/26.3.267

Dijksterhuis, G. B., Zandstra, E., De Wijk, R., and Smeets, M. A. M. (2013). *Smelly and Dirty: Valence, Not Semantics, of Odours Prompt Cleaning Behaviour.* Poster presentation in Pangborn Sensory Science Conference, Rio de Janeiro, 11–15 August 2013.

Doty, R. L., Cometto-Muniz, J. E., Jalowayski, A. A., Dalton, P., Kendal-Reed, M., and Hodgson, M. (2004). Assessment of upper respiratory tract and ocular irritative effects of volatile chemicals in humans. *Crit. Rev. Toxicol.* 34, 85–142. doi: 10.1080/10408440490269586

Engen, T. (1982). *The Perception of Odours.* New York: Academic Press.

Förster, J., and Liberman, N. (2007). "Knowledge activation," in *Social Psychology: Handbook of Basic Principles*, eds A. W. Kruglaski and E. Tory-Higgings (New York: The Guilford Press).

Gaillet, M., Sulmont-Rossé, C., Issanchou, S., Chabanet, C., and Chambaron, S. (2013). Priming effects of an olfactory food cue on subsequent food-related behaviour. *Food Qual. Prefer.* 30, 274–281. doi: 10.1016/j.foodqual.2013.06.008

Gilbert, A. N. (2008). "Recovered memories. Proust's soggy Madeleine," in *What the nose Knows. The Science of Scent in Everyday Life*, ed. A. Gilbert (New York, NY: Crown Publishers), 189–204.

Gottfried, J. A., and Dolan, R. J. (2003). The nose smells what the eye sees: crossmodal visual isual facilitation of human olfactory perception. *Neuron* 39, 375–386. doi: 10.1016/S0896-6273(03)00392-1

Gottfried, J. A., and Dolan, R. J. (2004). Human orbitofrontal cortex mediates extinction learning while accessing conditioned representations of value. *Nat. Neurosci.* 7, 1145–1153. doi: 10.1038/nn1314

Gross-Isseroff, R., and Lancet, D. (1988). Concentration-dependent changes of perceived odour quality. *Chem. Senses* 13, 191–204. doi: 10.1093/chemse/13.2.191

Herz, R. S. (2009). Aromatherapy facts and fictions: a scientific analysis of olfactory effects on mood, physiology and behaviour. *Int. J. Neurosci.* 119, 263–290. doi: 10.1080/00207450802333953

Herz, R. S., and von Clef, J. (2001). The influence of verbal labelling on the perception of odors: evidence for olfactory illusions? *Perception* 30, 381–391. doi: 10.1068/p3179

Holland, R. W., Hendriks, M., and Aarts, H. (2005). Smells like clean spirit: nonconsious effects of scent on cognition and behaviour. *Psychol. Sci.* 9, 689–693. doi: 10.1111/j.1467-9280.2005.01597.x

Hyde, R. J., and Witherly, S. A. (1993). Dynamic contrast: a sensory contribution to palatability. *Appetite* 21, 1–16. doi: 10.1006/appe.1993.1032

Jellinek, J. S. (2004). Proust remembered: has Proust's account of autobiographical odour-cued memory recall really been investigated? *Chem. Senses* 29, 455–458. doi: 10.1093/chemse/bjh043

Kaeppler, K., and Mueller, F. (2013). Odour classification: a review of factors influencing perception-based odour arrangements. *Chem. Senses* 38, 189–209. doi: 10.1093/chemse/bjs141

Karremans, J. C., Stroeber, W., and Claus, J. (2006). Beyond Vicary's fantasies: the impact of subliminal priming and brand choice. *J. Exp. Soc. Psychol.* 42, 792–798. doi: 10.1016/j.jesp.2005.12.002

Kermen, F., Chakirian, A., Sezille, C., Joussain, P., Le Goff, G., Ziessel, A., et al. (2011). Molecular complexity determines the number of olfactory notes and the pleasantness of smells. *Sci. Rep.* 1, 206. doi: 10.1038/srep00206

Klauer, K. C. (1997). Affective priming. *Eur. Rev. Soc. Psychol.* 8, 67–103. doi: 10.1080/14792779643000083

Knasko, S. C., Gilbert, A. N., and Sabini, J. (1990). Emotional state, physical well-being and performance in the present of a feigned ambient odour. *J. Appl. Soc. Psychol.* 20, 1345–1357. doi: 10.1111/j.1559-1816.1990.tb01476.x

Koenig, O., Bourron, G., and Royet, J. P. (2000). Evidence for separate perceptive and semantic memories for odours: a priming experiment. *Chem. Senses* 25, 703–708. doi: 10.1093/chemse/25.6.703

Köster, E. P. (2002). "The specific characteristics of the sense of smell," in *Olfaction, Taste and Cognition*, eds C. Rouby, B. Schaal, D. Dubois, R. Gervais, and A. Holley (Cambridge: University Press), 27–43. doi: 10.1017/CBO9780511546389.007

Köster, E. P., and Degel, J. (2000). Are weak odours stonger than strong odours? The influence of odour on human performance. *Aromachol. Rev.* 2, 9.

Lawless, H. T. (1977). The pleasantness of mixtures in taste and olfaction. *Sensory Process.* 1, 227–237.

Loersch, C., and Payne, C. B. (2011). The situated inference model: an integrative account of the effects of primes on perception, behaviour, and motivation. *Perspect. Psychol. Sci.* 6, 234–252. doi: 10.1177/1745691611406921

Melcher, J. M., and Schooler, J. W. (1996). The misremembrance of wines past: verbal and perceptual expertise differentially mediate verbal overshadowing of taste memory. *J. Mem. Lang.* 35, 231–245. doi: 10.1006/jmla.1996.0013

Miller, S. M., and Maner, J. K. (2011). Ovulation as a male mating prime: subtle signs ofwomen's omen's fertility influence men's mating cognition and behavior. *J. Personal. Soc. Psychol.* 100, 295–308. doi: 10.1037/a0020930

Olofsson, J. K., Rogalski, E., Harrison, T., Marsel Mesulam, M., and Gottfried, J. A. (2013). A cortical pathway to olfactory naming: evidence from primary progressive aphasia. *Brain* 136, 1245–1259. doi: 10.1093/brain/awt019

Olsson, M. J. (1999). Implicit testing of odor memory: instances of positive and negative repetition priming. *Chem. Senses* 24, 347–350. doi: 10.1093/chemse/24.3.347

Olsson, M. J., Faxbrink, M., and Jönsson, F. U. (2002). "Repetition priming in odour memory," in *Olfaction, Taste and Cognition*, eds B. Rouby, B. Schaal, D. Dubois, R. Gervais, and A. Holley (New York: Cambridge University Press), 246–260. doi: 10.1017/CBO9780511546389.022

O'Mahony, M. (1978). Smell illusions and suggestion: reports of smells contingent on tones played on television and radio. *Chem. Senses* 3, 183–189. doi: 10.1093/chemse/3.2.183

Proust, M. (1913). *A La Recherche du Temps perdu.* Paris: Bernard Grasset.

Schröder, T., and Thagard, P. (2013). The affective meanings of automatic social behaviours: three mechanisms that explain priming. *Psychol. Rev.* 12, 255–280. doi: 10.1037/a0030972

Schwarz, N., and Clore, G. L. (1983). Mood, misattribution, and judgments of well-being: informative, and directive functions of affective states. *J. Personal. Soc. Psychol.* 45, 513–523. doi: 10.1037/0022-3514.45.3.513

Schwarz, N., and Clore, G. L. (2003). Mood as information: 20 years later. *Psychol. Inquiry* 14, 296–303.

Smeets, M. A. M., Dubas, J., Jörg, N., and Aarts, H. (2010). *Odour Priming of (Infant) Nurturing Behaviour. Oral Presentation during Symposium: "More than Meets the Eye: Hidden Signals and Social Communication."* Annual meeting of Association for Psychological Science, Boston.

Smeets, M. A. M., Schifferstein, H. N. J., Boelema, S. R., and Lensvelt-Mulders, G. (2008). The odour awareness scale (OAS): a new scale for measuring positive and negative odour awareness. *Chem. Senses* 33, 725–734. doi: 10.1093/chemse/bjn038

Stevenson, R. J. (2010). An initial evaluation of the functions of human olfaction. *Chem. Senses* 35, 3–20. doi: 10.1093/chemse/bjp083

Stevenson, R. J., and Boakes, R. A. (2003). A mnemonic theory of odour perception. *Psychol. Rev.* 110, 340–364. doi: 10.1037/0033-295X.110.2.340

Stevenson, R. J., Rich, A., and Russell, A. (2012). The nature and origin of cross-model associations to odours. *Perception* 41, 606–609. doi: 10.1068/p7223

Stevenson, R. J., and Wilson, D. A. (2007). Odour perception: an object recognition approach. *Perception* 36, 1821–1833. doi: 10.1068/p5563

Toffolo, M. B. J., Smeets, M. A. M., and van den Hout, M. (2012). Proust phenomenon revisited: odours as triggers of aversive memories. *Cogn. Emot.* 26, 83–92. doi: 10.1080/02699931.2011.555475

Wilson, D. A., and Stevenson, R. J. (2006). *Learning to Smell: Olfactory Perception from Neurobiology to Behaviour.* Baltimore: John Hopkins University Press.

Wise, P. M., Olsson, M. J., and Cain, W. S. (2000). Quantification of odour quality. *Chem. Senses* 25, 429–443. doi: 10.1093/chemse/25.4.429

The influence of health-risk perception and distress on reactions to low-level chemical exposure

Linus Andersson, Anna-Sara Claeson, Lisa Ledin, Frida Wisting and Steven Nordin *

Department of Psychology, Umeå University, Umeå, Sweden

Correspondence:
Steven Nordin, Department of Psychology, Umeå University, SE-901 87 Umeå, Sweden
e-mail: steven.nordin@psy.umu.se

The general aim of the current study was to investigate how perceived health risk of a chemical exposure and self-reported distress are related to perceived odor intensity and odor valence, symptoms, cognitive performance over time as well as reactions to blank exposure. Based on ratings of general distress, 20 participants constituted a relatively low distress group, and 20 other participants a relatively high distress group. Health risk perception was manipulated by providing positively and negatively biased information regarding *n*-butanol. Participants made repeated ratings of intensity, valence and symptoms and performed cognitive tasks while exposed to 4.7 ppm *n*-butanol for 60 min (first 10 min were blank exposure) inside an exposure chamber. Ratings by the positive and negative bias groups suggest that the manipulation influenced perceived health risk of the exposure. The high distress group did not habituate to the exposure in terms of intensity when receiving negative information, but did so when receiving positive information. The high distress group, compared with the low distress group, rated the exposure as significantly more unpleasant, reported greater symptoms and performed worse on a cognitively demanding task over time. The positive bias group and high distress group rated blank exposure as more intense. The main findings suggest that relatively distressed individuals are negatively affected by exposures to a greater degree than non-distressed.

Keywords: health-risk perception, olfaction, environmental psychology, perception, sensitization, bias, distress, cognition

INTRODUCTION

In a series of seminal studies, Dalton and colleagues showed that the words used to describe a chemical significantly alters how individuals react when being exposed to it. Exposure described as harmful elicited higher ratings of intensity and sensory irritation over time, compared with identical exposure described in a positive or neutral fashion. Moreover, individuals receiving negative rather than positive or neutral information reported more symptoms after an exposure session (Dalton, 1996, 1999; Dalton et al., 1997). Dalton and colleagues utilized an exposure chamber, but similar effects have been found when using transient stimuli. Djordjevic et al. (2008) found that negative, compared with positive or neutral odor labels, result in significantly higher intensity ratings and lower ratings of pleasantness of odorants delivered in glass bottles. Ratings of hedonic value, argued to be the dominant dimension in olfaction (Richardson and Zucco, 1989), seems to be more easily influenced by differently phrased information than ratings of intensity (Djordjevic et al., 2008; Nordin et al., 2013). Providing differently phrased information about an exposure does not always seem to influence intensity ratings (Kobayashi et al., 2007), and the effect seems to be greater for chemicals eliciting trigeminal sensations (i.e., pungency; Dalton et al., 1997).

Nevertheless, the outcomes of these studies show that neither the perceived properties of an airborne chemical, nor its assumed health effects depend solely on the type and strength of the exposure. If the results are applicable outside the laboratory, they suggest that expectancy of possible health risks is a factor to consider when evaluating and setting exposure limits. This argument is corroborated by population-based studies emphasizing the importance of health-risk perception as an indicator of symptom reports (Shusterman et al., 1991; Claeson et al., 2013). Indeed, no exposure is actually necessary for people to report symptoms attributed to chemicals, as shown by sham exposure studies (Knasko et al., 1990; Lange and Fleming, 2005). In addition to the sensory and hedonic aspects reviewed above, Nordin et al. (2013) reported that negative health-risk perception has deleterious consequences for cognitive performance.

Reactions to chemicals are also influenced by the constitution or general well-being of the exposed individual. Negative affectivity is a trait that has been associated with greater unpleasantness ratings and symptom reports after chemical exposure (Dalton, 2002; Smeets and Dalton, 2005). Chen and Dalton (2005) reported that anxious women rated the intensity of both pleasant and unpleasant chemical stimuli as higher than did non-anxious women. Highly anxious, compared with non-anxious women, also report more symptoms when exposed to low levels of chemical solvents (Orbæk et al., 2005). Ihrig et al. (2006) found that positive and negative affectivity influences symptom reports from men as well–an effect most clearly seen with low-level exposure. At higher concentrations the impact of such traits was diminished. Several other traits or conditions associated with higher reactivity to chemical exposures have been reported in the literature, including chemical intolerance (Andersson et al.,

2009a,b), migraine (Sjöstrand et al., 2010) as well as neurologic and endocrine disorders (Spielman, 1998).

Situational circumstances and predisposing traits are not only relevant for short-term reactions to chemicals commonly investigated in exposure studies. They constitute two main factors in models of medically unexplained symptoms. In combination, they are assumed to increase the risk of developing long-term illness. Vulnerable individuals confronted with a deleterious exposure is at risk of developing a vicious cycle of responses that is maintained over time (Richardson and Engel, 2004; Deary et al., 2007; McEwen, 2007; Ganzel et al., 2010). The temporal aspect of the findings by Dalton and colleagues (Dalton, 1996, 1999; Dalton et al., 1997) becomes relevant in this context as sensitization (i.e., increased responses over time) can be seen as an indication of an illness generating cycle. For instance, sensitization has been hypothesized to be the characteristic feature of medically unexplained symptoms such as chemical intolerance or chronic pain (Overmier, 2002; Yunus, 2008). Habituation (i.e., decreased responses over time) is the opposite to sensitization. Investigating how situational and predisposing factors interact to generate sensitized responses may be relevant for occupational health issues and can assist in pinpointing individuals at risk of developing clinical conditions.

In this vein, the general aim of the current study was to investigate how health-risk perception, manipulated by biased information, and rated distress are related to sensitization/habituation in individuals exposed to low, non-toxic concentrations of an airborne chemical. Based on the literature reviewed above, our first hypothesis was that individuals reporting relatively high distress would sensitize to a weak chemical exposure described in a negative manner, whereas individuals reporting relatively low distress would habituate. Sensitization/habituation was assessed by ratings of perceived intensity and pleasantness/unpleasantness of the chemical *n*-butanol, as well as symptoms over time. The second hypothesis was that individuals receiving negative information bias and reporting higher distress would perform worse on cognitive tasks during exposure compared with negatively biased individuals reporting lower distress. We also investigated whether information bias and distress were related to a tendency of reacting to blanks, i.e., making false alarms.

METHOD

PARTICIPANTS

Forty non-smoking, non-pregnant participants aged between 18 and 35 years with a self-reported normal sense of smell were recruited through billboard advertisements on Umeå University campus and public areas such as the hospital, library, employment office and cafés. Prior to the exposure, participants were screened for anosmia (constituting an exclusion criterion) using a 0.44% v/v (336 ppm) concentration of n-butanol (99%, Merck) of the Connecticut Chemosensory Clinical Research Center Threshold Test (Cain, 1989).

Subsequent to the exposure, all participants filled out the SCL-90 inventory (Fridell et al., 2002). The SCL-90 is a widely used self-report symptom inventory covering nine symptom dimensions: somatization, obsessive-compulsive, interpersonal sensitivity, depression, anxiety, hostility, phobic anxiety, paranoid ideation, and psychotism (Derogatis et al., 1976). The mean score of all the items of the SCL-90 constitutes the Global Severity Index (GSI) and has been argued to be a good measure of general distress or well-being (Cyr et al., 1985; Fridell et al., 2002). We performed a median split to divide the participants into two groups based on the GSI. Those with a relatively low GSI constituted the low distress group. Those with a relatively high GSI constituted the high distress group. Importantly, the distress groups in this regard refer to non-pathological variations in the population. Descriptive data of the participants are given in **Table 1**. There was no significant difference between the two bias groups in terms of GSI score, age or sex, as assessed by independent samples t-tests and Mann-Whitney U-tests (all t and $Z < 0.9$; all $p > 0.38$).

All participants were given written and spoken information about the study. The study was conducted in accordance with the Helsinki Declaration and approved by the Ethics Committee at Umeå University (# 2012-154-31M). A signed informed consent was obtained from each participant. All participants were given 200 SEK (~20 EUR) for their participation.

MATERIALS AND PROCEDURES

Chemical exposure

Participants were exposed to *n*-butanol (99.4% Baker) at a concentration of 4.7 ppm while seated in a windowed exposure chamber. *n*-Butanol was chosen since it was considered relatively ambiguous and unfamiliar, which was expected to facilitate the information bias manipulation. The concentration was chosen to be clearly detectable (above the olfactory threshold 40 ppb; Nagata, 2003) but well–below the threshold for sensory irritation (24.5 ppm; Ruth, 1986). The intensity was also chosen based on pilot testing. The stimulus material was vaporized using a nebulizer. To ensure a consistent concentration in the exposure chamber a known amount of the odorant was fed through the nebulizer into a feed stream of filtered air monitored by a mass flow controller. The mixture was then diluted (by another stream of filtered air) to the desired concentration before it was fed

Table 1 | Descriptive data of the participants, clustered according to distress and bias group.

	Positive bias	Negative bias	Pos and neg bias
Low distress, *n*	10	10	20
Women / men, *n*	5/5	4/6	9/11
Age, *M* years (±*SD*)	25 (4.2)	24 (3.6)	25 (3.9)
GSI, *M* (±*SD*)	0.19 (0.08)	0.16 (0.07)	0.18 (0.07)
High distress, *n*	10	10	20
Women / men, *n*	5/5	6/4	11/9
Age, *M* years (±*SD*)	24 (4.3)	24 (4.9)	24 (4.5)
GSI, *M* (±*SD*)	0.65 (0.21)	0.64 (0.51)	0.64 (0.38)
Low and high distress, *n*	20	20	40
Women / men, *n*	10/10	10/10	20/20
Age, *M* years (±*SD*)	24 (4.2)	24 (4.2)	24 (4.2)
GSI, *M* (±*SD*)	0.42 (0.27)	0.40 (0.43)	0.41 (0.36)

GSI = Global Severity Index of the SCL-90.

into the exposure chamber. The vapor-phase concentration was measured inside the exposure chamber with a photoionization detector (PID, RAE Systems). The exposure chamber has a volume of 2.7 m^3 (height × width × depth: 200 × 90 × 150 cm). Air was exchanged at a rate of 7.8 times per hour. The mean temperature across participants at the end of testing was 22.3°C (*SD* ± 1.0), and the relative humidity was 18.9% (*SD* ± 2.5).

Information bias

Participants were given either positive or negative information regarding the chemical used for exposure. The negatively biased group was told that butanol is an industrial solvent that can produce symptoms at higher concentrations, and that the aim of the study was to assess possible negative effects on performance at levels below the toxicological threshold. When seated in the exposure chamber, the negatively biased group could see a poster showing hazard pictograms and risk phrases associated with *n*-butanol. The positively biased group was told that butanol is a natural extract found in many food products, and can be produced by fermenting, e.g., corn. These participants were told that the aim of the study was to investigate whether ambient *n*-butanol could diminish sleepiness, possibly resulting in greater cognitive performance. While seated in the chamber, the positively biased group could see a poster with chocolate bars and a text informing the reader that butanol is an important component in high quality chocolate. The posters were placed on the laboratory wall so that the participants could see them easily, but at such a distance that they did not seem directed to the person sitting in the chamber. The rationale for using the posters was to remind the participants of the biased information during the exposure, in a manner not obviously and suspiciously directed at them. Neither of the bias groups were misled, as both the positive and negative information are in fact true.

Apparatus

The sequence of psychophysical ratings and cognitive tasks was programmed using E-Prime 2.0 software (Psychology Software Tools, Pittsburgh, PA). A Windows 7 laptop computer (Compaq 8510) connected to a 24 inch screen (Asus VK246H) in front of the participants and a Microsoft Bluetooth Number Pad placed on a lap tray were used to present tasks and record responses.

TASKS

Ratings of intensity, valence and symptoms

Participants rated the chemosensory intensity and valence of the exposure using a Borg CR-100 scale (Borg and Borg, 2002).The CR-100 is a verbally anchored ratio scale (Borg, 1998; Borg and Borg, 2001) with descriptive adjectives that correspond to specific numbers on the scale: Nothing at all, 0; minimum, 1.5; extremely weak, 2.5; very weak, 6; weak, 12; moderate, 25; strong, 45; very strong, 70; extremely strong, 90; near maximal, 100. Numbers above 100 are not labeled, but approaches the label absolute maximum. For valence ratings the participants were prompted to add a plus sign before the rating if the exposure was judged as pleasant, and a minus sign before the rating if deemed unpleasant.

Ten symptoms were rated using the Borg CR-100 scale (Borg and Borg, 2002). These constituted eye irritation, nasal mucosal irritation, skin irritation, throat irritation, shortness of breath, concentration difficulties, dizziness, tiredness, headache and nausea. They were chosen since they have been shown to frequently (20–69%) be reported by persons with chemical intolerance (Andersson et al., 2009a), and since they together represent a broad range of symptoms (airway, mucosae, skin, cognitive, head-related, and gastrointestinal). The mean of these 10 symptoms were used as a composite score in the statistical analysis.

Plus/minus lists

Participants performed a plus/minus task based on Jersild (1927). Participants were prompted to add, subtract or alternate between adding and subtracting three from a random two-digit number ranging from 13 to 96. Each plus/minus list block consisted of one addition list, one subtraction list and one alternating list in which the task was to shift operation after each number. Participants were told to perform the tasks as quickly and correctly as possible. After each input, the screen either flashed green if the answer was correct, or red if incorrect. Each list had the duration of 60 s. The plus/minus lists were assumed to be related to general cognitive performance. The task was chosen based on a study by Nordin et al. (2013) in which biased information influenced the performance of this task. Task performance was analyzed based on the mean number of correct answers in the plus, minus and plus/minus lists within each block.

Updating task

Participants performed an additional cognitive task, assumed to be more difficult than the plus/minus lists. It was based on the letter memory task described in Miyake et al. (2000). In the current task, single numbers (1, 2, 3 or 4) were presented serially on the center of the screen for 2000 ms with a 1000 ms inter-stimulus interval. Participants were to recall and type in the last four numbers in the correct order after each list. Seven lists were presented in random order, with a length of 5, 7, 9, 11, 13, and 15 digits. The list length was unknown to the participants. Number of correctly recalled sequences was used as a measure of task performance.

PROCEDURE

An overview of the experimental procedure is provided in **Figure 1**. After giving the informed consent, receiving the biased information and passing the odor detection test, participants were seated in a chair inside the chamber with the door open. The participants received the lap tray with a numerical keyboard through which responses were recorded. Participants practiced the plus/minus lists, the updating task and how to rate intensity and valence. They also rated their baseline symptoms. After the approximately 15 min training/baseline session, participants were informed that the actual study would begin right after the chamber door was closed. They were told that the concentration of the chemical inside the chamber could vary during the session. Unknown to the participants, no chemical was delivered into the chamber during the first 10 min of testing. After the 10 min period of blank exposure, the *n*-butanol was released into the chamber and reached its peak concentration after about 8 min. The concentration remained at this peak level for the rest of the session. During the exposure, participants performed a total of 12 ratings of intensity and valence, eight blocks of plus/minus lists, two blocks of updating tasks and two symptom rating blocks (cf. **Figure 1**). At the end of the exposure session, the participants used a Borg CR-100 scale to rate to what degree they believed the exposure to be harmful or beneficial for health. Similar to the valence ratings, participants added a plus sign before the rating if the exposure was judged as beneficial, and a minus sign before the rating if deemed harmful. After the exposure session, participants filled out the SCL-90 questionnaire. Participants were then debriefed and told about the different information biases.

STATISTICAL ANALYSIS

Analyses were performed using full factorial mixed model analyses of variance (ANOVAs) in IBM SPSS Statistics 20. The α was set at 0.05, with values < 0.1 considered as tendencies. Significant interaction effects were further analyzed and discussed only if they pertained to the factors Bias or Distress, as per the hypotheses. Effects not associated with the hypotheses are reported in **Table 2**. Greenhouse-Geisser correction was applied in cases where df > 1. In such cases, uncorrected *dfs* are reported. Effect sizes are reported as eta sqared (η^2) and were calculated using Microsoft Office Excel, 2010.

RESULTS

MANIPULATION OF HEALTH RISK PERCEPTION

The participants' judgments of beneficial or harmful health effects of the exposure was analyzed using a 2 × 2 (Bias [positive, negative] × Distress [low, high]) ANOVA. As seen in **Figure 2**, the negative bias group rated the exposure as more harmful than did the positive bias group, $F_{(1, 36)} = 6.7$, $p = 0.014$, $\eta^2 = 0.11$. Distress did not affect the health risk judgments, $F_{(1, 36)} = 0.8$, $p = 0.375$.

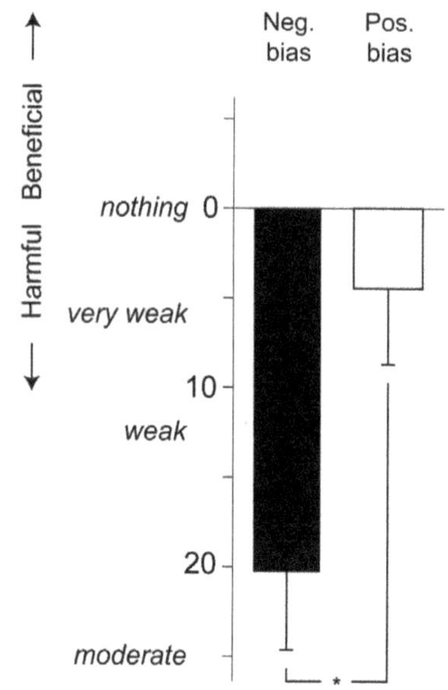

FIGURE 2 | Mean (+ standard error) ratings of harmful or beneficial health effects of the chemical exposure, using a Borg CR-100 scale. *P*-values refer to the ANOVA parameter estimates (*$p < 0.05$).

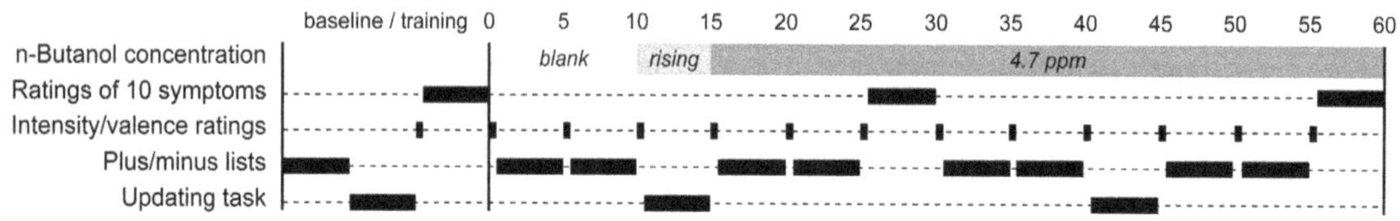

FIGURE 1 | Overview of experimental procedure. The exposure session began at min 0.

Table 2 | *F*-values (and, if statistically significant, eta-squared, η^2) for the full factorial mixed model ANOVAs.

	Blank exposure		Chemical exposure		Symptom ratings	Cognitive performance	
	Intensity	Valence	Intensity	Valence		Plus/minus	Updating
Time (T)	2.2	0.4	6.8 (0.13)***	0.4	25.1 (0.12)***	5.7 (0.04)**	16.9 (0.31)***
Bias (B)	7.2 (0.14)*	4.1(0.10)†	1.9	2.8	0.1	0.7	1.8
Distress (D)	6.2 (0.12)*	1.5	14.8 (0.28)***	8.5 (0.18)**	7.8 (0.17)**	1.9	4.0 (0.10)‡
T × B	0.3	0.2	1.2	0.1	1.5	1.2	0.5
T × D	1.3	2.4	2.9 (0.06)*	2.7 (0.07)*	4.2 (0.06)*	1.3	0.9
B × D	2.3	0.4	0.0	0.1	1.2	0.6	0.0
T × B × D	1.0	0.5	3.8 (0.07)**	1.3	0.4	1.6	0.2
Symptom (S)					18.3 (0.14)***		
T × S					6.3 (0.04)***		

No other significant effects involving the factors Symptom or Task (plus/minus lists); all F < 2.1.
$^*p < 0.05$; $^{**}p < 0.01$; $^{***}p < 0.001$; $^{\dagger}p = 0.052$; $^{\ddagger}p = 0.054$.

INTENSITY AND VALENCE RATINGS DURING BLANK EXPOSURE

Possible group differences of intensity ratings during blank exposure were investigated using a 2 × 2 × 2 (Time [first and second rating during blank exposure] × Bias [positive, negative] × Distress [low, high]) ANOVA. The positive bias group rated the blank exposure as more intense than did the negative bias group (cf. **Figure 3**) as seen by a main effect of Bias $F_{(1, 36)} = 6.2$, $p = 0.017$, $\eta^2 = 0.12$. Additionally, the high distress group rated the blanks as more intense than the low distress group (cf. **Figure 3**) as seen by a main effect of Distress, $F_{(1, 36)} = 7.2$, $p = 0.011$, $\eta^2 = 0.14$. An ANOVA with the same factors was performed on valence ratings, revealing a tendency of a main effect of Bias, $F_{(1, 36)} = 4.1$, $p = 0.052$, $\eta^2 = 0.10$. The tendency is that the positive bias group rated the blanks as more pleasant than did the negative bias group (cf. **Figure 3**).

INTENSITY AND VALENCE RATINGS DURING CHEMICAL EXPOSURE

A 9 × 2 × 2 (Time [nine ratings during chemical exposure] × Bias [positive, negative] × Distress [low, high]) ANOVA using intensity ratings during chemical exposure revealed a Time

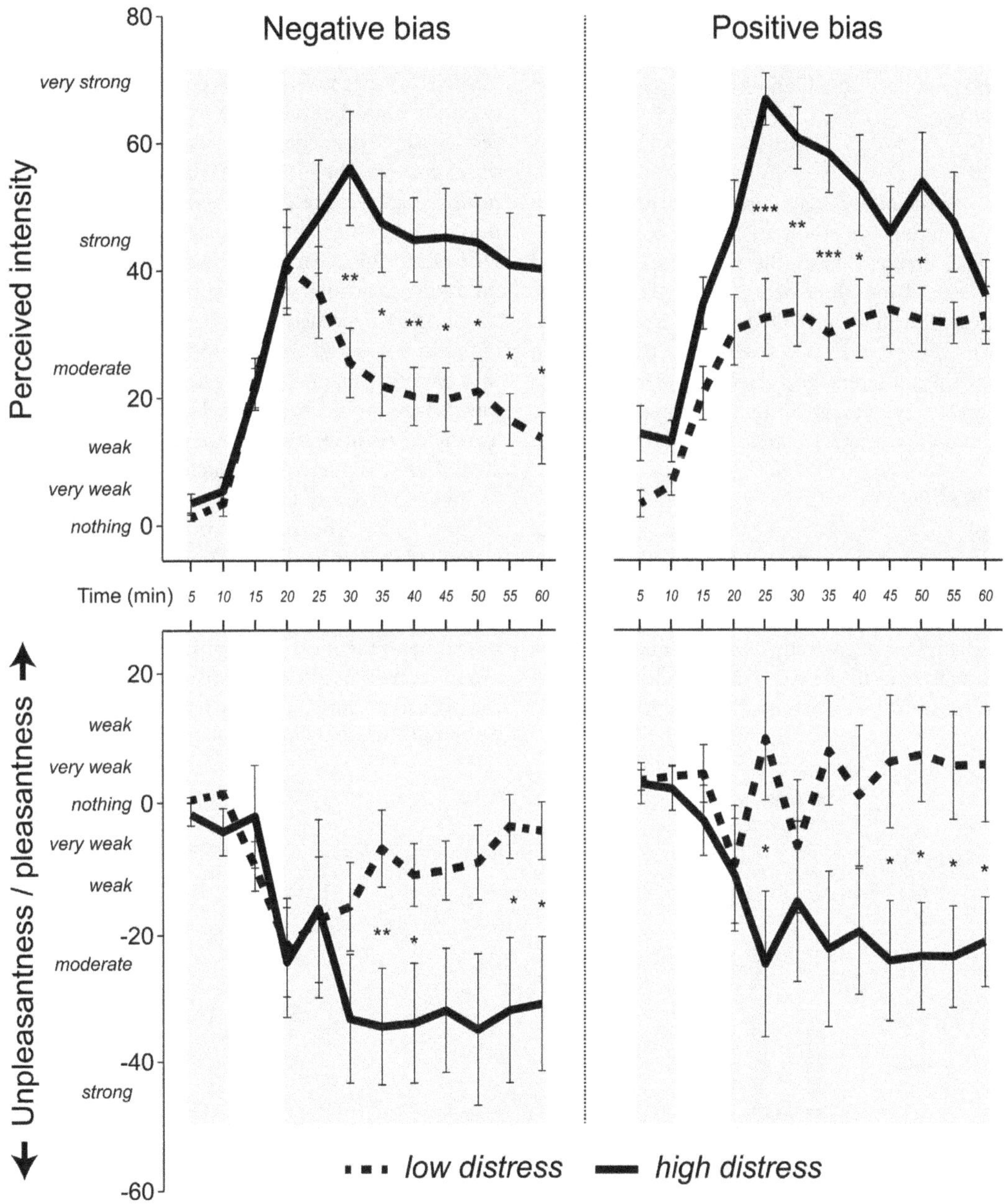

FIGURE 3 | Mean (± standard error) ratings of intensity and valence in 5 min intervals, using a Borg CR-100 scale. Pleasantness was rated as positive values and unpleasantness as negative values. Shaded areas indicate values used in the statistical analyses. The first two ratings were made during blank exposure. The last nine ratings were made when the *n*-butanol concentration was at a stable concentration. *P*-values refer to the ANOVA parameter estimates (* $p < 0.05$, ** $p < 0.01$, *** $p < 0.001$).

× Bias × Distress interaction, $F_{(8, 288)} = 3.8$, $p = 0.007$, $\eta^2 = 0.07$. *Post-hoc* ANOVAs separating the factors Bias and Distress revealed a significant effect of Time for the low distress group receiving negative bias, $F_{(8, 288)} = 5.5$, $p = 0.005$, ?$^2 = 0.38$, indicating that individuals in this group rated intensities as lower over time (cf. **Figure 3**). The high distress group receiving positive bias also reported lower intensities over time, as seen by a significant effect of Time, $F_{(8, 288)} = 4.8$, $p = 0.009$, $\eta^2 = 0.35$ (cf. **Figure 3**). There was no effect of Time in the high distress group receiving negative bias, or the low distress group receiving positive bias (see **Figure 3**). Valence ratings were analyzed using an ANOVA with the same factors, yielding a Time × Distress interaction $F_{(8, 288)} = 2.7$, $p = 0.048$, $\eta^2 = 0.07$. **Figure 3** reveals that the ratings of the low distress group approached zero over time, whereas the valence ratings of the high distress group remained negative over time.

SYMPTOM RATINGS

Symptom ratings (mean of eye irritation, nose irritation, skin irritation, throat irritation, shortness of breath, concentration difficulties, dizziness, tiredness, headache and nausea) were analyzed with a 3 × 2 × 2 (Time [three occasions] × Bias [positive, negative] × Distress [low, high]) ANOVA. There was a Time × Distress interaction, $F_{(2, 72)} = 4.2$ $p = 0.026$, $\eta^2 = 0.06$. As seen in **Figure 4**, the significant interaction refers to the high distress group reporting greater symptoms in the middle and end of the session. Notably, Bias did not affect symptom ratings (**Table 2**).

COGNITIVE PERFORMANCE

Mean number of correct answers in the plus, minus and plus/minus lists were analyzed with a 9 × 2 × 2 (Time [nine blocks] × Bias [positive, negative] × Distress [low, high]) ANOVA. There were no significant effects for the factors Bias or Distress (**Table 2**). Number of correctly recalled sequences in the updating task was analyzed with a 3 × 2 × 2 (Time [three blocks] × Bias [positive, negative] × Distress [low, high]) ANOVA. There was a tendency of a main effect of Distress, with a lower amount of correctly recalled sequences in the high distress group $F_{(1, 36)} = 4.0$ $p = 0.054$, $\eta^2 = 0.10$. Despite the lack of a Time × Distress interaction, parameter estimates nevertheless reveal that the Distress effect is greater at the end of the session. This is illustrated in **Figure 5**.

DISCUSSION

This study was conducted to investigate the effects of health-risk perception and self-reported distress on reactions to a low-level chemical exposure. Participants rated the perceived intensity and valence of blank stimuli and *n*-butanol, reported symptoms and performed cognitive tasks during the exposure session. Health-risk perception was manipulated by giving participants either positively or negatively phrased information regarding the compound used in the study. The manipulation was regarded as successful, as the participants receiving negative information judged the exposure to be more harmful compared with those receiving positive bias (**Figure 2**). Furthermore, participants were assigned into relatively high and low distress groups based on self-reports. Distress, in this regard, does not refer to pathological problems, but rather as normal variation in terms of rated well-being.

Our first hypothesis was that individuals reporting relatively high distress would sensitize to the chemical exposure described in a negative manner, whereas individuals reporting relatively low distress would habituate. Negative bias has previously been associated with increasing intensity ratings over time (Dalton, 1996, 1999). Similarly, traits such as anxiety have also been linked to higher perceived intensity of chemical exposure (Chen and Dalton, 2005). The analysis of the intensity ratings partly corroborated the first hypothesis by revealing an interaction between information bias, self-reported distress and time. The low distress group receiving negative bias reported intensities as decreasing over time to the invariant exposure (**Figure 3**). The high distress group receiving negative bias neither sensitized nor habituated to the exposure, but seemed to reach a stable plateau in terms of perceived intensity. Positive bias had the opposite effect on the

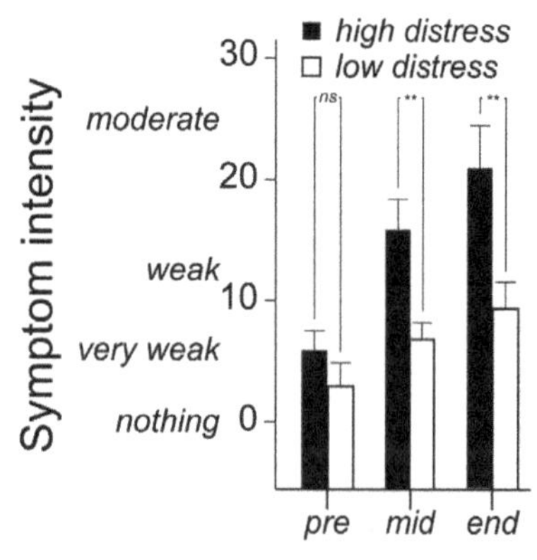

FIGURE 4 | Mean (+ standard error) ratings of eye irritation, nose irritation, skin irritation, throat irritation, shortness of breath, concentration difficulties, dizziness, tiredness, headache, and nausea before (pre), in the middle of (mid) and at the end of the *n*-butanol exposure session. Ratings are made on a Borg CR-100 scale. *P*-values refer to the ANOVA parameter estimates (** $p < 0.01$).

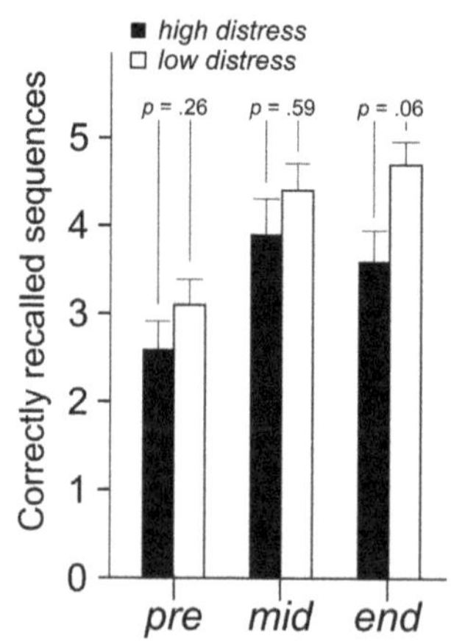

FIGURE 5 | Mean (+ standard error) number of correctly recalled sequences in the updating task. *P*-values refer to the ANOVA parameter estimates.

rated intensities in the high and low distress group. Analyses of the Bias × Distress × Time interaction revealed that the high distress group habituated over time, whereas the low distress group did not (cf. **Figure 3**).

Among the interpretations of these results, we would like to point out one result in particular. By the end of the session in which participants received positive information bias, the high and low distress group rated the exposure as similar in terms of mean intensity (**Figure 3**). The same result was not seen when participants received negative information. The differences in perceived intensities between the high distress and low distress group rather increased with time. The mean perceived intensity of the distressed group was "strong" throughout the exposure session when rated according to the Borg CR-100 scale. The negatively biased non-distressed group rated the exposure as "weak" by the end of the session. These results suggest rather large, time-dependent discrepancies in basic sensory judgments between distressed and non-distressed individuals, but only when the exposure is deemed unhealthy. The interactions between bias and distress can be seen as an expansion of previous studies revealing a bias effect on intensity ratings (Dalton, 1996, 1999). The result may also be relevant for occupational exposure limits by revealing the extent of differences in the ratings of basic properties of the surroundings (Smeets and Dalton, 2005).

The analyses of valence and symptom ratings revealed effects of distress, but no interactions including information bias and distress in combination. The high distress group did not habituate in terms of rated unpleasantness, whereas the low distress group did. Moreover, the high distress group reported greater symptoms over time compared with the low distress group. These results do not contradict the first hypothesis stating that negative bias will have more deleterious effects in distressed individuals. However, as the same results were found when a positive bias was given, information bias seems to be redundant for these measures. The lack of a bias effect is seemingly at odds with earlier reports of bias effects on valence ratings (Kobayashi et al., 2007; Djordjevic et al., 2008; Nordin et al., 2013). There are, however, differences in exposure conditions that should be considered before regarding the current results as contradictory to previous studies. The long exposure may for instance hide initial bias differences in valence ratings. Although not part of the statistical analyses, the ratings in **Figure 3** suggest possible bias effects in the beginning, but perhaps not at the end of the exposure. A hypothesis for future studies, based on this argument, would be that non-distressed individuals, to a greater degree than distressed, change their minds regarding the valence of extended exposures even if initially rating them as unpleasant.

The current study also revealed that the high distress group had a tendency of worse performance on the updating task, but not on plus/minus lists. In line with these results, trait anxiety has previously been associated with worse cognitive performance when exposed to chemicals, arguably due to greater distraction (Orbæk et al., 2005). The updating task used in the current study necessitates constant monitoring and updating of information in working memory (Miyake et al., 2000). A reasonable explanation for the worse performance in the high distress group is that the exposure, regarded as unpleasant and eliciting symptoms over time, interferes with this demanding task. The plus/minus lists are arguably less strenuous than the updating task, which might explain the lack of effects for this measure. Nordin et al. (2013) found a bias effect on plus/minus lists, a result that was not mirrored in the current study. The arithmetic task was, however, arguably easier in the current study, and consisted of adding and subtracting three from the presented number, instead of adding and subtracting seven as in the Nordin et al. study. The second hypothesis pertaining to worse performance in the high distress group is thus partly supported by current results.

Finally, the analyses revealed that the high distress group regarded the blank exposure as more intense than the low distressed group did. This may be seen as a higher false alarm rate in distressed individuals, parallel to that found in persons scoring high on somatization (Brown et al., 2012). Positive bias was also associated with higher intensity ratings of blanks, compared with the negative bias case. It is possible that this effect is due to the instructions, i.e., that the positive information referred to *n*-butanol as having a stimulating effect which may have been interpreted as being more intense. Moreover, there was a tendency of the positively biased group rating the blanks as more pleasant than did the negatively biased group, at least before the participants were exposed. Pleasantness is also the dimension that Knasko (1992) was able to manipulate by biased information during sham exposure.

Although investigated in a relatively small convenience sample calling for future replications, the tentative conclusion of this study is that traits, in this case self-reported distress, affects the reactions to low-level chemical exposure in terms of valence ratings, perceived symptoms and performance on a demanding cognitive task. Situational factors, i.e., health-risk perception interact with distress when making judgments of the intensity of the exposure. Relatively distressed individuals do not habituate in terms of intensity judgments when receiving negative information about an exposure, whereas relatively non-distressed individuals do. Generally, the lack of habituation in the distressed group could be seen as the first signs of the vicious cycle of responses that lead to the development of medically unexplained illnesses (Richardson and Engel, 2004; Deary et al., 2007; McEwen, 2007; Ganzel et al., 2010). Applied to e.g., occupational settings, the results could imply that individuals with normal sensory functioning, exposed to the same levels of ambient chemicals will over time differ significantly regarding how they experience their surroundings. A relatively non-distressed person will get used to the exposure. A relatively (albeit non-pathologically) distressed individual will perceive it as strong and unpleasant, as eliciting symptoms and affecting performance, especially if receiving negative information.

AUTHOR CONTRIBUTIONS

All authors contributed to the design of the study and interpretation of results. Steven Nordin supervised the project. Anna-Sara Claeson prepared the exposure chamber and conducted the chemical analyses. Lisa Ledin, Frida Wisting, and Linus Andersson collected and analyzed the data. Linus Andersson wrote most of the manuscript.

ACKNOWLEDGMENTS

This study was supported by grants from the Swedish Research Council for Health, Working Life and Welfare.

REFERENCES

Andersson, M. J. E., Andersson, L., Bende, M., Millqvist, E., and Nordin, S. (2009a). The idiopathic environmental intolerance symptom inventory: development, evaluation, and application. *J. Occup. Environ. Med.* 51, 838–847. doi: 10.1097/JOM.0b013e3181a7f021

Andersson, L., Bende, M., Millqvist, E., and Nordin, S. (2009b). Attention bias and sensitization in chemical sensitivity. *J. Psychosom. Res.* 66, 407–416. doi: 10.1016/j.jpsychores.2008.11.005

Borg, E., and Borg, G. (2002). A comparison of AME and CR100 for scaling perceived exertion. *Acta Psychol.* 109, 157–175. doi: 10.1016/S0001-6918(01)00055-5

Borg, G. (1998). *Borg's Perceived Exertion and Pain Scales.* Champaign, IL: Human Kinetics.

Borg, G., and Borg, E. (2001). A new generation of scaling methods: level-anchored ratio scaling. *Psychologica* 28, 15–45.

Brown, R. J., Skehan, D., Chapman, A., Perry, E. P., McKenzie, K. J., Lloyd, D. M., et al. (2012). Physical symptom reporting is associated with a tendency to experience somatosensory distortion. *Psychosom. Med.* 74, 648–655. doi: 10.1097/PSY.0b013e3182595358

Cain, W. S. (1989). Testing olfaction in a clinical setting. *Ear Nose Throat J.* 68, 322–328.

Chen, D., and Dalton, P. (2005). The effect of emotion and personality on olfactory perception. *Chem. Senses* 30, 345–351. doi: 10.1093/chemse/bji029

Claeson, A.-S., Lidén, E., Nordin, M., and Nordin, S. (2013). The role of perceived pollution and health risk perception in annoyance and health symptoms: a population-based study of odorous air pollution. *Int. Arch. Occup. Environ. Health* 86, 367–374. doi: 10.1007/s00420-012-0770-8

Cyr, J. J., McKenna-Foley, J. M., and Peacock, E. (1985). Factor structure of the SCL-90-R: is there one? *J. Person. Assess.* 49, 571–578. doi: 10.1207/s15327752jpa4906_2

Dalton, P. (1996). Odor perception and beliefs about risk. *Chem. Senses* 21, 447–458. doi: 10.1093/chemse/21.4.447

Dalton, P. (1999). Cognitive influences on health symptoms from acute chemical exposure. *Health Psychol.* 18, 579–590. doi: 10.1037/0278-6133.18.6.579

Dalton, P. (2002). Odor, irritation and perception of health risk. *Int. Arch. Occup. Environ. Health* 75, 283–290. doi: 10.1007/s00420-002-0312-x

Dalton, P., Wysocki, C. J., Brody, M. J., and Lawley, H. J. (1997). The influence of cognitive bias on the perceived odor, irritation and health symptoms from chemical exposure. *Int. Arch. Occup. Environ. Health* 69, 407–417. doi: 10.1007/s004200050168

Deary, V., Chalder, T., and Sharpe, M. (2007). The cognitive behavioural model of medically unexplained symptoms: a theoretical and empirical review. *Clin. Psychol. Rev.* 27, 781–797. doi: 10.1016/j.cpr.2007.07.002

Derogatis, L. R., Rickels, K., and Rock, A. F. (1976). The SCL-90 and the MMPI: a step in the validation of a new self-report scale. *Br. J. Psychiatry* 128, 280–289. doi: 10.1192/bjp.128.3.280

Djordjevic, J., Lundström, J. N., Clément, F. Boyle, J. A., Pouliot, S., and Jones-Gotman, M. (2008). A rose by any other name: would it smell as sweet? *J. Neurophysiol.* 99, 386–393. doi: 10.1152/jn.00896.2007

Fridell, M., Cesarec, Z., Johansson, M., and Thorsen, S. M. (2002). *SCL-90: Svensk Normering, Standardisering och Validering av Symtomskalan.* Stockholm: Statens Institutionsstyrelse SiS.

Ganzel, B. L., Morris, P. A., and Wethington, E. (2010). Allostasis and the human brain: integrating models of stress from the social and life sciences. *Psychol. Rev.* 117, 134–174. doi: 10.1037/a0017773

Ihrig, A., Hoffmann, J., and Triebig, G. (2006). Examination of the influence of personal traits and habituation on the reporting of complaints at experimental exposure to ammonia. *Int. Arch. Occup. Environ. Health* 79, 332–338. doi: 10.1007/s00420-005-0042-y

Jersild, A. T. (1927). Mental set and shift. *Arch. Psych.* 14, 1–81.

Knasko, S. C. (1992). Ambient odor's effect on creativity, mood, and perceived health. *Chem. Senses* 17, 27–35. doi: 10.1093/chemse/17.1.27

Knasko, S. C., Gilbert, A. N., and Sabini, J. (1990). Emotional state, physical well-being, and performance in the presence of feigned ambient odor. *J. Appl. Soc. Psychol.* 20, 1345–1357. doi: 10.1111/j.1559-1816.1990.tb01476.x

Kobayashi, T., Sakai, N., Kobayakawa, T., Akiyama, S., Toda, H., and Saito, S. (2007). Effects of cognitive factors on perceived odor intensity in adaptation/habituation processes: from 2 different odor presentation methods. *Chem. Senses* 33, 163–171. doi: 10.1093/chemse/bjm075

Lange, L. J., and Fleming, R. (2005). Cognitive influences on the perception of somatic change during a feigned chemical release. *J. Appl. Soc. Psychol.* 35, 463–486. doi: 10.1111/j.1559-1816.2005.tb02131.x

McEwen, B. S. (2007). Physiology and neurobiology of stress and adaptation: central role of the brain. *Physiol. Rev.* 87, 873–904. doi: 10.1152/physrev.00041.2006

Miyake, A., Friedman, N. P., Emerson, M. J., Witzki, A. H., Howerter, A., and Wager, T. D. (2000). The unity and diversity of executive functions and their contributions to complex "frontal lobe" tasks: a latent variable analysis. *Cogn. Psychol.* 41, 49–100. doi: 10.1006/cogp.1999.0734

Nagata, Y. (2003). Odor intensity and odor threshold value. *J. Jpn. Air Cleaning Ass.* 41, 17–25.

Nordin, S., Claeson, A.-S., Andersson, M. J. E., Sommar, L., Andrée, J., Lundqvist, K., et al. (2013). Impact of health-risk perception on odor perception and cognitive performance. *Chemosens. Percept.* doi: 10.1007/s12078-013-9153-0

Orbæk, P., Persson, R., and Österberg, K. (2005). Impact of trait anxiety and social conformity on responses to experimental chemical challenge. *Environ. Toxicol. Pharmacol.* 19, 659–664. doi: 10.1016/j.etap.2004.12.033

Overmier, J. B. (2002). Sensitization, conditioning, and learning: can they help us understand somatization and disability? *Scand. J. Psychol.* 43, 105–112. doi: 10.1111/1467-9450.00275

Richardson, J. T., and Zucco, G. M. (1989). Cognition and olfaction: a review. *Psychol. Bull.* 105, 352–360. doi: 10.1037/0033-2909.105.3.352

Richardson, R. D., and Engel, C. C. (2004). Evaluation and management of medically unexplained physical symptoms. *Neurologist* 10, 18–30. doi: 10.1097/01.nrl.0000106921.76055.24

Ruth, J. H. (1986). Odor thresholds and irritation levels of several chemical substances: a review. *Am. Ind. Hyg Ass. J.* 47, 142–151. doi: 10.1080/15298668691389595

Shusterman, D., Lipscomb, J., Neutra, R., and Satin, K. (1991). Symptom prevalence and odor-worry interaction near hazardous waste sites. *Environ. Health Perspect.* 94, 25–30. doi: 10.2307/3431288

Sjöstrand, C., Savic, I., Laudon-Meyer, E., Hillert, L., Lodin, K., and Waldenlind, E. (2010). Migraine and olfactory stimuli. *Curr. Pain Headache Rep.* 14, 244–251. doi: 10.1007/s11916-010-0109-7

Smeets, M. A. M., and Dalton, P. (2005). Evaluating the human response to chemicals: odor, irritation and non-sensory factors. *Environ. Toxicol. Pharmacol.* 19, 581–588. doi: 10.1016/j.etap.2004.12.023

Spielman, A. I. (1998). Chemosensory function and dysfunction. *Crit. Rev. Oral Biol. Med.* 9, 267–291. doi: 10.1177/10454411980090030201

Yunus, M. B. (2008). Central sensitivity syndromes: a new paradigm and group nosology for fibromyalgia and overlapping conditions, and the related issue of disease versus illness. *Semin. Arthritis Rheum.* 37, 339–352. doi: 10.1016/j.semarthrit.2007.09.003

21

The influences of age on olfaction

***Richard L. Doty*[1]* and Vidyulata Kamath*[1,2]**

[1] *Department of Otorhinolaryngology: Head and Neck Surgery, Smell and Taste Center, Perelman School of Medicine, University of Pennsylvania, Philadelphia, PA, USA*

[2] *Division of Medical Psychology, Department of Psychiatry and Behavioral Sciences, The Johns Hopkins University School of Medicine, Baltimore, MD, USA*

Correspondence:
Richard L. Doty, Department of Otorhinolaryngology: Head and Neck Surgery, Smell and Taste Center, Perelman School of Medicine, University of Pennsylvania, HUP-3400 Spruce Street, Philadelphia, PA 19104, USA
e-mail: richard.doty@uphs.upenn.edu

Decreased olfactory function is very common in the older population, being present in over half of those between the ages of 65 and 80 years and in over three quarters of those over the age of 80 years. Such dysfunction significantly influences physical well-being and quality of life, nutrition, the enjoyment of food, as well as everyday safety. Indeed a disproportionate number of the elderly die in accident gas poisonings each year. As described in this review, multiple factors contribute to such age-related loss, including altered nasal engorgement, increased propensity for nasal disease, cumulative damage to the olfactory epithelium from viral and other environmental insults, decrements in mucosal metabolizing enzymes, ossification of cribriform plate foramina, loss of selectivity of receptor cells to odorants, changes in neurotransmitter and neuromodulator systems, and neuronal expression of aberrant proteins associated with neurodegenerative disease. It is now well established that decreased smell loss can be an early sign of such neurodegenerative diseases as Alzheimer's disease and sporadic Parkinson's disease. In this review we provide an overview of the anatomy and physiology of the aging olfactory system, how this system is clinically evaluated, and the multiple pathophysiological factors that are associated with its dysfunction.

Keywords: age, Alzheimer's disease, anatomy, olfaction, Parkinson's disease, physiology, psychophysics, neurodegeneration

INTRODUCTION

The sense of smell determines our ability to perceive thousands of odors, including ones associated with such hazards as leaking natural gas, fire, and spoiled food. This important sense mediates, to a large degree, the flavor of foods and beverages and significantly enhances quality of life. We use this sense to confirm that our clothes, homes, and offices are clean, and to fully enjoy flowers, perfumes, festive occasions, personal care products, and nature (e.g., the mountains and the sea shore). It is perhaps not surprising, then, that smell loss or disordered smell function significantly impacts our safety, appetite, nutrition, and physical and mental well-being.

Cross-sectional studies suggest that about half of the United States population between 65 and 80 years of age has demonstrable smell loss and that, over the age of 80, approximately three-quarters experience such loss (Doty et al., 1984a; Duffy et al., 1995; Murphy et al., 2002). Somewhat lower prevalence estimates are seen in very healthy cohorts (Ship and Weiffenbach, 1993; Doty et al., 2011) and in some other populations (Bramerson et al., 2004; Karpa et al., 2010), although test methods and criteria for defining dysfunction vary considerably among studies. As a result of survivor bias and other factors, cross-sectional studies likely underestimate the prevalence of age-related olfactory dysfunction, and longitudinal studies are needed to determine incidence rates and individual changes that may occur over time from factors that damage the olfactory system (London et al., 2008). With rare exception (e.g., Schubert et al., 2011), few longitudinal studies have focused on olfactory function, *per se*, with most having the goal of detecting incipient dementia or other neurological disorders in older cohorts (Graves et al., 1999; Devanand et al., 2000; Wilson et al., 2007b; Herting et al., 2008; Olofsson et al., 2008, 2009; Ross et al., 2008; Schubert et al., 2008; Conti et al., 2013; Iranzo et al., 2013; Velayudhan et al., 2013). However, regardless of whether cross-sectional or longitudinal tests are employed, age-related decrements are robust and, as described later in this review, are detectable by any number of olfactory tests, including ones employing psychophysical, electrophysiological, and psychophysiological procedures. Results from most such tests are strongly correlated, reflecting, in large part, mutual dependence upon the integrity of common elements of the olfactory pathways.

The consequences of olfactory dysfunction are staggering. In addition to explaining why many older persons complain that food lacks flavor (Schiffman and Zervakis, 2002), decreased ability to smell is largely responsible for the disproportionate number of elderly who die in accidental gas poisonings and explosions each year. In Britain, ~10% of all accidental deaths in the home between 1931 and 1956 occurred from coal-gas poisoning, with the majority occurring in persons over the age of 60 years (Chalke et al., 1958). Stevens et al. have estimated that 45% of older adults are unable to detect petroleum gas diluted to the level dictated by safety standards, as compared to only 10% of younger adults (Stevens et al., 1987). In a 2004 study of 445 patients with chemosensory dysfunction, a number of whom were elderly, 37% of those with olfactory impairment reported having experienced an olfaction-related hazardous event at some point in their lives, as compared to only 19% of those with no such impairment. Cooking-related incidents were most common (45%), with ingestion of spoiled food (25%), lack of ability to detect leaking natural gas (23%), and inability to smell a fire (7%) being less frequent (Santos et al., 2004). One longitudinal study of 1162 older individuals without dementia found that the mortality risk was 36% higher in those with low scores on a smell test after adjusting for such variables as sex, age, and education (Wilson et al., 2011a).

This review addresses the functional and pathological changes that occur in the olfactory system as a result of age. The influences of age-related diseases on olfaction, such as Alzheimer's and Parkinson's disease, are briefly mentioned but not reviewed in detail; the reader is referred elsewhere for recent reviews of such influences (Barresi et al., 2012; Doty, 2012a,b). To provide a template for understanding the neural underpinnings of age-related changes in olfaction, we first provide an overview of basic olfactory anatomy and physiology. This is followed by the types of changes that are observed on a range of functional tests and their anatomical and neuropathological correlates.

BASIC ANATOMY AND PHYSIOLOGY OF THE NOSE AND OLFACTORY SYSTEM

The human nose is comprised of two separate nasal passages separated by a septum. An external opening, termed the naris or nostril, enters into each chamber. Extending from the lateral walls of the chambers are nasal turbinates, cartilaginous structures that are covered with a highly vascularized epithelium which serves to warm, humidify, and cleanse the air (Frye, 2003). The latter is achieved by creating turbulent flow, largely as a result of a narrowing of the cavity close to the aperture of each naris (the nasal valve). The turbulence drives particulate and other airborne matter onto the nasal mucus which is continuously moved to the gut via respiratory cilia that beat in unison (Schwab and Zenkel, 1998). Damage to respiratory cilia is associated with bacterial build-up and other problems that can impair nasal function and, ultimately, the ability to smell (Cohen, 2006).

Before an odorant is able to initiate the neural activity responsible for smell perception, it must first enter the nasal cavity from either the nares or from the nasal pharynx (i.e., from the mouth) and be absorbed into the mucus covering the olfactory epithelium. This mucus, which differs in composition from that of the mucus within the nasal cavity proper, is largely derived from specialized Bowman's glands (Getchell and Getchell, 1992). Among its secretions are odorant-binding proteins that shepherd the transit of hydrophobic odorants to the olfactory receptors (Pelosi, 1994), growth factors associated with mitosis and other cell-related processes (Federico et al., 1999), numerous immune factors (Gladysheva et al., 1986), and biotransformation enzymes involved in not only odorant clearance, but in destruction of viruses and bacteria, degradation of pro-inflammatory peptides, and toxicant metabolism (Ding and Dahl, 2003).

The cells of the olfactory epithelium are derived embryologically from both the olfactory placode and the neural crest (Katoh et al., 2011). This specialized epithelium, which lines the upper regions of the septum, cribriform plate, superior turbinate, and sectors of the middle turbinate (Leopold et al., 2000), is innervated not only by olfactory receptor cells, but by fibers from the trigeminal nerve, the nervus terminalis (Cranial Nerve 0), and autonomic fibers from the superior cervical ganglion (Zielinski et al., 1989). In addition to the receptor cells, whose cilia differ from those elsewhere in the nose in lacking dynein arms and intrinsic motility, this epithelium is comprised of sustentacular (supporting) cells, microvillar cells, basal cells, and duct cells from the Bowman's glands (Menco and Morrison, 2003). Sustentacular cells add structural support to the epithelium and, among other things, insulate receptor cells from one another. These cells are also involved in the biotransformation of noxious chemicals and maintenance of the ionic milieu that surrounds the olfactory receptor cell cilia (Vogalis et al., 2005). Two morphologically distinct types of basal cells are recognized—electron-dense horizontal cells that express cytokeratin and electron-lucent globose cells which do not express cytokeratin (Mackay-Sim, 2010). It is from these multipotent stem cells, most notably the horizontal cells, that the olfactory receptor and other cell types germinate (Iwai et al., 2008). When damaged, the olfactory epithelium can be reconstituted from these cells, although the success of such regeneration is influenced by age-related processes such as telomere shortening (Watabe-Rudolph et al., 2011) and the degree of cumulative damage from prior environmental insults, including those from pollution and viral and bacterial infections (Harkema et al., 2006). The rate of mitosis of the basal cells is regulated by multiple processes, including local cell density, resident macrophages, neural activity, and damage to olfactory sensory neurons (Camara and Harding, 1984; Mackay-Sim and Patel, 1984; Borders et al., 2007). Biochemical and mechanical stress contribute to the sensory neuron differentiation from the basal cells (Feron et al., 1999). A cross-section of the olfactory epithelium is depicted in **Figure 1A**, whereas the ciliated surface is depicted in **Figure 1B**.

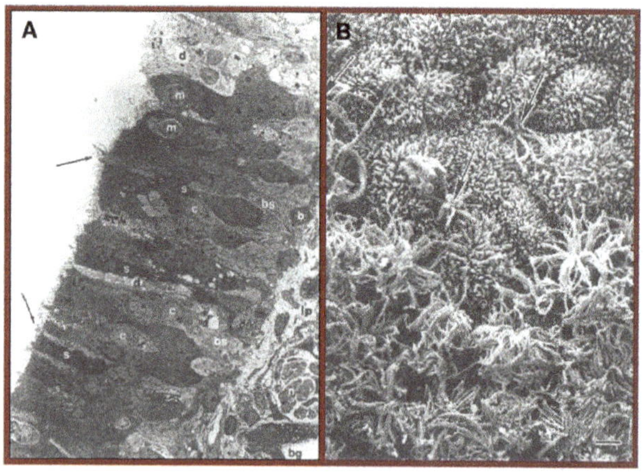

FIGURE 1 | (A) Cross-section of the human olfactory epithelium. Four main types of cells can be discerned: bipolar receptor cells (arrows point to largely denuded cilia at dendritic knobs); c, cell body, microvillar cells (m), sustentacular cells (s), and basal cells (b); bg, Bowman's gland; lp, lamina propria; n, collection of axons within an ensheathing cell; d, degenerating cell; bs, basal cell undergoing mitosis. Photo courtesy of Dr. David Moran, Longmont, Colorado. **(B)** A transition zone between the human olfactory epithelium (bottom) and the respiratory epithelium (top). Arrows signify two examples of olfactory receptor cell dendrites with cilia that have been cut off. Bar = 5 μm. From Menco and Morrison (2003), with permission.

Over 350 different functional receptor proteins are expressed in the cilia of human olfactory receptor cells (Rouquier et al., 2000). Only one type of receptor protein is embedded in the ciliary membrane of a given receptor cell (Chess et al., 1994), even though most such cells respond to a range of odorant ligands (Holley et al., 1974; Sicard and Holley, 1984). Thus, the peripheral "olfactory code" is made up of activated sets of overlapping receptor cells that can be viewed as spatial maps within both the epithelium and the olfactory bulbs (Johnson and Leon, 2007). However, coding is complex, given that more types of receptors are recruited as an odorant's concentration is increased (Malnic et al., 1999; Kajiya et al., 2001). The olfactory receptors themselves are members of the heptahelical G-protein-coupled receptor (GPCR) superfamily whose genes are distributed across all but two chromosomes, with most being on chromosome 11 and the majority of the others on chromosomes 1, 6, and 9 (Glusman et al., 2001). Odorants bind to receptor pockets located on receptor transmembrane domains 3, 5, and 6 (Saito et al., 2009). The bond is not tight, with dwell times less than a millisecond (Bhandawat et al., 2005). Transduction results from activating a GTP-binding protein which, in turn, activates type III adenylyl cyclase, catalyzing the production of 3′,5′-cyclic monophosphate (cAMP) and opening cyclic nucleotide-gated channels. This results in the cellular influx of sodium and calcium ions and depolarization of the cell (Breer, 1994). Further amplification occurs from the opening of calcium-activated chloride channels and the resultant efflux of Cl^- from the cell (Stephan et al., 2009). While members of the trace amine-associated receptor (TAAR) family (Liberles and Buck, 2006) have been identified in the olfactory epithelia of a range of mammals, including humans, their role is poorly understood and ligands that activate murine TAARs do not activate intact primate orthologs (Staubert et al., 2010).

Bundles of olfactory receptor axons ultimately form the olfactory fila which are ensheathed by Schwann cell-like mesaxons, astrocytes, and fibroblasts. These bundles, which collectively make up Cranial Nerve I, aggregate beneath the basement membrane in the connective tissue-rich lamina propria and then penetrate multiple openings (foramina) of the cribriform plate—the thin sector of the ethmoid bone that separates the nasal cavity from the brain (De Lorenzo, 1957). The ensheathing cells have unique properties, as they not only provide guidance to axons projecting from the nasal cavity into the brain, but, along with monocytic cells, phagocytize bacteria and other xenobiotics which might otherwise enter into the brain (Smithson and Kawaja, 2010; Panni et al., 2013). Once inside the cranial cavity, the receptor cell axons make up the first of several layers of the olfactory bulb (**Figure 2**) and individually ramify into the globe-like glomeruli that constitute the next layer of the bulb (Meisami et al., 1998). In young persons, there are more than a thousand glomeruli, but this number decreases with age, reflecting, in part, loss of neurotrophic factors from degenerating receptor cells.

Interestingly, receptor cells that express the same receptor protein project to the same glomeruli, making the glomeruli, in one sense, functional representatives of the receptor types. The transmitter of the olfactory receptor cells, glutamate, acts upon NMDA and AMPA receptors on dendrites of projection neurons, the mitral and tufted cells. Juxtaglomerular cells modulate glutamate release via presynaptic D_1 and $GABA_B$ receptors on the receptor cell axon terminals (O'Connor and Jacob, 2008). Similar post-synaptic modulation occurs via activation of GABA and serotonin (5HT) receptors on the mitral and tufted cell apical dendrites. Additional modulation of these cells occurs within the bulb's external plexiform layer, where their secondary dendrites form, for example, dendro-dendritic connections with GABAergic granule cells, the most numerous cells of the olfactory bulb (Shepherd, 1972). Granule cell activity is modulated primarily by centrifugal input from neurons whose cell bodies fall outside of the olfactory bulb and which are influenced by central processes, including metabolic states. Importantly, some centrifugal neurons modulate the activity of microglial cells within the bulb and elsewhere which, if not kept in check, can induce nerve cell injury via the expression of Toll-like receptors that promote pro-inflammatory and pro-apoptotic activity (Lehnardt et al., 2007; Tang et al., 2007; Ziegler et al., 2007).

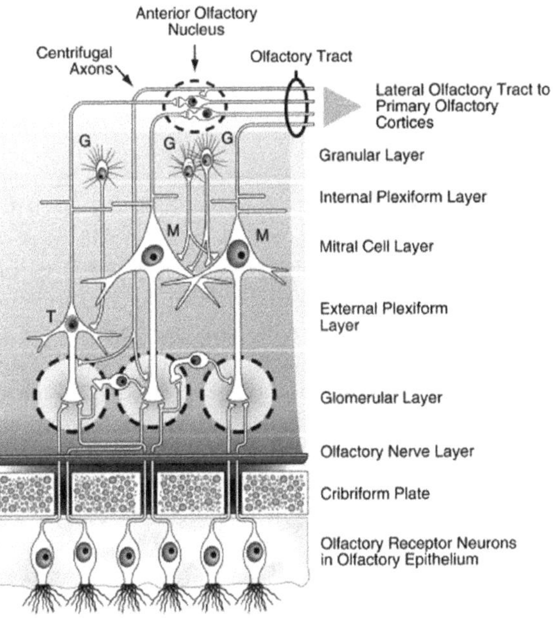

FIGURE 2 | Schematic drawing of the major layers of the olfactory bulb and the interactions between the different types of bulbar cells. Abbreviations: G, granule cells; M, mitral cells; T, tufted cells. Note that the largely GABAergic granule cells send projections into the mitral cell and external plexiform layers, and that some small cells extend projections into more than one glomerulus. Reprinted with permission from Duda (2010), with permission.

Like the olfactory neuroepithelium, a number of olfactory bulb cells, most notably periglomerular and granule cells, undergo periodic replacement (Bedard and Parent, 2004). There is evidence that considerable plasticity occurs within the glomerular region of the olfactory bulb throughout life, in addition to that which occurs during early post-natal development (LaMantia and Purves, 1989; Sawada et al., 2011). In humans, as in rodents and non-human primates, neural stem cells within the anterior portion of the subventricular zone (SVZ) of the brain generate neuroblasts even in adulthood. Some of these neuroblasts, in turn, migrate along the rostral migratory stream (a pathway extending from the SVZ to the olfactory bulb) to ultimately repopulate interneurons within the granule and glomerular layers of the bulb (Kam et al., 2009). There is some controversy, however, as the extent and nature of this migration in humans (Wang et al., 2011a).

The mitral and tufted cell axons project to more central olfactory structures, including the anterior olfactory nucleus, the piriform cortex, the rostral entorhinal cortex, and the corticobasal nuclei of the amygdala (Cleland and Linster, 2003). Since the afferent projections of the olfactory system to the cortex bypass the thalamus, some investigators have characterized the olfactory bulb as the "thalamus of the olfactory system" (Kay and Sherman, 2007). Although most bulbar projections to the aforementioned brain regions are ipsilateral, second order projections are made to the contralateral hemisphere via the anterior olfactory nucleus and anterior commissure. Subsequent connections are formed with the orbitofrontal cortex (OFC), hippocampus, thalamus, hypothalamus, and cerebellum (Cleland and Linster, 2003). The OFC, a multimodal structure, is thought to play a vital role in flavor perception, combining input from taste, texture, and smell (Rolls and Grabenhorst, 2008). Lesions in this area impair the identification of odors and flavors (Jones-Gotman and Zatorre, 1988). Because of these connections, one investigator has noted that "existing data suggest that [olfactory testing] may actually be among the most sensitive and selective measures of OFC dysfunction" (p. 464) (Zald, 2006).

AGE-RELATED OLFACTORY LOSS IN HUMANS AND ITS QUANTIFICATION

Quantitative testing of the sense of smell, which is easy to perform in the clinic, is critical for identifying the nature and degree of smell dysfunction experienced by older persons. Many elderly fail to recognize their deficit or, when they do so, either overestimate or underestimate its magnitude. Importantly, a significant number complain of taste loss, not recognizing the primary contribution of olfaction in determining the flavor of their food. Based on quantitative testing, the clinician can inform many patients that their function, while diminished in an absolute sense, is still well above that of most of their peers, a point that provides considerable solace to those groping with the multiple changes that accompany the aging process.

Age-related deficits in olfactory function are detected by a number of types of olfactory tests, including psychophysical tests (e.g., tests of odor detection, identification, discrimination, memory, and suprathreshold intensity), electrophysiological tests (e.g., odor event-related potentials), and psychophysiological tests (e.g., odor-related changes in heart rate and respiration). All such tests generally detect age-related decrements in the olfactory system. Since hundreds of studies have documented such decrements, only selected examples are presented here.

PSYCHOPHYSICAL TESTS

Deficits observed in older persons have been most commonly detected using psychophysical tests—tests that require a conscious response on the part of the patient. With the possible exception of some measures of suprathreshold intensity and pleasantness, the results from the majority of psychophysical tests are positively correlated with one another (Doty et al., 1994; Koskinen et al., 2004), with the size of the correlations between any two tests being bounded by the reliability coefficient of the less reliable test (Doty et al., 1995). Thus, the weight of the evidence suggests that individuals have a "general olfactory acuity" factor similar to the general intelligence factor proposed for various tests of intelligence (Yoshida, 1984; Doty et al., 1994). Despite this evidence, and the fact that comparison of results from nominally disparate olfactory tests is confounded by differing reliabilities, odorants, non-olfactory task demands, and operational procedures, for heuristic reasons age-related deficits are described below for nominally distinct classes of tests. As will be seen, age-related effects are found regardless of the employed measuring instrument, although, in general, longer tests are more reliable and, hence, more sensitive to such deficits (Doty et al., 1995).

The most widely used psychophysical tests are *identification tests*. A number of identification tests, such as the 40-item University of Pennsylvania Smell Identification Test (UPSIT; **Figure 3**) and its briefer 12-item version (the Brief Smell Identification Test or B-SIT), can be self-administered. In such tests familiar odorants are presented and the subject is required to identify the name of the odor from written alternatives or, in some cases, to choose a picture that depicts the source of the odor (Doty et al., 1984b, 1996; Richman et al., 1992; Kobal et al., 1996; Hummel et al., 1997; Nordin et al., 2002; Kobayashi et al., 2006; Krantz et al., 2009; Cameron and Doty, 2013). In addition to absolute determination of function (e.g., normal or mild, moderate, severe, or total loss), sex- and age-related normative data are available for some such tests, making it possible to determine a patient's percentile rank relative to peers (Doty, 1995). Odor identification tests are clearly sensitive to age-related

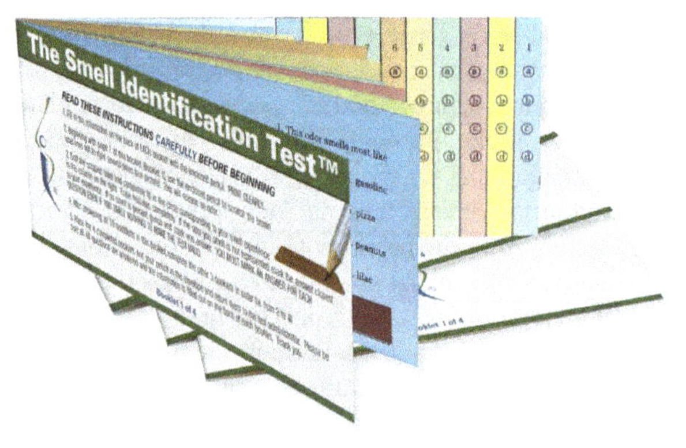

FIGURE 3 | The 40-item University of Pennsylvania Smell Identification Test (UPSIT). This test is comprised of four booklets, each containing 10 microencapsulated ("scratch and sniff") odors which are released by a pencil tip. The examinee is required to provide an answer on each test item (see columns on last page of each booklet) even if no odor is perceived or the perceived odor does not smell like one of the response alternatives (i.e., the test is forced-choice). This test has been administered to hundreds of thousands of subjects and is available in 15 different language versions. Photograph courtesy of Sensonics International, Haddon Heights, New Jersey USA.

decrements in the ability to smell (Doty et al., 1984a, 2011; Cain and Stevens, 1989; Cain and Gent, 1991; Schiffman, 1991; Ship et al., 1996; Griep et al., 1997; Kaneda et al., 2000; Larsson et al., 2000; Murphy et al., 2002; Larsson et al., 2004; Calhoun-Haney and Murphy, 2005; Schumm et al., 2009; Hedner et al., 2010a,b; Olofsson et al., 2010; Wong et al., 2010; Schubert et al., 2011, 2012; Wehling et al., 2011; Wilson et al., 2011a; Menon et al., 2013; Pinto et al., 2013). Because a number of odors are not universally recognized, identification tests are often adjusted to contain odorants and response alternatives familiar to those in a given culture. An example of the prototypical age-related decrement present in odor identification is shown in **Figure 4** (Doty et al., 1984a).

Odor threshold tests are conceptually analogous to pure-tone hearing threshold tests, except that the stimuli consist of a range of concentrations of an odorant, rather than a range of tones. Unlike most auditory threshold tests, forced-choice testing is usually employed. In a given test, a series of different concentrations of an odorant are presented to a subject via sniff bottles, squeeze bottles, felt-tip pens, or olfactometers, such as the one depicted in **Figure 5**. Dilutions are commonly made in half-log steps using mineral oil, propylene glycol, or other liquids as the dilution media. The goal of the test is to detect the lowest odorant concentration that can be reliably detected (detection threshold) or recognized (recognition threshold) (Cain et al., 1983; Doty et al., 1984b; Takagi, 1989; Doty, 1995; Hummel et al., 1997).

As with odor identification tests, significant age-related alterations are generally observed regardless of the psychophysical paradigm used to establish the threshold (Chalke et al., 1958; Fordyce, 1961; Joyner, 1963; Kimbrell and Furchtgott, 1963; Venstrom and Amoore, 1968; Strauss, 1970; Schiffman et al., 1976; Murphy, 1983; Van Toller and Dodd, 1987; Cain and Gent, 1991; Stuck et al., 2006; Larsson et al., 2009), with somewhat lower thresholds (greater sensitivity) in the healthiest cohorts (Griep et al., 1997). Studies that have explored a spectrum of ages typically report age-related performance functions similar to those depicted for odor identification (**Figure 3**), although such functions depend upon the involved odorant (Venstrom and Amoore, 1968; Deems and Doty, 1987).

Suprathreshold odor discrimination tests require the subject to discriminate among sets of odorants or odorant mixtures, for example by identifying the "odd" stimulus or set of stimuli from foils (Jehl et al., 1995; Kobal et al., 2000; Weierstall and Pause, 2012). In some instances, similarities among odorants are established and the similarity ratings or correlations subjected to statistical procedures such as multidimensional scaling, a procedure that aids in visualizing how well the stimuli can be differentiated from one another (Schiffman and Leffingwell, 1981). Older persons, on average, are less able than younger ones to discriminate between stimuli (Schiffman and Pasternak, 1979). Some match-to-sample discrimination tests intersperse differing delay intervals between the inspection odor and response set (Bromley and Doty, 1995; Choudhury et al., 2003). The goal is to assess the ability to remember the inspection odor and chose it from foils. However, the odor memory component of such tests can be confounded with semantic issues (e.g., labeling an odor with a name and then remembering the name of the odor whose memory is already present in long-term memory stores) (Jonsson et al., 2011). Such confounding can be overcome to some degree by using unfamiliar odorants that are difficult to consistently label or by employing incidental memory tasks (Møller et al., 2004, 2007).

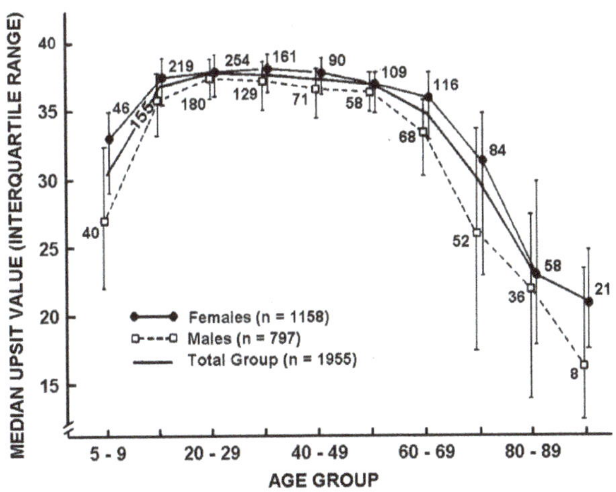

FIGURE 4 | Scores on the University of Pennsylvania Smell Identification Test (UPSIT) as a function of age and gender in a large heterogeneous group of subjects. Numbers by data points indicate sample sizes. From Doty et al. (1984a), with permission.

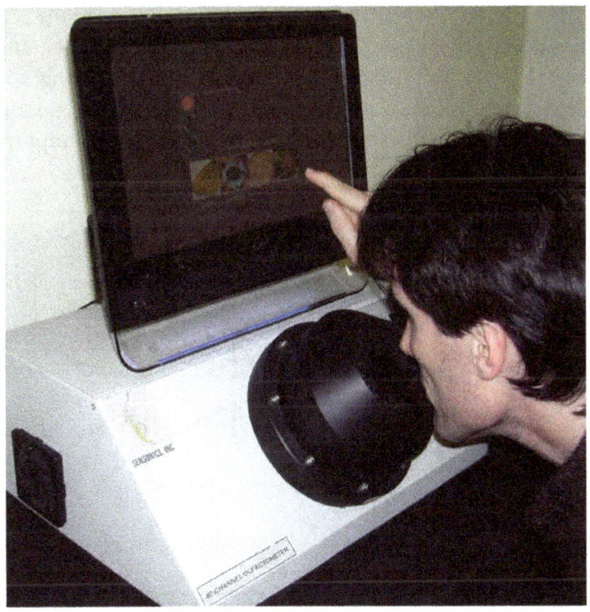

FIGURE 5 | The Self-administered Computerized Olfactory Testing System (SCOTS). This modern olfactometer allows for self-administration of olfactory threshold tests, among other types of tests, and automatically calculates the threshold value based upon subject responses. This system eliminates administrator error in the presentation of test stimuli and provides exacting control of stimulus duration, inter-stimulus intervals, and other factors. Photograph courtesy of Sensonics International, Haddon Heights, New Jersey USA.

An example of the influences of age and sex on an odor discrimination/memory test is presented in **Figure 6**. In this study, no effects of 10, 30, and 60 s delay intervals were observed, supporting the view that short-term odor memory is not affected in most persons and that performance differences in match-to-sample tests largely reflect discrimination, *per se* (Engen et al., 1973; Choudhury et al., 2003). It should be emphasized that it is probably impossible to completely disassociate memory processes from other nominal forms of odor perception, since memory is involved in most olfactory tasks and consciousness itself is, in effect, a form of memory. Importantly, age-related deficits in odor recognition may be a reflection of greater difficulties in recalling odor knowledge or names than in poorer ability to perceive or recognize the involved odors (Larsson et al., 2006).

Suprathreshold measures of the perceived strength of odors, as assessed using rating scales and magnitude estimates, have been shown to be sensitive to age in some, but not all, studies. Differences in procedures, odorants assessed, and sample sizes likely explain such discrepancies. In a study of over 26,000 respondents to a scratch-and-sniff odor survey of members of the National Geographic Society, ratings of the strength of single concentrations of six odorants were obtained using a 5-point rating scale (Wysocki and Gilbert, 1989). Age-related declines in the ratings were most noticeable for mercaptans (26% decline over the life span) and amyl acetate (22% decline), with less decline occurring for eugenol (14%), rose (13%), androstenone (10%), and Galaxolide (3%). Those odorants that showed the least decline were initially rated as less intense and were usually more difficult for older persons to identify. Importantly, when the data from the six stimuli were averaged, the age-related declines in the odor ratings began for males in their 20's and for females in their 40's.

Findings from studies assessing age-related changes in perceived intensities across multiple suprathreshold odorant concentrations have been variable. Most studies have employed magnitude estimation procedures to assess the build-up of stimulus intensity as odorant concentration is increased. In the classical magnitude estimation procedure, subjects are instructed to assign numbers in proportion to the relative perceived intensity of different concentrations of an odor (e.g., if a stimulus smells twice as strong as another, a number twice as large is assigned, and so on) (Doty and Laing, 2003). Each subject is allowed, in most instances, to choose the specific numbers they wish to employ (the "free modulus" method). In some cases, responses other than numbers are used, such as pulling a tape measure a distance proportional to the perceived intensity. Murphy (1983), using the mixed olfactory/trigeminal stimulant menthol, found the slope of the stimulus:response magnitude estimation function of 10 older persons to be less steep than that of 10 younger persons. However, other investigators have not observed such stark slope differences. In a study of 120 subjects ranging from 6 to 94 years of age, for example, magnitude estimates made to various concentrations of 1-propanol were unrelated to age, leading the authors to erroneously conclude that age did not influence olfaction (Rovee et al., 1975). Similarly unimpressive age-related effects were observed in a study of 137 subjects that assessed the intensities of phenyl ethyl alcohol and pyridine (Cowart, 1989). Stevens et al., in a study of 20 young and 20 old subjects, also found no strong evidence for meaningful age-related altered slopes in stimulus:response functions for amyl butyrate, a relatively non-pungent odorant, or CO_2, a strong trigeminal stimulant (Stevens et al., 1982). However, by using the method of cross-modal matching, the relative position of parallel stimulus:response functions was found to differ between the young and old subjects (**Figure 7**). In this procedure, low pitch broad-band tones were interspersed among the odorant concentration trials and the subjects were required to estimate the intensities of both the tones and the smells relative to one another. Under the assumption that the broad-band low frequency tones were not markedly influenced by age, differences in

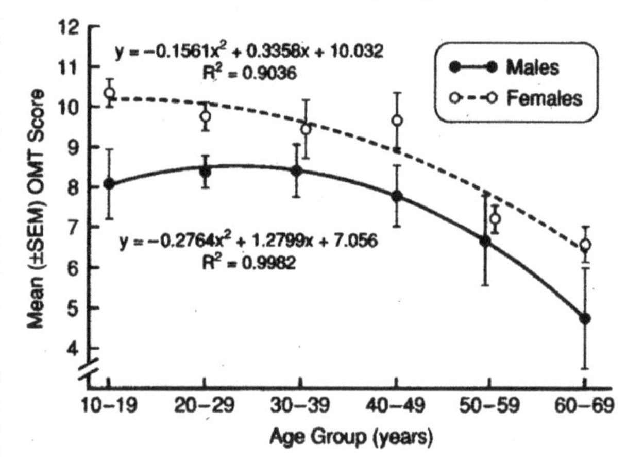

FIGURE 6 | Test scores for men and women on a 12-item odor discrimination/memory test as a function of age. Note age-related decline in performance and the fact that women outperform men at all ages. Data are collapsed over 0-, 30- and 60-s delay intervals. From Choudhury et al. (2003), with permission.

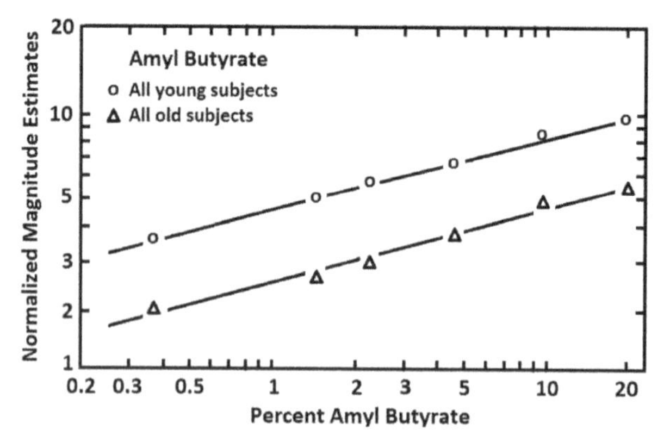

FIGURE 7 | Magnitude estimates given to six concentrations of amyl butyrate after adjustment for number usage by the employment of a cross-modal matching procedure. Each age group was comprised of 10 men and 10 women. The younger group ranged in age from 18 to 25 years, and the older group from 65 to 85 years. From Stevens et al. (1982), with permission.

idiosyncratic number usage could be taken into account, allowing an assessment of the magnitude of absolute odor intensity estimates. As is clear from **Figure 5**, the percentage decrement in strength observed in older subjects was uniform across concentrations. Similar findings have been noted in cross-modal matching studies for amyl acetate, amyl butyrate, benzaldehyde, ethyl alcohol, limonene, and pyridine (Stevens and Cain, 1985).

ELECTROPHYSIOLOGICAL TESTS

Odor-induced recordings have been obtained from electrodes placed near or on the olfactory epithelium, producing a summated negative potential termed the electro-olfactogram (EOG) (Hosoya and Yashida, 1937; Ottoson, 1956). EOG magnitude is proportional to stimulus concentration and is correlated with perceived intensity, although it can be present even after death, suggesting it alone cannot be relied upon as a measure of odor perception, *per se*. Recording can be tedious and activity in one area of the olfactory epithelium is not necessarily representative of activity in other areas. Although one can surmise from the age-related general decreases in the integrity of the olfactory epithelium that EOGs would be expected to be smaller, to our knowledge no such study has been performed. It is noteworthy, however, that EOG activity is found on the anterior surface of the middle turbinate and a few millimeters below the anterior insertion of the middle turbinate, suggesting, along with biopsy samples, that the olfactory epithelium extends farther forward in some people than traditionally believed (Leopold et al., 2000).

A more practical electrophysiological procedure is the measurement of odor-induced electrical activity at the level of the scalp (e.g., the odor event-related potential or OERP). This activity reflects odor-related changes induced in electrical fields generated by large populations of cortical neurons (Gevins and Remond, 1987). However, the signals are small ($<50\,\mu V$), can be difficult extract from the background EEG, and require complex stimulus presentation equipment (**Figure 8**). In one study, for example, OERPs were not identifiable in nearly a third of subjects with no olfactory deficits (Lotsch and Hummel, 2006). Nevertheless, age-related alterations in the latency and amplitude of OERPs have been observed, with older persons typically exhibiting longer N1 latencies and smaller N1 and P2 amplitudes (**Figure 9**) (Murphy et al., 1994; Evans et al., 1995; Hummel et al., 1998; Covington et al., 1999; Thesen and Murphy, 2001; Stuck et al., 2006; Morgan and Murphy, 2010). Although classic procedures analyze only time-locked potentials, recently developed procedures combine traditional EEG and OERP methodology to assess activity within both time and frequency domains (Huart et al., 2012; Osman and Silas, 2014). Age-related responses using these newer methods have yet to be assessed.

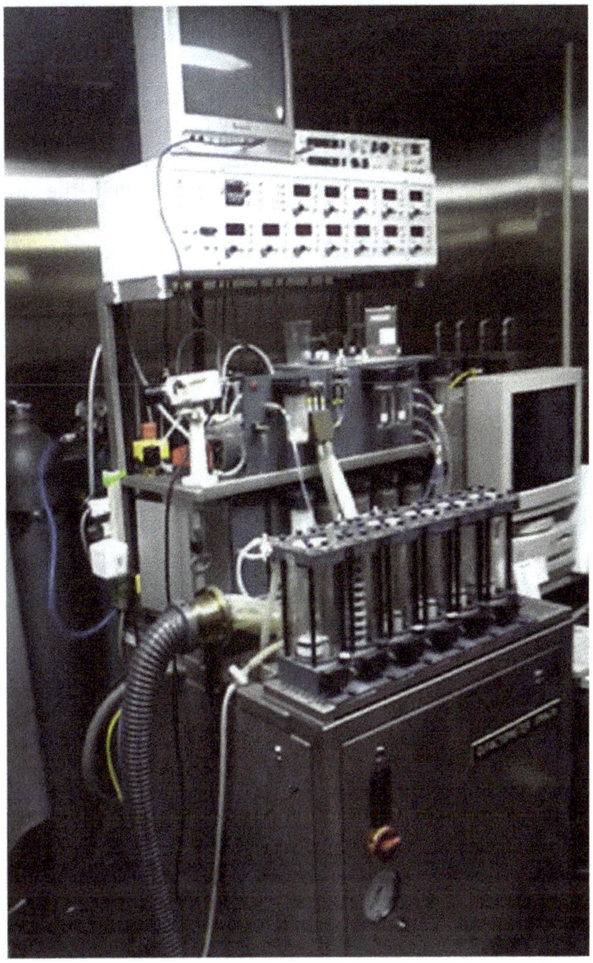

FIGURE 8 | Air-dilution olfactometer used to present pulses of odorants into a purified and humidified airstream directed through nares of a subject. This device ensures that the odor event-related potentials (OERPs) are not confounded by somatosensory artifacts due to alterations in stimulus pressure, temperature, or other factors. Photo courtesy of the University of Pennsylvania Smell and Taste Center, Philadelphia, PA.

PSYCHOPHYSIOLOGICAL TESTS

Psychophysiological tests are tests which measure mainly autonomic nervous system responses to stimuli, in this case odor. Among such measures are changes in heart rate (Bensafi et al., 2002), blood pressure (Nagai et al., 2000), respiration (Kleemann et al., 2009), and skin conductance (Møller and Dijksterhuis, 2003). In the case of the nose, cardiovascular and respiratory changes can reflect activity of the trigeminal nerve (CN V), rather than the olfactory nerve (CN I), limiting in some cases the usefulness of such tests (Allen, 1928).

A recently developed test measures a basic respiratory response to smelling an unpleasant odor (Frank et al., 2003, 2004, 2006). In this test, called the Sniff Magnitude Test, the subject sniffs a canister. Upon the initiation of the sniff, which is detected by air pressure changes sensed by cannulas positioned just inside the nose, the canister opens and either odorless air or a bad smelling odorant (e.g., methylthiobutyrate or ethyl 3-mercaptoproprionate) is released. Persons with a good sense of smell immediately stop sniffing, whereas those with a poor sense of smell take longer to inhibit their sniff or, if anosmic, may not inhibit their inhalation at all (Tourbier and Doty, 2007). The magnitude and duration of the sniff is assessed by a computer and a ratio computed between the area of the sniff pressure-time curve on odorant trials to that on blank air trials. Like other olfactory measures, this measure is sensitive to age-related olfactory changes (**Figure 10**) (Frank et al., 2006).

CAUSES OF AGE-RELATED OLFACTORY LOSS

It seems intuitive that structural changes would be present in the aging nose and olfactory system that would explain the functional declines observed in older persons. Indeed, as described below, a number of age-related alterations within the nose, olfactory epithelium, bulb, and higher brain structures have been associated to one degree or another with olfactory dysfunction. Moreover, several genes have been found to contribute, albeit to a modest degree, to the age-related decline in odor identification.

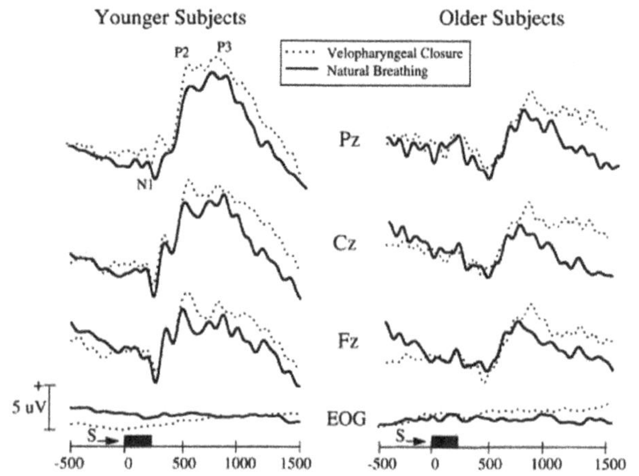

FIGURE 9 | Olfactory event-related potentials obtained from 12 younger (mean age: 24 years) and 12 older (mean age: 71 years) subjects using normal breathing or breathing after being trained to close the palate to minimize airflow from the mouth (velopharyngeal closure). Note the smaller amplitude and longer latency responses in the older group. From Thesen and Murphy (2001), with permission.

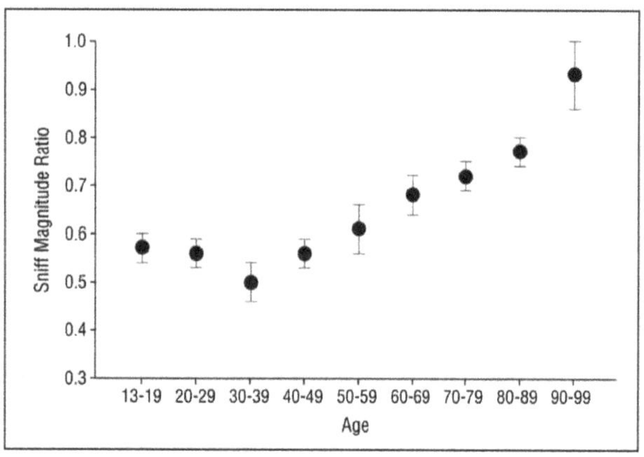

FIGURE 10 | Mean (s.e.m.) sniff magnitude ratios obtained from the Sniff Magnitude Test as a function of age. Sample size = 137 subjects, 74% of whom were female. From Frank et al. (2006), with permission.

For example, persons over the age of 70 who are homozygous for the val allele of the val66met polymorphism of brain derived neurotrohic factor (BDNF) exhibit a somewhat greater 5-year decline in odor identification performance than persons heterozygous for this allel (v/m) or homozygous for the met allel (m/m) (Hedner et al., 2010b). Older carriers of the ε4-allele of the human apolipoprotein E gene, a plasma protein involved in lipid transport, exhibit greater longitudinal declines in odor identification than non-carriers (Calhoun-Haney and Murphy, 2005). This occurs even after controlling for the effects of vocabulary and general cognitive status, suggesting that the influences of this allele on odor identification ability are independent of clinical dementia (Olofsson et al., 2010).

More recently, Doty et al. tested the odor identification ability of 1222 very old twins and singletons, including 91 centenarians (Doty et al., 2011). Unlike cognition, the sex- and age-adjusted heritability coefficients for odor identification from the two genetic models employed were quite low (i.e., 0.13 and 0.16 compared to 0.70 for cognition). These authors point out that nearly all twin studies looking at middle aged or older study cohorts report low heritability coefficients, in contrast to studies in which only young cohorts are assessed. One explanation for this observation is that the initial effects of heritability on function are eventually swamped by other factors in older persons, including the cumulative environmental insults to the olfactory epithelium, as described below.

CHANGES IN NON-OLFACTORY ELEMENTS OF THE NOSE

Odorant access to the olfactory receptors can be altered by age-related changes in nasal airflow patterns and mucous composition, including those associated with diseases which are more common in the elderly. The prevalence of chronic rhinosinusitis, nasal polyposis, and lessened mucocilliary clearance increases with age (Settipane, 1996; Cho et al., 2012), as does nasal resistance, as measured by rhinomanometry (Edelstein, 1996). The nasal epithelium undergoes age-related atrophy, decreases in mucosal blood flow, and decrements in elasticity (Somlyo and Somlyo, 1968; Bende, 1983). In general, older persons report experiencing more frequent episodes of postnasal drip, nasal drainage, sneezing, and coughing than younger ones (Edelstein, 1996). Interestingly, increased age is associated with a significant *decrease* in asthma (Jarvis et al., 2012) and a number of abnormalities of the nasopharynx, such as adenoidal hypertrophy, inflammation, cystic degeneration, or thick mucus discharge (Edelstein, 1996). Recently it has been shown that sleep apnea, a disorder associated with restriction of nasal airflow that increases in prevalence with age, has an adverse effect on smell function (Salihoglu et al., 2013).

It must not be forgotten that the nose is a dynamic organ. Airflow patterns are regularly shifting, reflecting multiple influences on nasal turbinate engorgement and secretory activity from air temperature, humidity, physical activity, psychological stress, and environmental xenobiotics such as allergens, nanoparticles, toxic chemicals, and infectious agents (Frye, 2003). Nasal engorgement is regulated in large degree by the autonomic nervous system. Thus, relative sympathetic/parasympathetic dominance influences the lateralized changes in engorgement of the nasal capillary bodies that occur over time. Although *reciprocal* and *cyclic* left:right fluctuations in relative airflow—termed the nasal cycle—are not as common as previously believed (Gilbert, 1989; Mirza et al., 1997), there is evidence that olfactory sensitivity is somewhat higher during the so-called sympathetic phase of this putative cycle, i.e., when the left side of the nose is relatively more engorged than the right (Frye and Doty, 1992). Since nearly three-quarters of adults over the age of 50 no longer exhibit this cycle (Mirza et al., 1997), a subtle lowering of olfactory sensitivity could mark the transition from the predominance of relative more sympathetic dominance to a more balanced sympathetic/parasympathetic mode. Age-related changes the suprachiasmatic nucleus, a brain center involved in the control of a number of biological rhythms, could conceivably account for this effect (Farajnia et al., 2014).

An important non-neural process that undoubtedly compromises smell function is the age-related decline in the size and number of patent foramina of the cribriform plate (Krmpotic-Nemanic, 1969; Kalmey et al., 1998). The occlusion or decrement in size of these holes can lead to a pinching off or elimination of olfactory receptor cell axons that enter into the brain from the olfactory epithelium (**Figure 11**). Kalmey et al. found a 47.3% reduction of the area of the foramina within the posterior centimeter of the cribriform plate in men older than 50 years relative to those younger than this age (7.19 vs. 3.79 mm^2) (Kalmey et al., 1998). The reduction in women was 28.8% (5.61 vs. 3.99 mm^2).

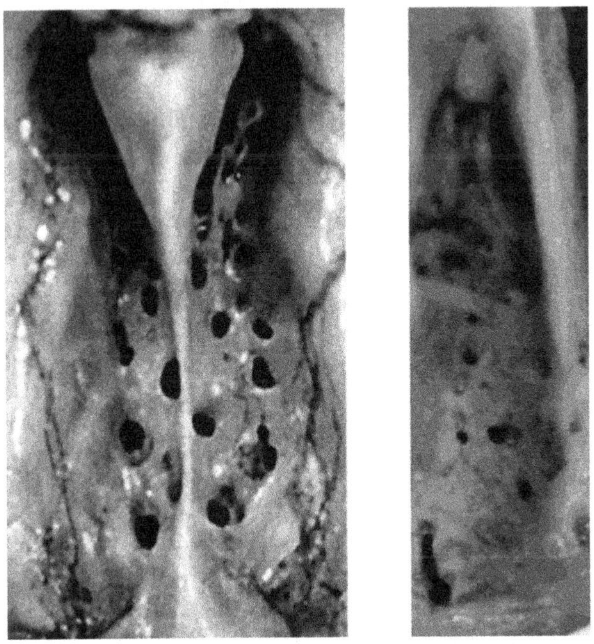

FIGURE 11 | Left: left and right halves of the cribriform plate of a 25-year-old female in superior view. **Right:** left half of cribriform plate of a 66-year-old male in superior view. Note the difference in size and number of patent foramina that transmit cranial nerve I between the young and old cribriform plates. Anterior is toward top. From Kalmey et al. (1998), with permission.

As described in the next section, the olfactory neuroepithelium becomes compromised as we age. While there are multiple reasons for this compromise, it is clear that the clearance of bacteria and other agents from the nasal cavity—clearance that depends in large part on the nature of the mucus and mucocilliary activity—changes across the lifespan. In one study of adults ranging in age from 18 to 100 years, for example, mucociliary function was found to be impaired in about 30% of those 60 years of age and older (Sakakura et al., 1983).

CHANGES IN THE OLFACTORY NEUROEPITHELIUM

Histological studies of the human olfactory epithelium have shown age-related changes in its nature and integrity, including decreased number of receptors, a thinning of the epithelium in general, and alterations in the cellular patterns and zonal distributions of the nuclei of the olfactory receptor and sustentacular cells. Intermingling of supporting and receptor cell nuclei are common, as is intercalation of respiratory epithelium with that of the olfactory epithelium, reflecting replacement of the olfactory epithelia with respiratory epithelia (Naessen, 1971; Nakashima et al., 1984; Morrison and Costanzo, 1990; Paik et al., 1992) (**Figure 12**). Similar alterations are noted in rodents exposed to olfactory toxins such as 3-methyl indole and 3-trifluoromethyl pyridine (Gaskell et al., 1990; Peele et al., 1991). In infancy and early childhood, the olfactory epithelium is highly vascularized, with blood capillaries being found in its basal layers and in close association with the perikarya of the receptor cells (Naessen, 1971). With age, these intraepithelial vessels regress and the epithelium becomes avascular. In adulthood, pigment granules are evident in the cytoplasm of sustentacular cells—granules that increase in number in the elderly (Naessen, 1971).

There are a number of reasons for the age-related decline in olfactory receptor cells and other elements of the olfactory epithelium. *First,* neurogenic processes appear to be compromised with age. In the rat, the ratio of dead or dying cells to the number of live receptor cells increases with aging (Mackay-Sim, 2003), suggesting the possibility that receptor cells from older individuals have less mitotic activity than those from younger individuals. This is in accord with the observation that following chemical destruction of the olfactory receptors of mice with zinc sulfate or methyl-formimino-methyl ester, morphological repair is slower or nonexistent in older animals (Matulionis, 1982; Rehn et al., 1986). *Second,* the aforementioned age-related decline in the size and number of patent foramina of the cribriform plate may result in necrosis of the olfactory receptor cells, eliminating them from the olfactory epithelium (Krmpotic-Nemanic, 1969; Kalmey et al., 1998). *Third,* immunologic and enzymatic defense mechanisms critical for maintaining the integrity of the epithelium become compromised with age. For example, age-related reductions have been found in the expression of phase I and phase II xenobiotic metabolizing enzymes, including carnosinase, glutathione, S-transferases, heat-shock protein 70, and isoforms of cytochrome P-450 (Kirstein et al., 1991; Getchell et al., 1995; Krishna et al., 1995). *Fourth,* age-related losses occur in the specificity of the responses of individual receptor cells. For example, electrophysiological tuning curves are broader in biopsied receptor cells from older than from younger persons (Rawson et al.,

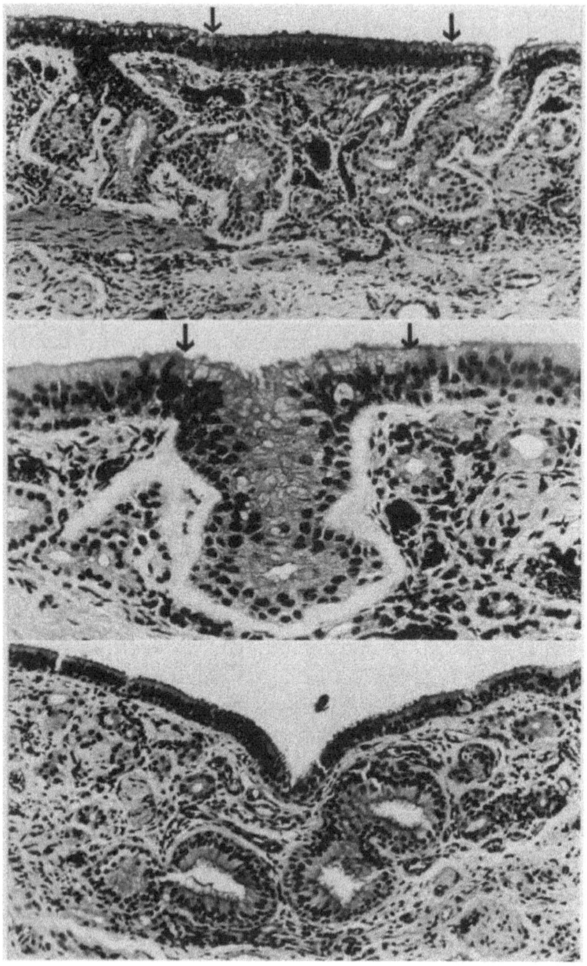

FIGURE 12 | Respiratory epithelium in the olfactory region of the adult human. Top: ciliated and goblet cell-containing respiratory epithelium has invaded degenerated olfactory neuroepithelium (between arrows). Arrows indicate junction of respiratory and olfactory epithelia (HandE, × 100). **Middle:** gland-like invagination (between arrows) of respiratory epithelium into the lamina propria (HandH, × 200). **Bottom:** gland-like respiratory epithelium with large lumina in the lamina propria (HandE, × 1000). From Nakashima et al. (1984), with permission.

1998). *Fifth*, exposures to air-borne environmental agents, including air pollution, cigarette smoke, viruses, bacteria, and other xenobiotics, damage regions of the olfactory epithelium, having more functional consequence in later years when their cumulative effects have taken a toll on the epithelium (Smith, 1942; Hirai et al., 1996; Loo et al., 1996). As mentioned earlier, environmental factors likely swamp age-related genetic factors in determining the degree of olfactory function in later life (Doty et al., 2011). Thus, Loo et al. found no age-related decrement in the number of mature olfactory neurons in the olfactory mucosa in rats reared in a pathogen-free environment, unlike the situation in rats reared in a normal laboratory environment (Loo et al., 1996).

CHANGES IN THE OLFACTORY BULB

In parallel with the integrity of the olfactory epithelium, the size of the olfactory bulb and a number of its laminae—most notably the glomerular layer—declines with age in humans and other animals (Bhatnagar et al., 1987; Yousem et al., 1998; Sama et al., 2008). While this decline may reflect, to some degree, generalized atrophy, loss of neuronal elements, and increases in astroglia, most of the decline appears to be secondary to damage to the olfactory neuroepithelium from nasal infections, chronic rhinitis, lack of airflow, and exposures to xenobiotics; (see Holt, 1917; Frühwald, 1935; Smith, 1935; Meurman, 1950; Liss and Gomez, 1958). Indeed, one can use the number of glomeruli of autopsy specimens to infer the amount of destruction of the olfactory epithelium. In a classic study, Smith (1942) did just that, counting the number of glomeruli to estimate age-related losses of human olfactory receptors. In his examination of 205 olfactory bulbs from 121 autopsy specimens, he concluded that the loss of the olfactory nerves begins soon after birth and continues throughout life at the rate of approximately 1% per year. However, considerable variability was noted at all ages and a reassessment of his data using medians rather than means suggests that glomerular loss is most evident after the fifth decade of life, more or less paralleling what is shown in **Figure 3** for odor identification.

Bhatnagar et al. (1987) quantitatively assessed the morphology of eight pairs of bulbs from women who died between the ages of 25 and 102 years. Corresponding bulb volumes, estimated for the ages of 25, 60, and 95 years by linear regression, were 50.02, 43.35, and 36.68 mm^3. Mean mitral cell numbers for these three age groups were 50,935, 32,718, and 14,501, respectively. Other cell types were not enumerated. As would be expected from the work of Smith (1942), the glomerular layer was markedly influenced by age and, in the older specimens, was discontinuous and evident only in the rostral areas of the bulb.

Some studies have noted, in brains from non-demented older persons, neurofibrillary tangles in the olfactory bulb that increase as a function of age. For example, Kishikawa et al. (1990) observed such tangles in 35.3% of olfactory bulbs from 133 individuals ranging from 40 to 91 years (mean = 64.3 years), only one of whom had dementia. Most of the tangles were within the anterior olfactory nucleus, although a few were found in mitral and tufted cells. This percentage increased to 40.5% when only those over the age of 50 years were included in the sample. Similar types of pathology have been noted in autopsied olfactory bulbs from young persons who had lived in highly polluted regions of Mexico City, in some cases in association with nanoparticles that have entered into the bulbs via the olfactory fila (Calderon-Garciduenas et al., 2010).

In the first of a series of important quantitative studies, Hinds and McNelly measured the volume of the glomerular, external plexiform, internal plexiform, and olfactory nerve layers of the olfactory bulb of Sprague Dawley rats at 3, 12, 24, 27, and 30 months of age (Hinds and McNelly, 1977). They also assessed the number of mitral cells and the volume of their nuclei, cell bodies, and dendritic trees, as well as the total length and mean cross-sectional area of the associated dendrites. Until the age of 24 months, a ~50% developmental increase in the volumes of each of the layers was observed, as was a doubling in the size of the volumes of the cell bodies and dendritic trees of the mitral cells. From 24 to 30 months, the volume of olfactory bulb layers decreased. Subsequently, the number of mitral cells also decreased. Although the total volume of mitral cell dendritic trees declined slightly from 24 to 27 months, the volume of individual mitral cell dendritic trees, as well as cell body and nuclear size, increased, presumably reflecting compensation for the decrease in mitral cell numbers.

In a subsequent study, these general findings were replicated in the Charles River rat strain (Hinds and McNelly, 1981), save for a lack of a decline in mitral cell number in the older animals. Concurrent assessment was also made of alterations in the olfactory epithelium. After 18 months, olfactory bulb volumes declined and, after 24 months, decreases in the average volumes of the mitral cell bodies and the glomerular dendrites were observed. A comparison of regression lines for changes in number of olfactory receptors on the septum with that of the size of mitral cell bodies suggested that the decline in receptor number began several months before the decline in mitral cell size. This implied that the bulbar changes were in response to the epithelial changes. In the remaining olfactory receptor cells, an increase in the number of synapses per cell within the glomeruli occurred in the oldest rats evaluated, implying compensatory responses.

Age-related changes in the volume of human olfactory bulbs have also been documented *in vivo* using magnetic resonance imaging (MRI) (Yousem et al., 1998; Buschhuter et al., 2008). However, such decrements are not specific to aging, are variable, and are plastic to some degree. Thus, olfactory bulb volume is reduced in cigarette smokers (Schriever et al., 2013) and in those with a number of neurological diseases or other disorders (Yousem et al., 1995b). These include acute depression (Negoias et al., 2010), Alzheimer's disease (Thomann et al., 2009), childhood abuse (Croy et al., 2013), chronic sinusitis (Rombaux et al., 2008), congential anosmia with and without Kallmann syndrome (Yousem et al., 1993, 1996; Abolmaali et al., 2002; Koenigkam-Santos et al., 2011; Levy et al., 2013), epilepsy (Hummel et al., 2012), head trauma (Yousem et al., 1995a; Doty et al., 1997; Landis et al., 2005; Jiang et al., 2009), multiple sclerosis (Goektas et al., 2011; Schmidt et al., 2011), Parkinson's disease (Wang et al., 2011b; Brodoehl et al., 2012), polyposis (Herzallah et al., 2013), schizophrenia (Turetsky et al., 2003; Nguyen et al., 2011), and prior upper respiratory infections associated with chronic smell loss (Rombaux et al., 2009). Such studies strongly suggest that olfactory bulb volume is a marker for olfactory function in general (Yousem et al., 1998; Turetsky et al., 2003; Buschhuter et al., 2008; Haehner et al., 2008; Hummel et al., 2011; Rombaux et al., 2012). Evidence of plasticity comes from observations that over time the shrinkage of olfactory bulbs in humans due to rhinosinusitis can be reversed as a result of treatment (Gudziol et al., 2009) and that rodent intrabulbar circuitry can recover from occlusion after reinstating nasal patency (Cummings and Belluscio, 2010).

CHANGES IN CENTRAL BRAIN REGIONS INVOLVED IN OLFACTORY PROCESSING

It is widely appreciated that aging is accompanied by decreased brain weight, cortical thickness, white matter integrity, and transmitter activity, and increased neuronal vulnerability, including early changes within brain structures associated with olfactory system processing (Kemper, 1984). Among such changes are disproportionate decrements in the volume of the hippocampus, amygdala, piriform cortex, anterior olfactory nucleus, and frontal poles of the brain. In a cohort of non-demented subjects ranging in age from 51 to 77 years, Segura et al. (2013) found that UPSIT scores were significantly correlated with the volume of the right amygdala and bilaterally with the volume of gray matter in the perirhinal and entorhinal cortices. Such scores were also inversely correlated with cortical thickness in the postcentral gyrus and with fractional anisotropy and mean diffusivity levels in the splenum of the corpus callosum and the superior longitudinal fasciculi.

A number of age-related neurodegenerative disease pathologies, including abnormal deposits of tau and α-synuclein, have been associated with olfactory dysfunction in older non-demented persons, suggesting that some age-related alterations may reflect "pre-clinical" neurodegenerative disease. For example, in a longitudinal clinicopathological study of 122 non-demented subjects, Wilson et al. (2007a) found inverse correlations between B-SIT scores obtained before death and the post-mortem density of neurofibrillary tangles in the entorhinal cortex, the CA1 subfield of the hippocampus, and the subiculum. Similar associations were found by this group between pre-mortem B-SIT scores and post-mortem measures of Lewy bodies within limbic and cortical brain regions (Wilson et al., 2011b), leading the authors to conclude that olfactory function is impaired in Lewy body disease even in otherwise asymptomatic individuals.

Persons with mild cognitive impairment (MCI) who convert to AD typically have more smell loss than MCI patients who do not convert (Croy et al., 2009). In AD, tau-related neurofibrillary pathology seems to be more closely linked to olfactory dysfunction than β-amyloid plaque pathology. Thus, some studies find no direct associations between the AD-related decrement in odor identification ability and brain β-amyloid, as measured by PET imaging of Pittsburgh compound B, an *in vivo* marker of brain amyloid levels (Bahar-Fuchs et al., 2010). This observation is consistent with post-mortem studies which, after controlling for the adverse influences of tau, find no strong associations between pre-mortem olfactory function and post-mortem levels of β-amyloid in olfactory eloquent brain regions of older individuals (Wilson et al., 2007a). It is noteworthy that anosmia, *per se*, is correlated with wide spread changes in gray matter within olfaction-related structures, including the piriform cortex, insular cortex, OFC, medial prefrontal cortex, hippocampus, parahippocampal gyrus, supramarginal gyrus, nucleus accumbens, subcallosal gyrus, and the medial and dorsolateral prefrontal cortices (Bitter et al., 2010).

Functional imaging studies, such as those employing fMRI and positron emission tomography (PET), also demonstrate age-related changes in the processing of olfactory information, as reflected by decrements in odor-induced activation in central olfactory pathways. It should be noted, however, that such decrements need not be indicative of the locus of dysfunction. This is because the activity of a given central brain region often depends upon input from other brain regions that themselves may be compromised. Nevertheless, such imaging does represent the overall functioning of the system. Yousem et al., in a pioneering fMRI study, found that odors activated fewer voxels within the right

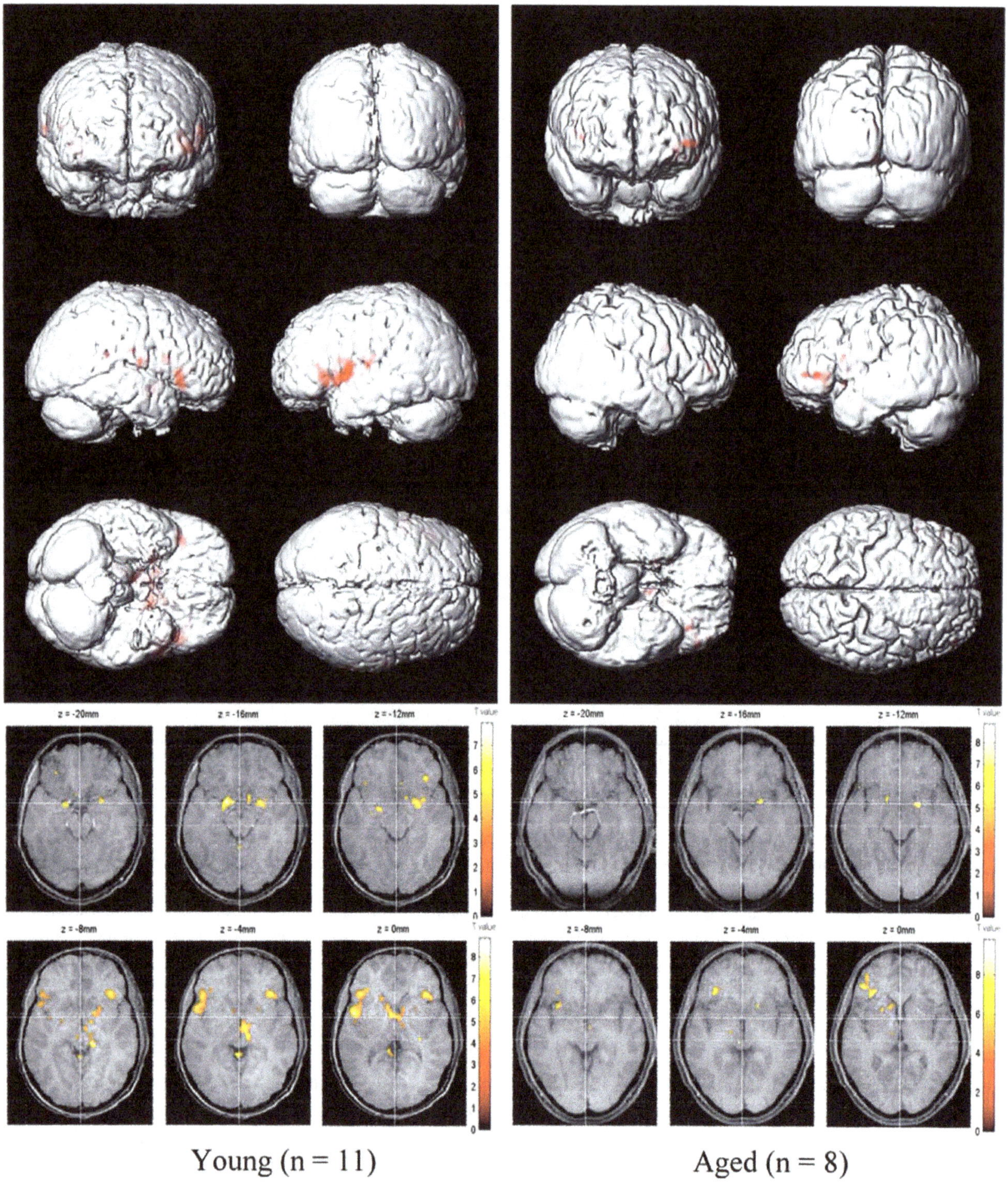

FIGURE 13 | Olfactory functional magnetic resonance imaging (fMRI) activation maps from 11 younger (left; mean age = 23.9 years) and 8 older (right; mean age = 66.4 years) persons to lavender and spearmint odors. Note greater activation in the younger subjects. From Wang et al. (2005), with permission.

inferior frontal and left and right superior frontal and perisylvian zones in old than in young persons (Yousem et al., 1999). Subsequently, Suzuki and his associates noted less fMRI odor-induced activation in 6 older persons than in 6 younger persons during an odor discrimination task in a region within the left orbital pole (Suzuki et al., 2001). Wang et al. (2005) found age-related decreases in activation in structures comprising the primary olfactory cortex, most notably in the right amygdala and piriform and periamygdaloid cortices (**Figure 13**). These investigators chose subjects whose UPSIT scores were within the normal age-adjusted range, although slightly lower scores were evident in the 11 young subjects (mean age = 23.9) than in the 8 older subjects (mean age = 66.4); respective UPSIT means = 37.3 and 34.1, $p = 0.0004$. More recently, Wong et al. (2010) found that a measure of nigrostriatal denervation in healthy elderly persons over the age 60 years, as determined by PET imaging of the brain dopamine transporter (DAT), was significantly correlated with UPSIT scores, suggesting that age-related declines in nigrostriatal function may account, in part, for age-related losses in smell ability.

NEUROCHEMICAL CHANGES IN THE BRAIN

It is well established that age-related changes occur in numerous enzyme, neurotransmitter, and neuromodulator systems within the brain. In many cases, the largest age-related decline occurs before the age of 60 years, as exemplified by enzymes involved in the synthesis of GABA (glutamate decarboxylase), acetylcholine (choline acetyltransferase), and both norepinephrine and dopamine (tyrosine hydroxylase) (Selkoe and Kosik, 1984). Hence, significant neurochemical changes are likely present prior to the onset of neuropathology and cognitive and motor phenotypes associated such age-related diseases as AD and PD. This implies that some such changes may "prime" the organism or lower the threshold for adverse influences from neural insults, mutations, and other deleterious factors in the elderly and could be, in fact, a critical substrate for the so-called "preclinical" stages of some age-related neurodegenerative diseases. Importantly, such neurochemical changes may be region specific, preferentially involving, for example, limbic structures early in the aging process (Strong, 1998). Imaging studies suggest that binding sites for a number of neurotransmitters are significantly decreased in the brains of older persons (Dewey et al., 1990; Rosier et al., 1996; Volkow et al., 2000).

While several age-related neurotransmitter deficiencies may contribute to the olfactory loss observed in elderly persons, one system stands out as being particularly prepotent—the cholinergic system. Acetylcholine is intimately involved in the modulation of olfactory function, such as increasing contrast and synchronization of odor-induced activity from the bulb to the piriform cortex and facilitating attention, odor learning, memory, and cortical plasticity (de Almeida et al., 2013). Cholinergic projections reach all sectors of the olfactory system from origins within the medial septum, the nucleus basalis of Meynert, and the horizontal and vertical diagonal band of Broca (Schliebs and Arendt, 2011). Patients with MCI exhibit olfactory deficits and cholinergic dysfunction prior to the onset of AD—dysfunction which is unaccompanied by significant cell loss (Schliebs and Arendt, 2011). Interestingly, cholinergic neurons directly modulate neural activity within the olfactory bulb and tonically inhibit, along with some other neurotransmitters, the activity of microglial cells critical for immune responses to brain damage and foreign agents (Doty, 2012a). When such modulation is significantly perturbed, the release of inhibition on the microglial cells can occur, resulting in the secretion of inflammatory mediators and other factors which, in extreme instances, can be deleterious to neurons (Tang et al., 2007; Lalancette-Hebert et al., 2009).

It is noteworthy that the relative magnitude of olfactory deficits of a number of neurodegenerative and neurodevelopmental diseases appears to be associated with the relative damage to the basal cholinergic system. Such disorders include AD, PD, Down syndrome, Parkinson-Dementia complex of Guam, Korsakoff syndrome, amyotrophic lateral sclerosis, schizophrenia, and progressive supranuclear palsy (for olfactory test scores, see, e.g., Mair et al., 1986; Doty et al., 1987, 1988, 1991, 1993; Kopala et al., 1994; Sajjadian et al., 1994; Wenning et al., 1995; McKeown et al., 1996; for quantitative assessments of basal cholinergic cell losses or volumes, see Arendt et al., 1983; Nakano and Hirano, 1983, 1984; Casanova et al., 1985; Rogers et al., 1985; Vogels et al., 1990; Yoshida et al., 1992; Kasashima and Oda, 2003). Age-related damage to the nucleus basalis has also been observed, although its magnitude is not generally as marked as that seen in AD and PD.

CONCLUSION

This review addressed the functional and pathophysiological changes that occur in the human olfactory system as a result of age. Basic information about the anatomy, physiology, and measurement of this primary sensory system was provided, along with a general overview of the nature of age-related changes that occur in olfactory perception. Numerous factors that likely contribute to such changes were assessed, including changes in autonomic control of nasal engorgement, increased propensity for nasal disease, cumulative damage to the olfactory epithelium from environmental insults, decrements in protective metabolizing enzymes in the olfactory mucosa, occlusion of the foramina of the cribriform plate, loss of selectivity of olfactory receptor neurons to odorants, changes in neurotransmitter and neuromodulator systems, and neuropathological processes such as the expression of aberrant proteins associated with such neurodegenerative diseases as AD and PD. As apparent from the research examined in this review, it is likely that there are multiple determinants of the olfactory loss of older persons, although the relative importance of each is yet to be established.

AUTHOR CONTRIBUTIONS

Dr. Doty wrote the first draft of the manuscript. Dr. Kamath contributed to the literature review and to the writing of two subsequent drafts. Both authors were involved in the writing of the final manuscript.

ACKNOWLEDGMENTS

This research was supported by the following contract: DOD W81XWH-09-1-0467.

REFERENCES

Abolmaali, N. D., Hietschold, V., Vogl, T. J., Huttenbrink, K. B., and Hummel, T. (2002). MR evaluation in patients with isolated anosmia since birth or early childhood. *Am. J. Neuroradiol.* 23, 157–164.

Allen, W. F. (1928). Effect on respiration, blood pressure, and carotid pulse of various inhaled and insufflated vapors when stimulating one cranial nerve and various combinations of cranial nerves. *Amer. J. Physiol.* 87, 319–325.

Arendt, T., Bigl, V., Arendt, A., and Tennstedt, A. (1983). Loss of neurons in the nucleus basalis of Meynert in Alzheimer's disease, paralysis agitans and Korsakoff's disease. *Acta Neuropathol.* 61, 101–108. doi: 10.1007/BF00697388

Bahar-Fuchs, A., Chetelat, G., Villemagne, V. L., Moss, S., Pike, K., Masters, C. L., et al. (2010). Olfactory deficits and amyloid-beta burden in Alzheimer's disease, mild cognitive impairment, and healthy aging: a PiB PET study. *J. Alzheimers. Dis.* 22, 1081–1087.

Barresi, M., Ciurleo, R., Giacoppo, S., Foti, C. V., Celi, D., Bramanti, P., et al. (2012). Evaluation of olfactory dysfunction in neurodegenerative diseases. *J. Neurol. Sci.* 323, 16–24. doi: 10.1016/j.jns.2012.08.028

Bedard, A., and Parent, A. (2004). Evidence of newly generated neurons in the human olfactory bulb. *Dev. Brain Res.* 151, 159–168. doi: 10.1016/j.devbrainres.2004.03.021

Bende, M. (1983). Blood flow with 133Xe in human nasal mucosa in relation to age, sex and body position. *Acta Otolaryngol.* 96, 175–179. doi: 10.3109/00016488309132889

Bensafi, M., Rouby, C., Farget, V., Bertrand, B., Vigouroux, M., and Holley, A. (2002). Influence of affective and cognitive judgments on autonomic parameters during inhalation of pleasant and unpleasant odors in humans. *Neurosci. Lett.* 319, 162–166. doi: 10.1016/S0304-3940(01)02572-1

Bhandawat, V., Reisert, J., and Yau, K. W. (2005). Elementary response of olfactory receptor neurons to odorants. *Science* 308, 1931–1934. doi: 10.1126/science.1109886

Bhatnagar, K. P., Kennedy, R. C., Baron, G., and Greenberg, R. A. (1987). Number of mitral cells and the bulb volume in the aging human olfactory bulb: a quantitative morphological study. *Anat. Rec.* 218, 73–87. doi: 10.1002/ar.1092180112

Bitter, T., Gudziol, H., Burmeister, H. P., Mentzel, H. J., Guntinas-Lichius, O., and Gaser, C. (2010). Anosmia leads to a loss of gray matter in cortical brain areas. *Chem. Senses* 35, 407–415. doi: 10.1093/chemse/bjq028

Borders, A. S., Hersh, M. A., Getchell, M. L., van, R. N., Cohen, D. A., Stromberg, A. J., et al. (2007). Macrophage-mediated neuroprotection and neurogenesis in the olfactory epithelium. *Physiol. Genomics* 31, 531–543. doi: 10.1152/physiolgenomics.00008.2007

Bramerson, A., Johansson, L., Ek, L., Nordin, S., and Bende, M. (2004). Prevalence of olfactory dysfunction: the skovde population-based study. *Laryngoscope* 114, 733–737. doi: 10.1097/00005537-200404000-00026

Breer, H. (1994). Odor recognition and second messenger signaling in olfactory receptor neurons. *Sem. Cell Biol.* 5, 25–32. doi: 10.1006/scel.1994.1004

Brodoehl, S., Klingner, C., Volk, G. F., Bitter, T., Witte, O. W., and Redecker, C. (2012). Decreased olfactory bulb volume in idiopathic Parkinson's disease detected by 3.0-Tesla magnetic resonance imaging. *Mov. Disord.* 27, 1019–1025. doi: 10.1002/mds.25087

Bromley, S. M., and Doty, R. L. (1995). Odor recognition memory is better under bilateral than unilateral test conditions. *Cortex* 31, 25–40. doi: 10.1016/S0010-9452(13)80103-7

Buschhuter, D., Smitka, M., Puschmann, S., Gerber, J. C., Witt, M., Abolmaali, N. D., et al. (2008). Correlation between olfactory bulb volume and olfactory function. *Neuroimage* 42, 498–502. doi: 10.1016/j.neuroimage.2008.05.004

Cain, W. S., Gent, J., Catalanotto, F. A., and Goodspeed, R. B. (1983). Clinical evaluation of olfaction. *Am. J. Otolaryngol.* 4, 252–256. doi: 10.1016/S0196-0709(83)80068-4

Cain, W. S., and Gent, J. F. (1991). Olfactory sensitivity: reliability, generality, and association with aging. *J. Exp. Psychol. Hum Percept. Perform.* 7, 382–391. doi: 10.1037/0096-1523.17.2.382

Cain, W. S., and Stevens, J. C. (1989). Uniformity of olfactory loss in aging. *Ann. N.Y. Acad. Sci.* 561, 29–38. doi: 10.1111/j.1749-6632.1989.tb20967.x

Calderon-Garciduenas, L., Franco-Lira, M., Henriquez-Roldan, C., Osnaya, N., Gonzalez-Maciel, A., Reynoso-Robles, R., et al. (2010). Urban air pollution: influences on olfactory function and pathology in exposed children and young adults. *Exp. Tox. Pathol.* 62, 91–102. doi: 10.1016/j.etp.2009.02.117

Calhoun-Haney, R., and Murphy, C. (2005). Apolipoprotein epsilon4 is associated with more rapid decline in odor identification than in odor threshold or dementia rating scale scores. *Brain Cogn.* 58, 178–182. doi: 10.1016/j.bandc.2004.10.004

Camara, C. G., and Harding, J. W. (1984). Thymidine incorporation in the olfactory epithelium of mice: early exponential response induced by olfactory neurectomy. *Brain Res.* 308, 63–68. doi: 10.1016/0006-8993(84)90917-X

Cameron, E. L., and Doty, R. L. (2013). Odor identification testing in children and young adults using the smell wheel. *Int. J. Pediatr. Otorhinolaryngol.* 77, 346–350. doi: 10.1016/j.ijporl.2012.11.022

Casanova, M. F., Walker, L. C., Whitehouse, P. J., and Price, D. L. (1985). Abnormalities of the nucleus basalis in Down's syndrome. *Ann. Neurol.* 18, 310–313. doi: 10.1002/ana.410180306

Chalke, H. D., Dewhurst, J. R., and Ward, C. W. (1958). Loss of smell in old people. *Public Health* 72, 223–230. doi: 10.1016/S0033-3506(58)80053-0

Chess, A., Simon, I., Cedar, H., and Axel, R. (1994). Allelic inactivation regulates olfactory receptor gene expression. *Cell* 78, 823–834. doi: 10.1016/S0092-8674(94)90562-2

Cho, S. H., Hong, S. J., Han, B., Lee, S. H., Suh, L., Norton, J., et al. (2012). Age-related differences in the pathogenesis of chronic rhinosinusitis. *J. Allergy Clin. Immunol.* 129, 858–860. doi: 10.1016/j.jaci.2011.12.002

Choudhury, E. S., Moberg, P., and Doty, R. L. (2003). Influences of age and sex on a microencapsulated odor memory test. *Chem. Senses* 28, 799–805. doi: 10.1093/chemse/bjg072

Cleland, T. A., and Linster, C. (2003). "Central olfactory structures," in *Handbook of Olfaction and Gustation.* 2nd Edn., ed R. L. Doty (New York, NY: Marcel Dekker), 165–180.

Cohen, N. A. (2006). Sinonasal mucociliary clearance in health and disease. *Ann. Otol. Rhinol. Laryngol. Suppl* 196, 20–26.

Conti, M. Z., Vicini-Chilovi, B., Riva, M., Zanetti, M., Liberini, P., Padovani, A., et al. (2013). Odor identification deficit predicts clinical conversion from mild cognitive impairment to dementia due to Alzheimer's disease. *Arch. Clin. Neuropsychol.* 28, 391–399. doi: 10.1093/arclin/act032

Covington, J. W., Geisler, M. W., Polich, J., and Murphy, C. (1999). Normal aging and odor intensity effects on the olfactory event-related potential. *Int. J. Psychophysiol.* 32, 205–214. doi: 10.1016/S0167-8760(99)00012-4

Cowart, B. J. (1989). Relationships between taste and smell across the adult life span. *Ann. N.Y. Acad. Sci.* 561, 39–55. doi: 10.1111/j.1749-6632.1989.tb20968.x

Croy, I., Lange, K., Krone, F., Negoias, S., Seo, H. S., and Hummel, T. (2009). Comparison between odor thresholds for phenyl ethyl alcohol and butanol. *Chem. Senses.* 34, 523–527. doi: 10.1093/chemse/bjp029

Croy, I., Negoias, S., Symmank, A., Schellong, J., Joraschky, P., and Hummel, T. (2013). Reduced olfactory bulb volume in adults with a history of childhood maltreatment. *Chem. Senses* 38, 679–684. doi: 10.1093/chemse/bjt037

Cummings, D. M., and Belluscio, L. (2010). Continuous neural plasticity in the olfactory intrabulbar circuitry. *J. Neurosci.* 30, 9172–9180. doi: 10.1523/JNEUROSCI.1717-10.2010

de Almeida, L., Idiart, M., and Linster, C. (2013). A model of cholinergic modulation in olfactory bulb and piriform cortex. *J. Neurophysiol.* 109, 1360–1377. doi: 10.1152/jn.00577.2012

Deems, D. A., and Doty, R. L. (1987). Age-related changes in the phenyl ethyl alcohol odor detection threshold. *Trans. Pa. Acad. Ophthalmol. Otolaryngol.* 39, 646–650.

De Lorenzo, A. J. (1957). Electron microscopic observations of the olfactory mucosa and olfactory nerve. *J. Biophys. Biochem. Cytol.* 3, 839–850. doi: 10.1083/jcb.3.6.839

Devanand, D. P., Michaels-Marston, K. S., Liu, X., Pelton, G. H., Padilla, M., Marder, K., et al. (2000). Olfactory deficits in patients with mild cognitive impairment predict Alzheimer's disease at follow-up. *Am. J. Psychiatry* 157, 1399–1405. doi: 10.1176/appi.ajp.157.9.1399

Dewey, S. L., Volkow, N. D., Logan, J., MacGregor, R. R., Fowler, J. S., Schlyer, D. J., et al. (1990). Age-related decreases in muscarinic cholinergic receptor binding in the human brain measured with positron emission tomography (PET). *J. Neurosci. Res.* 27, 569–575. doi: 10.1002/jnr.490270418

Ding, X., and Dahl, A. R. (2003). "Olfactory mucosa: composition, enzymatic localization, and metabolism," in *Handbook of Olfaction and Gustation.* 2nd Edn., ed R. L. Doty (New York, NY: Marcel Dekker), 51–73.

Doty, R. L. (1995). *The Smell Identification TestTM Administration Manual.* 3rd Edn. Haddon Heights, NJ: Sensonics, Inc.

Doty, R. L. (2012a). Olfaction in Parkinson's disease and related disorders. *Neurobiol. Dis.* 46, 527–552. doi: 10.1016/j.nbd.2011.10.026

Doty, R. L. (2012b). Olfactory dysfunction in Parkinson disease. *Nat. Rev. Neurol.* 8, 329–339. doi: 10.1038/nrneurol.2012.80

Doty, R. L., Deems, D. A., and Stellar, S. (1988). Olfactory dysfunction in parkinsonism: a general deficit unrelated to neurologic signs, disease stage, or disease duration. *Neurology* 38, 1237–1244. doi: 10.1212/WNL.38.8.1237

Doty, R. L., Golbe, L. I., McKeown, D. A., Stern, M. B., Lehrach, C. M., and Crawford, D. (1993). Olfactory testing differentiates between progressive supranuclear palsy and idiopathic Parkinson's disease. *Neurology* 43, 962–965. doi: 10.1212/WNL.43.5.962

Doty, R. L., and Laing, D. A. (2003). "Psychophysical measurement of human olfactory function, including odorant mixture assessment," in *Handbook of Olfaction and Gustation*. 2nd Edn., ed R. L. Doty (New York, NY: Marcel Dekker), 203–228. doi: 10.1201/9780203911457

Doty, R. L., Marcus, A., and Lee, W. W. (1996). Development of the 12-item cross-cultural smell identification test (CC-SIT). *Laryngoscope* 106, 353–356. doi: 10.1097/00005537-199603000-00021

Doty, R. L., McKeown, D. A., Lee, W. W., and Shaman, P. (1995). A study of the test-retest reliability of ten olfactory tests. *Chem. Senses* 20, 645–656. doi: 10.1093/chemse/20.6.645

Doty, R. L., Perl, D. P., Steele, J. C., Chen, K. M., Pierce, J. D. Jr., Reyes, P., et al. (1991). Odor identification deficit of the parkinsonism-dementia complex of Guam: equivalence to that of Alzheimer's and idiopathic Parkinson's disease. *Neurology* 41, 77–80. doi: 10.1212/WNL.41.5_Suppl_2.77

Doty, R. L., Petersen, I., Mensah, N., and Christensen, K. (2011). Genetic and environmental influences on odor identification ability in the very old. *Psychol. Aging* 26, 864–871. doi: 10.1037/a0023263

Doty, R. L., Reyes, P. F., and Gregor, T. (1987). Presence of both odor identification and detection deficits in Alzheimer's disease. *Brain Res. Bull.* 18, 597–600. doi: 10.1016/0361-9230(87)90129-8

Doty, R. L., Shaman, P., Applebaum, S. L., Giberson, R., Siksorski, L., and Rosenberg, L. (1984a). Smell identification ability: changes with age. *Science* 226, 1441–1443. doi: 10.1126/science.6505700

Doty, R. L., Shaman, P., and Dann, M. (1984b). Development of the University of Pennsylvania smell identification test: a standardized microencapsulated test of olfactory function. *Physiol. Behav.* 32, 489–502. doi: 10.1016/0031-9384(84)90269-5

Doty, R. L., Smith, R., McKeown, D. A., and Raj, J. (1994). Tests of human olfactory function: principal components analysis suggests that most measure a common source of variance. *Percept. Psychophys.* 56, 701–707. doi: 10.3758/BF03208363

Doty, R. L., Yousem, D. M., Pham, L. T., Kreshak, A. A., Geckle, R., and Lee, W. W. (1997). Olfactory dysfunction in patients with head trauma. *Arch. Neurol.* 54, 1131–1140. doi: 10.1001/archneur.1997.00550210061014

Duda, J. E. (2010). Olfactory system pathology as a model of Lewy neurodegenerative disease. *J. Neurol. Sci.* 289, 49–54. doi: 10.1016/j.jns.2009.08.042

Duffy, V. B., Backstrand, J. R., and Ferris, A. M. (1995). Olfactory dysfunction and related nutritional risk in free-living, elderly women. *J. Am. Diet. Assoc.* 8, 879–884. doi: 10.1016/S0002-8223(95)00244-8

Edelstein, D. R. (1996). Aging of the normal nose in adults. *Laryngoscope* 106, 1–25. doi: 10.1097/00005537-199609001-00001

Engen, T., Kuisma, J. E., and Eimas, P. D. (1973). Short-term memory of odors. *J. Exp. Psychol.* 99, 222–225. doi: 10.1037/h0034645

Evans, W. J., Cui, L., and Starr, A. (1995). Olfactory event-related potentials in normal human subjects: effects of age and gender. *EEG Clin. Neurophysiol.* 95, 293–301. doi: 10.1016/0013-4694(95)00055-4

Farajnia, S., Deboer, T., Rohling, J. H., Meijer, J. H., and Michel, S. (2014). Aging of the suprachiasmatic clock. *Neuroscientist* 20, 44–55. doi: 10.1177/1073858413 498936

Federico, G., Maremmani, C., Cinquanta, L., Baroncelli, G. I., Fattori, B., and Saggese, G. (1999). Mucus of the human olfactory epithelium contains the insulin-like growth factor-I system which is altered in some neurodegenerative diseases. *Brain Res.* 835, 306–314. doi: 10.1016/S0006-8993(99)01614-5

Feron, F., Mackay-Sim, A., Andrieu, J. L., Matthaei, K. I., Holley, A., and Sicard, G. (1999). Stress induces neurogenesis in non-neuronal cell cultures of adult olfactory epithelium. *Neuroscience.* 88, 571–583. doi: 10.1016/S0306-4522(98)00233 -4

Fordyce, I. D. (1961). Olfaction tests. *Br. J. Ind. Med.* 18, 213–215.

Frank, R. A., Dulay, M. F., and Gesteland, R. C. (2003). Assessment of the sniff magnitude test as a clinical test of olfactory function. *Physiol. Behav.* 78, 195–204. doi: 10.1016/S0031-9384(02)00965-4

Frank, R. A., Dulay, M. F., Niergarth, K. A., and Gesteland, R. C. (2004). A comparison of the sniff magnitude test and the University of Pennsylvania smell identification test in children and nonnative english speakers. *Physiol. Behav.* 81, 475–480. doi: 10.1016/j.physbeh.2004.02.020

Frank, R. A., Gesteland, R. C., Bailie, J., Rybalsky, K., Seiden, A., and Dulay, M. F. (2006). Characterization of the sniff magnitude test. *Arch. Otolaryngol. Head Neck Surg.* 132, 532–536. doi: 10.1001/archotol.132.5.532

Frühwald, V. (1935). Die Folgen des einseitigen Nasenverschlusses auf die Riechschleimhaut und auf den Bulbus und Tractus olfactorius. *Archiv. fur Ohren Nasen und Kehlkopfheilkunde* 139, 153–173. doi: 10.1007/BF01586653

Frye, R. E. (2003). "Nasal patency and the aerodynamics of nasal airflow: measurement by rhinomanometry and acoustic rhinometry, and the influence of pharmacological agents," in *Handbook of Olfaction and Gustation*. 2nd Edn., ed R. L. Doty (New York, NY: Marcel Dekker), 439–460.

Frye, R. E., and Doty, R. L. (1992). *Chemical Signals in Vertebrates*, Vol. VI, eds R. L. Doty and D. Müller-Schwarze. (New York, NY: Plenum), 595–596. doi: 10.1007/978-1-4757-9655-1_91

Gaskell, B. A., Hext, P. M., Pigott, G. H., Doe, J. E., and Hodge, M. C. (1990). Olfactory and hepatic changes following a single inhalation exposure of 3-trifluoromethyl pyridine in rats: concentration and temporal aspects. *Toxicology* 62, 35–51. doi: 10.1016/0300-483X(90)90029-G

Getchell, M. L., and Getchell, T. V. (1992). Fine structural aspects of secretion and extrinsic innervation in the olfactory mucosa. *Microsc. Res. Tech.* 23, 111–127. doi: 10.1002/jemt.1070230203

Getchell, T. V., Krishna, N. S., Dhooper, N., Sparks, D. L., and Getchell, M. L. (1995). Human olfactory receptor neurons express heat shock protein 70: age-related trends. *Ann. Otol. Rhinol. Laryngol.* 104, 47–56.

Gevins, A. S., and Remond, A. (1987). *Methods of Analysis of Brain Electrical and Magnetic Signals*. New York, NY: Elsevier.

Gilbert, A. N. (1989). Reciprocity versus rhythmicity in spontaneous alternations of nasal airflow. *Chronobiol. Int.* 6, 251–257. doi: 10.3109/07420528909056926

Gladysheva, O., Kukushkina, D., and Martynova, G. (1986). Glycoprotein composition of olfactory mucus in vertebrates. *Acta Histochem.* 78, 141–146. doi: 10.1016/S0065-1281(86)80047-2

Glusman, G., Yanai, I., Rubin, I., and Lancet, D. (2001). The complete human olfactory subgenome. *Genome Res.* 11, 685–702. doi: 10.1101/gr.171001

Goektas, O., Schmidt, F., Bohner, G., Erb, K., Ludemann, L., Dahlslett, B., et al. (2011). Olfactory bulb volume and olfactory function in patients with multiple sclerosis. *Rhinology* 49, 221–226. doi: 10.4193/Rhino10.136

Graves, A. B., Bowen, J. D., Rajaram, L., McCormick, W. C., McCurry, S. M., Schellenberg, G. D., et al. (1999). Impaired olfaction as a marker for cognitive decline: interaction with apolipoprotein E epsilon4 status. *Neurology* 53, 1480–1487. doi: 10.1212/WNL.53.7.1480

Griep, M. I., Mets, T. F., Collys, K., Vogelaere, P., Laska, M., and Massart, D. L. (1997). Odour perception in relation to age, general health, anthropometry and dental state. *Arch. Gerontol. Geriatr.* 25, 263–275. doi: 10.1016/S0167-4943(97)00017-4

Gudziol, V., Buschhuter, D., Abolmaali, N., Gerber, J., Rombaux, P., and Hummel, T. (2009). Increasing olfactory bulb volume due to treatment of chronic rhinosinusitis–a longitudinal study. *Brain* 132, 3096–3101. doi: 10.1093/brain/awp243

Haehner, A., Rodewald, A., Gerber, J. C., and Hummel, T. (2008). Correlation of olfactory function with changes in the volume of the human olfactory bulb. *Arch. Otolaryngol. Head Neck Surg.* 134, 621–624. doi: 10.1001/archotol.134. 6.621

Harkema, J. R., Carey, S. A., and Wagner, J. G. (2006). The nose revisited: a brief review of the comparative structure, function, and toxicologic pathology of the nasal epithelium. *Toxicol. Pathol.* 34, 252–269. doi: 10.1080/01926230600713475

Hedner, M., Larsson, M., Arnold, N., Zucco, G. M., and Hummel, T. (2010a). Cognitive factors in odor detection, odor discrimination, and odor identification tasks. *J. Clin. Exp. Neuropsychol.* 32, 1062–1067. doi: 10.1080/1380339100 3683070

Hedner, M., Nilsson, L. G., Olofsson, J. K., Bergman, O., Eriksson, E., Nyberg, L., et al. (2010b). Age-related olfactory decline is associated with the BDNF Val66met polymorphism: evidence from a population-based study. *Front. Aging Neurosci.* 2:24. doi: 10.3389/fnagi.2010.00024

Herting, B., Schulze, S., Reichmann, H., Haehner, A., and Hummel, T. (2008). A longitudinal study of olfactory function in patients with idiopathic Parkinson's disease. *J. Neurol.* 255, 367–370. doi: 10.1007/s00415-008-0665-5

Herzallah, I. R., Askar, S. M., Amer, H. S., Ahmed, A. F., El-Anwar, M. W., and Eesa, M. H. (2013). Olfactory bulb volume changes in patients with sinonasal polyposis: a magnetic resonance imaging study. *Otolaryngol. Head Neck Surg.* 148, 689–693. doi: 10.1177/0194599813477606

Hinds, J. W., and McNelly, N. A. (1977). Aging of the rat olfactory bulb: growth and atrophy of constituent layers and changes in size and number of mitral cells. *J. Comp. Neurol.* 72, 345–367. doi: 10.1002/cne.901710304

Hinds, J. W., and McNelly, N. A. (1981). Aging in the rat olfactory system: correlation of changes in the olfactory epithelium and olfactory bulb. *J. Comp. Neurol.* 203, 441–453. doi: 10.1002/cne.902030308

Hirai, T., Kojima, S., Shimada, A., Umemura, T., Sakai, M., and Itakura, C. (1996). Age-related changes in the olfactory system of dogs. *Neuropathol. Appl. Neurobiol.* 22, 531–539. doi: 10.1111/j.1365-2990.1996.tb01132.x

Holley, A., Duchamp, A., Revial, M. F., and Juge, A. (1974). Qualitative and quantitative discrimination in the frog olfactory receptors: analysis from electrophysiological data. *Ann. N.Y. Acad. Sci.* 237, 102–128. doi: 10.1111/j.1749-6632.1974.tb49847.x

Holt, C. M. (1917). Studies on the olfactory bulbs of the albino rat. I. Experiments to determine the effect of a defective diet and of exercise upon the weight of the olfactory bulbs. *J. Comp. Neurol.* 27, 201–234. doi: 10.1002/cne.900270203

Hosoya, Y., and Yashida, H. (1937). Über die bioelektrische Erscheinungen an der Riechschleimhaut. *Jpn. J. Med. Sci. III. Biophys.* 5, 22–23.

Huart, C., Legrain, V., Hummel, T., Rombaux, P., and Mouraux, A. (2012). Time-frequency analysis of chemosensory event-related potentials to characterize the cortical representation of odors in humans. *PLoS ONE* 7:e33221. doi: 10.1371/journal.pone.0033221

Hummel, T., Barz, S., Pauli, E., and Kobal, G. (1998). Chemosensory event-related potentials change with age. *Electroencephalogr. Clin. Neurophysiol.* 108, 208–217. doi: 10.1016/S0168-5597(97)00074-9

Hummel, T., Henkel, S., Negoias, S., Galvan, J. R., Bogdanov, V., Hopp, P., et al. (2012). Olfactory bulb volume in patients with temporal lobe epilepsy. *J. Neurol.* 260, 1004–1008. doi: 10.1007/s00415-012-6741-x

Hummel, T., Sekinger, B., Wolf, S. R., Pauli, E., and Kobal, G. (1997). "Sniffin' sticks": olfactory performance assessed by the combined testing of odor identification, odor discrimination and olfactory threshold. *Chem. Senses* 22, 39–52. doi: 10.1093/chemse/22.1.39

Hummel, T., Smitka, M., Puschmann, S., Gerber, J. C., Schaal, B., and Buschhuter, D. (2011). Correlation between olfactory bulb volume and olfactory function in children and adolescents. *Exp. Brain Res.* 214, 285–291. doi: 10.1007/s00221-011-2832-7

Iranzo, A., Serradell, M., Vilaseca, I., Valldeoriola, F., Salamero, M., Molina, C., et al. (2013). Longitudinal assessment of olfactory function in idiopathic REM sleep behavior disorder. Parkinsonism *Relat. Disord.* 19, 600–604. doi: 10.1016/j.parkreldis.2013.02.009

Iwai, N., Zhou, Z., Roop, D. R., and Behringer, R. R. (2008). Horizontal basal cells are multipotent progenitors in normal and injured adult olfactory epithelium. *Stem Cells* 26, 1298–1306. doi: 10.1634/stemcells.2007-0891

Jarvis, D., Newson, R., Lotvall, J., Hastan, D., Tomassen, P., Keil, T., et al. (2012). Asthma in adults and its association with chronic rhinosinusitis: the GA2LEN survey in Europe. *Allergy* 67, 91–98. doi: 10.1111/j.1398-9995.2011.02709.x

Jehl, C., Royet, J. P., and Holley, A. (1995). Odor discrimination and recognition memory as a function of familiarization. *Percept. Psychophys.* 57, 1002–1011. doi: 10.3758/BF03205459

Jiang, R. S., Chai, J. W., Chen, W. H., Fuh, W. B., Chiang, C. M., and Chen, C. C. (2009). Olfactory bulb volume in Taiwanese patients with posttraumatic anosmia. *Am. J. Rhinol. Allergy* 23, 582–584. doi: 10.2500/ajra.2009.23.3370

Johnson, B. A., and Leon, M. (2007). Chemotopic odorant coding in a mammalian olfactory system. *J. Comp. Neurol.* 503, 1–34. doi: 10.1002/cne.21396

Jones-Gotman, M., and Zatorre, R. J. (1988). Olfactory identification deficits in patients with focal cerebral excision. *Neuropsychologia* 26, 387–400. doi: 10.1016/0028-3932(88)90093-0

Jonsson, F. U., Moller, P., and Olsson, M. J. (2011). Olfactory working memory: effects of verbalization on the 2-back task. *Mem. Cogn.* 39, 1023–1032. doi: 10.3758/s13421-011-0080-5

Joyner, R. E. (1963). Olfactory acuity in an industrial population. *J. Occup. Med.* 5, 37–42.

Kajiya, K., Inaki, K., Tanaka, M., Haga, T., Kataoka, H., and Touhara, K. (2001). Molecular bases of odor discrimination: reconstitution of olfactory receptors that recognize overlapping sets of odorants. *J. Neurosci.* 21, 6018–6025.

Kalmey, J. K., Thewissen, J. G., and Dluzen, D. E. (1998). Age-related size reduction of foramina in the cribriform plate. *Anat. Rec.* 251, 326–329. doi: 10.1002/(SICI)1097-0185(199807)251:3<326::AID-AR7>3.3.CO;2-#

Kam, M., Curtis, M. A., McGlashan, S. R., Connor, B., Nannmark, U., and Faull, R. L. (2009). The cellular composition and morphological organization of the rostral migratory stream in the adult human brain. *J. Chem. Neuroanat.* 37, 196–205. doi: 10.1016/j.jchemneu.2008.12.009

Kaneda, H., Maeshima, K., Goto, N., Kobayakawa, T., Ayabe-Kanamura, S., and Saito, S. (2000). Decline in taste and odor discrimination abilities with age, and relationship between gustation and olfaction. *Chem. Senses* 25, 331–337. doi: 10.1093/chemse/25.3.331

Karpa, M. J., Gopinath, B., Rochtchina, E., Jie, J. W., Cumming, R. G., Sue, C. M., et al. (2010). Prevalence and neurodegenerative or other associations with olfactory impairment in an older community. *J. Aging Health* 22, 154–168. doi: 10.1177/0898264309353066

Kasashima, S., and Oda, Y. (2003). Cholinergic neuronal loss in the basal forebrain and mesopontine tegmentum of progressive supranuclear palsy and corticobasal degeneration. *Acta Neuropathol.* 105, 117–124. doi: 10.1007/s00401-002-0621-x

Katoh, H., Shibata, S., Fukuda, K., Sato, M., Satoh, E., Nagoshi, N., et al. (2011). The dual origin of the peripheral olfactory system: placode and neural crest. *Mol. Brain* 4:34. doi: 10.1186/1756-6606-4-34

Kay, L. M., and Sherman, S. M. (2007). An argument for an olfactory thalamus. *Trends Neurosci.* 30, 47–53. doi: 10.1016/j.tins.2006.11.007

Kemper, T. (1984). "Neuroanatomical and neuropathological changes during age and dementia," in *Clinical Neurology of Aging*, ed M. L. Albert (New York, NY: Oxford University Press), 3–67.

Kimbrell, G. M., and Furchtgott, E. (1963). The effect of aging on olfactory threshold. *J. Gerontol.* 18, 364–365. doi: 10.1093/geronj/18.4.364

Kirstein, C. L., Coopersmith, R., Bridges, R. J., and Leon, M. (1991). Glutathione levels in olfactory and non-olfactory neural structures of rats. *Brain Res.* 543, 341–346. doi: 10.1016/0006-8993(91)90047-Y

Kishikawa, M., Iseki, M., Nishimura, M., Sekine, I., and Fujii, H. (1990). A histopathological study on senile changes in the human olfactory bulb. *Acta Pathol. Jpn.* 40, 255–260. doi: 10.1111/j.1440-1827.1990.tb01559.x

Kleemann, A. M., Kopietz, R., Albrecht, J., Schopf, V., Pollatos, O., Schreder, T., et al. (2009). Investigation of breathing parameters during odor perception and olfactory imagery. *Chem. Senses* 34, 1–9. doi: 10.1093/chemse/bjn042

Kobal, G., Hummel, T., Sekinger, B., Barz, S., Roscher, S., and Wolf, S. (1996). "Sniffin' sticks": screening of olfactory performance. *Rhinology* 34, 222–226.

Kobal, G., Klimek, L., Wolfensberger, M., Gudziol, H., Temmel, A., Owen, C. M., et al. (2000). Multicenter investigation of 1,036 subjects using a standardized method for the assessment of olfactory function combining tests of odor identification, odor discrimination, and olfactory thresholds. *Eur. Arch. Otorhinolaryngol.* 257, 205–211. doi: 10.1007/s004050050223

Kobayashi, M., Saito, S., Kobayakawa, T., Deguchi, Y., and Costanzo, R. M. (2006). Cross-cultural comparison of data using the odor stick identification test for Japanese (OSIT-J). *Chem Senses* 31, 335–342. doi: 10.1093/chemse/bjj037

Koenigkam-Santos, M., Santos, A. C., Versiani, B. R., Diniz, P. R., Junior, J. E., and de Castro, M. (2011). Quantitative magnetic resonance imaging evaluation of the olfactory system in Kallmann syndrome: correlation with a clinical smell test. *Neuroendocrinology* 94, 209–217. doi: 10.1159/000328437

Kopala, L. C., Good, K. P., and Honer, W. G. (1994). Olfactory hallucinations and olfactory identification ability in patients with schizophrenia and other psychiatric disorders. *Schizophr. Res.* 12, 205–211. doi: 10.1016/0920-9964(94)90030-2

Koskinen, S., Vento, S., Malmberg, H., and Tuorila, H. (2004). Correspondence between three olfactory tests and suprathreshold odor intensity ratings. *Acta Otolaryngol. (Stockh)* 124, 1072–1077. doi: 10.1080/00016480410015776

Krantz, E. M., Schubert, C. R., Dalton, D. S., Zhong, W., Huang, G. H., Klein, B. E., et al. (2009). Test-retest reliability of the San Diego odor identification test and comparison with the brief smell identification test. *Chem. Senses* 34, 435–440. doi: 10.1093/chemse/bjp018

Krishna, N. S., Getchell, T. V., Dhooper, N., Awasthi, Y. C., and Getchell, M. L. (1995). Age- and gender-related trends in the expression of glutathione S-transferases in human nasal mucosa. *Ann. Otol. Rhinol. Laryngol.* 104, 812–822.

Krmpotic-Nemanic, J. (1969). Presbycusis, presbystasis and presbyosmia as consequences of the analogous biological process. *Acta Otolaryngol. (Stockh)* 67, 217–223. doi: 10.3109/00016486909125446

Lalancette-Hebert, M., Phaneuf, D., Soucy, G., Weng, Y. C., and Kriz, J. (2009). Live imaging of Toll-like receptor 2 response in cerebral ischaemia reveals a role of olfactory bulb microglia as modulators of inflammation. *Brain* 132, 940–954. doi: 10.1093/brain/awn345

LaMantia, A. S., and Purves, D. (1989). Development of glomerular pattern visualized in the olfactory bulbs of living mice. *Nature* 341, 646–649. doi: 10.1038/341646a0

Landis, B. N., Beutner, D., Frasnelli, J., Huttenbrink, K. B., and Hummel, T. (2005). Gustatory function in chronic inflammatory middle ear diseases. *Laryngoscope* 115, 1124–1127. doi: 10.1097/01.MLG.0000163750.72441.C3

Larsson, M., Farde, L., Hummel, T., Witt, M., Lindroth, N. E., and Backman, L. (2009). Age-related loss of olfactory sensitivity: association to dopamine transporter binding in putamen. *Neuroscience* 161, 422–426. doi: 10.1016/j.neuroscience.2009.03.074

Larsson, M., Finkel, D., and Pedersen, N. L. (2000). Odor identification: influences of age, gender, cognition, and personality. *J. Gerontol. Psychol. Sci. Soc. Sci.* 55, 304–310. doi: 10.1093/geronb/55.5.P304

Larsson, M., Nilsson, L. G., Olofsson, J. K., and Nordin, S. (2004). Demographic and cognitive predictors of cued odor identification: evidence from a population-based study. *Chem. Senses* 29, 547–554. doi: 10.1093/chemse/bjh059

Larsson, M., Oberg, C., and Backman, L. (2006). Recollective experience in odor recognition: influences of adult age and familiarity. *Psychol. Res.* 70, 68–75. doi: 10.1007/s00426-004-0190-9

Lehnardt, S., Lehmann, S., Kaul, D., Tschimmel, K., Hoffmann, O., Cho, S., et al. (2007). Toll-like receptor 2 mediates CNS injury in focal cerebral ischemia. *J. Neuroimmunol.* 190, 28–33. doi: 10.1016/j.jneuroim.2007.07.023

Leopold, D. A., Hummel, T., Schwob, J. E., Hong, S. C., Knecht, M., and Kobal, G. (2000). Anterior distribution of human olfactory epithelium. *Laryngoscope* 110, 417–421. doi: 10.1097/00005537-200003000-00016

Levy, L. M., Degnan, A. J., Sethi, I., and Henkin, R. I. (2013). Anatomic olfactory structural abnormalities in congenital smell loss: magnetic resonance imaging evaluation of olfactory bulb, groove, sulcal, and hippocampal morphology. *J. Comput. Assist. Tomogr.* 37, 650–657. doi: 10.1097/RCT.0b013e31829bfa3b

Liberles, S. D., and Buck, L. B. (2006). A second class of chemosensory receptors in the olfactory epithelium. *Nature.* 442, 645–650. doi: 10.1038/nature05066

Liss, L., and Gomez, F. (1958). The nature of senile changes of the human olfactory bulb and tract. *AMA Arch. Otolaryngol.* 67, 167–171. doi: 10.1001/archotol.1958.00730010173006

London, B., Nabet, B., Fisher, A. R., White, B., Sammel, M. D., and Doty, R. L. (2008). Predictors of prognosis in patients with olfactory disturbance. *Ann. Neurol.* 63, 159–166. doi: 10.1002/ana.21293

Loo, A. T., Youngentob, S. L., Kent, P. F., and Schwob, J. E. (1996). The aging olfactory epithelium: neurogenesis, response to damage, and odorant-induced activity. *Int. J. Dev. Neurosci.* 14, 881–900. doi: 10.1016/S0736-5748(96)00046-9

Lotsch, J., and Hummel, T. (2006). The clinical significance of electrophysiological measures of olfactory function. *Behav. Brain. Res.* 170, 78–83. doi: 10.1016/j.bbr.2006.02.013

Mackay-Sim, A. (2003). "Neurogenesis in the olfactory neuroepithelium," in *Handbook of Olfaction and Gustation.* 2nd Edn., ed R. L. Doty (New York, NY: Marcel Dekker), 93–113.

Mackay-Sim, A. (2010). Stem cells and their niche in the adult olfactory mucosa. *Arch. Ital. Biol.* 148, 47–58.

Mackay-Sim, A., and Patel, U. (1984). Regional differences in cell density and cell genesis in the olfactory epithelium of the salamander, *Ambystoma tigrinum. Exp. Brain Res.* 57, 99–106. doi: 10.1007/BF00231136

Mair, R. G., Doty, R. L., Kelly, K. M., Wilson, C. S., Langlais, P. J., McEntee, W. J., et al. (1986). Multimodal sensory discrimination deficits in Korsakoff's psychosis. *Neuropsychologia* 24, 831–839. doi: 10.1016/0028-3932(86)90082-5

Malnic, B., Hirono, J., Sato, T., and Buck, L. B. (1999). Combinatorial receptor codes for odors. *Cell* 96, 713–723. doi: 10.1016/S0092-8674(00)80581-4

Matulionis, D. H. (1982). "Effects of the aging process on olfactory neuron plasticity," in *Olfaction and Endocrine Regulation,* ed W. Breipohl (London: IRL Press), 299–308.

McKeown, D. A., Doty, R. L., Perl, D. P., Frye, R. E., Simms, I., and Mester, A. (1996). Olfactory function in young adolescents with Down's syndrome. *J. Neurol. Neurosurg. Psychiatry* 61, 412–414. doi: 10.1136/jnnp.61.4.412

Meisami, E., Mikhail, L., Baim, D., and Bhatganar, K. (1998). Observations on glomeruli and mitral cell numbers and accessory olfactory bulb in adult and aging human olfactory bulbs. *Proc. N.Y. Acad. Sci.* 855, 708–715. doi: 10.1111/j.1749-6632.1998.tb10649.x

Menco, B. P. M., and Morrison, E. E. (2003). "Morphology of the mammalian olfactory epithelium: form, fine structure, function, and pathology," in *Handbook of Olfaction and Gustation.* 2nd Edn., ed R. L. Doty (New York, NY: Marcel Dekker), 17–49.

Menon, C., Westervelt, H. J., Jahn, D. R., Dressel, J. A., and O'Bryant, S. E. (2013). Normative Performance on the brief smell identification test (BSIT) in a multi-ethnic bilingual cohort: a project FRONTIER study. *Clin. Neuropsychol.* 27, 946–961. doi: 10.1080/13854046.2013.796406

Meurman, O. H. (1950). Experimental studies of the effect of pathological changes in the nasal mucous membrane on the olfactory bulb. *Acta Otolaryngol.* 38, 477–483. doi: 10.3109/00016485009118408

Mirza, N., Kroger, H., and Doty, R. L. (1997). Influence of age on the "nasal cycle." *Laryngoscope* 107, 62–66. doi: 10.1097/00005537-199701000-00014

Møller, P., and Dijksterhuis, G. (2003). Differential human electrodermal responses to odours. *Neurosci. Lett.* 346, 129–132. doi: 10.1016/S0304-3940(03)00498-1

Møller, P., Mojet, J., and Koster, E. P. (2007). Incidental and intentional flavor memory in young and older subjects. *Chem. Senses* 32, 557–567. doi: 10.1093/chemse/bjm026

Møller, P., Wulff, C., and Koster, E. P. (2004). Do age differences in odour memory depend on differences in verbal memory? *Neuroreport* 15, 915–917. doi: 10.1097/00001756-200404090-00036

Morgan, C. D., and Murphy, C. (2010). Differential effects of active attention and age on event-related potentials to visual and olfactory stimuli. *Int. J. Psychophysiol.* 78, 190–199. doi: 10.1016/j.ijpsycho.2010.07.008

Morrison, E. E., and Costanzo, R. M. (1990). Morphology of the human olfactory epithelium. *J. Comp. Neurol.* 297, 1–13. doi: 10.1002/cne.902970102

Murphy, C. (1983). Age-related effects on the threshold, psychophysical function, and pleasantness of menthol. *J. Gerontol.* 38, 217–222. doi: 10.1093/geronj/38.2.217

Murphy, C., Nordin, S., de, W. R., Cain, W. S., and Polich, J. (1994). Olfactory-evoked potentials: assessment of young and elderly, and comparison to psychophysical threshold. *Chem. Senses* 19, 47–56. doi: 10.1093/chemse/19.1.47

Murphy, C., Schubert, C. R., Cruickshanks, K. J., Klein, B. E., Klein, R., and Nondahl, D. M. (2002). Prevalence of olfactory impairment in older adults. *JAMA* 288, 2307–2312. doi: 10.1001/jama.288.18.2307

Naessen, R. (1971). An enquiry on the morphological characteristics and possible changes with age in the olfactory region of man. *Acta Otolaryngol.* 71, 49–62. doi: 10.3109/00016487109125332

Nagai, M., Wada, M., Usui, N., Tanaka, A., and Hasebe, Y. (2000). Pleasant odors attenuate the blood pressure increase during rhythmic handgrip in humans. *Neurosci. Lett.* 289, 227–229. doi: 10.1016/S0304-3940(00)01278-7

Nakano, I., and Hirano, A. (1983). Neuron loss in the nucleus basalis of Meynert in parkinsonism-dementia complex of Guam. *Ann. Neurol.* 13, 87–91. doi: 10.1002/ana.410130118

Nakano, I., and Hirano, A. (1984). Parkinson's disease: neuron loss in the nucleus basalis without concomitant Alzheimer's disease. *Ann. Neurol.* 15, 415–418. doi: 10.1002/ana.410150503

Nakashima, T., Kimmelman, C. P., and Snow, J. B. Jr. (1984). Structure of human fetal and adult olfactory neuroepithelium. *Arch. Otolaryngol.* 110, 641–646. doi: 10.1001/archotol.1984.00800360013003

Negoias, S., Croy, I., Gerber, J., Puschmann, S., Petrowski, K., Joraschky, P., et al. (2010). Reduced olfactory bulb volume and olfactory sensitivity in patients with acute major depression. *Neuroscience* 169, 415–421. doi: 10.1016/j.neuroscience.2010.05.012

Nguyen, A. D., Pelavin, P. E., Shenton, M. E., Chilakamarri, P., McCarley, R. W., Nestor, P. G., et al. (2011). Olfactory sulcal depth and olfactory bulb volume in patients with schizophrenia: an MRI study. *Brain Imag. Behav.* 5, 252–261. doi: 10.1007/s11682-011-9129-0

Nordin, S., Nyroos, M., Maunuksela, E., Niskanen, T., and Tuorila, H. (2002). Applicability of the scandinavian odor identification test: a Finnish-Swedish comparison. *Acta Otolaryngol.* 122, 294–297. doi: 10.1080/000164802753648187

O'Connor, S., and Jacob, T. J. (2008). Neuropharmacology of the olfactory bulb. *Curr. Mol. Pharmacol.* 1, 181–190. doi: 10.2174/1874467210801030181

Olofsson, J., Ronnlund, M., Nordin, S., Hedner, M., Nilsson, L. G., Nyberg, L., et al. (2008). Odor identification impairment predicts cognitive decline and Alzheimer's disease. *Int. J. Psychol.* 43, 469.

Olofsson, J. K., Nordin, S., Wiens, S., Hedner, M., Nilsson, L. G., and Larsson, M. (2010). Odor identification impairment in carriers of ApoE-varepsilon4 is independent of clinical dementia. *Neurobiol. Aging* 31, 567–577. doi: 10.1016/j.neurobiolaging.2008.05.019

Olofsson, J. K., Ronnlund, M., Nordin, S., Nyberg, L., Nilsson, L. G., and Larsson, M. (2009). Odor identification deficit as a predictor of five-year global cognitive change: interactive effects with age and ApoE-epsilon4. *Behav. Genet.* 39, 496–503. doi: 10.1007/s10519-009-9289-5

Osman, A., and Silas, J. (2014). "Electrophysiological measurement of olfactory function," in *Handbook of Olfaction and Gustation, 3rd Edn.*, ed R. L. Doty (New York, NY: Wiley-Liss).

Ottoson, D. (1956). Analysis of the electrical activity of the olfactory epithelium. *Acta Physiol. Scand.* 35, 1–83.

Paik, S. I., Lehman, M. N., Seiden, A. M., Duncan, H. J., and Smith, D. V. (1992). Human olfactory biopsy. The influence of age and receptor distribution. Arch. Otolaryngol. *Head Neck Surg.* 118, 731–738. doi: 10.1001/archotol.1992.01880070061012

Panni, P., Ferguson, I. A., Beacham, I., Mackay-Sim, A., Ekberg, J. A., and St. John, J. A. (2013). Phagocytosis of bacteria by olfactory ensheathing cells and Schwann cells. *Neurosci. Lett.* 539, 65–70. doi: 10.1016/j.neulet.2013.01.052

Peele, D. B., Allison, S. D., Bolon, B., Prah, J. D., Jensen, K. F., and Morgan, K. T. (1991). Functional deficits produced by 3-methylindole-induced olfactory mucosal damage revealed by a simple olfactory learning task. *Toxicol. Appl. Pharmacol.* 107, 191–202. doi: 10.1016/0041-008X(91)90202-P

Pelosi, P. (1994). Odorant-binding proteins. *Crit. Rev. Biochem. Mol. Biol.* 29, 199–228. doi: 10.3109/10409239409086801

Pinto, J. M., Schumm, L. P., Wroblewski, K. E., Kern, D. W., and McClintock, M. K. (2013). Racial disparities in olfactory loss among older adults in the United States. *J. Gerontol. A Biol. Sci. Med. Sci.* doi: 10.1093/gerona/glt063. [Ebub ahead of print].

Rawson, N. E., Gomez, G., Cowart, B., and Restrepo, D. (1998). The use of olfactory receptor neurons (ORNs) from biopsies to study changes in aging and neurodegenerative diseases. *Ann. N.Y. Acad. Sci.* 855, 701–707. doi: 10.1111/j.1749-6632.1998.tb10648.x

Rehn, B., Breipohl, W., Mendoza, A. S., and Apfelbach, R. (1986). Changes in granule cells of the ferret olfactory bulb associated with imprinting on prey odours. *Brain Res.* 373, 114–125. doi: 10.1016/0006-8993(86)90321-5

Richman, R. A., Post, E. M., Sheehe, P. R., and Wright, H. N. (1992). Olfactory performance during childhood. I. Development of an odorant identification test for children. *J. Pediatr.* 121, 908–911. doi: 10.1016/S0022-3476(05)80337-3

Rogers, J. D., Brogan, D., and Mirra, S. S. (1985). The nucleus basalis of Meynert in neurological disease: a quantitative morphological study. *Ann. Neurol.* 17, 163–170. doi: 10.1002/ana.410170210

Rolls, E. T., and Grabenhorst, F. (2008). The orbitofrontal cortex and beyond: from affect to decision-making. *Prog. Neurobiol.* 86, 216–244. doi: 10.1016/j.pneurobio.2008.09.001

Rombaux, P., Huart, C., Deggouj, N., Duprez, T., and Hummel, T. (2012). Prognostic value of olfactory bulb volume measurement for recovery in postinfectious and posttraumatic olfactory loss. *Otolaryngol. Head Neck Surg.* 147, 1136–1141. doi: 10.1177/0194599812459704

Rombaux, P., Martinage, S., Huart, C., and Collet, S. (2009). Post-infectious olfactory loss: a cohort study and update. *B-ENT*, 5(Suppl. 13), 89–95.

Rombaux, P., Potier, H., Bertrand, B., Duprez, T., and Hummel, T. (2008). Olfactory bulb volume in patients with sinonasal disease. *Am. J. Rhinol.* 22, 598–601. doi: 10.2500/ajr.2008.22.3237

Rosier, A., Dupont, P., Peuskens, J., Bormans, G., Vandenberghe, R., Maes, M., et al. (1996). Visualisation of loss of 5-HT2A receptors with age in healthy volunteers using [18F]altanserin and positron emission tomographic imaging. *Psychiat. Res.* 68, 11–22. doi: 10.1016/S0925-4927(96)02806-5

Ross, G. W., Petrovitch, H., Abbott, R. D., Tanner, C. M., Popper, J., Masaki, K., et al. (2008). Association of olfactory dysfunction with risk for future Parkinson's disease. *Ann. Neurol.* 63, 167–173. doi: 10.1002/ana.21291

Rouquier, S., Blancher, A., and Giorgi, D. (2000). The olfactory receptor gene repertoire in primates and mouse: evidence for reduction of the functional fraction in primates. *Proc. Natl. Acad. Sci. U.S.A.* 97, 2870–2874. doi: 10.1073/pnas.040580197

Rovee, C. K., Cohen, R. Y., and Shlapack, W. (1975). Life-span stability in olfactory sensitivity. *Dev. Psychol.* 11, 311–318. doi: 10.1037/h0076566

Saito, H., Chi, Q., Zhuang, H., Matsunami, H., and Mainland, J. D. (2009). Odor coding by a Mammalian receptor repertoire. *Sci. Signal.* 2, ra9. doi: 10.1126/scisignal.2000016

Sajjadian, A., Doty, R. L., Gutnick, D. N., Chirurgi, R. J., Sivak, M., and Perl, D. (1994). Olfactory dysfunction in amyotrophic lateral sclerosis. *Neurodegeneration* 3, 153–157.

Sakakura, Y., Ukai, K., Majima, Y., Murai, S., Harada, T., and Miyoshi, Y. (1983). Nasal mucociliary clearance under various conditions. *Acta Otolaryngol.* 96, 167–173. doi: 10.3109/00016488309132888

Salihoglu, M., Kendirli, M. T., Altundag, A., Tekeli, H., Saglam, M., Cayonu, M., et al. (2013). The effect of obstructive sleep apnea on olfactory functions. *Laryngoscope.* doi: 10.1002/lary.24565. [Epub ahead of print].

Sama, U. H., Tahir, M., and Lone, K. P. (2008). Age and gender-related differences in mitral cells of olfactory bulb. *J. Coll. Physicians Surg. Pak.* 18, 669–673.

Santos, D. V., Reiter, E. R., DiNardo, L. J., and Costanzo, R. M. (2004). Hazardous events associated with impaired olfactory function. *Arch. Head Neck Surg.* 130, 317–319. doi: 10.1001/archotol.130.3.317

Sawada, M., Kaneko, N., Inada, H., Wake, H., Kato, Y., Yanagawa, Y., et al. (2011). Sensory input regulates spatial and subtype-specific patterns of neuronal turnover in the adult olfactory bulb. *J. Neurosci.* 31, 11587–11596. doi: 10.1523/JNEUROSCI.0614-11.2011

Schiffman, S., and Pasternak, M. (1979). Decreased discrimination of food odors in the elderly. *J. Gerontol.* 34, 73–79. doi: 10.1093/geronj/34.1.73

Schiffman, S. S. (1991). Taste and smell losses with age. *Bol. Asoc. Med. P.R.* 83, 411–414.

Schiffman, S. S., and Leffingwell, J. C. (1981). Perception of odors of simple pyrazines by young and elderly subjects: a multidimensional analysis. *Pharmacol. Biochem. Behav.* 14, 787–798. doi: 10.1016/0091-3057(81)90362-2

Schiffman, S. S., Moss, J., and Erickson, R. P. (1976). Thresholds of food odors in the elderly. *Exp. Aging Res.* 2, 389–398. doi: 10.1080/03610737608257997

Schiffman, S. S., and Zervakis, J. (2002). Taste and smell perception in the elderly: effect of medication and disease. *Adv. Food Nutr. Res.* 44, 247–346. doi: 10.1016/S1043-4526(02)44006-5

Schliebs, R., and Arendt, T. (2011). The cholinergic system in aging and neuronal degeneration. *Behav. Brain Res.* 221, 555–563. doi: 10.1016/j.bbr.2010.11.058

Schmidt, F. A., Goktas, O., Harms, L., Bohner, G., Erb, K., Dahlslett, B., et al. (2011). Structural correlates of taste and smell loss in encephalitis disseminata. *PLoS ONE* 6:e19702. doi: 10.1371/journal.pone.0019702

Schriever, V. A., Reither, N., Gerber, J., Iannilli, E., and Hummel, T. (2013). Olfactory bulb volume in smokers. *Exp. Brain Res.* 225, 153–157. doi: 10.1007/s00221-012-3356-5

Schubert, C. R., Carmichael, L. L., Murphy, C., Klein, B. E., Klein, R., and Cruickshanks, K. J. (2008). Olfaction and the 5-year incidence of cognitive impairment in an epidemiological study of older adults. *J. Am. Geriatr. Soc.* 56, 1517–1521. doi: 10.1111/j.1532-5415.2008.01826.x

Schubert, C. R., Cruickshanks, K. J., Fischer, M. E., Huang, G. H., Klein, B. E., Klein, R., et al. (2012). Olfactory impairment in an adult population: the Beaver Dam Offspring Study. *Chem. Senses* 37, 325–334. doi: 10.1093/chemse/bjr102

Schubert, C. R., Cruickshanks, K. J., Klein, B. E., Klein, R., and Nondahl, D. M. (2011). Olfactory impairment in older adults: five-year incidence and risk factors. *Laryngoscope* 121, 873–878. doi: 10.1002/lary.21416

Schumm, L. P., McClintock, M., Williams, S., Leitsch, S., Lundstrom, J., Hummel, T., et al. (2009). Assessment of sensory function in the national social life, health, and aging project. *J. Gerontol. B Psychol. Sci. Soc. Sci.* 64B (Suppl. 1), i76–i85. doi: 10.1093/geronb/gbp048

Schwab, J. A., and Zenkel, M. (1998). Filtration of particulates in the human nose. *Laryngoscope* 108, 120–124. doi: 10.1097/00005537-199801000-00023

Segura, B., Baggio, H. C., Solana, E., Palacios, E. M., Vendrell, P., Bargallo, N., et al. (2013). Neuroanatomical correlates of olfactory loss in normal aged subjects. *Behav. Brain Res.* 246, 148–153. doi: 10.1016/j.bbr.2013.02.025

Selkoe, D., and Kosik, K. (1984). "Neurochemical changes with aging," in *Clinical Neurology of Aging*, ed M. L. Albert (New York, NY: Oxford University Press), 53–75.

Settipane, G. A. (1996). Nasal polyps and immunoglobulin E (IgE). *Allergy Asthma Proc.* 17, 269–273. doi: 10.2500/108854196778662237

Shepherd, G. M. (1972). Synaptic organization of the mammalian olfactory bulb. *Physiol. Rev.* 52, 864–917.

Ship, J. A., Pearson, J. D., Cruise, L. J., Brant, L. J., and Metter, E. J. (1996). Longitudinal changes in smell identification. *J. Gerontol. A Biol. Sci. Med. Sci.* 51, M86–M91. doi: 10.1093/gerona/51A.2.M86

Ship, J. A., and Weiffenbach, J. M. (1993). Age, gender, medical treatment, and medication effects on smell identification. *J. Gerontol. A. Biol. Sci. Med. Sci.* 48, M26–M32. doi: 10.1093/geronj/48.1.M26

Sicard, G., and Holley, A. (1984). Receptor cell responses to odorants: similarities and differences among odorants. *Brain Res.* 292, 283–296. doi: 10.1016/0006-8993(84)90764-9

Smith, C. G. (1935). The change in volume of the olfactory and accessory olfactory bulbs of the albino rat during postnatal life. *J. Comp. Neurol.* 61, 477–508. doi: 10.1002/cne.900610305

Smith, C. G. (1942). Age incidence of atrophy of olfactory nerves in man. *J. Comp. Neurol.* 77, 589–594. doi: 10.1002/cne.900770306

Smithson, L. J., and Kawaja, M. D. (2010). Microglial/macrophage cells in mammalian olfactory nerve fascicles. *J. Neurosci. Res.* 88, 858–865. doi: 10.1002/jnr.22254

Somlyo, A. P., and Somlyo, A. V. (1968). Vascular smooth muscle. I. Normal structure, pathology, biochemistry, and biophysics. *Pharmacol. Rev.* 20, 197–272.

Staubert, C., Boselt, I., Bohnekamp, J., Rompler, H., Enard, W., and Schoneberg, T. (2010). Structural and functional evolution of the trace amine-associated receptors TAAR3, TAAR4 and TAAR5 in primates. *PLoS ONE* 5:e11133. doi: 10.1371/journal.pone.0011133

Stephan, A. B., Shum, E. Y., Hirsh, S., Cygnar, K. D., Reisert, J., and Zhao, H. (2009). ANO2 is the cilial calcium-activated chloride channel that may mediate olfactory amplification. *Proc. Natl. Acad. Sc.i U.S.A.* 106, 11776–11781. doi: 10.1073/pnas.0903304106

Stevens, J. C., and Cain, W. S. (1985). Age-related deficiency in the perceived strength of 6 odorants. *Chem. Senses* 10, 517–529. doi: 10.1093/chemse/10.4.517

Stevens, J. C., Cain, W. S., and Weinstein, D. E. (1987). Agining impairs the ability to detect gas odor. *Fire Technol.* 23, 198–204. doi: 10.1007/BF01036936

Stevens, J. C., Plantinga, A., and Cain, W. S. (1982). Reduction of odor and nasal pungency associated with aging. *Neurobiol. Aging* 3, 125–132. doi: 10.1016/0197-4580(82)90008-2

Strauss, E. L. (1970). A study on olfactory acuity. *Ann. Otol. Rhinol. Laryngol.* 79, 95–104.

Strong, R. (1998). Neurochemical changes in the aging human brain: implications for behavioral impairment and neurodegenerative disease. *Geriatrics* 53(Suppl. 1), S9–S12.

Stuck, B. A., Frey, S., Freiburg, C., Hormann, K., Zahnert, T., and Hummel, T. (2006). Chemosensory event-related potentials in relation to side of stimulation, age, sex, and stimulus concentration. *Clin. Neurophysiol.* 117, 1367–1375. doi: 10.1016/j.clinph.2006.03.004

Suzuki, Y., Critchley, H. D., Suckling, J., Fukuda, R., Williams, S. C., Andrew, C., et al. (2001). Functional magnetic resonance imaging of odor identification: the effect of aging. *J. Gerontol. A Biol. Sci. Med. Sci.* 56, M756–M760. doi: 10.1093/gerona/56.12.M756

Takagi, S. F. (1989). Standardized olfactometries in Japan – a review over ten years. *Chem. Senses* 14, 25–46. doi: 10.1093/chemse/14.1.25

Tang, S. C., Arumugam, T. V., Xu, X., Cheng, A., Mughal, M. R., Jo, D. G., et al. (2007). Pivotal role for neuronal Toll-like receptors in ischemic brain injury and functional deficits. *Proc. Natl. Acad. Sci. U. S. A* 104, 13798–13803. doi: 10.1073/pnas.0702553104

Thesen, T., and Murphy, C. (2001). Age-related changes in olfactory processing detected with olfactory event-related brain potentials using velopharyngeal closure and natural breathing. *Internat J. Psychophysiol.* 40, 119–127. doi: 10.1016/S0167-8760(00)00157-4

Thomann, P. A., Dos, S. V., Seidl, U., Toro, P., Essig, M., and Schroder, J. (2009). MRI-derived atrophy of the olfactory bulb and tract in mild cognitive impairment and Alzheimer's disease. *J. Alzheimers Dis.* 17, 213–221. doi: 10.3233/JAD-2009-1036

Tourbier, I. A., and Doty, R. L. (2007). Sniff magnitude test: relationship to odor identification, detection, and memory tests in a clinic population. *Chem. Senses* 32, 515–523. doi: 10.1093/chemse/bjm020

Turetsky, B. I., Moberg, P. J., Arnold, S. E., Doty, R. L., and Gur, R. E. (2003). Low olfactory bulb volume in first-degree relatives of patients with schizophrenia. *Am. J. Psychiatry* 160, 703–708. doi: 10.1176/appi.ajp.160.4.703

Van Toller, S., and Dodd, G. H. (1987). Presbyosmia and olfactory compensation for the elderly. *Brit. J. Clin. Pract.* 41, 725–728.

Velayudhan, L., Pritchard, M., Powell, J. F., Proitsi, P., and Lovestone, S. (2013). Smell identification function as a severity and progression marker in Alzheimer's disease. *Int. Psychogeriatr.* 25, 1157–1166. doi: 10.1017/S1041610213000446

Venstrom, D., and Amoore, J. E. (1968). Olfactory threshold in relation to age, sex or smoking. *J. Food Sci.* 33, 264–265. doi: 10.1111/j.1365-2621.1968.tb01364.x

Vogalis, F., Hegg, C. C., and Lucero, M. T. (2005). Ionic conductances in sustentacular cells of the mouse olfactory epithelium. *J. Physiol* 562, 785–799. doi: 10.1113/jphysiol.2004.079228

Vogels, O. J., Broere, C. A., ter Laak, H. J., ten Donkelaar, H. J., Nieuwenhuys, R., and Schulte, B. P. (1990). Cell loss and shrinkage in the nucleus basalis Meynert complex in Alzheimer's disease. *Neurobiol. Aging* 11, 3–13. doi: 10.1016/0197-4580(90)90056-6

Volkow, N. D., Logan, J., Fowler, J. S., Wang, G. J., Gur, R. C., Wong, C., et al. (2000). Association between age-related decline in brain dopamine activity and impairment in frontal and cingulate metabolism. *Am. J. Psychiatry* 157, 75–80. doi: 10.1176/appi.ajp.157.10.1709

Wang, C., Liu, F., Liu, Y. Y., Zhao, C. H., You, Y., Wang, L., et al. (2011a). Identification and characterization of neuroblasts in the subventricular zone and rostral migratory stream of the adult human brain. *Cell Res.* 21, 1534–1550. doi: 10.1038/cr.2011.83

Wang, J., Eslinger, P. J., Smith, M. B., and Yang, Q. X. (2005). Functional magnetic resonance imaging study of human olfaction and normal aging. *J. Gerontol. A Biol. Sci. Med. Sci.* 60, 510–514. doi: 10.1093/gerona/60.4.510

Wang, J., You, H., Liu, J. F., Ni, D. F., Zhang, Z. X., and Guan, J. (2011b). Association of olfactory bulb volume and olfactory sulcus depth with olfactory function in patients with Parkinson disease. *AJNR Am. J. Neuroradiol.* 32, 677–681. doi: 10.3174/ajnr.A2350

Watabe-Rudolph, M., Begus-Nahrmann, Y., Lechel, A., Rolyan, H., Scheithauer, M. O., Rettinger, G., et al. (2011). Telomere shortening impairs regeneration of the olfactory epithelium in response to injury but not under homeostatic conditions. *PLoS ONE* 6:e27801. doi: 10.1371/journal.pone.0027801

Wehling, E., Nordin, S., Espeseth, T., Reinvang, I., and Lundervold, A. J. (2011). Unawareness of olfactory dysfunction and its association with cognitive functioning in middle aged and old adults. *Arch. Clin Neuropsychol.* 26, 260–269. doi: 10.1093/arclin/acr019

Weierstall, R., and Pause, B. M. (2012). Development of a 15-item odour discrimination test (Dusseldorf Odour Discrimination Test). *Perception* 41, 193–203. doi: 10.1068/p7113

Wenning, G. K., Shephard, B., Hawkes, C., Petruckevitch, A., Lees, A., and Quinn, N. (1995). Olfactory function in atypical parkinsonian syndromes. *Acta Neurol. Scand.* 91, 247–250. doi: 10.1111/j.1600-0404.1995.tb06998.x

Wilson, R. S., Arnold, S. E., Schneider, J. A., Tang, Y., and Bennett, D. A. (2007a). The relationship between cerebral Alzheimer's disease pathology and odour identification in old age. *J. Neurol. Neurosurg. Psychiatry* 78, 30–35. doi: 10.1136/jnnp.2006.099721

Wilson, R. S., Schneider, J. A., Arnold, S. E., Tang, Y., Boyle, P. A., and Bennett, D. A. (2007b). Olfactory identification and incidence of mild cognitive impairment in older age. *Arch. Gen. Psychiatry* 64, 802–808. doi: 10.1001/archpsyc.64.7.802

Wilson, R. S., Yu, L., and Bennett, D. A. (2011a). Odor identification and mortality in old age. *Chem. Senses* 36, 63–67. doi: 10.1093/chemse/bjq098

Wilson, R. S., Yu, L., Schneider, J. A., Arnold, S. E., Buchman, A. S., and Bennett, D. A. (2011b). Lewy bodies and olfactory dysfunction in old age. *Chem. Senses* 36, 367–373. doi: 10.1093/chemse/bjq139

Wong, K. K., Muller, M. L., Kuwabara, H., Studenski, S. A., and Bohnen, N. I. (2010). Olfactory loss and nigrostriatal dopaminergic denervation in the elderly. *Neurosci. Lett.* 484, 163–167. doi: 10.1016/j.neulet.2010.08.037

Wysocki, C. J., and Gilbert, A. N. (1989). National geographic smell survey. Effects of age are heterogenous. *Ann. N.Y. Acad. Sci.* 561, 12–28. doi: 10.1111/j.1749-6632.1989.tb20966.x

Yoshida, M. (1984). Correlation analysis of detection threshold data for "standard test" odors. *Bull. Fac. Sci. Eng. Cho. Univ.* 27, 343–353.

Yoshida, M., Murakami, N., Hashizume, Y., and Takahashi, A. (1992). A clinicopathological study on 13 cases of motor neuron disease with dementia. *Rinsho Shinkeigaku* 32, 1193–1202.

Yousem, D. M., Geckle, R., and Doty, R. L. (1995a). MR of patients with post-traumatic olfactory deficits. *Chem. Senses* 20, 338.

Yousem, D. M., Geckle, R. J., and Doty, R. L. (1995b). Evaluation of olfactory deficits in neurodegenerative disorders. *Radiology* 197, 173.

Yousem, D. M., Geckle, R. J., Bilker, W. B., and Doty, R. L. (1998). Olfactory bulb and tract and temporal lobe volumes. Normative data across decades. *Ann. N.Y. Acad. Sci.* 855, 546–555. doi: 10.1111/j.1749-6632.1998.tb10624.x

Yousem, D. M., Geckle, R. J., Bilker, W., McKeown, D. A., and Doty, R. L. (1996). MR evaluation of patients with congenital hyposmia or anosmia. *Am. J. Roentgenol.* 166, 439–443. doi: 10.2214/ajr.166.2.8553963

Yousem, D. M., Maldjian, J. A., Hummel, T., Alsop, D. C., Geckle, R. J., Kraut, M. A., et al. (1999). The effect of age on odor-stimulated functional MR imaging. *AJNR Am. J. Neuroradiol.* 20, 600–608.

Yousem, D. M., Turner, W. J., Li, C., Snyder, P. J., and Doty, R. L. (1993). Kallmann syndrome: MR evaluation of olfactory system. *AJNR Am. J. Neuroradiol.* 14, 839–843.

Zald, D. H. (2006). "Neuropsychological assessment of the orbitofrontal cortex," in *The Orbitofrontal Cortex*, eds D. H. Zald and S. L. Rauch (New York, NY: Oxford University Press), 449–480. doi: 10.1093/acprof:oso/9780198565741.001.0001

Ziegler, G., Harhausen, D., Schepers, C., Hoffmann, O., Rohr, C., Prinz, V., et al. (2007). TLR2 has a detrimental role in mouse transient focal cerebral ischemia. *Biochem. Biophys. Res Commun.* 359, 574–579. doi: 10.1016/j.bbrc.2007.05.157

Zielinski, B. S., Getchell, M. L., Wenokur, R. L., and Getchell, T. V. (1989). Ultrastructural localization and identification of adrenergic and cholinergic nerve terminals in the olfactory mucosa. *Anat. Rec.* 225, 232–245. doi: 10.1002/ar.1092250309

22

Crossmodal effect of music and odor pleasantness on olfactory quality perception

Carlos Velasco[1]*, Diana Balboa[1], Fernando Marmolejo-Ramos[2] and Charles Spence[1]

[1] Crossmodal Research Laboratory, Department of Experimental Psychology, University of Oxford, Oxford, Oxfordshire, UK
[2] School of Psychology, Faculty of Health Sciences, University of Adelaide, Adelaide, SA, Australia

***Correspondence:**
Carlos Velasco, Crossmodal Research Laboratory, Department of Experimental Psychology, University of Oxford, 9 South Parks Road, Oxford OX1 3UD, Oxfordshire, UK
e-mail: carlos.velasco@psy.ox.ac.uk

Previous research has demonstrated that ratings of the perceived pleasantness and quality of odors can be modulated by auditory stimuli presented at around the same time. Here, we extend these results by assessing whether the hedonic congruence between odor and sound stimuli can modulate the perception of odor intensity, pleasantness, and quality in untrained participants. Unexpectedly, our results reveal that broadband white noise, which was rated as unpleasant in a follow-up experiment, actually had a more pronounced effect on participants' odor ratings than either the consonant or dissonant musical selections. In particular, participants rated the six smells used as being less pleasant and less sweet when they happened to be listening to white noise, as compared to any one of the other music conditions. What is more, these results also add evidence to support the existence of a close relationship between an odor's hedonic character and the perception of odor quality. So, for example, independent of the sound condition, pleasant odors were rated as sweeter, less dry, and brighter than the unpleasant odors. These results are discussed in terms of their implications for the understanding of crossmodal correspondences between olfactory and auditory stimuli.

Keywords: crossmodal correspondences, olfaction, audition, pleasantness, white noise

INTRODUCTION

Researchers have demonstrated that olfactory perception can be influenced by inputs from the other senses presented prior to and/or at the same time (see Calvert et al., 2004; Stein, 2012 for reviews). In fact, a variety of crossmodal correspondences—the name given to the tendency for people to match the information presented in one sensory modality to that presented in another (see Spence, 2011, for a review)—have been documented between olfaction and the other senses (e.g., Stevenson et al., 2012; Deroy et al., 2013). So, for example, to date, crossmodal associations have been demonstrated between odors and pitch (Belkin et al., 1997; Deroy et al., 2013), brightness (Kemp and Gilbert, 1997), colors (e.g., Schifferstein and Tanudjaja, 2004; Demattè et al., 2006a; Maric and Jacquot, 2013), basic tastes (Urdapilleta et al., 2006), and even tactile stimuli (Demattè et al., 2006b).

Deroy et al. (2013) recently suggested that people may use descriptors or attributes that are normally associated with other sensory modalities such as pitch, brightness, and sweetness to describe olfactory stimuli/percepts because of the various crossmodal correspondences that exist between the senses. It is interesting to note, though, that the crossmodal interactions that link olfactory and auditory stimuli have received far less attention than, for example, those that exist between vision and audition (Seo and Hummel, 2011). Nonetheless, over the last couple of decades, researchers have started to document the existence of a number of crossmodal correspondences between olfactory and auditory stimuli. For instance, Belkin et al. (1997) provided one of the first examples of olfactory–auditory correspondences, showing that people would match a series of odors varying in quality, to sounds that differed in terms of their pitch (cf. Piesse, 1891). These results were later extended by Crisinel and Spence (2012) who also found that people tended to match certain odors to the timbres of particular musical instruments (see also Crisinel et al., 2013).

While the crossmodal correspondence between specific olfactory stimuli and, say, particular colors could be explained by their co-occurrence in foodstuffs (think only of the red color of strawberries and the associated aroma), it is far harder to think of an environmental explanation that could explain why people would reliably (or consistently) associate specific musical parameters with particular olfactory stimuli and why these associations would, in turn, influence information processing (see Belkin et al., 1997; Deroy et al., 2013). In their recent review, Deroy et al. (2013) suggested that one potential explanation for the existence of crossmodal correspondences between auditory and olfactory stimuli may sometimes be related to the hedonic properties of the stimuli presented in the two modalities (see also Stevenson et al., 2012). As Marks (1978, p. 181) indicated, sensory qualities "*talk over their common feeling.*" This notion has also been supported by recent research pointing to the idea that the emotional (hedonic) similarity between olfactory and auditory information may be crucial to both crossmodal correspondences and multisensory information processing (see

Seo and Hummel, 2011; Crisinel and Spence, 2012; Hanson-Vaux et al., 2013).

Seo and Hummel (2011) reported two experiments in which they assessed the effect of auditory stimulation on the perceived pleasantness and intensity of odors. In their first study, they investigated whether auditory cues that were semantically congruent with the olfactory stimuli (sounds that were crossmodally better matched to the odors, i.e., the smell of potato chips while listening to the sound of crunching crisps) would modulate the perceived intensity and pleasantness of the odor. In their second experiment, the authors evaluated whether odor intensity and pleasantness could be influenced simply by manipulating the hedonic valence of the auditory stimuli.

Seo and Hummel (2011) reported that olfactory stimuli (such as the smell of coffee) were rated as more pleasant when paired with congruent sounds (i.e., when listening to the sound of drinking coffee in this example) as compared to incongruent sounds, and that the hedonic valence associated with the sounds can be transferred crossmodally, and thus influence people's odor evaluations. Interestingly, however, no crossmodal effect on the perceived intensity of the odors was reported. Seo and Hummel (2011) suggested that the results of their first study may have been attributable to the existence of a crossmodal congruency effect (e.g., Shams and Seitz, 2008), while the results of their second experiment could be explained in terms of some form of halo/horn effect (e.g., see Thorndike, 1920; Kappes et al., 2006). This evidence points to a hedonic similarity account. It may be the case that there is a crossmodal transfer of the hedonic evaluation of the information presented in one sensory modality onto the information processed in the other.

Seo et al. (2014) recently extended Seo and Hummel's (2011) results to more abstract auditory cues. In three experiments, the authors demonstrated that people match a variety of odors and background music, that congruent (to odors) background music (i.e., Christmas carols) would enhance the rated pleasantness of certain odors, and that congruent sounds had an impact upon odor familiarity and identification. For example, participants liked the smell of cinnamon more when it was presented together with (congruent) Christmas carols as compared to incongruent sounds. The authors suggested that the association between cinnamon and Christmas is very typical for the German participants whom they tested. The statistical regularities of the environment and co-occurrence of multisensory stimuli can thus lead to specific crossmodal associations (Shams and Seitz, 2008).

Further research is still needed in order to clarify the potential influence of auditory cues in odor perception, and its underlying mechanisms, since the crossmodal interactions between these senses are likely to operate at various different levels of human information processing (see Deroy et al., 2013). In the present study, we aimed to assess any effect of the pleasantness of the music on the perceived pleasantness and/or intensity of the odors. In addition, we also wanted to assess whether having congruent (vs. incongruent, in terms of the perceived pleasantness) auditory and olfactory stimuli would influence the perception of other odor qualities such as sweetness, brightness, acidity, and dryness, which are attributes commonly used to describe fragrances (e.g., in the context of perfumery; Zarzo and Stanton, 2009) and have been shown to be crossmodally associated to odors (Stevenson et al., 2012).

In the present study, we manipulated the crossmodal congruency based on a matching of the hedonic qualities of the stimuli. There is an intriguing question here as to whether and why changing what one hears can change an observer's experience of an olfactory stimulus. There is a need to clarify both the nature of the specific associations that exist between odors and sounds, and the influence that auditory cues may exert on the perception of odor attributes in, for example, the case of fine fragrances.

MATERIALS AND METHODS

PARTICIPANTS

Thirty-three untrained participants (20 females, M_{age} = 31.9 years, SD_{age} = 10.65, range = 18–58 years) took part in this experiment, which was approved by the Central University Research Ethics Committee of the University of Oxford. The experiment was conducted in accordance with the ethical guidelines laid down by the Department of Experimental Psychology, at the University of Oxford.

The participants gave their informed consent and completed two questionnaires in order to assess any potential sensory dysfunction prior to their taking part in the study: an adapted version of the Hearing Handicap Inventory for the Elderly (HHIE-S) for auditory functioning (Ventry and Weinstein, 1983) and the Multi-Clinic Smell and Taste Questionnaire (MCSTQ-Sc, olfactory section) for olfactory dysfunction (see Nordin et al., 2003) were used, and only those participants who did not report any dysfunction were included. The experiment lasted for approximately 40–50 min. The participants were compensated for their time with £8.

APPARATUS AND MATERIALS

Six odors, one from *Le Nez du Café* (Brizard and Co, Dorchester, UK) and five from *Le Nez du Vin* kits (Brizard and Co, Dorchester, UK), were selected as the olfactory stimuli. These kits have been designed to help those who would like to learn more about coffee/wine to experience a number of the characteristic odors commonly found in the different kinds of coffee/wine. In addition, they have been previously used in research involving crossmodal associations to odors (e.g., Crisinel and Spence, 2012; Hanson-Vaux et al., 2013). The samples were selected based on a preliminary experiment (see below) and consisted of odors identified as lemon, orange, and bilberry (all rated as pleasant), and musk, dark chocolate, and smoked (all rated as unpleasant).

In the preliminary study, 12 participants (seven females and five males, M_{age} = 24.9 years, SD_{age} = 5.7 range = 19–40) rated both the pleasantness and intensity of a variety of odors from Le Nez du Café (Coffee Blossom, Garden Peas, and Smoke) and Le Nez du Vin (Apricot, Bilberry, Cinnamon, Dark Chocolate, Orange, Lemon, Musk, Smoked, and Toast) kits. The ratings were made on visual analog scales (VAS) anchored between *not at all* (0) and *very* (100), which were presented using the E-Prime 2.0 software (Psychology Software Tools, Inc.). A summary of the results for the perceived pleasantness and intensity ratings are shown in **Figures 1A,C**, respectively. It is important to note here

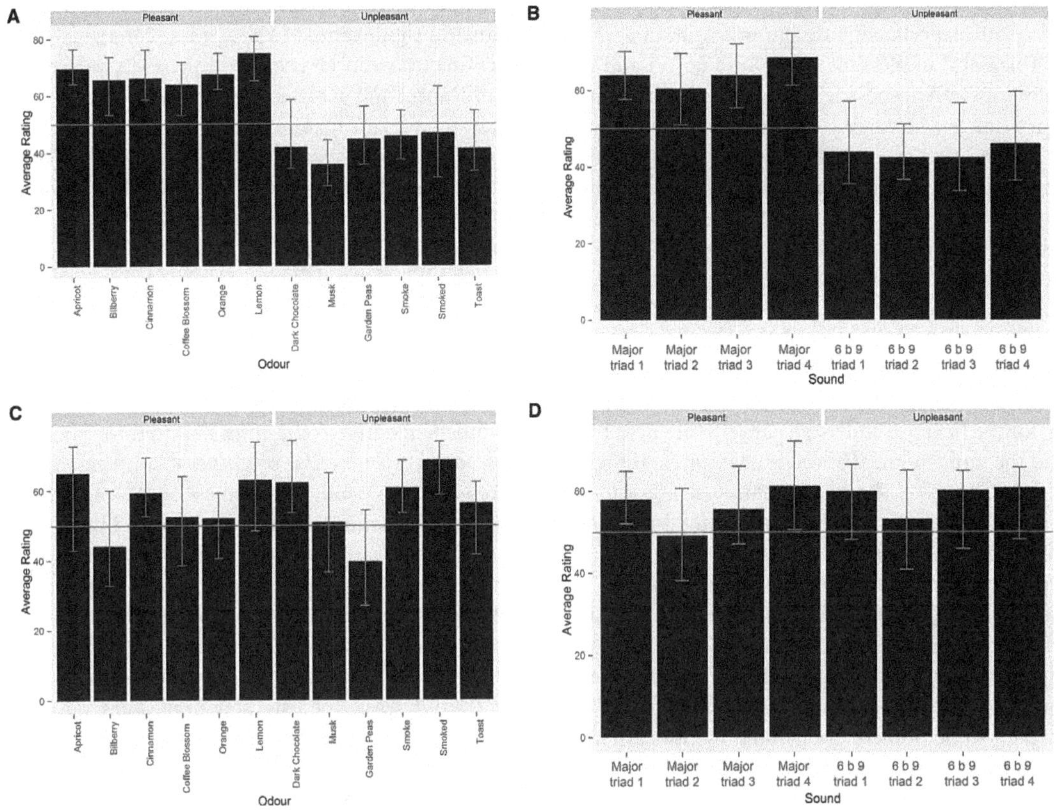

FIGURE 1 | Participants' average (Harrell–Davis estimator of the median; Vélez and Correa, 2014) pleasantness ratings for the odors (A) and for the sounds (B), and intensity ratings for the odors (C) and sounds (D). The ratings were performed on a scale ranging from 0 (not at all) to 100 (very). The error bars represent 95% bias-corrected-and-accelerated bootstrap confidence intervals.

that, although it may seem surprising to find that the participants found the smell of dark chocolate to be unpleasant, previous research has also documented that certain odors (e.g., parmesan cheese, truffle, and pepper, see Seo et al., 2010), when presented out of (a food-related) context, can be perceived as unpleasant (Deroy et al., 2013).

The selected odors were those that were given the most extreme hedonic ratings (in terms of either their pleasantness or unpleasantness). The intensity ratings of the selected odors were analyzed by means of a repeated measures analysis of variance (ANOVA) in order to determine whether participants perceived the intensity of the odors differently. The ANOVA did not reveal any statistically significant difference between the ratings.

In addition to the selected odors, a no-odor (baseline) condition was also included, which consisted of participants sniffing an odorless empty bottle. All of the samples were presented in small glass bottles, covered with opaque paper, and hidden in black containers in order to prevent the participants from seeing the color of the sample liquids (cf. Crisinel and Spence, 2012).

The auditory stimuli were created with the software Finale (Finale, 2012; MakeMusic®, Inc.). They consisted of three musical fragments played on the piano with the very same melodies but different, in terms of their dissonance (i.e., pleasantness), triad chords accompaniments. The dissonance of the triads went from the most consonant fragment (major triad) to the most dissonant fragment (6 ♭9 triad), giving rise to six musical fragments (three consonant, three dissonant). These musical fragments can be heard at https://soundcloud.com/xmodal/sets/sounds-odours. The sounds were designed on the basis of previous research suggesting the existence of an association between different dissonant and consonant musical pieces and pleasantness/unpleasantness (see Blood et al., 1999; Sammler et al., 2007). White noise (70 dB) was used as a putatively neutral stimulus. The sounds were edited in Audacity (Audacity®, the Free, Cross-Platform Sound Editor) to last for exactly 10 s, and were presented over headphones (Sony MDR-NC6 Noise Canceling) at a loudness level of 70 dB.

The consonant and dissonant auditory stimuli were assessed in a preliminary study in order to determine whether they were rated as expected; either pleasant (consonant) or unpleasant (dissonant). The same participants who had taken part in the odor pre-test also took part in this pre-test (the order was counterbalanced). The participants rated the pleasantness of the odors using a VAS (from 0 = not at all, to 100 = very). The mean pleasantness and intensity ratings are highlighted in **Figures 1B,D**, respectively. The participants rated each of the musical pieces as either pleasant or unpleasant as expected.

PROCEDURE

A within-participants experimental design was utilized with two factors: music (pleasant, unpleasant, and white noise) and odor (pleasant, unpleasant, and no-odor). The participants sat approximately 60 cm from a computer (with a screen resolution of 1366 × 768 pixels, and a screen refresh rate of 60 Hz), in order to perform the task. The instructions and response scales were presented on the computer monitor, and were also presented verbally in order to avoid any confusion.

Forty-nine different combinations of olfactory and auditory cues (seven odors and seven sounds, including the no-odor and white noise conditions) were presented in a random order to the participants. The auditory stimuli were presented for 10 s. Approximately 5 s after the onset of the auditory stimuli, the odor was presented, for the next 5 s, under the participant's nose by the experimenter at the same moment as an instruction on the screen said *Please sniff the odor once*. The participants were asked to sniff the odor just once in order to control that the total number of sniffs per session was the same across participants.

After the presentation of the stimuli, the participants had to rate a number of odor attributes (pleasantness, intensity, sweetness, brightness, acidity, and dryness) on VASs anchored between *not at all* and *very much*. Note that participants were not instructed about how they should interpret the different attributes included. However, some of these are commonly used attributes when describing fragrances (e.g., in the context of perfumery; Zarzo and Stanton, 2009) or have been shown, in the olfactory domain, to be crossmodally matched to odors (Stevenson et al., 2012). What is more, there has been growing interest in odors taking on gustatory properties such as sweetness or sourness (Stevenson and Boakes, 2004), and dryness (Zarzo and Stanton, 2009), while brightness has been shown to be crossmodally associated to odors of different qualities (see von Hornbostel, 1931; Cohen, 1934; Kemp and Gilbert, 1994, 1997). To minimize any olfactory desensitization, there was a 15 s gap between the odor presentations, which together with the time participants took to respond to the scales made approximately 25 s between odor presentations. White noise was presented during this time (cf. Seo and Hummel, 2011).

RESULTS

Average ratings obtained by participants for each odor–music combination were estimated using the Harrell–Davis estimator of the median (Vélez and Correa, 2014). Note that a number of assumptions for parametric tests were violated (e.g., the data was not normally distributed), thus, a robust analysis, the rank-based ANOVA-type statistic[1] (see Noguchi et al., 2012), was used to analyze the results. Average ratings were submitted to this ANOVA with the factors of music (pleasant, unpleasant, or white noise), and odor (pleasant, unpleasant, or odorless) for each of the odor attributes that the participants had to rate (pleasantness, intensity, sweetness, brightness, acidity, and dryness). **Figure 2** displays the average ratings obtained and **Table 1** shows the results of the analyses.

Pairwise comparisons for the music factor failed to reach statistical significance. Although less conservative multiple comparisons tests can be used (and these do indeed reach statistical significance) the analyses are kept since they evidenced a statistically significant main effect of music on the pleasantness (p = 0.016), sweetness (p = 0.046), and dryness (p = 0.031) ratings. It is then possible to assert that the odors that were presented after white noise were rated as less pleasant, less sweet, and drier, as compared to the other conditions.

In addition, Kendall tau correlations were performed between the different scores for each attribute for pleasant odors in the pleasant music and white noise conditions, and for unpleasant odors, in the unpleasant music and white noise conditions (see **Figure 3** for a summary of the results).

Independently of the music condition, positive correlations were observed between brightness and pleasantness, brightness and sweetness, and pleasantness and sweetness. Moreover, a positive correlation was also documented between intensity and pleasantness in the pleasant music and white noise conditions for the pleasant odors, while a negative correlation was found between these attributes in the unpleasant music and white noise conditions, for the unpleasant odors. A positive correlation was found between acidity and brightness in all conditions except for the unpleasant music and unpleasant odors condition. In addition, a negative correlation was found between intensity and sweetness in the unpleasant music and white noise conditions for unpleasant odors, while a positive correlation between these attributes was found in the white noise condition for the pleasant odor. Taken together, then, these results suggest that although certain relationships seem to be unaffected by the music condition (e.g., the relationship between pleasantness and sweetness), certain others may change as a function of the condition (e.g., the relationship between intensity and pleasantness).

DISCUSSION

The main aim of the present study was to assess whether musical pieces rated as pleasant or unpleasant would influence odors rated as either pleasant or unpleasant. Interestingly, when white noise was played in the background, a significant effect on participants' ratings of the odor (relative to the other music conditions) was observed. When the odors were presented together with the white noise they were rated as less pleasant, as less sweet, and drier than in the other auditory conditions. This result provides evidence for the idea that white noise can have an effect on odor perception (when compared to a condition in which background music was played) and in particular it can influence participants' hedonic ratings and perceived odor quality (e.g., sweetness).

Although, to the best of our knowledge, little previous research has been conducted to assess the influence of white noise on olfactory perception, suggestive evidence from its influence on the other senses may shed some light on its effects in the present study. Ferber and Cabanac (1987), for instance, conducted a study in the taste domain in which the hedonic valence of sucrose (but not of sodium chloride) solutions were shown to increase (meaning that people reported liking the solutions more) when listening to either loud noise or music. The sweet solutions were

[1] Note that effect sizes have not yet been proposed for this type of ANOVAs.

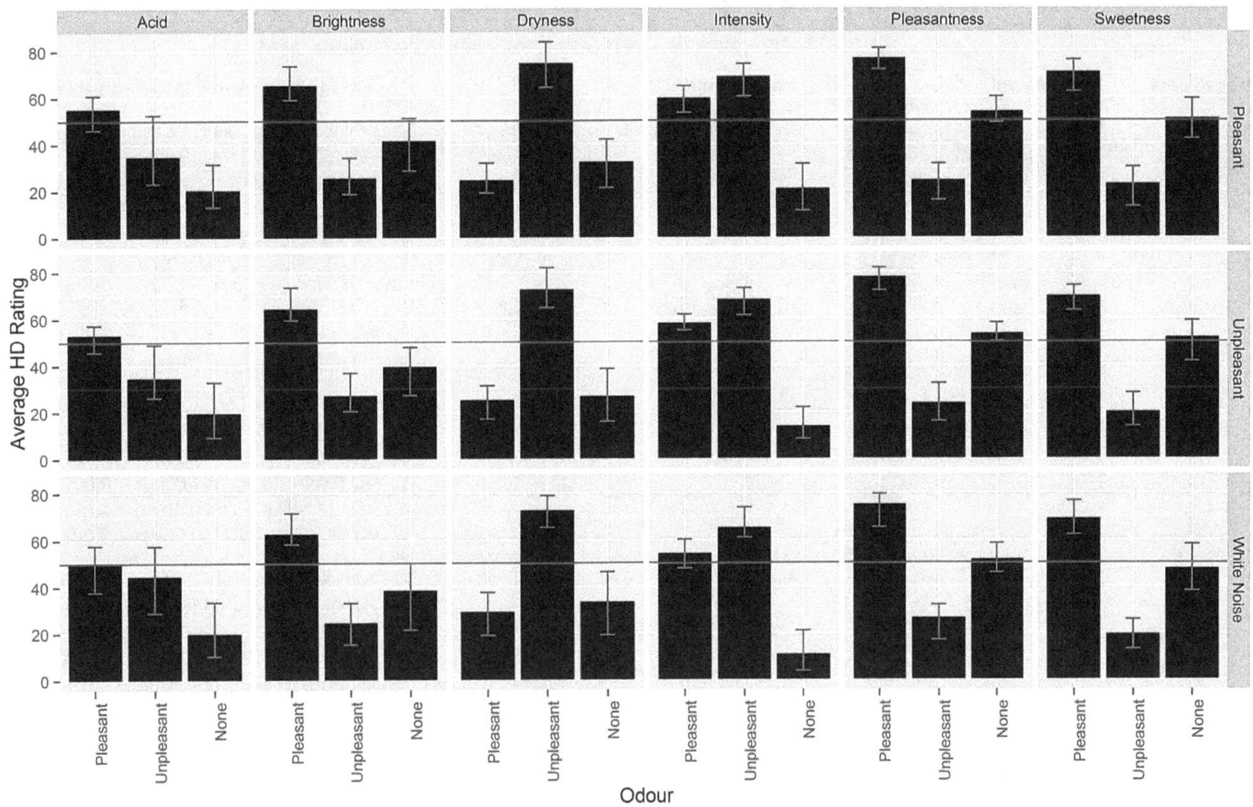

FIGURE 2 | Average ratings (Harrell–Davis estimator of the median) for each attribute in each odor and musical condition. The error bars represent 95% bias-corrected-and-accelerated bootstrap confidence intervals (Efron, 1987).

rated as significantly more pleasant when the participants were in the presence of the loud background noise or music (both presented at 90 dB over headphones) than when tasting in silence or while listening to quiet music (70 dB) instead. Interestingly, despite the fact that each person was allowed to listen to the music that they liked (that is, they were encouraged to bring their own preferred music into the study), it was the presumably unpleasant white noise that actually gave rise to the largest sweetness enhancement effects. Ferber and Cabanac (1987) suggested that this particular crossmodal effect may have been mediated indirectly via the modulatory effect of noise on participants' arousal/stress levels which, in turn, may have affected their taste perception. It is important to note that this study only used 10 participants.

On the other hand, Masuda et al. (2008) reported that white noise had an effect on people's ratings of the perceived moistness of pretzels. In addition, and more relevant to the aims of the present study, Woods et al. (2011) conducted two experiments designed to assess the effect of background noise on food perception and found that the perceived sweetness and saltiness of a variety of different foodstuffs, were lower in the white noise condition as compared to the other sound condition. Woods et al. (2011) concluded that background noise reduced the perception of gustatory attributes (see also Spence et al., 2014). It may be the case, then, that background white noise, or the hedonic value associated with it, not only affects the perception of gustatory but also olfactory attributes (Spence, 2014).

It is worth noting that white noise has been used as a neutral sound condition in previous studies on odor–sound interactions (Seo and Hummel, 2011; Seo et al., 2014). It may be the case that context can play an important role in guiding participants' ratings (c.f., Martino and Marks, 2001); in other words, the combination of auditory stimuli that are used in the very same experiment may influence the way in which participants evaluate the different odors. That said, although people perceived the consonant and dissonant musical selections as respectively pleasant and unpleasant in the pre-test, the relative hedonic value of each musical piece may have changed when also including white noise (as shown in the follow-up experiment). This in turn, may have been reflected in the way in which white noise affected odor perception. Moreover, it may be the case that the consonant and dissonant pieces utilized were not sufficient to evoke a distinctive hedonic response, as compared to white noise (more salient).

In a follow-up study, we had participants rate the consonant and dissonant musical pieces on a hedonic scale (as done in the preliminary experiment) but in this case white noise was included, in order to assess whether participants' ratings would be the same. The sounds were presented randomly four times to a group of 20 participants (eight females, M_{age} = 36.5 years, SD_{age} = 9.9, range = 23–55 years) who rated both their intensity and pleasantness on

Table 1 | Results of the ATS performed on each of the attributes assessed in the experiment.

	ANOVA-type statistic analyses and two-sample permutation tests		
Odor attributes	**Main effects**	**Interactions**	**Pairwise comparisons (M_{HD}) [*p*-value $_{FDR}$]**
Pleasantness	M: $F_{(1.69,\infty)} = 4.41$, $p = 0.016$ O: $F_{(1.87,\infty)} = 89.28$, $p < 0.001$	M × O: $F_{(2.81,\infty)} = 0.74$, $p = 0.519$ (ns)	M: WN (50.23) vs. PM (54.04): $p = 0.18$ [0.33] O: WN (50.23) vs. UM (53.42): $p = 0.22$ [0.33] PM (54.04) vs. UM (53.42): $p = 0.41$ [0.41] NO (52.69) vs. PO (76.74): $p < 0.001$ [0.001] NO (52.69) vs. UO (25.50): $p < 0.001$ [0.001] PO (76.74) vs. UO (25.50): $p < 0.001$ [0.001]
Intensity	M: $F_{(1.77,\infty)} = 1.07$, $p = 0.33$ O: $F_{(1.53,\infty)} = 81.94$, $p < 0.001$	M × O: $F_{(3.57,\infty)} = 1.15$, $p = 0.32$ (ns)	O: NO (13.96) vs. PO (57.61): $p < 0.001$ [0.001] NO (13.96) vs. UO (67.54): $p < 0.001$ [0.001] PO (57.61) vs. UO (67.54): $p < 0.001$ [0.001]
Sweetness	M: $F_{(1.83,\infty)} = 3.16$, $p = 0.046$ O: $F_{(1.81,\infty)} = 57.12$, $p < 0.001$	M × O: $F_{(2.85,\infty)} = 1.12$, $p = 0.33$ (ns)	M: WN (44.21) vs. PM (47.61): $p = 0.28$ [0.42] O: WN (44.21) vs. UM (47.90): $p = 0.22$ [0.42] PM (47.61) vs. UM (47.90): $p = 0.51$ [0.51] NO (50.14) vs. PO (69.65): $p < 0.001$ [0.001] NO (50.14) vs. UO (20.55): $p < 0.001$ [0.001] PO (69.65) vs. UO (20.55): $p < 0.001$ [0.001]
Dryness	M: $F_{(1.68,\infty)} = 3.70$, $p = 0.031$ O: $F_{(1.71,\infty)} = 63.75$, $p < 0.001$	M × O: $F_{(1.76,\infty)} = 1.05$, $p = 0.34$ (ns)	M: WN (42.85) vs. PM (41.06): $p = 0.36$ [0.79] O: WN (42.85) vs. UM (38.46): $p = 0.79$ [0.79] PM (41.06) vs. UM (38.46): $p = 0.68$ [0.79] NO (31.34) vs. PO (25.71): $p = 0.89$ [0.89] NO (31.34) vs. UO (73.14): $p < 0.001$ [0.001] PO (25.71) vs. UO (73.14): $p < 0.001$ [0.001]
Acidity	M: $F_{(1.97,\infty)} = 0.74$, $p = 0.47$ O: $F_{(1.52,\infty)} = 11.27$, $p < 0.001$	M × O: $F_{(2.89,\infty)} = 2.29$, $p = 0.07$ (ns)	O: NO (19.61) vs. PO (53.80): $p < 0.001$ [0.001] NO (19.61) vs. UO (36.85): $p < 0.001$ [0.001] PO (53.80) vs. UO (36.85): $p < 0.001$ [0.001]
Brightness	M: $F_{(1.94,\infty)} = 1.56$, $p = 0.21$ O: $F_{(1.92,\infty)} = 42.63$, $p < 0.001$	M × O: $F_{(2.30,\infty)} = 0.33$, $p = 0.74$ (ns)	O: NO (40.13) vs. PO (63.54): $p < 0.001$ [0.001] NO (40.13) vs. UO (25.59): $p = 0.002$ [0.002] PO (63.54) vs. UO (25.59): $p < 0.001$ [0.001]

M, music; O, odor; WN, white noise; PM, pleasant music; UN, unpleasant music; NO, no-odor; PO, pleasant odor; UO, unpleasant odor; FDR, false discovery rate (Bejamini and Hochberg, 1995); M_{HD}, Harrell–Davis estimator of the median. The p-value of the FDR should be taken as the adjusted final p-value obtained.

VAS scales anchored with *not at all* and *very much*. A repeated measures ANOVA (Greenhouse–Geisser-corrected) indicated a significant difference between the ratings, $F_{(2.248,42.721)} = 53.751$, $p < 0.001$, $\eta_p^2 = 0.739$. Pairwise comparisons using the Bonferroni correction revealed that participants rated white noise as significantly more unpleasant as compared to any of the other musical pieces ($p < 0.001$, for all comparisons). Importantly, no significant difference between the intensity ratings was found. Note that these results contrast with the preliminary experiment in which a difference was found between consonant and dissonant sounds, though white noise was not included. The aforementioned results point to the fact that the context created by particular sets of stimuli can influence participants' ratings of those stimuli, which is consistent with the idea that context plays a key role in crossmodal correspondences.

Why should music and background sounds influence the perception of olfactory stimuli? As mentioned before, one possibility here is that the hedonic value (Kenneth, 1923; Marks, 1978; Deroy et al., 2013) of a stimulus presented to one sensory channel extends to the information presented in another (e.g., "halo effect," see Seo and Hummel, 2011; Spence and Piqueras-Fiszman, 2014). Another possibility is that the information presented to one sensory modality captures more attention and thus influences the perception of the information in another modality (e.g., Boyle et al., 2006; Woods et al., 2011). These accounts are not necessarily incompatible in that participants may attend to information in one modality and if it is hedonically congruent with the other modality being evaluated, this may then strengthen its hedonic value. If it is not congruent (neither semantically nor hedonically), it may then interfere. Notably, this research is at an early stage, and thus further research is still needed in order to clarify the mechanisms underlying such phenomena.

Elsewhere, Spence and Shankar (2010) conducted a study in which they found that people's rating of chocolate samples was unaffected by listening to consonant vs. dissonant triads. It is also plausible that under certain circumstances, particular consonant and dissonant sounds may not influence participants' perception of odors/flavors (though see Sammler et al., 2007 for a study on how music can influence emotion).

Our results also contribute to the existing body of research suggesting that there is a relationship between pleasantness and odor qualities (e.g., Dravnieks et al., 1984; Stevenson and Boakes, 2004). That is, unpleasant odors were rated as dryer and more

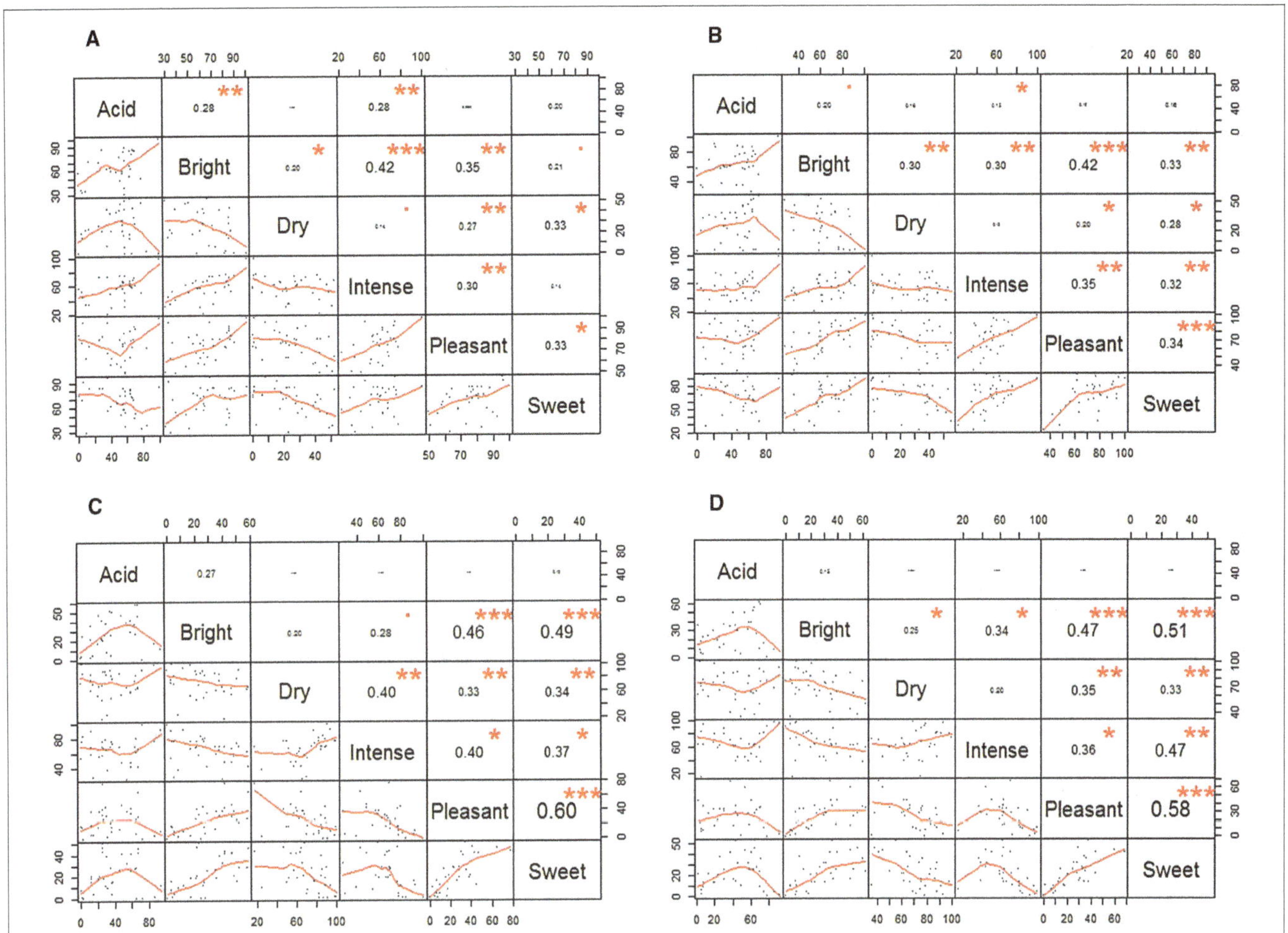

FIGURE 3 | Correlations between the ratings for the attributes of the pleasant music and pleasant odors (A), the white noise and pleasant odors (B), the unpleasant music and unpleasant odors (C), and the white noise and unpleasant odors (D) conditions. The value within each box represents the Kendall tau coefficient and the *p*-values should be interpreted as follows: $^{\bullet}p < 0.5$, $^{*}p < 0.05$, $^{**}p < 0.01$, $^{***}p < 0.001$. In order to be coherent with the non-parametric tests used, locally weighted scatterplot smoothing (LOESS) lines (a non-parametric regression method) are shown instead of the traditional parametric straight lines (parametric regression method). Note, however, that interpretation of these lines is different from traditional ones. For example, the fitting lines in the scatterplot of intense-sweet **(D)** seem to indicate that there is a negative quadratic relationship, but this curvature is caused by only a few data points. The same occurs with intense-pleasant negative quadratic relationship.

intense, as compared to the other odors, while pleasant odors were rated as sweeter and brighter, as compared to the others (see Zarzo and Stanton, 2009, for opposite uses of the descriptors sweet and dry when describing odors). Although the results presented here are limited in that only three odors per condition were included, they may nevertheless shed lights on how different olfactory percepts can be associated to the hedonic properties of odors. For instance, our results are in line with previous research (see Henion, 1971; Distel et al., 1999 for examples) suggesting that unpleasant odors are perceived as more intense (though matched in terms of their intensity in the pre-test); however, the association between pleasantness and intensity can be complex, and can vary as a function of the odors (e.g., Rouby et al., 2009); in other words, pleasantness and intensity can vary together and the direction of this variation depends upon the nature of the stimuli used, and the perceiver. On the other hand, previous research has suggested that people generally tend to prefer sweet smells (i.e., the smell of caramel, strawberry, vanilla, etc.; Stevenson and Boakes, 2004), which is also reflected in our results.

Notably, although our results contribute to the growing literature on the crossmodal influences in odor perception, a number of limitations should be mentioned. First, the main experiment did not include a no-sound condition, which limits the results to white noise as compared to dissonant and consonant sounds. Moreover, since participants were not explicitly informed about how to interpret each of the attributes used in this study (e.g., bright, dry), it is possible that their interpretation was not the same (e.g., Kaeppler and Mueller, 2013; though see Koulakov et al., 2011). In addition, although it has been documented that white noise can influence olfactory perception and that this may be attributed to its hedonic value (as compared to consonant and dissonant sounds), it is still an open question as to whether these effects are a product of some kind of "halo effect," an attentional shift, or a combination of both. Future research may help to address this element and to extend the results to other food-related and non-food odors.

As a final note, it is worth mentioning that suggestive evidence from Wesson and Wilson (2010) indicates that the rat's olfactory tubercle responds to tones, and that certain units in this structure show superadditive or suppressive responses when tones and odors are presented at the same time. Interestingly, animal studies suggest that there may be a strong evolutionary relationship between olfaction and audition (e.g., Cohen et al., 2011). This has been explained in terms of the idea that in natural environments animals may experience both olfactory and auditory stimuli at the same time in a variety of situations (e.g., think, for example, of the noise that can be heard when opening a fruit, while its smell is released). While the neural mechanisms that underlie olfactory–auditory interactions in humans remain largely unknown, scientists are now starting to point to the fact that auditory–olfactory crossmodal integration can potentially serve a variety of heretofore little considered functions (e.g., social perception of action, see Aglioti and Pazzaglia, 2011).

ACKNOWLEDGMENTS

Carlos Velasco would like to thank COLFUTURO, Colombia, for financial help toward funding his PhD. Charles Spence would like to acknowledge the Rethinking the Senses grant from the AHRC (UK; AH/L007053/1). We would also like to thank Dr. Jorge Vélez for his thoughtful suggestions on the statistical analysis. We would also like to thank the helpful comments of both reviewers.

REFERENCES

Aglioti, S. M., and Pazzaglia, M. (2011). Sounds and scents in (social) action. *Trends Cogn. Sci.* 15, 47–55. doi: 10.1016/j.tics.2010.12.003

Bejamini, Y., and Hochberg, Y. (1995). Controlling the false discovery rate: a practical and powerful approach to multiple testing. *J. R. Stat. Soc. Ser. B Stat. Methodol.* 57, 289–300.

Belkin, K., Martin, R., Kemp, S. E., and Gilbert, A. N. (1997). Auditory pitch as a perceptual analogue to odor quality. *Psychol. Sci.* 8, 340–342. doi: 10.1111/j.1467-9280.1997.tb00450.x

Blood, A. J., Zatorre, R. J., Bermudez, P., and Evans, A. C. (1999). Emotional responses to pleasant and unpleasant music correlate with activity in paralimbic brain regions. *Nat. Neurosci.* 2, 382–287. doi: 10.1038/7299

Boyle, Y., Bentley, D. E., Watson, A., and Jones, A. K. P. (2006). Acoustic noise in functional magnetic resonance imaging reduces pain unpleasantness ratings. *Neuroimage* 31, 1278–1283. doi: 10.1016/j.neuroimage.2006.01.025

Calvert, G., Spence, C., and Stein, B. E. (eds). (2004). *The Handbook of Multisensory Processing*. Cambridge, MA: MIT Press.

Cohen, L., Rothschild, G., and Mizrahi, A. (2011). Multisensory integration of natural odors and sounds in the auditory cortex. *Neuron* 72, 357–369. doi: 10.1016/j.neuron.2011.08.019

Cohen, N. E. (1934). Equivalence of brightnesses across modalities. *Am. J. Psychol.* 46, 117–119. doi: 10.2307/1416240

Crisinel, A.-S., Jacquier, C., Deroy, O., and Spence, C. (2013). Composing with cross-modal correspondences: music and odors in concert. *Chemosens. Percept.* 6, 45–52. doi: 10.1007/s12078-012-9138-4

Crisinel, A.-S., and Spence, C. (2012). A fruity note: crossmodal associations between odors and musical notes. *Chem. Senses* 37, 151–158. doi: 10.1093/chemse/bjr085

Demattè, M. L., Sanabria, D., and Spence, C. (2006a). Cross-modal associations between odors and colors. *Chem. Senses* 31, 531–538. doi: 10.1093/chemse/bjj057

Demattè, M. L., Sanabria, D., Sugarman, R., and Spence, C. (2006b). Cross-modal interactions between olfaction and touch. *Chem. Senses* 31, 291–300. doi: 10.1093/chemse/bjj031

Deroy, O., Crisinel, A.-S., and Spence, C. (2013). Crossmodal correspondences between odors and contingent features: odors, musical notes, and geometrical shapes. *Psychon. Bull. Rev.* 20, 878–896. doi: 10.3758/s13423-013-0397-0

Distel, H., Ayabe-Kanamura, S., Martínez-Gómez, M., Schicker, I., Kobayakawa, T., Saito, S., et al. (1999). Perception of everyday odors: correlation between intensity, familiarity and strength of hedonic judgement. *Chem. Senses* 24, 191–199. doi: 10.1093/chemse/24.2.191

Dravnieks, A., Masurat, T., and Lamm, R. A. (1984). Hedonics of odors and odor descriptors. *J. Air Pollut. Control Assoc.* 34, 752–755. doi: 10.1080/00022470.1984.10465810

Efron, B. (1987). Better bootstrap confidence intervals [with discussion]. *J. Am. Stat. Assoc.* 82, 171–200. doi: 10.1080/01621459.1987.10478410

Ferber, C., and Cabanac, M. (1987). Influence of noise on gustatory affective ratings and preference for sweet or salt. *Appetite* 8, 229–235. doi: 10.1016/0195-6663(87)90022-5

Hanson-Vaux, G., Crisinel, A. S., and Spence, C. (2013). Smelling shapes: cross-modal correspondences between odors and shapes. *Chem. Senses* 38, 161–166. doi: 10.1093/chemse/bjs087

Henion, K. E. (1971). Odor pleasantness and intensity: a single dimension? *J. Exp. Psychol.* 90, 275–279. doi: 10.1037/h0031549

Kaeppler, K., and Mueller, F. (2013). Odor classification: a review of factors influencing perception-based odor arrangements. *Chem. Senses* 38, 189–209. doi: 10.1093/chemse/bjs141

Kappes, S. M., Schmidt, S. J., and Lee, S.-Y. (2006). Color halo/horns and halo-attribute dumping effects within descriptive analysis of carbonated beverages. *J. Food Sci.* 71, S590–S595. doi: 10.1111/j.1750-3841.2006.00161.x

Kemp, S. E., and Gilbert, A. N. (1994). The cross-modal relationship between vision and olfaction is dimensional: color value varies inversely with odor intensity. *Chem. Senses* 19, 495.

Kemp, S. E., and Gilbert, A. N. (1997). Odor intensity and color lightness are correlated sensory dimensions. *Am. J. Psychol.* 110, 35–46. doi: 10.2307/1423699

Kenneth, J. H. (1923). Mental reactions to smell stimuli. *Psychol. Rev.* 30, 77–79. doi: 10.1037/h0068405

Koulakov, A. A., Kolterman, B. E., Enikolopov, A. G., and Rinberg, D. (2011). In search of the structure of human olfactory space. *Front. Syst. Neurosci.* 5:65. doi: 10.3389/fnsys.2011.00065

Maric, Y., and Jacquot, M. (2013). Contribution to understanding odour–colour associations. *Food Qual. Prefer.* 27, 191–195. doi: 10.1016/j.foodqual.2012.05.001

Marks, L. E. (1978). *The Unity of the Senses: Interrelations Among the Modalities*. New York, NY: Academic Press.

Martino, G., and Marks, L. E. (2001). Synesthesia: strong and weak. *Curr. Dir. Psychol. Sci.* 10, 61–65. doi: 10.1111/1467-8721.00116

Masuda, M., Yamaguchi, Y., Arai, K., and Okajima, K. (2008). Effect of auditory information on food recognition. *IEICE Tech. Rep.* 108, 123–126.

Noguchi, K., Gel, Y. R., Brunner, E., and Konietschke, F. (2012). nparLD: an R software package for the nonparametric analysis of longitudinal data in factorial experiments. *J. Stat. Softw.* 50, 1–23.

Nordin, S., Brämerson, A., Murphy, C., and Bende, M. (2003). A Scandinavian adaptation of the multi-clinic smell and taste questionnaire: evaluation of questions about olfaction. *Acta Otolaryngol.* 123, 536–542. doi: 10.1080/00016480310001411

Piesse, C. H. (1891). *Piesse's Art of Perfumery*, 5th Edn. London: Piesse and Lubin. Available at: http://www.gutenberg.org/files/16378/16378-h/16378-h.htm

Rouby, C., Pouliot, S., and Bensafi, M. (2009). Odor hedonics and their modulators. *Food Qual. Prefer.* 20, 545–549. doi: 10.1016/j.foodqual.2009.05.004

Sammler, D., Grigutsch, M., Fritz, T., and Koelsch, S. (2007). Music and emotion: electrophysiological correlates of the processing of pleasant and unpleasant music. *Psychophysiology* 44, 293–304. doi: 10.1111/j.1469-8986.2007.00497.x

Schifferstein, H. N. J., and Tanudjaja, I. (2004). Visualizing fragrances through colors: the mediating role of emotions. *Perception* 33, 1249–1266. doi: 10.1068/p5132

Seo, H.-S., Arshamian, A., Schemmer, K., Scheer, I., Sander, T., Ritter, G., et al. (2010). Cross-modal integration between odors and abstract symbols. *Neurosci. Lett.* 175–178. doi: 10.1016/j.neulet.2010.05.011

Seo, H.-S., and Hummel, T. (2011). Auditory–olfactory integration: congruent or pleasant sounds amplify odor pleasantness. *Chem. Senses* 39, 215–228. doi: 10.1093/chemse/bjt070

Seo, H.-S., Lohse, F., Luckett, C. R., and Hummel, T. (2014). Congruent sound can modulate odor pleasantness. *Chem. Senses* 39, 215–228. doi: 10.1093/chemse/bjt070

Shams, L., and Seitz, A. R. (2008). Benefits of multisensory learning. *Trends Cogn. Sci.* 12, 411–417. doi: 10.1016/j.tics.2008.07.006

Spence, C. (2011). Crossmodal correspondences: a tutorial review. *Atten. Percept. Psychophys.* 73, 971–995. doi: 10.3758/s13414-010-0073-7

Spence, C. (2014). Noise and its impact on the perception of food and drink. *Flavour* 3:9. doi: 10.1186/2044-7248-3-9

Spence, C., Michel, C., and Smith, B. (2014). Airplane noise and the taste of umami. *Flavour* 3, 2. doi: 10.1186/2044-7248-3-2

Spence, C., and Piqueras-Fiszman, B. (2014). *The Perfect Meal: The Multisensory Science of Food and Dining.* Chichester: John Wiley & Sons.

Spence, C., and Shankar, M. U. (2010). The influence of auditory cues on the perception of, and responses to, food and drink. *J. Sens. Stud.* 25, 406–430. doi: 10.1111/j.1745-459X.2009.00267.x

Stein, B. E. (ed.). (2012). *The New Handbook of Multisensory Processes.* Cambridge, MA: MIT Press.

Stevenson, R. J., and Boakes, R. A. (2004). "Sweet and sour smells: learned synaesthesia between the senses of taste and smell," *The Handbook of Multisensory Processing*, eds G. A. Calvert, C. Spence, and B. E. Stein (Cambridge, MA: MIT Press), 69–83.

Stevenson, R. J., Rich, A., and Russell, A. (2012). The nature and origin of cross-modal associations to odors. *Perception* 41, 606–619. doi: 10.1068/p7223

Thorndike, E. L. (1920). A constant error in psychological ratings. *J. Appl. Psychol.* 4, 25–29. doi: 10.1037/h0071663

Urdapilleta, I., Giboreau, A., Manetta, C., Houix, O., and Richard, J. F. (2006). The mental context for the description of odors: a semantic space. *Eur. Rev. Appl. Psychol.* 56, 261–271. doi: 10.1016/j.erap.2005.09.013

Vélez, J. I., and Correa, J. C. (2014). Should we think of a different median estimator? *Comun. Estad.* 7, 11–17.

Ventry, I. M., and Weinstein, B. E. (1983). Identification of elderly people with hearing problems. *ASHA* 25, 37–42.

von Hornbostel, E. M. (1931). Über Geruchshelligkeit [On odor/smell brightness]. *Pflugers Arch. Gesamte Physiol. Menschen Tiere* 227, 517–538. doi: 10.1007/BF01755351

Wesson, D. W., and Wilson, D. A. (2010). Smelling sounds: olfactory–auditory sensory convergence in the olfactory tubercle. *J. Neurosci.* 30, 3013–3021. doi: 10.1523/JNEUROSCI.6003-09.2010

Woods, A. T., Poliakoff, E., Lloyd, D. M., Kuenzel, J., Hodson, R., Gonda, H., et al. (2011). Effect of background noise on food perception. *Food Qual. Prefer.* 22, 42–47. doi: 10.1016/j.foodqual.2010.07.003

Zarzo, M., and Stanton, D. T. (2009). Understanding the underlying dimensions in perfumers' odor perception space as a basis for developing meaningful odor maps. *Atten. Percept. Psychophys.* 71, 225–247. doi: 10.3758/APP.71.2.225

Permissions

All chapters in this book were first published by Frontiers; hereby published with permission under the Creative Commons Attribution License or equivalent. Every chapter published in this book has been scrutinized by our experts. Their significance has been extensively debated. The topics covered herein carry significant findings which will fuel the growth of the discipline. They may even be implemented as practical applications or may be referred to as a beginning point for another development.

The contributors of this book come from diverse backgrounds, making this book a truly international effort. This book will bring forth new frontiers with its revolutionizing research information and detailed analysis of the nascent developments around the world.

We would like to thank all the contributing authors for lending their expertise to make the book truly unique. They have played a crucial role in the development of this book. Without their invaluable contributions this book wouldn't have been possible. They have made vital efforts to compile up to date information on the varied aspects of this subject to make this book a valuable addition to the collection of many professionals and students.

This book was conceptualized with the vision of imparting up-to-date information and advanced data in this field. To ensure the same, a matchless editorial board was set up. Every individual on the board went through rigorous rounds of assessment to prove their worth. After which they invested a large part of their time researching and compiling the most relevant data for our readers.

The editorial board has been involved in producing this book since its inception. They have spent rigorous hours researching and exploring the diverse topics which have resulted in the successful publishing of this book. They have passed on their knowledge of decades through this book. To expedite this challenging task, the publisher supported the team at every step. A small team of assistant editors was also appointed to further simplify the editing procedure and attain best results for the readers.

Apart from the editorial board, the designing team has also invested a significant amount of their time in understanding the subject and creating the most relevant covers. They scrutinized every image to scout for the most suitable representation of the subject and create an appropriate cover for the book.

The publishing team has been an ardent support to the editorial, designing and production team. Their endless efforts to recruit the best for this project, has resulted in the accomplishment of this book. They are a veteran in the field of academics and their pool of knowledge is as vast as their experience in printing. Their expertise and guidance has proved useful at every step. Their uncompromising quality standards have made this book an exceptional effort. Their encouragement from time to time has been an inspiration for everyone.

The publisher and the editorial board hope that this book will prove to be a valuable piece of knowledge for researchers, students, practitioners and scholars across the globe.

List of Contributors

Ella Pagliarini and Monica Laureati
Department of Food, Environmental and Nutritional Sciences (DeFENS), Università degli Studi di Milano, Milano, Italy

Davide Gaeta
Dipartimento di Economia Aziendale, Università degli Studi di Verona, Verona, Italy

M. Luisa Demattè, Isabella Endrizzi and Flavia Gasperi
Department of Food Quality and Nutrition, Research and Innovation Centre, Fondazione Edmund Mach, San Michele all'Adige, Italy

Pauline Joussain, Catherine Rouby and Moustafa Bensafi
Lyon Neuroscience Research Center, CNRS UMR5292, INSERM U1028, University of Lyon, Lyon, France

Han-Seok Seo, Suji Lee and Sungeun Cho
Department of Food Science, University of Arkansas, Fayetteville, AR, USA

Chantal Triscoli
Clinical Neuroscience and Rehabilitation, Institute of Neuroscience and Physiology, University of Gothenburg, Gothenburg, Sweden
Department of Psychology, University of Gothenburg, Gothenburg, Sweden

Ilona Croy and Håkan Olausson
Clinical Neuroscience and Rehabilitation, Institute of Neuroscience and Physiology, University of Gothenburg, Gothenburg, Sweden

Uta Sailer
Clinical Neuroscience and Rehabilitation, Institute of Neuroscience and Physiology, University of Gothenburg, Gothenburg, Sweden
Department of Psychology, University of Gothenburg, Gothenburg, Sweden

Thierry Thomas-Danguin, Sébastien Romagny, Fouzia El Mountassir, Anne-Marie Le Bon and Gérard Coureaud
Centre des Sciences du Goût et de l'Alimentation, CNRS UMR6265, INRA UMR1324, Université de Bourgogne, Dijon, France

Charlotte Sinding
Smell and Taste Clinic, Department of Otorhinolaryngoly, TU Dresden, Dresden, Germany

Boriana Atanasova
INSERM U930, Université François Rabelais, Tours, France

Elodie Le Berre
Unilever R&D, Vlaardingen, Netherlands

Elena V. Ignatieva
Laboratory of Evolutionary Bioinformatics and Theoretical Genetics, Institute of Cytology and Genetics, Siberian Branch, Russian Academy of Sciences, Novosibirsk, Russia
Department of Natural Science, Novosibirsk State University, Novosibirsk, Russia

Victor G. Levitsky
Department of Natural Science, Novosibirsk State University, Novosibirsk, Russia
Laboratory of Molecular-Genetic Systems, Institute of Cytology and Genetics, Siberian Branch, Russian Academy of Sciences, Novosibirsk, Russia

Nikolay S. Yudin
Department of Natural Science, Novosibirsk State University, Novosibirsk, Russia
Laboratory of Human Molecular Genetics, Institute of Cytology and Genetics, Siberian Branch, Russian Academy of Sciences, Novosibirsk, Russia

Mikhail P. Moshkin
Department of Natural Science, Novosibirsk State University, Novosibirsk, Russia
Laboratory of Mammalian Ecological Genetics, Institute of Cytology and Genetics, Siberian Branch, Russian Academy of Sciences, Novosibirsk, Russia

Nikolay A. Kolchanov
Department of Natural Science, Novosibirsk State University, Novosibirsk, Russia
Department of Systems Biology, Institute of Cytology and Genetics, Siberian Branch, Russian Academy of Sciences, Novosibirsk, Russia
National Research centre "Kurchatov Institute", Moscow, Russia

Pierre Maurage
Laboratory for Experimental Psychopathology, Psychological Sciences Research Institute, Université catholique de Louvain, Louvain-la-Neuve, Belgium

Philippe Rombaux
Department of Otorhinolaryngology, St Luc Hospital and Institute of Neuroscience, Université catholique de Louvain, Brussels, Belgium

Philippe de Timary
Laboratory for Experimental Psychopathology, Psychological Sciences Research Institute, Université catholique de Louvain, Louvain-la-Neuve, Belgium
Department of Adult Psychiatry, St Luc Hospital and Institute of Neuroscience, Université catholique de Louvain, Brussels, Belgium

Caroline Sezille, Arnaud Fournel, Catherine Rouby and Moustafa Bensafi
CNRS, UMR5292, INSERM1028, Lyon Neuroscience Research Center, University of Lyon, Lyon, France

Fanny Rinck
Lidilem Laboratory, University of Grenoble, Grenoble, France

Sylvia Schablitzky and Bettina M. Pause
Department of Experimental Psychology, Heinrich-Heine-University, Düsseldorf, Germany

Jean-Pierre Royet, Jane Plailly, Anne-Lise Saive and Alexandra Veyrac
Olfaction: From Coding to Memory Team, Centre de Recherche en Neurosciences de Lyon, CNRS UMR 5292, INSERM U1028, Université Lyon 1, Lyon, France

Chantal Delon-Martin
INSERM, U836, NeuroImagerie Fonctionnelle et Perfusion Cerebrale, Grenoble, France
Université Joseph Fourier, Grenoble Institut des Neurosciences, Grenoble, France

Sandra T. Glass
Division of Clinical Pharmacy and Diagnostics, Department of Pharmaceutical Chemistry, University of Vienna, Vienna, Austria
Department of Health Sciences and Technology, Institute for Human Movement Sciences and Sport, ETH Zurich, Zurich, Switzerland

Elisabeth Lingg
Division of Clinical Pharmacy and Diagnostics, Department of Pharmaceutical Chemistry, University of Vienna, Vienna, Austria

Maria Larsson and Artin Arshamian
Gösta Ekman Laboratory, Department of Psychology, Stockholm University, Stockholm, Sweden
Department of Psychology, Stockholm University, Stockholm, Sweden

Eva Heuberger
Division of Clinical Pharmacy and Diagnostics, Department of Pharmaceutical Chemistry, University of Vienna, Vienna, Austria
Division of Clinical Psychology and Psychotherapy, Department of Psychology, Saarland University, Saarbruecken, Germany
Pharmaceutical Biology, Department of Pharmacy, Saarland University, Saarbruecken, Germany

Johan Willander and Kristina Karlsson
Department of Psychology, Stockholm University, Stockholm, Sweden

E. Leslie Cameron
Department of Psychological Science, Carthage College, Kenosha, WI, USA

Egon P. Köster
Psychological Laboratory, Helmholtz Institute, Utrecht University, Utrecht, Netherlands

Per Møller
Department of Food Science, University of Copenhagen, Frederiksberg, Denmark

Jozina Mojet
Wageningen – UR, Food and Biobased Research, Wageningen, Netherlands

Matthieu Ischer, Naëm Baron, David Sander and Sylvain Delplanque
Swiss Center for Affective Sciences, University of Geneva, Geneva, Switzerland
Department of Psychology, University of Geneva, Geneva, Switzerland

Christophe Mermoud
Department of Medicine, University of Geneva, Geneva, Switzerland

Alexander Toet and Martin G. van Schaik
TNO, Soesterberg, Netherlands
Department of Information and Computing Sciences, University Utrecht, Utrecht, Netherlands

Wei He
Consumer Science and Intelligent Systems, Food and Biobased Research, Wageningen University and Research Centre, Wageningen, Netherlands
Division of Human Nutrition, Sensory Science and Eating Behaviour, Wageningen University, Wageningen, Netherlands

Sanne Boesveldt and Cees de Graaf
Division of Human Nutrition, Sensory Science and Eating Behaviour, Wageningen University, Wageningen, Netherlands

René A. de Wijk
Consumer Science and Intelligent Systems, Food and Biobased Research, Wageningen University and Research Centre, Wageningen, Netherlands

M. A. M. Smeets
Unilever R&D, Vlaardingen, Netherlands
Faculty of Social and Behavioural Sciences, Utrecht University, Utrecht, Netherlands

G. B. Dijksterhuis
Unilever R&D, Vlaardingen, Netherlands
Section for Sensory and Consumer Science, Faculty of Science (FOOD), University of Copenhagen, Copenhagen, Denmark

Linus Andersson, Anna-Sara Claeson, Lisa Ledin, Frida Wisting and Steven Nordin
Department of Psychology, Umeå University, Umeå, Sweden

Richard L. Doty
Department of Otorhinolaryngology: Head and Neck Surgery, Smell and Taste Center, Perelman School of Medicine, University of Pennsylvania, Philadelphia, PA, USA

Vidyulata Kamath
Department of Otorhinolaryngology: Head and Neck Surgery, Smell and Taste Center, Perelman School of Medicine, University of Pennsylvania, Philadelphia, PA, USA
Division of Medical Psychology, Department of Psychiatry and Behavioral Sciences, The Johns Hopkins University School of Medicine, Baltimore, MD, USA

Isabelle Cayeux and Christelle Porcherot
Firmenich, S.A., Geneva, Switzerland

Carlos Velasco, Diana Balboa and Charles Spence
Crossmodal Research Laboratory, Department of Experimental Psychology, University of Oxford, Oxford, Oxfordshire, UK

Fernando Marmolejo-Ramos
School of Psychology, Faculty of Health Sciences, University of Adelaide, Adelaide, SA, Australia

Index

www.ingramcontent.com/pod-product-compliance
Lightning Source LLC
LaVergne TN
LVHW082212200926
848484LV00008B/2242